Thompson & Thompson
GENETICS IN MEDICINE

Fifth Edition

MARGARET W. THOMPSON, Ph.D.

Professor Emeritus
Department of Genetics
The Hospital for Sick Children
Department of Molecular and Medical Genetics
University of Toronto
Toronto, Ontario, Canada

RODERICK R. McINNES, M.D., Ph.D.

Associate Professor
Departments of Genetics and Pediatrics
The Hospital for Sick Children
Department of Molecular and Medical Genetics
University of Toronto
Toronto, Ontario, Canada

HUNTINGTON F. WILLARD, Ph.D.

Associate Professor
Department of Genetics
Stanford University School of Medicine
Stanford, California

W.B. SAUNDERS COMPANY
A Division of Harcourt Brace & Company
Philadelphia   London   Toronto   Montreal   Sydney   Tokyo

W.B. SAUNDERS COMPANY
A Division of
Harcourt Brace & Company

The Curtis Center
Independence Square West
Philadelphia, Pennsylvania 19106-3399

Library of Congress Cataloging-in-Publication Data

Thompson, Margaret W. (Margaret Wilson)
    Thompson & Thompson: Genetics in Medicine, Fifth Edition / by Margaret W. Thompson,
Roderick R. McInnes, Huntington F. Willard. — 5th ed.
        p.   cm.
    Rev. ed. of: Thompson & Thompson Genetics in medicine / by James S.
Thompson, Margaret W. Thompson. 4th ed. 1986.
    Includes bibliographical references and indexes.
    ISBN 0-7216-2817-6
    1. Medical genetics. I. McInnes, Roderick R. II. Willard,
Huntington F. III. Thompson, James S. (James Scott), 1919–1982
Genetics in medicine. IV. Title. V. Title: Genetics in medicine.
VI. Title: Thompson and Thompson: Genetics in Medicine, Fifth Edition.
    [DNLM: 1. Genetics, Medical. QZ 50 T474t]
RB155.T52   1991
616'.042 — dc20
DNLM/DLC   91-21907

Listed here are the latest translated edition of this book together
with the language of the translation and the publisher.

Persian (*4th Edition*) — Ali Farazmand, Allameh Tabata'I University, Tehran, Iran
Portuguese (*4th Edition*) — Editora Guanabara-Koogan, S. A., Rio de Janeiro, Brazil
Slovak (*4th Edition*) — Osveta, Martin, Czechoslovakia
Japanese (*3rd Edition*) — Kodansha Ltd., Tokyo, Japan
Spanish (*3rd Edition*) — Salvat Editores, S. A., Barcelona, Spain

Editor: Martin J. Wonsiewicz

Designer: Maureen Sweeney

Cover Designer: Michael Maystead

Production Manager: Peter Faber

Manuscript Editor: W. B. Saunders Staff

Illustration Specialist: Brett MacNaughton

Indexer: Anne Cope

Thompson & Thompson: Genetics in Medicine, Fifth Edition   ISBN 0–7216–2817–6
                                                                             International ISBN 0–7216–3113–4

Copyright © 1991, 1986, 1980, 1973, 1966 by W. B. Saunders Company

Printed in the United States of America.

Last digit is the print number: 9   8   7   6   5

PREFACE

The preface to the first edition of *Genetics in Medicine*, published at a time when genetics was just beginning to take its place as an accepted part of the medical curriculum, emphasized its fundamental role in the basic medical sciences and its important applications to clinical medicine, public health, and medical research. Today, some 25 years later, the role of genetics in medicine has expanded greatly. On the scientific level, the generation of new knowledge about human genes, unprecedented in its nature and extent, has redefined the scope of genetics in the analysis, diagnosis, treatment, and prevention of disease. On a practical plane, genetics is now recognized officially as a clinical and laboratory science, thus reflecting awareness within the medical profession of its expanded significance in medical education and practice. Indeed, today genetics is indispensable to virtually every branch of medical science, whether basic or clinical.

The primary aim of this edition, as of the previous ones, is to introduce the principles of medical genetics to medical students and to other students in the health professions who require a working knowledge of modern medical genetics: students in genetic counseling programs, graduate and advanced undergraduate students in molecular and human genetics, and fellows and residents, especially those preparing for certification in medical genetics or a related field. The text will provide students with a background for understanding and applying the new advances that are sure to be made during their professional years. It should also be useful to physicians, nurses, and others involved in any aspect of the management of genetic disease.

The book is designed for use as a textbook to accompany a one-semester course in human or medical genetics. However, it can also be used as a reference, and many of its new features, such as the boxes, which emphasize certain important topics in brief form, and the Appendices, in which reference material has been separated from the main text, are intended to enhance this aspect of the book.

This edition differs from earlier ones in that its focus has been enlarged to encompass the major recent advances in knowledge of the molecular aspects of genetics and the clinical applications of this new knowledge. Thus our aim has been to present molecular genetics in the context of classic human and medical genetics. To this end, new chapters have been added, and the book in its entirety has been extensively revised. As a consequence, some chapters may exceed the scope of a one-semester course. However, these chapters, most of which deal with specialized topics, can be skimmed or used only for reference, without interrupting the flow of the text. We are well aware of the information load faced by students and have tried to make the book as clear and elementary as the subject allows, stressing principles rather than details and medical rather than basic scientific aspects. We strongly believe, however, that the physicians of the next decade and their colleagues in clinical genetics will need as extensive a knowledge of genetics as can be provided.

As in earlier editions, each chapter ends with a set of problems (with answers provided at the end of the book). These problems, for the most part, illustrate the major concepts of human and medical genetics and give the student an opportunity to come to terms with the sometimes unfamiliar terminology. A glossary of the technical terms used in the book is provided.

Many of our colleagues in genetics have contributed to the preparation of this book by providing copies of unpublished material or figures or by reading various sections of the manuscript; it is a pleasure to record our indebtedness to them. Those who contributed figures are individually acknowledged in the figure legends, and others who have given us substantial assistance are named in the following list of acknowledgments. We have done our best to be accurate and to give appropriate credit, but the responsibility for errors or omissions is ours, not theirs. Most of the many new illustrations have been prepared by Mike Maystead of the Stanford Publication Services. Martin Wonsiewicz, Senior Editor, Medical Books, W.B. Saunders Company, and his colleagues have given us continuing encouragement and good will.

Last, we thank our laboratories and especially our families, most of all Danièle and Vicki, for their tolerance and support.

MARGARET W. THOMPSON
RODERICK R. McINNES
HUNTINGTON F. WILLARD

ACKNOWLEDGMENTS

The authors wish to express their appreciation to the people listed below, who have helped immeasurably in the preparation of this edition by providing unpublished material or by reading sections of the manuscript. Unfortunately, the list cannot include the many others who have contributed less directly, through informal discussions, especially the members of our laboratories and scores of medical students over many years of teaching.

Joanna Amberger
Arthur L. Beaudet
Carolyn J. Brown
Manuel Buchwald
Peter H. Byers
Patricia L. Chang
Joe T. R. Clarke
David R. Cox
Diane Wilson Cox
Ronald G. Crystal
Louis J. Elsas II
R. Alan B. Ezekowitz
Wayne A. Fenton
Uta Francke
Brenda Gallie
Joseph L. Goldstein
Stephen I. Goodman

Denis M. Grant
Roy A. Gravel
Michael S. Hershfield
Mark R. Hughes
Elaine M. Hutton
Haig H. Kazazian Jr.
Bert N. LaDu
David H. Ledbetter
Mark Leppert
David Lillicrap
Donald Mahuran
Victor A. McKusick
Ann B. Moser
Hugo W. Moser
Nancy Olivieri
Robert A. Phillips
Vicki E. Powers

Peter N. Ray
Neil J. Risch
Johanna Rommens
David S. Rosenblatt
Charles R. Scriver
Cheryl T. Shuman
Jacqueline Siegel-Bartelt
Katherine A. Siminovitch
Mark H. Skolnick
Stephen P. Spielberg
Grant R. Sutherland
Ikuko E. Teshima
Lap-Chee Tsui
David Valle
Bert Vogelstein
Dorothy Warburton
Ronald G. Worton

CONTENTS

INTRODUCTION

This is a special time in medical genetics, when it has achieved a recognized role as a core discipline that deals with human variability and human heredity and at the same time has developed approaches that allow new insight into many diseases and promise to provide far more in the near future. To give patients and their families the full benefit of expanding genetic knowledge, physicians and their colleagues in the health professions need to understand the underlying concepts of human genetics and the role of genes and environment in normal and abnormal development and in disease.

ROLE OF GENETICS IN MEDICINE

The place of genetics in medicine was not always as obvious as it is today. Although its significance both for the conceptual basis of medicine and for clinical practice is now fully recognized, not many years ago the subject was thought to be concerned only with the inheritance of trivial, superficial, and rare characteristics; the fundamental role of the gene in basic life processes was not understood. The discovery of the principles of heredity by the Austrian monk Gregor Mendel in 1865 received virtually no recognition from biologists and none at all from other scientists. Instead, his reports lay unnoticed in the scientific literature for 35 years.

Charles Darwin, whose great book *The Origin of Species* (published in 1859) emphasized the hereditary nature of variability among members of a species as an important factor in evolution, had no idea how inheritance operated. At that time heredity was thought to involve blending of the traits of the two parents, and Jean Baptiste Lamarck's idea of the inheritance of acquired characteristics was still accepted. Mendel's work could have clarified Darwin's concept of the mechanism of inheritance of variability, but although Mendel was aware of Darwin's work, Darwin seems never to have known of the significance of Mendel's work or even of its existence. Darwin's cousin Francis Galton, one of the titans of early medical genetics, also remained ignorant of Mendel's work despite its relevance to his own studies of "nature and nurture." Mendel himself, perhaps discouraged by the results of later, less favorably designed experiments, eventually abandoned experimental research, although his interest in biological science remained strong throughout his life.

Mendel's laws, which form the cornerstone of the science of genetics, were derived from his experiments with garden peas, in which he crossed pure lines differing in one or more clear-cut characteristics and followed the progeny of the crosses for at least two generations. The laws he derived from the results of his experiments may be stated as follows:

1. Unit inheritance. Mendel clearly stated that blending of the characteristics of the parents did not occur but that, although they might not be expressed in the first-generation offspring, the parental traits could reappear unchanged in a later generation. Modern teaching in genetics places little stress on this law, but in Mendel's time it was an entirely new concept. The word **gene** to denote the unit of inheritance was not used until 1909, when it was introduced by Wilhelm Johannsen.

2. Segregation. The two members of a single gene pair, known today as **alleles,** are never found in the same gamete but always segregate and pass to different gametes. In exceptional circumstances, when this rule is broken and the members of a chromosome pair fail to segregate normally, the typical consequence is severe abnormality in the offspring.

3. Independent assortment. Members of different gene pairs assort to the gametes independently of one another. In other words, there is random recombination of paternal and maternal chromosomes in the gametes. As described later, there is an important exception to this rule, not recognized by Mendel: genes closely linked on the same chromosome do not assort independently, but tend to remain together from generation to generation.

At the beginning of the 20th century, the rest of the biological community was ready to catch up with Mendel. By a curious coincidence, three workers (Hugo De Vries in Holland, Carl Correns in Germany, and Erich von Tschermak in Austria) independently and simultaneously rediscovered Mendel's laws. The development of genetics as a science dates not from Mendel's own paper but from the papers that reported the rediscovery.

The universal nature of Mendel's laws was soon recognized. As early as 1902 Archibald Garrod, who ranks with Francis Galton as a founder of medical genetics, could report the disorder alkaptonuria as the first human example of what is now known as Mendelian inheritance. In his paper, Garrod generously admitted his debt to the biologist William Bateson, who had seen the genetic significance of consanguineous marriage in the parents of some patients with what Garrod called "inborn errors of metabolism" and of the fact that if more than one family member was affected, the other affected members were virtually always sibs of the index patient, not parents, offspring, or other relatives. Bateson recognized this pattern as just what one would expect if alkaptonuria were inherited as a recessive trait in accordance with Mendel's laws. This is the first clear evidence of interaction in research between medical and nonmedical geneticists, which has continued to the present day and has contributed greatly to the rapid expansion of the field. It predated the introduction of the term **genetics** for the new science, which was also a contribution of Bateson, in 1906.

A growing understanding of the universal nature of the biological structure and function of living organisms led inevitably to recognition of the crucial role of genes in life processes. The concept, which was foreshadowed in Garrod's work, was formulated clearly by Beadle and Tatum in 1941 as the "one gene–one enzyme" hypothesis, now more generally phrased as "one gene–one protein." Today, human biochemical genetics is one of the dominant themes in medical genetics.

During the early 1940s, the molecular analysis of the genetic material made rapid progress, beginning with the discovery that genes are composed of deoxyribonucleic acid (DNA). In 1953, James Watson and Francis Crick described the molecular structure of DNA for which they were awarded the Nobel prize in 1962. Other outstanding discoveries in the early days of molecular genetics included the recognition that the DNA of the genes is transcribed into ribonucleic acid (RNA), which is in turn translated into protein, and the elucidation of the genetic code, by which the amino acid sequence of proteins is recorded in DNA.

By the late 1950s, techniques for the scientific study of human chromosomes had been developed, and researchers began to explore the role of chromosomes in sexual development and of chromosome abnormalities as causes of abnormal physical and mental development and reproductive problems. Even though human cytogenetics, the study of human chromosomes, has been a field of intensive research for many years, it still holds many challenging problems. Significant new findings about normal and abnormal chromosome structure and function continue to be reported, especially now that chromosome analysis goes hand in hand with molecular analysis in the study of the human genome.

Since the mid-1970s, with the aid of powerful

new technologies for the manipulation and analysis of DNA, the field of medical genetics has been transformed. Scientists are now able to locate and identify genes responsible for essential human proteins, characterize their mutations, and learn the nature of their protein products, thus gaining a deeper understanding of many poorly understood or previously unknown causes of disease. Because the molecular approach was so different from earlier ones, and its potential so great, it was called "the new genetics." More recently, the terms **reverse genetics** and **positional cloning** have been used to denote the cloning of genes of unknown function by gene mapping techniques. Some of the many examples of the molecular genetic approach to human diseases are described in later chapters.

For many years, although there was great interest in the mapping of human genes to their chromosomal locations, progress was relatively slow. A major reason for the difficulty was the unsuitability of human beings for gene mapping because of small family size, long generation time, and the impossibility of making the planned matings that can be used with experimental organisms. By means of cytogenetic and molecular genetic analysis together with family studies, however, human gene mapping has become a leading field of human genetic research. The Human Genome Project, an international project to map the entire human genome by the year 2005, seems sure to be one of the major research programs in genetics and is expected to have important medical benefits (Watson, 1990).

The expansion and application of genetic knowledge has already had fruitful consequences for clinical medicine. Today at least one third of the children in pediatric hospitals are there because of genetic disorders. This is a great change from the early years of the century and even from before the antibiotic era. Before the days of immunization, improved nutrition, and antibiotics, most hospitalized children had infectious diseases or nutritional disorders such as rickets. Today some of those with infections have genetic defects that impair their resistance, and, at least in developed countries, most cases of rickets are due not to faulty nutrition but to deleterious genes. Life-saving advances in clinical and surgical medicine increase the probability of survival and thus tend to raise the prevalence of genetic defects.

Disciplines Within Human and Medical Genetics

Genetics is a diverse subject, concerned with variation and heredity in all living organisms. Within this broad field, human genetics is the science of variation and heredity in human beings, and medical genetics deals with human genetic variation of medical significance. The two areas have extensive overlap, and in fact to many geneticists they are one and the same.

Within human and medical genetics, there are many fields of interest, as indicated by the various directions in which genetics has developed, as outlined earlier. Major recognized areas of specialization are the study of chromosomes (cytogenetics), the study of the structure and function of individual genes (molecular and biochemical genetics), and the application to diagnosis and patient care (clinical genetics). The literal meaning of *clinical* is *bedside* (*klinikos,* Greek for bedside), and a clinical geneticist is an appropriately qualified physician-geneticist directly involved in the diagnosis of genetic diseases and the care of patients with such diseases.

Other fields of human genetics such as population genetics, genetic epidemiology, developmental genetics, and immunogenetics also have medical relevance, especially in relation to the understanding and prevention of human disease.

In addition to clinical practice, medical genetics is applied to the care of patients in the fields of genetic counseling, population screening to identify persons at risk of developing or transmitting a genetic disorder, and prenatal diagnosis. Genetic counseling, which combines the provision of risk information with a support function, is maturing into a new health profession. Population screening for genetic disease has become an important public health initiative. Prenatal diagnosis, which makes use of many clinical and laboratory specialties in addition to genetics, is probably today the chief area in which genetics is applied to patient care.

Although it has always been most closely associated with pediatrics, medical genetics is also relevant to many other clinical specialties. In obstetrics, prenatal diagnosis of certain genetic defects has become a standard aspect of prenatal care. In adult medicine, it is recognized that many common disorders, such as coronary artery disease, hypertension, and diabetes mellitus, have important genetic components and that preventive medicine could be much more effective if it could be directed toward special genetically defined high-risk groups rather than toward the general population. Applications to many other fields, especially neurology, hematology, and oncology, are referred to in later chapters.

Although much of medical genetics is within the medical mainstream, genetics is unlike other medical specialties in that it is often oriented to prevention as well as to treatment and in that its focus is often not only the patient but the entire family.

Ethical Principles in Medical Genetics

The principles of medical ethics apply to genetics as to other medical disciplines, but some of the ethical dilemmas that can arise in medical genetics are rarely if ever seen in other branches of clinical practice. One type of difficulty is created by physicians' growing ability to perform presymptomatic testing — that is, to identify a disease-causing gene in a person before the condition has become clinically expressed. Physicians can also now recognize certain genetic predispositions associated with an additional risk of developing a particular disease; for example, they are aware that people with an inherited deficiency of alpha$_1$-antitrypsin (see Table 1 – 1) have an increased risk of lung disease, especially pronounced in smoky environments.

Huntington disease (HD; also listed in Table 1 – 1) is a neuropsychiatric disorder with onset in midlife, inherited from an affected parent as an autosomal dominant. In many cases, geneticists can determine, long before the disease becomes manifest, whether a relative of a patient with HD has inherited the gene. As described in Chapters 4 and 8, the test requires analysis of DNA markers close to the HD gene, in blood samples from family members. However, if presymptomatic testing is to be done, the patient must give consent to have his or her relatives informed about the diagnosis and its implications for them and their families, and the relatives must agree to provide blood samples for analysis. Each member has the right to make an informed decision whether to participate in the study, without coercion and after receiving full information from the physician or genetic counselor about the implications of the decision. Participants have a right *not* to know whether they are at risk, and in some circumstances this right is in conflict with the right of other family members to have such information. Confidentiality, a cardinal principle of medical ethics, can be especially difficult to maintain when one is dealing with presymptomatic testing on related persons. Family members who have agreed to participate in providing blood samples may find it difficult to understand why they are not entitled to access to one another's test results. Moreover, testing can provide unexpected information; for example, it can reveal cases of nonpaternity. Identification of nonpaternity raises the additional question of whether the person who provided the sample wants to receive such information, and it emphasizes the fact that the possibility of such an eventuality should be dealt with beforehand and covered in the consent form that each participant is asked to sign. These brief examples illustrate some of the difficulties that are encountered in predictive testing for genetic disease (Huggins et al., 1990).

CLASSIFICATION OF GENETIC DISORDERS

In clinical practice, the chief significance of genetics is its role in the causation of a large number of disorders. Virtually any disease is the result of the combined action of genes and environment, but the relative role of the genetic component may be large or small.

Among disorders caused wholly or partly by genetic factors, three main types are recognized:

1. Single-gene disorders
2. Chromosome disorders
3. Multifactorial disorders

Single-gene defects are caused by mutant genes. The mutation may be present on only one chromosome of a pair (matched with a normal allele on the homologous chromosome) or on both chromosomes of the pair. In either case, the cause is a single critical error in the genetic information.

Such disorders usually exhibit obvious and characteristic pedigree patterns. Most such defects are rare, with a frequency that may be as high as 1 in 500 but is usually much less (Table 1 – 1). How-

Table 1–1. Selected Examples of Significant Genetic Disorders

Disorder	Significance	Incidence	Chapter(s)*
Single-Gene Disorders			
Adenosine deaminase deficiency	Autosomal recessive enzyme defect that causes immunodeficiency; first condition to be approved for human gene therapy	Rare	13
Alpha₁-antitrypsin deficiency	Autosomal recessive deficiency of a major plasma protease inhibitor, leading to obstructive lung disease in homozygotes (more severe in smokers) and liver disease in some affected children	~1/3000 to 1/20,000	6, 12, 13
Cystic fibrosis	Common autosomal recessive disorder affecting regulation of membrane transport of ions in exocrine cells; first gene to be identified without prior knowledge of gene product or structural chromosomal aberration	~1/2000 in some Caucasian populations, very rare in Asians	4, 8, 12, 13
Duchenne muscular dystrophy	Common X-linked recessive disorder of muscle; gene identified by structural chromosomal aberration without prior knowledge of protein product; very large gene that is thus a frequent target for mutation	~1/3000 to 1/3500 males	4, 8, 12, 13
Familial hypercholesterolemia	Autosomal dominant defect of receptor for plasma low-density lipoprotein (LDL); associated with an increased frequency of coronary artery disease	~1/500 heterozygotes	4, 12, 13
Fragile X syndrome	Common form of X-linked mental retardation, associated with fragile site on X chromosome; unique genetic features; ~1/3 of carrier females show mild retardation	~1/1500 males, ~1/2000 to 1/3000 females	4
Glucose-6-phosphate dehydrogenase deficiency	Pharmacogenetic disorder; X-linked; many variants but two are common, one in Mediterranean, one in Africa; heterozygote advantage due to resistance to malaria	Ethnic variation, very common (1/4 to 1/20 males) in some populations	12
Hemophilia A	Common X-linked coagulation defect	~1/10,000 males	4
Huntington disease	Neurodegenerative disease, classic autosomal dominant of late onset, predictable by molecular testing at presymptomatic stage; first gene to be localized to a chromosome by DNA linkage analysis	Variable, 4 to 8/100,000, much higher in some small, isolated populations	4, 8
Myotonic dystrophy	Autosomal dominant, variable onset age and severity; maternal effect: patients with congenital onset typically have affected mothers	Most common autosomal dominant muscular dystrophy, ~1/10,000 up to ~1/1000 in some populations	4, 8
Neurofibromatosis type 1	Common autosomal dominant disorder with variable expression, high mutation rate, risk of malignancy; high proportion of new mutations (~50%); very large gene	~1/3000 to 1/5000	4, 8, 16
Osteogenesis imperfecta	Heterogeneous group of molecular defects of collagen; the prototypes of defects in structural proteins	~1/15,000 for most common type	12

Table continued on following page

Table 1−1. **Selected Examples of Significant Genetic Disorders** *Continued*

Disorder	Significance	Incidence	Chapter(s)*
Phenylketonuria	Autosomal recessive deficiency of phenylalanine hydroxylase, can cause mental retardation; prototype of diseases that can be detected by neonatal screening, with prevention of retardation by prompt dietary treatment	Variable, 1/5000 to 1/200,000; most common in Western Europeans	4, 12, 13
Retinoblastoma	Embryonic neoplasm of retina, associated with mutation or deletion of a pair of alleles on chromosome 13; both inherited and sporadic forms	~1/14,000	16
Sickle cell anemia	Defect in gene for β-globin chain of hemoglobin; first molecular disease to be identified; common in Africa; high frequency related to heterozygote advantage due to malaria resistance	Common mutation in equatorial Africa; ~1/400 American Blacks affected	4, 11, 13
Tay-Sachs disease	Autosomal recessive deficiency of hexosaminidase A; very common in Ashkenazi Jewish population	~1/3000 in Ashkenazi Jews; much lower in other populations	4, 7, 12
Thalassemia	Numerous defects of gene for either α- or β-globin chain of hemoglobin, leading to imbalance in relative amounts of the chains; very common in Mediterranean and Southern Asia	Most common single-gene disease; found in regions where malaria is endemic	4, 6, 11
Wilms tumor	Renal tumor of childhood, associated with deletion of chromosome 11p13; may be part of contiguous gene syndrome with aniridia, genitourinary problems, and retardation (WAGR syndrome); normal allele involved in development of urogenital system	~1/10,000	16
Cytogenetic Disorders			
Down syndrome	Trisomy 21, most common cause of moderate mental retardation; risk related to late maternal age	~1/800	9, 19
Trisomy 18	Extra autosome with characteristic phenotype of severe, multiple congenital malformations in liveborn infants	~1/8000	9
Trisomy 13	Extra autosome with characteristic phenotype of severe, multiple congenital malformations in liveborn infants	~1/25,000	9
Klinefelter syndrome	Male phenotype and characteristic abnormalities, usually associated with 47,XXY karyotype	~1/1000 males	10
Turner syndrome	Female phenotype and characteristic abnormalities, usually associated with 45,X karyotype	~1/5000 females	10
XXX syndrome	Common abnormal karyotype; may be associated with learning difficulties and infertility; often phenotypically normal	~1/1000 females	10
XYY syndrome	Common abnormal karyotype; may be associated with behavioral difficulties; often phenotypically normal	~1/1000 males	10

Table 1–1. Selected Examples of Significant Genetic Disorders *Continued*

Disorder	Significance	Incidence	Chapter(s)*
Prader-Willi syndrome	Dysmorphic syndrome with obesity and cognitive impairment; example of genomic imprinting, often due to cytogenetic deletion of chromosome 15q11-q13 on the paternally inherited chromosome	~1/10,000 to 1/25,000	4, 9
Multifactorial Disorders			
Congenital Malformations			
Cleft lip with or without cleft palate	Cleft of lip, with or without cleft palate, unilateral or bilateral	1/250 to 1/600, ethnic variation	15
Congenital heart diseases	Group of congenital heart defects, some partly genetic	1/125 to 1/250	15
Neural tube defects	Anencephaly, spina bifida, and less common forms	1/100 to 1/500, ethnic variation	15
Adult Diseases			
Cancer, some forms	Role of heredity in many forms of cancer incompletely understood, but often of major importance	>1/3 (exclusive of skin cancer)	16
Coronary artery disease	Disorder with multiple causes, including genetic predisposition	Heterogeneous, variable frequency, up to 1/15 in Western populations, currently declining	15
Diabetes mellitus	Failure of insulin production by beta cells of pancreas; certain human leukocyte antigen genes are major determinants of risk	Heterogeneous, 1/10 to 1/20 adults, less common in children	15
Mitochondrial Disorders			
Leber's hereditary optic neuropathy	First disease demonstrated to be due to a defect in the mitochondrial genome; maternally inherited	Rare	4

* Location of chief descriptions; see index also.

ever, there are many different kinds; about 4000 single-gene phenotypes, some 3000 of which are genetic disorders, have been described (McKusick, 1990), and their combined impact is significant. In several hundred of these diseases, the basic biochemical defect has been recognized, and in many the affected gene has been isolated and cloned (Beaudet et al., 1989).

The role of mitochondrial, as well as nuclear, genes as causes of disease is now recognized, and a defect in a mitochondrial gene has been identified in several disorders, including Leber's hereditary optic neuropathy. Mitochondrially transmitted diseases must therefore be recognized as a special type of single-gene disorder.

In **chromosome disorders,** the defect is due not to a single mistake in the genetic blueprint but to an excess or deficiency of the genes contained in whole chromosomes or chromosome segments.

For example, the presence of an extra copy of one chromosome, chromosome 21, produces a specific disorder, Down syndrome (Table 1–1), even though no individual gene on the chromosome is abnormal. As a group, chromosome disorders are quite common, affecting about 7 of 1000 liveborn infants and accounting for about half of all spontaneous first-trimester abortions.

Multifactorial inheritance is responsible for a number of developmental disorders resulting in congenital malformations and for many common disorders of adult life. Again, there appears to be no single error in the genetic information, but rather a combination of small variations that together can produce or predispose to a serious defect. Environmental factors may also be involved. Multifactorial disorders tend to recur in families but do not show the characteristic pedigree patterns of single-gene traits.

How Can a Physician Recognize that a Disorder Is Genetic?

One of the ironic characteristics of genetic disease is that affected persons usually seek out, not a geneticist, but rather a primary care physician. Because patients do not come in complaining that "my genes are killing me!" or that "I have a pain in my genes," the primary care physician must recognize that the symptoms have or may have a genetic explanation and must refer the patient to a geneticist's care. Thus it is the responsibility of primary care physicians to recognize the first clinical signs of genetic disease and to ask themselves, as a matter of routine, whether genetics has a role. This is what is meant by the genetic approach to medicine or by "genetic medicine."

If a disorder appears more than once in a family, it may have a genetic cause, and one of the purposes of this textbook is to describe ways to identify the various patterns of genetic disease in families. However, not all disorders that affect more than one member of a family are genetic, and not all genetic disorders affect more than one member of a family. How can the practicing physician recognize that a disorder in a given patient is genetic in nature, with all that such recognition implies for the patient and family members?

There is no simple answer to this question. One major clue is, of course, the diagnosis. Even though many genetic disorders lack specific diagnostic tests, the task of diagnosis is facilitated today by the many excellent descriptions of genetic disorders in the medical literature. Computer software is also contributing to genetic diagnosis, particularly to the diagnosis of dysmorphic syndromes.

To illustrate the variety of genetic problems that a physician might face, the accompanying box contains four brief histories of patients with relatively common genetic disorders. Each of the conditions is discussed in further detail elsewhere in the text.

Risk

One of the primary considerations in genetic medicine is evaluation of the recurrence risk — that is,

the risk that a genetic disorder in a patient will also affect other family members. Many people are unaware, however, that in *any* pregnancy there is an appreciable risk of an unfavorable outcome; for example, the risk of a congenital abnormality in any child of any parents is about 1 in 30 and, as the following section shows, the risk of a significant genetic disease making its appearance before the age of 25 is even higher. Table 1–2 summarizes the baseline risks faced by any couple contemplating a pregnancy. Risks for specific genetic defects in relatives of index patients may be based on the pattern of inheritance or may simply be empiric risks, based on experience. The estimation of recurrence risks in different situations is the basis of genetic counseling, and is considered in several later chapters.

The Load of Genetic Disease

Information on the frequency of genetic disorders in the population as a whole is needed both to allow health care planning and to provide a baseline against which possible future changes can be measured. There have been efforts in several countries to provide frequency estimates but, because of differences in ascertainment and classification, estimates for different populations are not strictly comparable. According to a report based on more than 1 million live births over 40 years, more than 5 percent of live-born persons under 25 years of age had a genetic disorder of single-gene, cytogenetic or multifactorial causation (Baird et al., 1988). The breakdown by disease category was as

Table 1–2. **Baseline Risks of Abnormal Outcome of Pregnancy**

Risk of some congenital abnormality present at birth	1 in 30
Risk of a severe physical or mental handicap	1 in 50
Risk of a serious physical or mental handicap in child of cousin parents	1 in 30
Risk of spontaneous abortion	1 in 8
Risk of stillbirth (North America)	1 in 125
Risk of perinatal death (North America)	1 in 150
Risk of death in first year of life after first week (North America)	1 in 200
Risk that a couple will be infertile	1 in 10

Based on Harper PS (1988) Practical genetic counselling, 3rd ed. Butterworth's, London.

Examples of Genetics in Medicine

1. A pregnant woman aged 37 presents to her primary care physician for prenatal care. Is her fetus at greater risk for a genetic disorder than would be the case if the woman's age was 27? If so, what is the risk, and what is the physician's responsibility in such a case?
Answer: When a woman is 37 years of age, the risk that her fetus will be born with a chromosome defect such as Down syndrome is about 1 in 225, whereas at age 27 the risk is only 1 in 1100. The woman should be advised of the risk and of the availability of prenatal diagnosis and be given the option of referral to a prenatal diagnosis program (see Chapters 9 and 19).

2. A physician is notified that routine prenatal screening for phenylketonuria (PKU) has shown that an infant in her care has tested positive for hyperphenylalaninemia. What is her responsibility?
Answer: The first step is to confirm the abnormal test and to determine the biochemical defect (in this example, PKU), and then to begin appropriate treatment. Support and genetic counseling are necessary, and prenatal diagnosis should be made available. The physician needs to be aware of special programs for the management of PKU and the problems associated with it. (See Chapters 4, 12, and 13.)

3. A 3-year-old child is seen on routine physical examination to have café-au-lait spots on the trunk. Is the child at risk for a genetic disorder? If so, how serious might it be? What is the physician's responsibility?
Answer: A possible diagnosis is neurofibromatosis, type 1. If this is confirmed, the clinical and genetic aspects of the situation both require attention. Regular evaluation is clinically important because of the numerous complications of the condition. Genetically, the disorder may have arisen by new mutation or may have been inherited. The genetic risks in the two situations differ. To distinguish between them, evaluation of the family history and examination of other family members are required. Genetic counseling is needed, and referral for prenatal diagnosis may also be appropriate. (See Chapter 4.)

4. A 46-year-old male is found by his primary care physician to have hyperlipidemia, which is a known risk factor for coronary artery disease. Family history reveals that a brother died at age 48 of coronary artery disease. What is the physician's responsibility?
Answer: The physician must first evaluate the significance of the hyperlipidemia, make a specific diagnosis on the basis of clinical examination and further laboratory tests, and make sensible recommendations to the patient. Many forms of primary hyperlipidemia are genetic, with either a single-gene or a multifactorial basis, but it may not be possible to establish a genetic diagnosis without determination of the lipid levels in first-degree relatives. Because the patient's family history suggests a genetic cause for the hyperlipidemia, the physician has a responsibility to give him full information about the possible genetic basis of hyperlipidemia and to recommend that his relatives be given this information. However, for ethical reasons, it is inappropriate for the physician to approach the relatives directly, because the patient has the responsibility for deciding whether to inform his relatives of his diagnosis and the implications for their own health.

follows:

Category	Frequency (%)	
Single-gene		
Autosomal dominant	0.14	
Autosomal recessive	0.17	
X-linked	0.05	
Total single-gene		0.36
Chromosomal		0.19
Multifactorial		
Congenital	2.3	
Other	2.4	
Total multifactorial		4.70
Unclassified genetic		0.12
Total		5.37

These figures, derived from a Health Surveillance Registry, may be underestimates. For example, the estimate of the frequency of chromosome disorders given here is only one third of that obtained from cytogenetic analysis of extensive series of newborns (see Chapter 9). Although probably minimal, the estimates are valuable indicators of the population incidence of genetic diseases with major health consequences and relatively early onset.

Family History

Taking a comprehensive family history is an important first step in the analysis of any disorder, whether or not the disorder is known to be genetic. According to Childs (1982), "to fail to take a good family history is bad medicine and someday will be criminal negligence." A family history is important because it can be helpful in diagnosis, can often show that a disorder is genetic, can provide information about the natural history of a disease and variation in its expression, and can clarify the pattern of inheritance, allowing the recurrence risk in other family members to be estimated.

Single-gene disorders have characteristic pedigree patterns, as described in Chapter 4. Single-gene inheritance can be simulated by several different mechanisms, especially by multifactorial inheritance but also by other processes, such as some types of chromosomal rearrangement or prenatal exposure of more than one child to a teratogen used by the mother. Cytogenetic disorders usually do not recur in families, but when they do, there is a need to investigate the basis of the recurrence, which may be a structural chromosomal abnormality or undetected mosaicism in a parent. Multifactorial disorders have patterns that are less characteristic but allow most multifactorial traits to be distinguished from single-gene traits in population studies, though not in individual pedigrees. An adequate family history should include information about the patient's relatives in the various family branches at least as far as the grandparents and their sibs, the parents and their sibs, and the patient's first cousins. The information should include such details as names, dates of birth and death, medical conditions, early infant deaths, stillbirths, and spontaneous abortions. Consanguinity of the parents and geographic or ethnic background should be documented. If the patient is a child, the mother's pregnancy history is important, especially with respect to very early events. *Information about unaffected family members is just as important as information about affected ones.* The history can be recorded in the form of a pedigree, which is essentially a diagram that records genetic information in unambiguous shorthand form, as described in Chapter 4.

Examples of Genetic Diseases

Table 1–1 is a partial list of some of the more significant genetic diseases discussed in this book. The disorders in the list have been selected because they are common or prominent genetic conditions that are used in the following chapters to illustrate a variety of important genetic principles. In some cases a disease has been selected primarily because of its important contributions to the expansion of molecular genetic knowledge, and in others because of a unique population distribution, but these are not the only reasons for inclusion. For example, PKU is the prototype disease for neonatal screening programs aimed at prevention of the serious sequelae of the inborn defect and for dietary treatment of metabolic disease. Retinoblastoma represents a single-gene form of cancer. Among the cytogenetic disorders, those listed are the most frequent and clinically significant types. Two main kinds of multifactorial disorders are included: (1) common congenital malformations and (2) common disorders of adult life with significant but often poorly understood genetic components. Finally, there is one example of a mitochondrial disease. These and other disorders considered in subsequent chapters by no means provide a complete overview in medical genetics but should give some understanding of the broad nature of genetic disease and how genetic knowledge and technology can be applied in the clinical setting.

During the 40-year professional life of today's medical students, extensive changes are likely to take place in the role of genetics in medicine. It is hard to imagine that any 40-year period could encompass changes greater than those of the years 1950 to 1990, in which both human cytogenetics and molecular genetics began, numerous genetic disorders were defined and characterized, and prenatal diagnosis of genetic disorders became very nearly routine. It is likely that the next major steps will be great expansion in the detection and prevention of genetic disease, correction of some defective genes by gene therapy, and mapping of the entire human genome. The basis of susceptibility to many common disorders, probably including malignancy, will be elucidated, allowing many such conditions to become predictable and even preventable. An introduction to the language and concepts of genetics and an appreciation of the genetic perspective of health and disease will form a framework for the lifelong learning that is part of any physician's career.

General References

Emery AEH (1986) Methodology in medical genetics, 2nd ed. Churchill Livingstone, Edinburgh.

Emery AEH, Rimoin DL (eds) (1990) Principles and practice of medical genetics, 2nd ed. Churchill Livingstone, Edinburgh.

Graham JM Jr, Rotter JI, Riccardi VM, et al (1989) Report of the task force on teaching human genetics in North American medical schools. Am J Hum Genet 44: 161–165.

Harper PS (1988) Practical genetic counselling, 3rd ed. Butterworth's, London.

McKusick VA (1990) Mendelian inheritance in man: catalogs of autosomal dominant, autosomal recessive, and X-linked phenotypes, 9th ed. Johns Hopkins University Press, Baltimore.

Scriver CR, Beaudet AL, Sly WS, Valle D (eds) (1989) The metabolic basis of inherited disease, 6th ed. McGraw-Hill, New York.

Vogel F, Motulsky AG (1986) Human genetics: problems and approaches, 2nd ed. Springer-Verlag, Berlin.

Weatherall DJ (1991) The new genetics and clinical practice, 3rd ed. Oxford University Press, Oxford, England.

CHAPTER
2

CHROMOSOMAL BASIS OF HEREDITY

When a cell divides, its nuclear material (**chromatin**) loses the relatively homogeneous appearance characteristic of nondividing cells and condenses to appear as a number of rod-shaped organelles, which are called **chromosomes** (*chroma*, color; *soma*, body) because they stain deeply with certain biological dyes. Although chromosomes are visible as discrete structures only in dividing cells, they retain their integrity between cell divisions. Chromatin is composed of deoxyribonucleic acid (**DNA**) and a complex class of chromosomal proteins. **Genes**, which at this point we define simply as units of genetic information, are encoded in the chromosomal DNA.

Each species has a characteristic chromosome complement (**karyotype**) in terms of the number and the morphology of its chromosomes. The genes are in linear order along the chromosomes, each gene having a precise position or **locus**. The **gene map**, the map of the chromosomal location of the genes, is also characteristic of each species and is, as far as we know, the same in all individuals within a species. The relative position of some genes appears to have been highly conserved in recent evolution, even among species as diverse as man and mouse.

The study of chromosomes, their structure, and their inheritance is called **cytogenetics**. The science of modern human cytogenetics dates from 1956, when Tjio and Levan developed effective techniques for chromosome analysis and established that the normal human chromosome number is 46. Since that time, much has been learned about human chromosomes, their normal structure, their molecular composition, the locations of the genes that they contain, and their numerous and varied abnormalities. Chromosome analysis has become an important diagnostic procedure in clinical medicine. As described in several subsequent chapters, chromosome anomalies are major causes of reproductive loss and birth defects and are common in many forms of cancer. The ability to interpret a chromosome report and some knowledge of the methodology, the scope, and the limitations of chromosome studies are essential skills for physicians and others working with patients with birth defects, mental retardation, disorders of sexual development, and many types of cancer.

THE HUMAN CHROMOSOMES

The 46 chromosomes of human somatic cells constitute 23 pairs. Of those 23 pairs, 22 are alike in males and females and are called **autosomes**. The remaining pair comprises the **sex chromosomes**: XX in females and XY in males. Members of a pair (described as **homologous chromosomes** or **homologs**) carry matching genetic information; that is, they have the same gene loci in the same sequence, though at any specific locus they may have either identical or slightly different forms, which are called **alleles**. One member of each pair of chromosomes is inherited from the father, the other from the mother. Normally, the members of a pair of autosomes are microscopically indistinguishable from one another. In females the sex chromosomes, the two **X chromosomes**, are likewise indistinguishable. In males, however, the sex chromosomes differ. One is an X, identical to the Xs of the female, inherited by a male from his mother and transmitted to his daughters; the other, the **Y chromosome**, is inherited from his father and transmitted to his sons. Later, we look at some exceptions to the simple and almost universal rule that human females are XX and human males are XY.

There are two kinds of cell division: mitosis and meiosis. **Mitosis** is ordinary somatic cell division, by which the body grows, differentiates, and effects repair. Mitotic division normally results in two daughter cells, each with chromosomes and genes identical to those of the parent cell. There may be dozens or even hundreds of successive mitoses in a line of somatic cells. **Meiosis** occurs only in cells of the germline and only once in a generation. It results in the formation of reproductive cells (**gametes**), each of which has only 23 chromosomes: one of each kind of autosome and either an X or a Y. Somatic cells have the **diploid** (*diploos*, double) or the 2n chromosome complement (i.e., 46 chromosomes), whereas gametes have the **haploid** (*haploos*, single) or the n complement (i.e., 23 chromosomes). Abnormalities of chromosome number or structure, which are usually clinically significant, can arise in both somatic cells and gametes by errors in cell division.

Techniques of Chromosome Analysis

The chromosomes of a dividing human cell are most readily analyzed at the metaphase or the prometaphase stage of mitosis. At these stages, the chromosomes appear under the microscope as a **chromosome spread** (Fig. 2–1), and each chro-

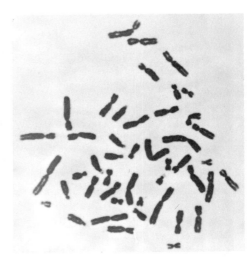

Figure 2–1. A chromosome spread prepared from a lymphocyte culture and stained by a "solid staining" technique. (Photomicrograph courtesy of R. G. Worton, The Hospital for Sick Children, Toronto.)

mosome is seen to consist of two **chromatids**, joined at the **centromere** (Fig. 2–2). Each chromatid is a double helix of DNA.

The centromere, or **primary constriction**, plays a key function in cell division as the region at which spindle fibers attach. It is a standard cytological landmark, dividing the chromosome into two **arms**, designated **p** (for *petit*) for the short arm and **q** for the long arm. Arms of individual chromosomes are indicated by the chromosome number followed by p or q; for example, 11p is the short arm of the chromosome designated as chromosome 11, and Yq is the long arm of the Y chromosome. Human chromosomes are classified by centromere position into three types (see Fig. 2–2): **metacentric**, with a more or less central centromere and arms of approximately equal length; **submetacentric**, with an off-center centromere and arms of clearly different lengths; and **acrocentric**, with the centromere near one end. A potential fourth type, **telocentric,** with the centromere at one end and only a single arm, does not occur in man, but it is a common type in other species; mouse chromosomes, for example, are telocentric.

The human acrocentric chromosomes (chromosomes 13, 14, 15, 21, and 22) have small masses of chromatin known as **satellites** attached to their short arms by narrow stalks (secondary constrictions). The stalks of these five chromosome pairs

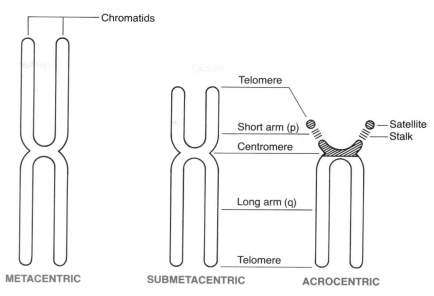

Figure 2-2. Chromosome types and landmarks, as described in the text.

contain the genes for 18S and 28S ribosomal RNA (rRNA). (See further discussion in Chapter 3.)

Cell Culture

Cells for chromosome analysis must be capable of growth and rapid division in culture. The most readily accessible cells that meet this requirement are white blood cells, specifically T lymphocytes. In order to prepare a short-term culture of these cells suitable for analysis, a sample of peripheral blood is obtained, usually by venipuncture, and mixed with heparin to prevent clotting. It is then centrifuged at a speed that allows the white cells to sediment out as a distinct layer, the buffy coat. The white cells are collected, placed in tissue culture medium, and stimulated to divide by the addition of a mitogenic (mitosis-stimulating) agent, **phytohemagglutinin**. The culture is incubated for about 72 hours until the cells are multiplying rapidly. A very dilute solution of **colchicine** is added next, to prevent completion of cell division by inhibiting spindle formation and delaying the separation of centromeres. As a result, cells arrested in metaphase accumulate in the culture. A **hypotonic solution** is then added to cause swelling of the cells, lysing them and releasing the chromosomes while keeping the centromeres intact. Chromosomes are fixed, spread on slides, and stained by one of several techniques. They are then ready for analysis.

Although ideal for fairly rapid clinical analysis, cell cultures prepared from peripheral blood have the disadvantage of being short-lived (3 to 4 days). Long-term cultures can be derived from a variety of other tissues (see Chapter 8). Skin biopsy, a minor surgical procedure, can provide samples of tissue that in culture produce **fibroblasts**, spindle-shaped cells that are capable of continuous growth in culture for many generations and can be used for a variety of biochemical and molecular studies, as well as for chromosome analysis. White blood cells can also be transformed in culture by the addition of Epstein-Barr virus, forming **lymphoblastoid** cell lines that are potentially immortal. **Bone marrow** can be obtained only by the relatively invasive procedure of marrow biopsy, but it has the advantage of containing a high proportion of dividing cells, so that little if any culturing is required. Its main use is in the diagnosis of suspected hematological malignancies. Its disadvantage is that the chromosome preparations obtained from marrow are relatively poor, with short, fuzzy chromosomes that are hard to band. **Fetal cells** derived from amniotic fluid (amniocytes) or obtained by chorionic villus biopsy can also be cultured successfully for cytogenetic, biochemical, or molecular analysis (see Chapter 19 for further discussion).

Chromosome Identification

The staining methods originally available for human cytogenetic analysis did not allow all 24 types of chromosome (22 autosomes, X, and Y) to be individually identified. Instead, the chromosomes could only be classified into seven groups,

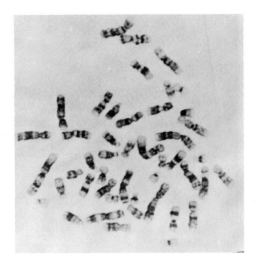

Figure 2–3. The chromosome spread shown in Figure 2–1, which has been destained and restained by a G banding technique. (Photomicrograph courtesy of R. G. Worton, The Hospital for Sick Children, Toronto.)

named by the letters A to G, on the basis of their overall length and the position of the centromere. With techniques now in common use, however, all the chromosomes can be individually identified.

Figures 2–1 and 2–3 show the same chromosome spread stained by two techniques. In Figure 2–1, the chromosomes have been stained with a so-called solid stain, which stains the chromosomes uniformly; different chromosomes can be only partially distinguished. In Figure 2–3, the same cell is shown after the chromosomes have been destained and restained by the Giemsa-staining (G-banding) method (to be described) in order to demonstrate their characteristic patterns of transverse bands. With this and other so-called banding techniques that are now in common use, all the chromosome types can be individually distinguished. The autosomes are numbered 1 to 22 on the basis of their overall length. (Actually, chromosome 21 is an exception to the rule, being slightly shorter than chromosome 22. However, before its smaller size was recognized, it was already well known as chromosome 21, which is

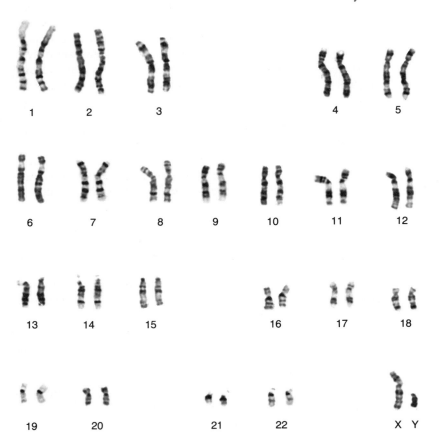

Figure 2–4. A human male karyotype with Giemsa banding (G banding). The chromosomes are at the prometaphase stage of mitosis and are arranged in a standard classification, numbered 1 to 22 in order of length and with the X and Y chromosomes shown separately. (Photomicrograph courtesy of Chin Ho, The Hospital for Sick Children, Toronto.)

present in three copies in most cases of a common chromosome abnormality, Down syndrome.)

Although experts can often analyze chromosome spreads directly under the microscope, a common procedure is to cut out the chromosomes from a photomicrograph and arrange them in pairs in a standard classification, as shown in Figure 2–4. The completed picture is a **karyotype**. The same term, karyotype, is also used for the standard chromosome set of an individual ("a normal male karyotype") or of a species ("the human karyotype"), as well as for the process of preparing such a standard figure ("karyotyping"). Researchers have developed computerized karyotyping systems that are capable of automatically selecting cells suitable for analysis, analyzing the stained chromosomes of the cell, and constructing a karyotype.

A uniform system of chromosome classification is internationally accepted. This system was originally formulated at a conference in Paris in 1971; later, some revision became necessary in order to describe the chromosomes as seen in more elongated prophase and prometaphase preparations (described later). The karyotype shown in Figure 2–4 shows chromosomes at the prometaphase stage, stained by the G-banding technique (see the following section). Figure 2–5 is a diagram of the banding pattern of a set of normal human chromosomes at approximately the same stage of condensation as the karyotype in Figure 2–4. A more detailed diagram, with the numbering system used to designate the individual bands, is provided in Appendix I.

STAINING METHODS FOR ROUTINE ANALYSIS

A number of banding methods are used routinely in cytogenetic laboratories for chromosomal identification and analysis of chromosome structure.

G Banding (see Figs. 2–3 and 2–4). This is the technique most widely used. The chromosomes are treated with trypsin, to denature the chromosomal proteins, and then with Giemsa stain. Each chromosome pair stains in a characteristic pattern of light and dark bands (G bands).

Q Banding (Fig. 2–6). This method requires staining with quinacrine mustard or related compounds and examination by fluorescence microscopy. The chromosomes stain in a specific pattern of bright and dim bands (Q bands), the bright Q bands correspond almost exactly to the dark G bands.

R Banding (Fig. 2–7). If the chromosomes receive heat pretreatment before Giemsa staining, the resulting dark and light bands (R bands) are the reverse of those produced by G or Q banding. In some cases, R banding provides information in addition to that given by G or Q banding. It is the standard method in many laboratories, especially in Europe.

SPECIAL PROCEDURES

For special situations, a number of techniques of chromosome culture and staining can be used:

C Banding. This method specifically involves staining the centromeric region of each chromosome and other regions containing **heterochromatin**: namely, sections of chromosomes 1q, 9q, and 16q adjacent to the centromere and the distal part of Yq. Heterochromatin is the type of chromatin defined by its property of remaining in the condensed state and staining darkly in nondividing (interphase) cells.

High-Resolution Banding (also called **prophase** or **prometaphase banding**). This type of banding is achieved through G-banding or R-banding techniques to stain chromosomes that have been prepared at an early stage of mitosis (prophase or prometaphase), when they are still in a relatively uncondensed state. Prophase banding (Fig. 2–8) is not a routine procedure in clinical cytogenetics but is used when a subtle structural abnormality of a chromosome is suspected; many laboratories, however, routinely use prometaphase banding, as shown in Figures 2–4, 2–6, and 2–7. Prometaphase and prophase chromosomes reveal 550 to 850 bands or even more in a haploid set, whereas standard metaphase preparations show only about 400 (see Appendix I). The technique requires arresting DNA synthesis in a cell culture so as to synchronize the cells and then releasing the block and harvesting the culture at a time when numerous cells are in late prophase or early metaphase, before they are maximally condensed.

Fragile Sites. Nonstaining gaps, known as fragile sites, are occasionally observed in characteristic sites on several chromosomes. Many such sites are known to be heritable variants. The only fragile site known to be clinically significant is seen near the end of Xq both in males with a specific

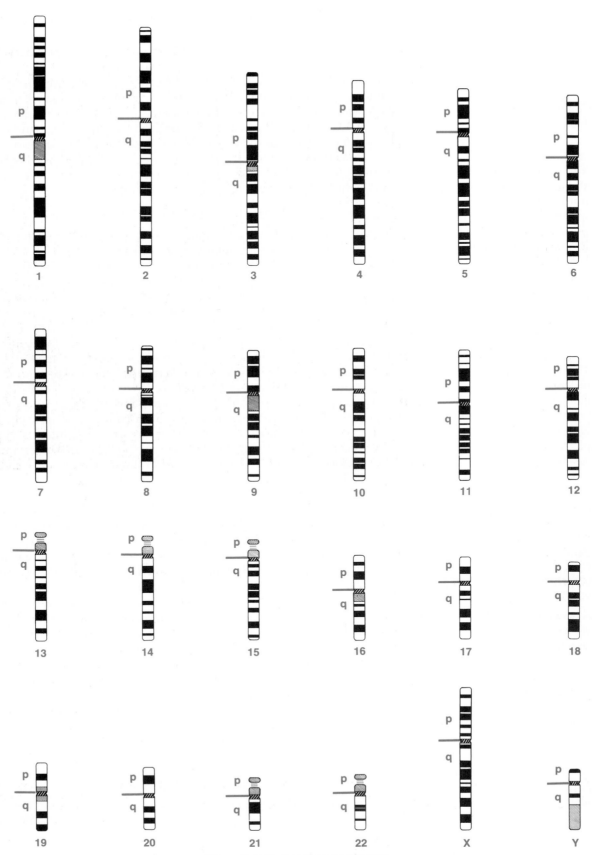

Figure 2–5. *See legend on opposite page*

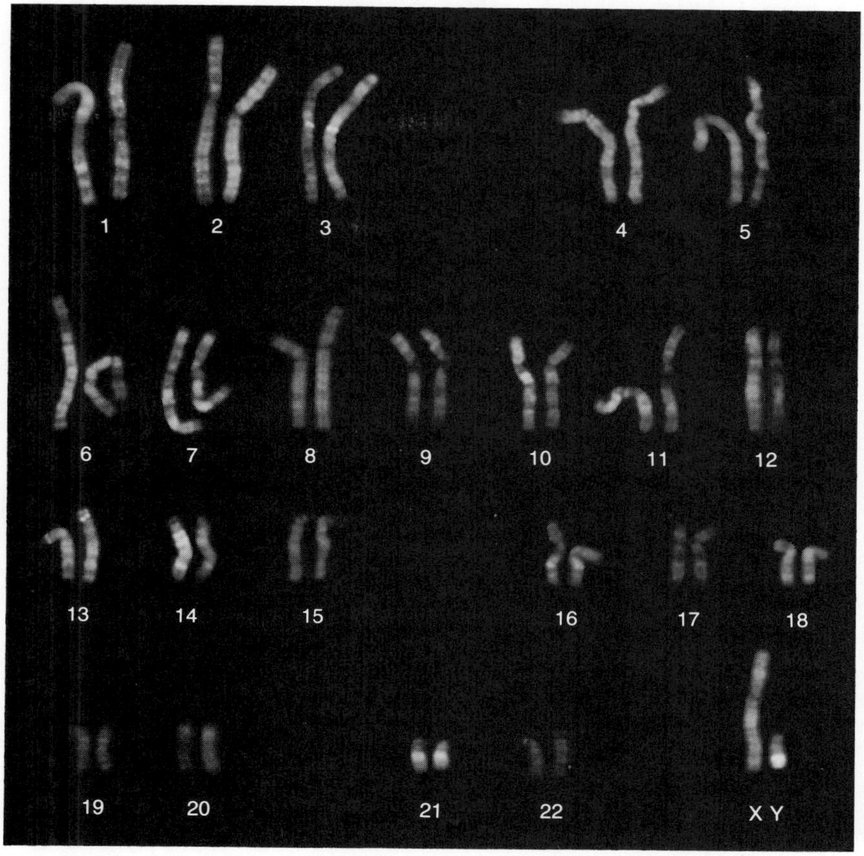

Figure 2-6. A Q-banded human male karyotype at the prometaphase stage. The chromosomes have been stained with quinacrine dihydrochloride and photographed under fluorescent light to show the Q bands. The bright Q bands are almost identical to the dark G bands. (Photomicrograph courtesy of Jeanette Holden, Kingston Psychiatric Hospital, Kingston, Ontario.)

and quite common form of X-linked mental retardation and in some female carriers of the same genetic defect (see discussion of the fragile X syndrome, Chapter 4). In order to demonstrate fragile sites, it is often necessary to culture the cells under unusual growth conditions. In the fragile X syndrome, the fragile site is visualized only in cells that have been cultured under conditions of thymidine deprivation. This is achieved either through a culture medium low in thymidine and folic acid or through the addition of an inhibitor of the enzyme thymidine synthetase to the medium. Because the fragile sites are often difficult to see in banded chromosome preparations, solid staining is required in addition to the special culture conditions. Detection of the fragile site on the X chromosome is a key diagnostic procedure specific for the fragile X syndrome.

Molecular Cytogenetics. The use of cloned DNA probes (prepared by recombinant DNA techniques; see Chapter 5) to examine chromosomes is called molecular cytogenetics. DNA probes specific for individual chromosomes or for chromosomal regions can be used to identify particular chromosomal rearrangements or to rapidly diagnose the existence of an abnormal chromosome number (i.e., not 46) in clinical material. This is a relatively specialized area now, but it may well become part of routine clinical cytogenetics practice in the future.

Figure 2-5. Diagram to show G-banding pattern for human chromosomes at the prometaphase stage of condensation, with about 550 bands per haploid karyotype. The chromosomes are represented as single-chromatid structures rather than as the two-chromatid structures seen in mitotic chromosomes under the microscope. (Redrawn from ISCN, 1985.) See also Appendix I.

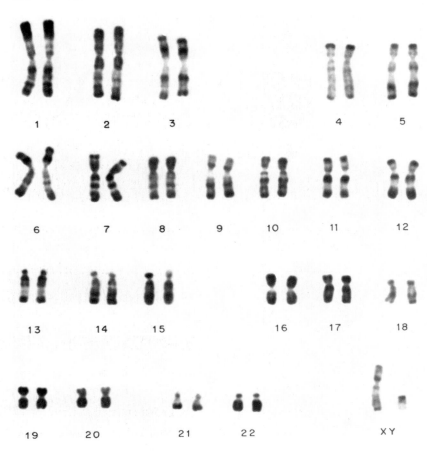

Figure 2-7. An R-banded human male karyotype at the prometaphase stage. The chromosomes have been stained by the reverse banding technique; the light bands are almost exactly equivalent to the dark G bands. (Photomicrograph courtesy of Claude-Lise Richer, University of Montreal.)

THE LIFE CYCLE OF A SOMATIC CELL

A human being begins life as a fertilized ovum (zygote), a diploid cell from which all the cells of the body (estimated at about 10^{14} in number) are

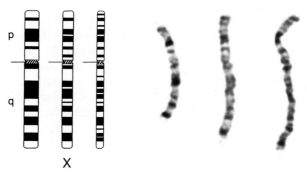

Figure 2-8. The X chromosome: idiograms and photomicrographs at three stages of resolution, metaphase, prometaphase, and prophase (*left to right*). Idiograms redrawn from ISCN (1985). (Photomicrographs courtesy of Yim Kwan Ng, The Hospital for Sick Children, Toronto.)

derived by a series of dozens or even hundreds of mitoses. Mitosis is obviously crucial for growth and differentiation, but it takes up only a small part of the life cycle of a cell. What goes on in **interphase**, the period between two successive mitoses?

As Figure 2-9 shows, mitosis is the shortest of the four stages of the cell cycle. Immediately after mitosis, the cell enters a phase in which there is no DNA synthesis, G_1 (Gap 1). Some cells spend a very long time, days or even years, in G_1; others pass through this stage in hours. Although the molecular mechanisms governing the length of the cell cycle and the timing of mitosis are not well understood, it appears that late in G_1 the cell passes a "restriction point," after which it will proceed through the rest of the cell cycle at a standard rate.

G_1 is followed by the **S phase**, the stage of DNA synthesis. During this stage, each chromosome, which in G_1 has been a single double-helical DNA molecule, replicates and becomes the typical

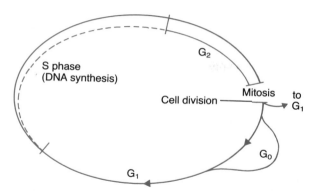

Figure 2–9. The mitotic cell cycle, described in the text.

two-chromatid chromosome that is familiar in metaphase preparations. DNA synthesis is not synchronous throughout the chromosome set or even within a single chromosome; rather, it begins at probably hundreds to thousands of sites along each chromosome, and individual chromosome segments have their own characteristic patterns of replication. Homologous pairs of chromosomes usually replicate synchronously. The same is not true, however, for the sex chromosomes. One of the two X chromosomes of female somatic cells is genetically inactivated in order to achieve dosage equivalence with male somatic cells, which have only a single X. The inactive X is late-replicating (in comparison with its active homolog) and eventually becomes the **sex chromatin** (Barr body) visible in female somatic cells during interphase. The molecular basis and the clinical significance of X inactivation are discussed later (see Chapters 4 and 10).

By the end of S phase, the DNA content of the cell has doubled, and during the next stage, called G_2 (Gap 2), each chromosome consists of two identical DNA molecules, the two sister chromatids. Throughout the whole cell cycle, though DNA synthesis is restricted, ribonucleic acids and proteins are produced and the cell gradually enlarges, eventually doubling its total mass before the next mitosis. G_2 is ended by mitosis, which begins when individual chromosomes begin to condense and become visible under the microscope as thin, extended threads.

The G_1, S, and G_2 phases together constitute interphase. In a typical growing cell culture, the three phases take a total of 16–24 hours, whereas mitosis lasts only 1 to 2 hours (see Fig. 2–9). However, there is great variation in the length of the

cell cycle, which ranges from a few hours in rapidly dividing cells, such as those of the dermis of the skin or the intestinal mucosa, to months in other cell types. In fact, some cell types, such as neurons and red blood cells, do not divide at all once they are fully differentiated but are permanently stopped during G_1 in a phase known as G_0. Other cells may enter G_0 but eventually return to continue through the cell cycle.

Mitosis

When a cell enters mitosis, each of its chromosomes consists of a pair of identical sister chromatids, joined at the centromere. During mitosis, an elaborate apparatus is brought into play to ensure that each of the two daughter cells receives a complete set of genetic information. This is achieved by a mechanism that distributes one chromatid of each chromosome to each daughter cell and is illustrated schematically in Figure 2–10.

The process of mitosis is continuous, but five stages are distinguished: prophase, prometaphase, metaphase, anaphase, and telophase.

Prophase. This stage initiates mitosis and is marked by gradual condensation of the chromosomes, disintegration, and eventual disappearance of the nucleolus and the beginning of the formation of the **mitotic spindle**. The **centrioles**, pairs of cytoplasmic organelles, form centers from which microtubules radiate. The centrioles gradually move to take up positions at the poles of the cell.

Prometaphase. The cell enters prometaphase when the nuclear membrane breaks up, allowing the chromosomes to disperse within the cell and to become attached to microtubules of the mitotic spindle by means of specialized structures called **kinetochores** (Fig. 2–11) that are located at each side of the centromere of each chromosome. At this stage the chromosomes have contracted further, though not maximally.

Metaphase. At metaphase the chromosomes reach maximal contraction. They become arranged at the equatorial plane of the cell, probably by means of the microtubules attached to their kinetochores. In living cells, the chromosomes can be seen to move actively as they are drawn to their positions, but the molecular basis of their move-

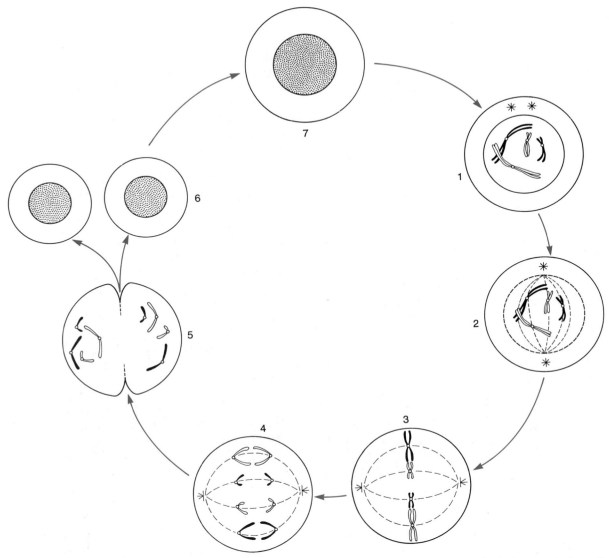

Figure 2-10. Mitosis. Diagrammatic representation, showing only two chromosome pairs. 1, prophase; 2, prometaphase; 3, metaphase; 4, anaphase; 5, telophase; 6,7 interphase. For further details, see text.

ment, like many other details about mitosis, remains unknown.

Anaphase. Anaphase begins abruptly when the chromosomes separate at the centromere, allowing the two chromatids of each chromosome (now independent **daughter chromosomes**) to move to opposite poles of the cell.

Telophase. In telophase, the chromosomes begin to decondense from their highly contracted state, a nuclear membrane begins to form around each of the two daughter nuclei, and each nucleus gradually resumes its interphase appearance.

To complete the process of cell division, the cytoplasm cleaves by a process known as **cytokinesis**, which is concurrent with the later stages of mitosis. Eventually there are two complete daughter cells, each with a nucleus containing all the genetic information of the original cell and approximately half the cytoplasm of the parent cell. The important difference between a cell entering mitosis and one that has just completed the process is that the parent cell's chromosomes each have a pair of chromatids, but the chromosomes of the daughter cell each consist of only one double

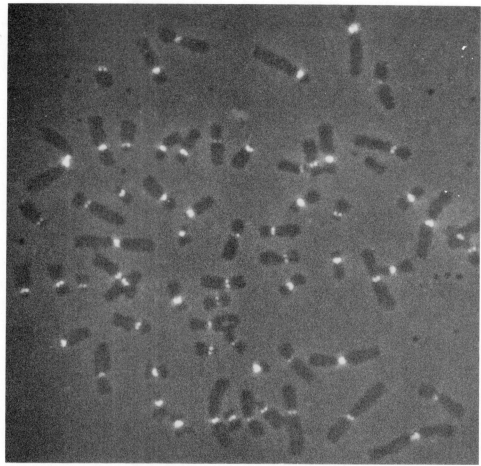

Figure 2–11. Kinetochores, structures by which chromosomes are attached to the mitotic spindle at prometaphase of mitosis (see text). Human chromosomes stained by indirect immunofluorescence with anticentromere (kinetochore) antibodies. (Photomicrograph courtesy of William Earnshaw, The Johns Hopkins University, Baltimore.)

helix, which will not be duplicated until the daughter cell in its turn reaches the S phase of the new cell cycle (see Fig. 2–9).

MEIOSIS

Meiosis is the type of cell division by which the diploid cells of the germline give rise to haploid gametes. The embryonic cells that are ancestral to the reproductive cells begin their differentiation in the wall of the yolk sac, from which they migrate to the genital ridges and become incorporated into the developing gonad. A primary spermatocyte or a primary oocyte, in which the first of the two meiotic divisions occurs, is derived from the zygote by a long series of mitoses.

Male and female gametes have different histories, but although the timing of events is very different, the sequence is the same. There are two successive meiotic divisions. Meiosis I is known as the **reduction division** because it is the division in which the chromosome number is reduced from diploid to haploid by the pairing of homologs in prophase and their segregation at anaphase. The X and Y chromosomes are not homologs but do have homologous segments at the tip of their short arms, and they pair in that region only. Meiosis II follows meiosis I without an intervening step of DNA replication. As in ordinary mitosis, the chromatids disjoin, and one chromatid of each chromosome passes to each daughter cell. Some of the stages distinguished in meiosis are shown in Figure 2–12.

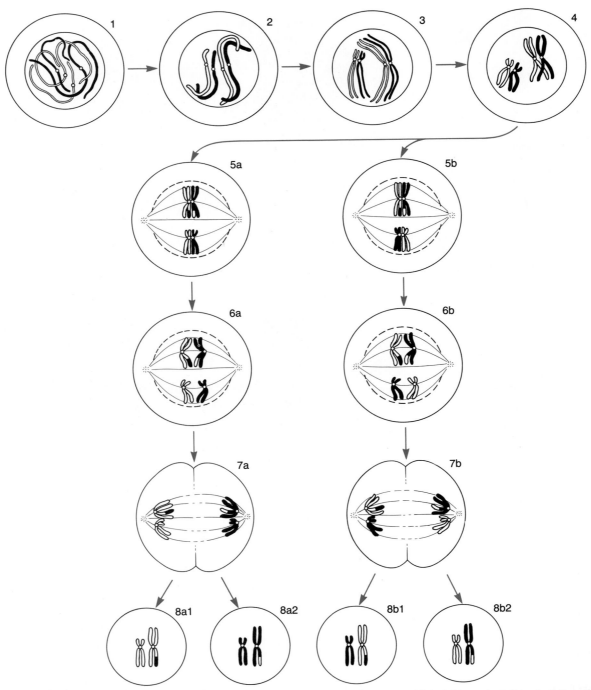

Figure 2–12. Meiosis. Diagrammatic representation of the process and its consequences. Meiosis I is on the left, meiosis II on the right. Two chromosome pairs and a single crossover in one chromosome pair are shown, allowing for eight arrangements in the gametes. *Meiosis I*: 1 to 4, stages of prophase I; 5a and 5b, alternative arrangements of the chromosome pairs at metaphase I; 6a and 6b, anaphase I; 7a and 7b, telophase I; 8a1, 8a2, 8b1, 8b2, the four possible distributions of the parental chromosome pairs at the end of meiosis I. *Meiosis II*: 9a1, 9a2, 9b1, 9b2, metaphase II; 10a1, 10a2, 10b1, 10b2, anaphase II; 11a1, 11a2, 11b1, 11b2, the eight combinations of the genetic material possible in the gametes.

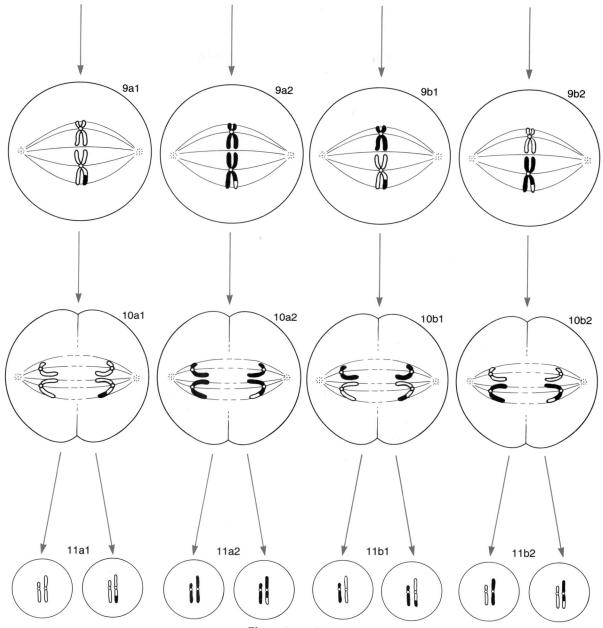

Figure 2-12. *Continued*

The First Meiotic Division (Meiosis I)

PROPHASE I

The prophase of meiosis I is a complicated process that differs from mitotic prophase in a number of ways, with important genetic consequences. Several stages are defined. Throughout all the stages, the chromosomes continually condense and become shorter and thicker.

Leptotene. The chromosomes, which have already replicated during the preceding S phase, become visible as thin threads that are beginning to condense. At this early stage, the two sister chromatids of each chromosome are so closely aligned that they cannot be distinguished. Unlike mitotic chromosomes, which are of uniform thickness (see Fig. 2–1), meiotic chromosomes have alternating thicker and thinner regions; the thick regions (**chromomeres**) have a characteristic pattern for each chromosome.

Zygotene. At this stage, homologous chromosomes begin to pair closely along their entire length. The process of pairing or **synapsis** is normally very precise, bringing corresponding DNA sequences into alignment along the length of the entire chromosomes.

Although the molecular basis of synapsis is not yet understood, electron microscopy reveals that the chromosomes are held together in some regions, but not throughout their entire length, by a **synaptonemal complex**, a ribbonlike tripartite structure containing protein. As shown in Figure 2–13, the synaptonemal complex has two lateral elements each 30 to 40 nm in diameter and a central element about 120 nm wide; these elements are connected by a series of transverse filaments. **Recombination nodules** form in association with the central element, and chromatin fibrils loop out from the lateral elements. The synaptonemal complex is essential to the phenomenon of crossing over, the exchange of homologous segments between nonsister chromatids of a pair of homologous chromosomes. Crossing over, which occurs during the next stage of meiosis, pachytene, is a biologically and clinically significant phenomenon and is described in more detail in Chapter 8.

Pachytene. During this stage, the chromosomes become much more tightly coiled, with more pronounced chromomeres. Synapsis is complete, and each pair of homologs appears as a **bivalent** (sometimes called a **tetrad** because it contains four chromatids). This is the stage at which crossing over takes place (Fig. 2–14).

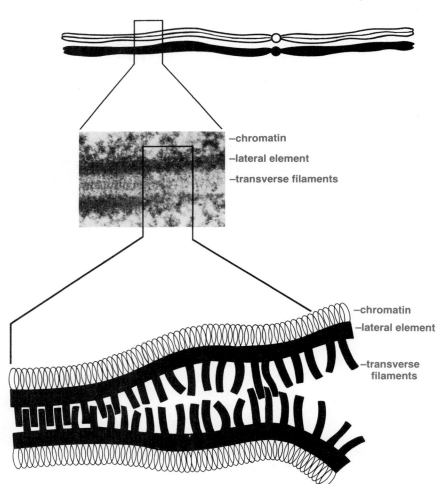

–chromatin

–lateral element

–transverse filaments

–chromatin

–lateral element

–transverse filaments

Figure 2–13. The synaptonemal complex (SC), which holds chromosomes together during synapsis (pairing). Diagrams show the relation of the SC to a pair of chromosomes at prophase (above) and details of the structure of the SC (below). (Photomicrograph courtesy of Peter Moens, York University, Toronto.)

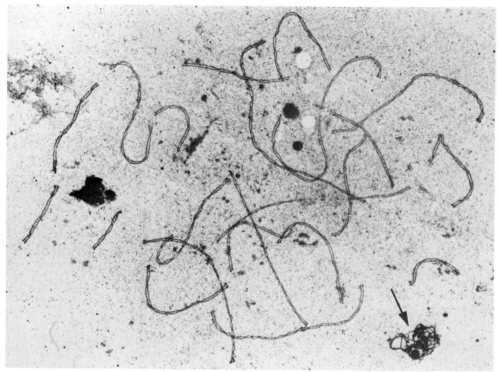

Figure 2-14. Electron micrograph of a human primary spermatocyte in meiosis, showing the 22 autosomal synaptonemal complexes and the XY pair (arrow). (Photomicrograph courtesy of A. C. Chandley, Western General Hospital, Edinburgh.)

Diplotene. The two components of each bivalent now begin to repel one another. Although the homologous chromosomes separate, their centromeres remain intact, so that each set of sister chromatids initially remains joined. Eventually the two homologs of each bivalent are held together only at points called **chiasmata** (crosses), which are believed to mark the locations of crossovers. The average number of chiasmata seen in human spermatocytes is about 50 (see Fig. 2-14).

Diakinesis. In this stage, the chromosomes reach maximal condensation.

METAPHASE I

Metaphase I begins, as in mitosis, when the nuclear membrane disappears. A spindle has formed, and the paired chromosomes align themselves on the equatorial plane with their centromeres oriented toward different poles.

ANAPHASE I

The two members of each bivalent disjoin, and their respective centromeres with the attached sister chromatids are drawn to opposite poles of the cell. Thus the chromosome number is halved, and each product has the haploid chromosome number. The bivalents assort independently of one another, and as a result the original paternal and maternal set are sorted into random combinations (see Fig. 2-12). The possible number of combinations of the 23 chromosome pairs that can be present in the gametes is 2^{23} (more than 8 million). The variety of genetic material that can be transmitted from parent to child is actually much greater than this because of the process of crossing over. As a result of this process each chromatid typically contains segments derived from each member of the parental chromosome pair; for example, at this stage a typical chromosome 1 is composed of three to five segments, alternately paternal and maternal in origin. (See further discussion in Chapter 8.)

Many errors can occur in cell division, and anaphase of meiosis I is the most error-prone step. Some of the consequences of meiotic irregularities are discussed in Chapters 9 and 10.

TELOPHASE I

By telophase the two haploid sets of chromosomes have grouped at the opposite poles of the cell.

Cytokinesis

After telophase I, the cell divides into two haploid daughter cells and enters interphase. In spermatogenesis the cytoplasm is more or less equally divided between the two daughter cells (Fig. 2–15), but in oogenesis one product (the secondary oocyte) receives almost all the cytoplasm, and the reciprocal product becomes the first polar body (Fig. 2–16). In contrast to mitosis, the interphase is brief, and the chromosomes condense only a little. The genetically important point is, however, that there is no S phase (i.e., no DNA synthesis) between the first and second meiotic divisions. After interphase, the chromosomes again decondense, and meiosis II begins.

The Second Meiotic Division (Meiosis II)

The second meiotic division is similar to an ordinary mitosis except that the chromosome number of the cell entering meiosis II is haploid. The end result is four haploid cells, each containing 23 chromosomes. As mentioned earlier, because of crossing over in meiosis I, the chromosomes of the products are not identical. Segregation of the different paternal and maternal forms of each gene takes place during either the first or the second meiotic division, depending on whether they have been involved in a crossover event in meiosis I.

Genetic Consequences of Meiosis

1. **Reduction of the chromosome number** from diploid to haploid, the essential step in the formation of gametes.

2. **Segregation of alleles**, at either meiosis I or meiosis II, in accordance with Mendel's first law.

3. Shuffling of the genetic material by **random assortment of the homologs**, in accordance with Mendel's second law.

4. Additional shuffling of the genetic material by **crossing over**, which is thought to have evolved as a mechanism for substantially increasing genetic variation.

Human Gametogenesis

The human primordial germ cells are recognizable by the 4th week of development outside the embryo proper, in the endoderm of the yolk sac. From there they migrate during the 6th week to the genital ridges and associate with somatic cells to form the primitive gonads, which soon differentiate into testes or ovaries, almost always in accordance with the cells' chromosome constitution (XY or XX). Both spermatogenesis and oogenesis require meiosis but have important differences in detail and timing that may have clinical and genetic consequences for the offspring.

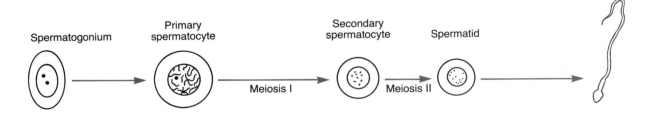

Spermatogonium   Primary spermatocyte   Secondary spermatocyte   Spermatid

Meiosis I   Meiosis II

~64 days

Figure 2–15. Diagram to illustrate human spermatogenesis in relation to the two meiotic divisions.

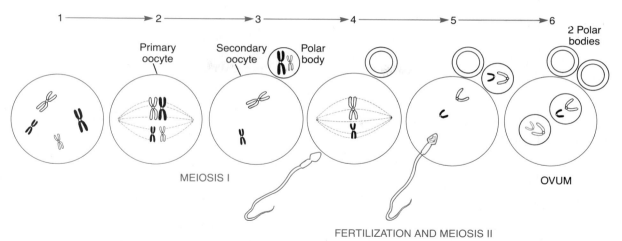

Figure 2–16. Diagram to illustrate human oogenesis and fertilization in relation to the two meiotic divisions. The stages labeled represent: oogonia (1), primary oocyte in early meiosis I (2), secondary oocyte at end of meiosis I (3), early meiosis II at time of fertilization (4), completion of meiosis II after fertilization (5), and fertilized ovum (6).

It is very difficult to study human meiosis directly. In the female, successive stages of meiosis take place in the fetal ovary, in the oocyte near the time of ovulation, and after fertilization. Although postfertilization stages can be studied in vitro, access to the earlier stages is limited. Material for the study of male meiosis is less difficult to obtain, inasmuch as testicular biopsy is included in the assessment of many men attending infertility clinics. In spite of recent technical advances, however, much remains to be learned about the cytogenetic, biochemical, and molecular mechanisms involved in normal meiosis and about the causes and consequences of meiotic irregularities.

Spermatogenesis

The stages of spermatogenesis are shown in Figure 2–15. **Sperm** (spermatozoa) are formed in the seminiferous tubules of the testes from the time of sexual maturity on. The tubules are lined with **spermatogonia**, which are in different stages of differentiation. These cells have developed from the primordial germ cells by a long series of mitoses. The last cell type in the developmental sequence is the **primary spermatocyte**, which undergoes meiosis I to form two haploid **secondary spermatocytes**. Secondary spermatocytes rapidly undergo meiosis II, each forming two **spermatids**, which differentiate without further division into **sperm**. In humans, the entire process takes about

64 days. The enormous number of sperm produced, typically about 200 million per ejaculate and an estimated 10^{12} in a lifetime, requires several hundred successive mitoses.

Oogenesis

In contrast to spermatogenesis, which is ongoing throughout life, oogenesis is largely complete at birth. The process is shown in Figure 2–16. The ova develop from **oogonia**, cells in the ovarian cortex that have descended from the primordial germ cells by a series of about 30 mitoses. Each oogonium is the central cell in a developing follicle. By about the 3rd month of prenatal development, the oogonia of the embryo have begun to develop into **primary oocytes**, some of which have already entered prophase of meiosis I. The process is not synchronized, and both early and late stages coexist in the fetal ovary. There are about 2.5 million oocytes at the time of birth, but most degenerate, and only about 400 eventually mature. The primary oocytes have all reached suspended prophase I (**dictyotene**) by the time of birth, and those that do not degenerate remain in that stage for many years.

After a woman has reached sexual maturity and as each individual follicle matures and ovulation occurs, the oocyte rapidly completes meiosis I, dividing in such a way that one cell becomes the secondary oocyte, containing most of the cytoplasm with its organelles, and the other becomes the first polar body. Meiosis II begins promptly and proceeds to the metaphase stage during ovulation, but it is completed only if fertilization occurs.

Fertilization and Early Embryonic Development

Fertilization usually takes place in the uterine tube within a day or so of ovulation. Although very large numbers of sperm may be present, the penetration of a single sperm into the ovum sets up a series of biochemical events that prevent the entry of other sperm.

Fertilization is followed by the completion of meiosis II, with the formation of the **ovum** and a second polar body. The chromosomes of the ovum and sperm become **pronuclei**, each surrounded by a nuclear membrane. The pronuclei approach and fuse, forming the diploid **zygote** (see Fig. 2–16). Although DNA synthesis is shut off in meiosis, the chromosomes of the zygote replicate soon after fertilization, and the zygote divides by mitosis to form two diploid daughter cells. This is the first of the series of cleavage divisions that initiate the process of embryonic development.

Although development begins with the formation of the zygote (conception), in clinical medicine the stage and duration of pregnancy are usually measured as the "menstrual age," dating from the beginning of the mother's last menstrual period, about 14 days before conception.

MEDICAL APPLICATIONS OF CHROMOSOME ANALYSIS

Chromosome analysis has a number of important medical applications, which are listed here and discussed further in later chapters:

Clinical Diagnosis. Numerous medical disorders, including some that are quite common, are associated with microscopically visible changes in chromosome number or structure and require chromosome analysis for diagnosis and genetic counseling (Chapters 9 and 10).

Linkage and Mapping. A major goal of medical genetics today is the mapping of specific genes to chromosomes. This topic is referred to repeatedly but discussed in detail in Chapter 8.

Cancer Cytogenetics. Chromosomal changes in somatic cells are involved in the initiation and progression of many types of cancer (Chapter 16).

Prenatal Diagnosis. Chromosome analysis is an essential procedure in prenatal diagnosis (Chapter 19).

General References

Chandley AC (1988) Meiosis in man. Trends Genet 4: 79–83.

ISCN (1985) An international system for human cytogenetic nomenclature. Karger Medical and Scientific Publishers, Basel.

McIntosh JR, McDonald KL (1989) The mitotic spindle. Sci Am 261: 48–56.

Moore KL (1988) The developing human: clinically oriented embryology, 4th ed. WB Saunders, Philadelphia.

Therman E (1986) Human chromosomes: structure, behavior, effects, 2nd ed. Springer-Verlag, New York.

Verma RS, Babu A (1989) Human chromosomes: manual of basic techniques. Pergamon Press, New York.

Problems

1. At a certain locus, a person is heterozygous, having the genotype A/a.
   a) What are the genotypes of this person's gametes?
   b) When do A and a segregate i) if there is no crossing over between the locus and the centromere of the chromosome? ii) if there is a single crossover between the locus and the centromere?

2. How many different genotypes are possible in the ova of a woman who is
   a) Heterozygous at a single locus?
   b) Heterozygous at four independent loci?
   c) Heterozygous at n independent loci?

3. Disregarding crossing over, which increases the amount of genetic variability, estimate the probability that all your chromosomes have come to you from your father's mother and your mother's mother. Would you be male or female?

4. A chromosome entering meiosis is composed of two chromatids, each of which is a double-stranded DNA molecule.
   a) In our species, at the end of meiosis I, how many chromosomes are there per cell? How many chromatids? How many DNA strands?
   b) At the end of meiosis II, how many chromosomes are there per cell? How many chromatids? How many DNA strands?
   c) When is the diploid chromosome number restored? When is the two-chromatid structure of a typical metaphase chromosome restored?

STRUCTURE AND FUNCTION OF CHROMOSOMES AND GENES

In the 1980s, remarkable progress was made in gaining knowledge of the structure and function of chromosomes and genes at the molecular level. This came about chiefly through the discovery and the widespread application of recombinant DNA (deoxyribonucleic acid) technology, which has provided the tools for a distinctive new approach to medical genetics and has already been usefully applied in many clinical situations. In this chapter we present an overview of the aspects of molecular genetics that are required for an understanding of the genetic approach to medicine. This chapter is not intended to provide an extensive description of the wealth of new information about gene structure and regulation. To supplement the information discussed in this chapter, Chapter 5 describes many experimental procedures of modern molecular genetics that are becoming critical to the practice and understanding of human and medical genetics.

ORGANIZATION OF THE HUMAN GENOME

The human genome, in its diploid form, consists of approximately 6 to 7 billion base pairs (or 6 to 7

million kilobase pairs (kb)) of DNA organized linearly into 23 pairs of chromosomes. The genome contains, by current estimates, 50,000 to 100,000 genes (encoding, therefore, an equal number of proteins) that control all aspects of embryogenesis, development, growth, reproduction, and metabolism—essentially all aspects of what makes a human being a functional organism. Thus the influence of genes and genetics on states of health and disease is widespread, and its roots are the information encoded in the DNA found in the human genome. We understand the role of only a small percentage of the total number of genes. Nonetheless, the general molecular and structural framework of the genome, of its chromosomes, and of its genes is becoming clear. Analysis of the organization of the human genome is an area of considerable excitement in human and medical genetics today; it is anticipated that much, if not all, of the genetic information in the genome will in the near future be identified and examined at the molecular level as part of what has been called the Human Genome Project, an international effort to map and sequence the entire human genome.

The characterization and understanding of

31

genes and their organization in the genome have an enormous impact on the understanding of physiological processes in the human organism in both health and disease, and consequently on the practice of medicine in general. As Nobel laureate Paul Berg stated,

> Just as our present knowledge and practice of medicine relies on a sophisticated knowledge of human anatomy, physiology, and biochemistry, so will dealing with disease in the future demand a detailed understanding of the molecular anatomy, physiology, and biochemistry of the human genome. . . . We shall need a more detailed knowledge of how human genes are organized and how they function and are regulated. We shall also have to have physicians who are as conversant with the molecular anatomy and physiology of chromosomes and genes as the cardiac surgeon is with the structure and workings of the heart. (Berg, 1981, p. 302.)

DNA Structure: A Brief Review

DNA is a polymeric nucleic acid macromolecule composed of three types of units: a five-carbon sugar, deoxyribose; a nitrogen-containing base; and a phosphate group (Fig. 3–1). The bases are of two types, purines and pyrimidines. In DNA, there are two purine bases, adenine (A) and guanine (G), and two pyrimidines, thymine (T) and

cytosine (C). Nucleotides, each composed of a base, a phosphate, and a sugar moiety, polymerize into long polynucleotide chains by 5'-3' phosphodiester bonds formed between adjacent deoxyribose units (Fig. 3–2). In the case of intact human chromosomes, these polynucleotide chains (in their double-helix form) can stretch hundreds of millions of nucleotides long.

The anatomical structure of DNA carries the chemical information that allows the exact transmission of genetic information from one cell to its daughter cells and from one generation to the next. At the same time, the primary structure of DNA specifies the amino acid sequences of the polypeptide chains of proteins, as described later in this chapter. DNA has special features that give it these properties. The native state of DNA, as elucidated by James Watson and Francis Crick in 1953, is a double helix (Fig. 3–3). The helical structure resembles a right-handed spiral staircase in which its two polynucleotide chains run in opposite directions, held together by hydrogen bonds between pairs of bases: A of one chain paired with T of the other, and G with C (Fig. 3–3). Consequently, knowledge of the sequence of nucleotide bases on one strand automatically allows one to determine the sequence of bases on the

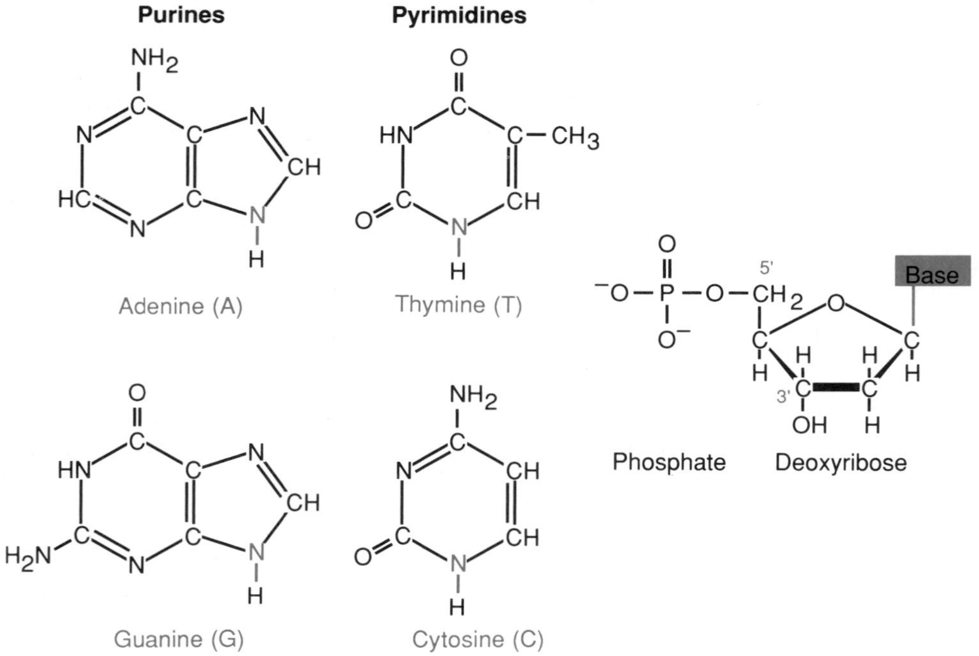

Figure 3–1. The four bases of DNA and the general structure of a nucleotide in DNA. Each of the four bases bonds with deoxyribose and a phosphate group to form the corresponding nucleotides.

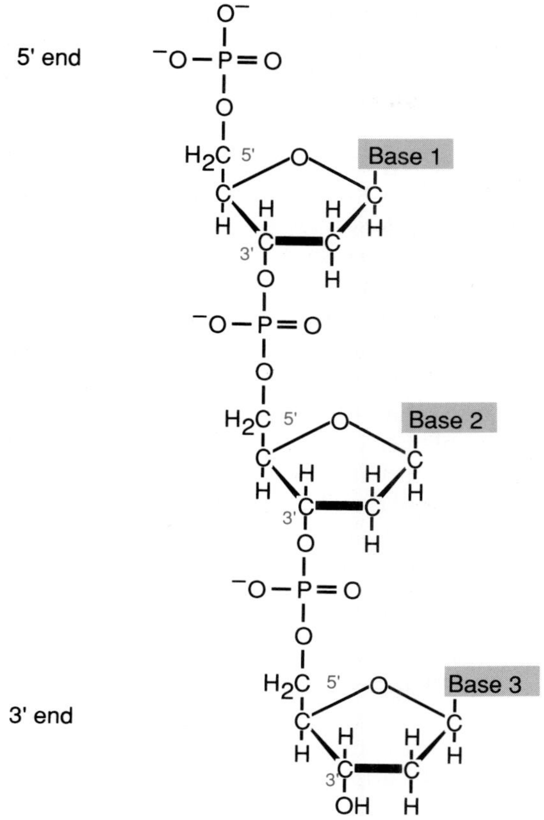

other strand. Thus a double-stranded DNA molecule can replicate precisely by separation of the two strands and synthesis of two new complementary strands, in accordance with the sequence of the original template strands (Fig. 3–4). Similarly, when necessary, the base complementarity allows efficient and correct repair of damaged DNA molecules.

Structure of Human Chromosomes

Each human chromosome is believed to consist of a single, continuous DNA double helix; that is, each chromosome is a long, linear double-stranded DNA molecule. (The only exception to this is the small circular mitochondrial chromosome, discussed later in this section.) In the human genome, these linear molecules range in size from approximately 50 million base pairs (for the smallest chromosome, chromosome 21) to 250 million base pairs (for the largest chromosome, chromosome 1). Chromosomes are not naked DNA double helices, however. The DNA molecule of a chromosome exists as a complex with a family of basic chromosomal proteins called **histones** and with a heterogeneous group of acidic, nonhistone proteins that are much less well characterized.

Figure 3–2. A portion of a DNA polynucleotide chain, showing the 3′–5′ phosphodiester bonds that link adjacent nucleotides.

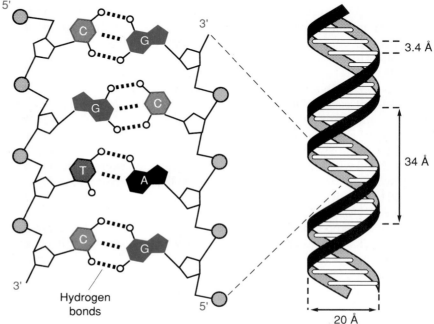

Figure 3–3. The structure of DNA. On the left is a two-dimensional representation of the two complementary strands of DNA, showing the AT and GC base pairs. Note that the orientation of the two strands is antiparallel. On the right is the double-helix model of DNA, as proposed by Watson and Crick. The horizontal "rungs" represent the paired bases. The helix is said to be right-handed because the strand going from lower left to upper right crosses over the opposite strand. (Based on Watson JD, Crick FHC [1953] Molecular structure of nucleic acids—A structure for deoxyribose nucleic acid. Nature 171:737–738.)

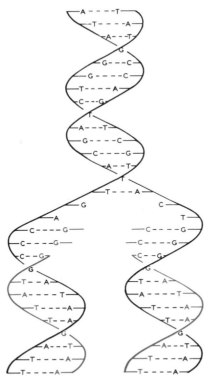

Figure 3–4. Replication of a DNA double helix, resulting in two identical daughter molecules, each composed of one parental strand (black) and one newly synthesized strand (red).

This complex of DNA and protein is called **chromatin.** There are five major types of histones, termed H1, H2A, H2B, H3, and H4. They play a critical role in the proper packaging of the chromatin fiber, as evidenced by the remarkable conservation of the amino acid sequences of H2A, H2B, H3, and H4 through evolution, even between species as diverse as chickens and humans. Two copies of each of these four histones constitute an octamer, around which a segment of DNA double helix winds, like thread around a spool (Fig. 3–5). Approximately 140 base pairs of DNA are associated with each histone core, making just under two turns around the octamer. After a short (20 to 60 base-pair) "spacer" segment of DNA, the next core DNA complex forms, and so on, giving chromatin the appearance of beads on a string. Each complex of DNA with core histones is called a **nucleosome,** the basic structural unit of chromatin. Histone H1, whose amino acid sequence varies more between species than do those of the core histones, appears to bind to DNA at the edge of

each nucleosome, in the internucleosomal spacer region. The amount of DNA associated with each unit of chromatin, including both the core nucleosome and the spacer region, is about 200 base pairs.

During the cell cycle, as described briefly in Chapter 2, chromosomes go through orderly stages of condensation and decondensation (Fig. 3–6). In the interphase nucleus, chromosomes and chromatin are quite decondensed in relation to the highly condensed state of chromatin in metaphase. Nonetheless, even in interphase chromosomes, DNA in chromatin is substantially more condensed than it would be as a native, protein-free double helix. Most if not all DNA in the nucleus interacts with histones to form nucleosomes. At this stage, the DNA is condensed to about a tenth of its native length. Thus, in more concrete terms, the DNA of human chromosome 1, which would be about 15 cm long as a naked double helix, is only about 1.5 cm long when complexed with chromosomal proteins.

The long strings of nucleosomes themselves are further compacted into a helical, secondary chromatin structure called a **solenoid** (see Fig. 3–5), which appears under the electron microscope as a thick, 30-nm-diameter fiber (about three times thicker than the nucleosomal fiber). This fiber appears to be the fundamental unit of chromatin organization. Each turn of the solenoid contains about six nucleosomes. Thus at this level of compaction in an interphase nucleus, the chromatin that makes up chromosome 1 is about 0.3 cm long. The solenoids are themselves packed into **loops** or domains attached at intervals of about 10 to 100 kb to a nonhistone protein **scaffold** or matrix. It has been speculated that loops are, in fact, functional units of DNA replication or gene transcription, or both, and that the attachment points of each loop are fixed along the chromosomal DNA. Thus one level of control of gene expression may depend on how DNA and genes are packaged into chromosomes and on their association with chromosomal proteins in the packaging process; unlike the chromosomes seen in stained preparations under the microscope or in photographs, the chromosomes of living cells are fluid and dynamic structures. The various hierarchical levels of packaging seen in an interphase chromosome are illustrated schematically in Figure 3–5.

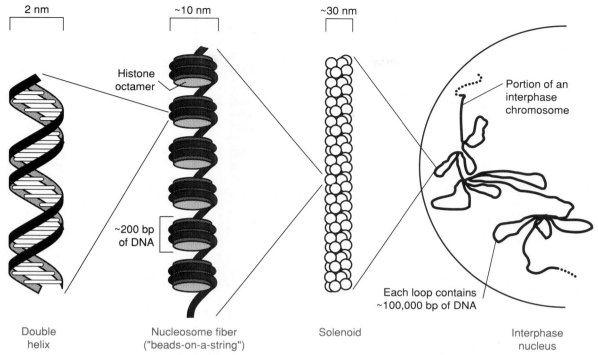

2 nm

~10 nm

~30 nm

Histone
octamer

~200 bp
of DNA

Portion of an
interphase
chromosome

Each loop contains
~100,000 bp of DNA

Double
helix

Nucleosome fiber
("beads-on-a-string")

Solenoid

Interphase
nucleus

Figure 3–5. Hierarchical levels of chromatin packaging in a human chromosome.

The loops may be the beginning of the knob-like thickenings (called **chromomeres**) observable under the microscope in early prophase chromosomes, as mitosis begins (see Fig. 3–6). As chromosomes condense further, adjacent chromomeres merge into larger ones. These clusters of chromomeres eventually become the dark-staining bands of G-banded prophase or metaphase chromosomes. At prophase, chromosomes are easily visible under the light microscope. As discussed in Chapter 2, 1000 or more bands can at this stage be recognized in stained chromosome preparations (high-resolution banding), and each band therefore contains several million base pairs of DNA (and, as described later, perhaps 50–100 genes). At prophase, chromosome 1 has condensed to an overall length of about 50 μm (condensed to about 1/3000 of the length of a naked double helix). When maximally condensed, at metaphase, DNA in chromosomes is about 1/10,000 of its native length. Therefore, each band recognized cytogenetically in metaphase preparations contains, on average, about 10 to 20 million base pairs of DNA. After metaphase, as cells complete mitosis or meiosis, chromosomes decondense and return to their relaxed state as chromatin in the interphase nucleus, ready to begin the cycle again (Fig. 3–6).

The precise behavior of individual chromosomes during the cell cycle is determined by a number of functional elements that are critical for the correct expression, duplication, and segregation of chromosomes. Among these, the most extensively characterized are **origins of DNA replication, telomeres,** and **centromeres.** Telomeres and centromeres were introduced in Chapter 2. We briefly discussed replication of a DNA double helix earlier (see Fig. 3–4). The considerable length of a human chromosome (as with all eukaryotic chromosomes) requires that replication initiate at several thousand locations in order to complete synthesis of the entire molecule within the S phase of the cell cycle. The points of initiation of DNA synthesis, called **origins,** may be specific DNA sequences located at intervals of several hundred kilobases along the length of a chromosome.

The enormous amount of DNA packaged into a metaphase chromosome can be appreciated when chromosomes are treated to remove most of the chromatin proteins in order to observe the protein scaffold (Fig. 3–7). When DNA is released

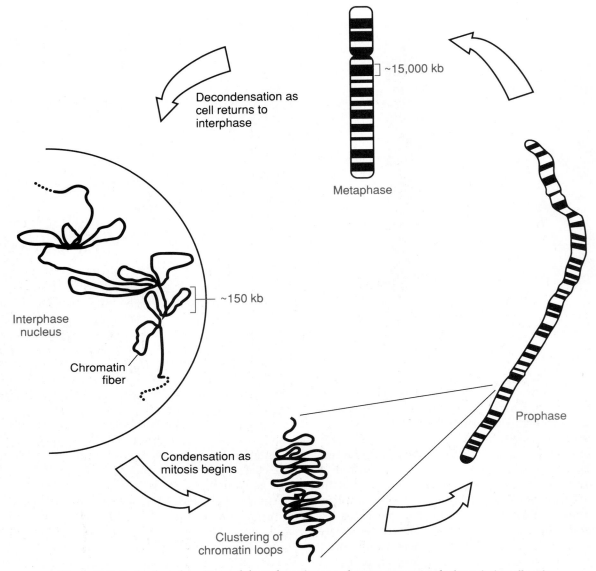

Figure 3-6. Cycle of condensation and decondensation as a chromosome proceeds through the cell cycle.

from chromosomes treated this way, long loops of DNA can be visualized, and the residual scaffolding can be seen to reproduce the outline of a typical metaphase chromosome.

The Mitochondrial Chromosome

Although the vast majority of genes are located in the nucleus, a small but important subset resides in the cytoplasm in the mitochondria. Mitochondrial genes exhibit exclusively maternal inheritance (see Chapter 4). All human cells have hundreds of mitochondria, each containing a number of copies of a small circular molecule, the mitochondrial chromosome. The mitochondrial DNA molecule is only 16 kb in length (less than 0.03 percent of the length of the smallest nuclear chromosome) and encodes 13 key structural genes, as well as a number of structural ribonucleic acid (RNA) genes. Mutations in mitochondrial genes have been demonstrated in several neuromuscular disorders, including the maternally transmitted Leber's hereditary optic neuropathy (see Chapter 4).

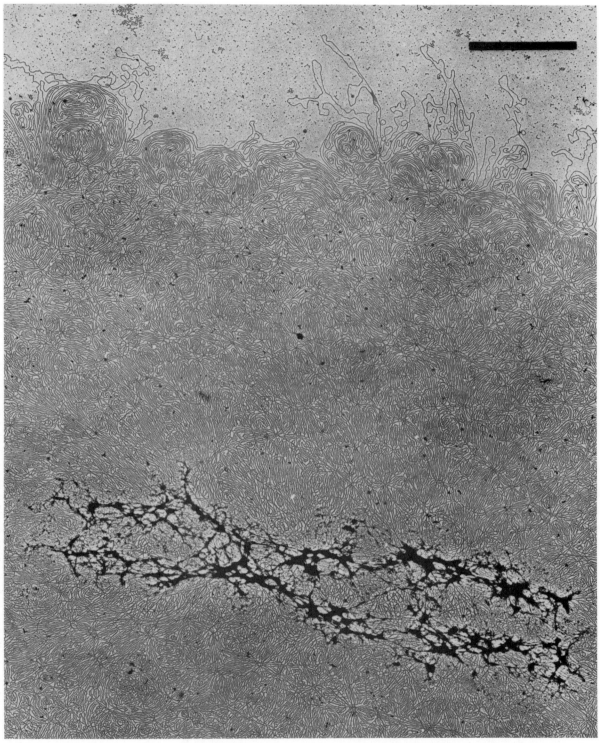

Figure 3-7. Electron micrograph of a protein-depleted human metaphase chromosome, showing the residual chromosome scaffold and loops of DNA. Individual DNA fibers can be best seen at the edge of the DNA loops. Bar = 2 microns. (From Paulson JR, Laemmli UK [1977] The structure of histone-depleted metaphase chromosomes. Cell 12:817–828. Reprinted by permission of the authors and Cell Press.)

Table 3-1. DNA in the Human Genome

Type of DNA	Proportion of Genome	Features
Unique or single-copy DNA	~75%	Includes most genes Located throughout genome
Repetitive DNA Dispersed	~15%	Interspersed with genes and other single-copy DNA Two major families (*Alu* and L1) Located throughout genome
Satellite DNA	~10%	Highly repeated sequences Several major families Highly localized in specific sites (centromeres, telomeres)

Classes of DNA in the Human Genome

The organization of DNA in the human genome is far more complex than was foreseen even as recently as 1980. Of the DNA in the genome, less than 10 percent actually encodes genes. Only about three quarters of the total linear length of the genome consists of so-called **single-copy** or **unique DNA** — that is, DNA whose nucleotide sequence is represented only once (or at most a few times) per haploid genome. The rest of the genome consists of several classes of **repetitive DNA** and includes DNA whose nucleotide sequence is repeated, either perfectly or with some variation, hundreds to millions of times in the genome. Whereas most (but not all) of the estimated 50,000 to 100,000 genes in the genome are represented in single-copy DNA, the repetitive DNA fraction is believed to play a role in maintaining chromosome structure or perhaps to play no essential role whatsoever (Table 3-1).

Single-Copy DNA Sequences

Although single-copy DNA makes up most of the DNA in the genome, much of its function remains a mystery because, as just mentioned, sequences actually encoding proteins (i.e., the coding portion of genes) constitute only a small proportion of all the single-copy DNA. Long stretches of unique DNA sequences (> 25 kb) are quite rare in the genome. Most single-copy DNA is found in short stretches (several kilobases or less), interspersed with members of various repetitive DNA families.

Satellite DNA Families

Several different categories of repetitive DNA are recognized (see Table 3-1). A useful distinguish-ing feature is whether the repeated sequences ("repeats") are clustered in one or a few locations or whether they are dispersed throughout the genome, interspersed with single-copy sequences along the chromosome. Clustered repeated sequences constitute an estimated 10 to 15 percent of the genome and consist of arrays of various short repeats organized tandemly in a head-to-tail fashion. The different types of such tandem repeats are collectively called **satellite DNAs**, so named because many of the original tandem repeat families could be purified by density centrifugation from the rest of the genome as "satellite" fractions of DNA. Use of the term "satellite" is widespread in human genetics today, and one has to be careful not to confuse satellite DNAs with the cytological satellites seen on the acrocentric chromosomes, referred to in Chapter 2.

Satellite DNA families vary with regard to their location in the genome, the total length of the tandem array, and the length of the constituent repeat units that make up the array. Some human satellite sequences are based on repetitions or variations, or both, of a short sequence such as a pentanucleotide. Long arrays of such repeats are found in heterochromatic regions on the proximal long arms of chromosomes 1, 9, and 16 and on nearly the entire long arm of the Y chromosome. Other satellite DNAs are based on somewhat longer basic repeats. For example, the α-satellite family of DNA is composed of tandem arrays of different copies of an approximately 171 base-pair unit, found at the centromeric region of each human chromosome. In general, satellite arrays can stretch several million base pairs or more in length and constitute up to several percent of the DNA content of an individual human chromosome.

A particular subgroup of satellite DNAs in

the human genome includes sequences referred to as **minisatellites** because their total array length seems far more limited. Each minisatellite is based on head-to-tail repetitions of an intermediate-length monomer (approximately 15 to 65 base pairs) and usually spans only a few kilobases (up to 20 kb or so) in total. Unlike the highly localized satellite arrays just considered, minisatellites are distributed more or less along the length of each chromosome. Many minisatellite sequences are important as molecular tools to examine the considerable variation that exists between genomes of different individuals (see Chapters 6 and 8). As a class, these "DNA markers," as they are called, are revolutionizing many areas of genetics such as mapping of the human genome, chromosome analysis, forensic medicine, and the diagnosis of inherited disease through molecular techniques.

Dispersed Repetitive DNA Families

In addition to tandemly repeated satellite DNAs, another major class of repetitive DNA in the genome consists of related sequences that are dispersed throughout the genome rather than localized (Table 3–1). Although many small DNA families meet this general description, two in particular warrant discussion because together they make up a significant proportion of the genome and because they have been implicated in genetic diseases.

The best-studied dispersed repetitive elements belong to the *Alu* **family,** so named because most members of the family are cleaved by a particular bacterial restriction endonuclease called *Alu*I, which was used in the initial purification of this DNA. (Restriction endonucleases are enzymes that recognize and cleave double-stranded DNA at specific sequences. These enzymes are major tools of modern molecular biology and recombinant DNA technology, as discussed in greater detail in Chapter 5.) The members of this family are about 300 base pairs in length and are recognizably related to each other although not identical in sequence. In total, there are about 500,000 *Alu* family members in the genome, making up an estimated 3 percent of human DNA. *Alu* sequences are found throughout the genome and are of medical significance because (as discussed in Chapter 6) aberrant recombination events between different *Alu* family members can be a cause of mutation in some genetic diseases.

The origin and distribution of *Alu* sequences throughout the genome has been a subject of interest. It is thought that *Alu* family members originated from one or a few copies of a primordial gene many millions of years ago by a process involving copying and integration of such copies into the genome at various locations. Because these extra copies were no longer required to be functional, they presumably were free to accumulate numerous nucleotide base changes during evolution. The present-day function, if any, of all these *Alu* family members is unknown. Why this particular DNA family has been so prolific in generating additional members remains an intriguing question.

A second major dispersed, repetitive DNA family is called the **L1 family.** L1 elements are long, repetitive sequences (up to 6 kb in length) that are found in about 10,000 copies per genome. Thus although there are many fewer copies in this family than in the *Alu* family, they are much longer, and the total contribution to the makeup of the genome is about the same: approximately 3 percent (Table 3–1). As with the *Alu* family, L1 sequences have been implicated as the cause of several mutations in hereditary disease (see Chapter 6), although the role, if any, of normal L1 sequences in the genome is unknown.

In a genome as complex and sophisticated as ours, it is interesting that such a large proportion of chromosomal DNA (including all of the satellite and dispersed repetitive DNAs and some of the single-copy DNA as well) has no identified or obvious function. Indeed, although the idea is anathema to some, it has been proposed that many such sequences (sometimes called "selfish" or "junk" DNA) have no function at all but are maintained in the genome simply because they can exploit cellular processes to ensure their own propagation.

Sequence Organization and Metaphase Chromosome Banding

Regions of the genome with similar characteristics of organization, replication, and expression are not arranged randomly but, rather, tend to be clustered together. This functional organization of the genome correlates remarkably well with its structural organization as revealed by metaphase chromosome banding (discussed in Chapter 2;

Table 3–2). The overall significance of this manner of genome organization is unclear; however, what is certain is that chromosomes are not a random collection of different types of genes and other DNA sequences.

G bands and Q bands (see Figs. 2–4 and 2–6) contain DNA that is, in general, slightly more AT-rich than the GC-rich DNA of R bands (Fig. 2–7). G and Q bands tend to replicate their DNA later in the S phase of the cell cycle than do R bands. There is a suggestion that this compositional dichotomy also extends to genes. About two thirds of human genes that have been localized to a specific band in the genome are located in R bands; relatively few have been precisely localized to G bands. Although the number of genes examined is still small, chromosomal abnormalities involving "gene-rich" R bands may have more clinical significance than those that involve "gene-poor" G bands.

Similarly, the two major families of dispersed repetitive DNA are not distributed at random throughout the genome. *Alu* family members (themselves somewhat GC-rich) are predominantly (but not exclusively) located in the GC-rich R bands. L1 family members, on the other hand, are somewhat AT-rich and localize to the AT-rich G and Q bands seen in metaphase chromosomes.

THE CENTRAL DOGMA: DNA → RNA → PROTEIN

Genetic information is contained in DNA in the chromosomes within the cell nucleus, but protein synthesis, during which the information encoded in the DNA is used, takes place in the cytoplasm. This compartmentalization reflects the fact that the human organism is a **eukaryote.** This means that human cells, like those of many other organisms (including protozoa and fungi), have a genuine nucleus containing the DNA, which is separated by a nuclear membrane from the cytoplasm. In contrast, in prokaryotes such as *Escherichia coli* (the intestinal bacterium that is also important for its wide use in molecular biology research; see Chapter 5), DNA is not enclosed within a nucleus. Because of the compartmentalization of eukaryotic cells, information transfer from the nucleus to the cytoplasm is a very complex process that has

Table 3–2. Composition of Metaphase Chromosome Bands

Banding Pattern	Properties
G bands, Q bands	Contain AT-rich DNA (55%–60%) Replicate late in S phase Contain few genes (mostly tissue specific) Rich in L1 family members
R bands	Contain GC-rich DNA (50%–60%) Replicate early in S phase Contain most genes (both housekeeping and tissue specific) Rich in *Alu* family members Rich in CpG islands

Based on Bickmore and Sumner (1989); Bernardi (1989); Holmquist (1987); Korenberg and Rykowski (1988).

been a focus of attention among molecular and cellular biologists.

The molecular link between these two related types of information (the DNA code of genes and the amino acid code of proteins) is **RNA (ribonucleic acid).** The chemical structure of RNA is similar to that of DNA, except that each nucleotide in RNA has a ribose sugar component instead of a deoxyribose; in addition, uracil (U) instead of thymine is one of the pyrimidines of RNA (Fig. 3–8). An additional difference between RNA and DNA is that RNA in most organisms exists as a single-stranded molecule, whereas DNA exists as a double helix (except transiently during DNA replication).

The informational relationships among DNA, RNA, and protein are circular: DNA directs the synthesis and sequence of RNA; RNA directs the synthesis and sequence of polypeptides; and specific proteins are involved in the synthesis and metabolism of DNA and RNA. This flow of infor-

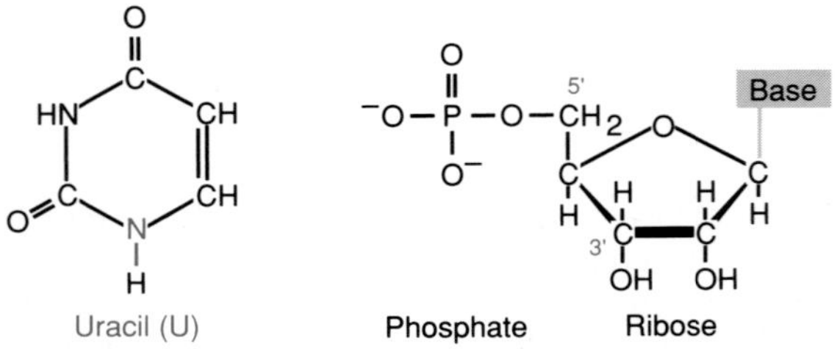

Figure 3–8. The pyrimidine uracil and the structure of a nucleotide in RNA. Note that the sugar ribose replaces the sugar deoxyribose of DNA.

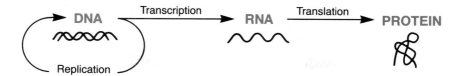

mation is often called the "central dogma" of molecular biology.

Genetic information is stored in DNA by means of a code (the **genetic code,** discussed later) in which the sequence of adjacent bases ultimately determines the sequence of amino acids in the encoded polypeptide. First, RNA is synthesized from the DNA template through a process known as **transcription.** The RNA, carrying the coded information in a form called **messenger RNA (mRNA),** is then transported from the nucleus to the cytoplasm, where the RNA sequence is decoded, or translated, to determine the sequence of amino acids in the protein being synthesized. This process of **translation** occurs on **ribosomes,** which are cytoplasmic organelles with binding sites for all of the interacting molecules, including the mRNA, involved in protein synthesis. Ribosomes are themselves made up of many different structural proteins in association with a specialized type of RNA known as **ribosomal RNA (rRNA).** Translation involves yet a third type of RNA, **transfer RNA (tRNA),** which provides the molecular link between the coded base sequence of the mRNA and the amino acid sequence of the protein.

Because of the interdependent flow of information represented by the central dogma, one can begin discussion of the molecular genetics of gene expression at any of its three informational levels: DNA, RNA, or protein. We begin by examining the structure of genes and defer discussion of the genetic code, transcription, and translation until later (see the "Fundamentals of Gene Expression" section later in this chapter).

Gene Structure and Organization

Until the late 1970s, the gene was visualized simply as a segment of a DNA molecule containing the code for the amino acid sequence of a polypeptide chain and the regulatory sequences necessary for expression. This is now known to be an incomplete description of genes in the human genome (and indeed in most eukaryotic genomes). In fact, very few genes exist as continuous coding sequences; rather, the vast majority of genes are interrupted by one or more noncoding regions. These so-called intervening sequences, or **introns,** are initially transcribed into RNA in the nucleus but are not present in the mature mRNA in the cytoplasm and are thus not represented in the final protein product. Introns alternate with coding sequences, or **exons,** that ultimately encode the amino acid sequence of the product (Fig. 3–9). Although a few genes in the human genome have no introns, most genes contain at least one and usually several. In many genes, the cumulative length of introns makes up a far greater proportion of a gene's total length than do the exons. Whereas some genes are less than 1 kb in length, others, such as the factor VIII gene shown in Figure 3–9, stretch on for hundreds of kilobases. One exceptional gene, the dystrophin gene on the X chromosome (mutations of which lead to Duchenne muscular dystrophy), spans more than 2000 kb.

Structural Features of a Typical Human Gene

A schematic representation of a stretch of chromosomal DNA containing a typical gene is shown in Figure 3–9, along with the structure of several specific genes. Together, they illustrate the range of features that characterize human genes. In Chapters 1 and 2, we briefly defined "gene" in general terms. At this point, we can now provide a molecular definition of a gene. In general usage, we define a gene as *a sequence of chromosomal DNA that is required for production of a functional product,* be it a polypeptide or a functional RNA molecule. As is clear from Figure 3–9, a gene includes not only the actual coding sequences but also adjacent nucleotide sequences required for the proper expression of the gene — that is, for the production of a normal mRNA molecule.

These adjacent regions provide the molecular "start" and "stop" signals for the synthesis of mRNA transcribed from the gene. At the 5′ end of

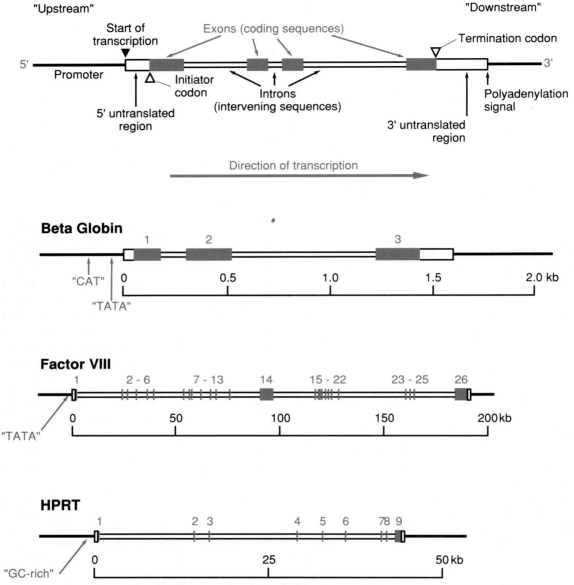

Figure 3–9. General structure of a typical human gene. Individual features are labeled in the figure and discussed in the text. Examples of three specific human genes are presented at the bottom of the figure. Individual exons are numbered. (Modified from Lawn et al., 1980; Gitschier et al., 1984; and Patel et al., 1986.)

the gene (sometimes called the "upstream flanking region") lies a **promoter** region, which includes sequences responsible for the proper initiation of transcription. Within the 5′ region are several DNA elements whose sequence is conserved among many different genes. This conservation, together with functional studies of gene expression in many laboratories, indicates that these particular sequence elements play an impor-

tant role in regulation. The roles of individual conserved promoter elements, identified in Figure 3–9, are discussed in greater detail in the section on "Fundamentals of Gene Expression." At the 3′ end of the gene (also called the "downstream flanking region") lies an untranslated region of importance that contains a signal for addition of a sequence of polyadenosine residues (the so-called polyA tail) to the end of the mature mRNA. Al-

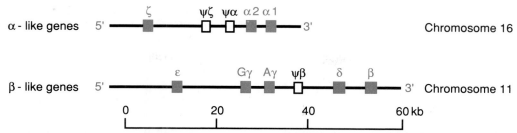

Figure 3-10. Chromosomal organization of the two clusters of human globin genes. Functional genes are indicated in red. Pseudogenes are indicated by the open boxes. (Redrawn from Nienhuis AW, Maniatis T [1987] Structure and expression of globin genes in erythroid cells. *In* Stamatoyannopoulos G, Nienhuis AW, Leder P, Majerus PW (eds) The molecular basis of blood diseases. WB Saunders, Philadelphia, pp. 28–65.)

though it is generally accepted that such closely neighboring regulatory sequences are located within the limits of what is called a "gene," the actual precise dimensions of any particular gene will remain somewhat uncertain until the potential functions of more distant sequences are fully characterized.

Gene Families

Many genes belong to families of closely related DNA sequences, recognized as families because of similarity in the nucleotide sequence of the genes themselves or in the amino acid sequence of the encoded polypeptides.

Several such gene families are diagrammed schematically in Figures 3–10 and 3–11. The α-globin and β-globin gene clusters, on chromosomes 16 and 11, respectively, are believed to have arisen by duplication of a primitive precursor gene about 500 million years ago. These two clusters contain genes coding for closely related globin chains expressed at different developmental stages, from embryo to adult. The individual genes within each cluster are more similar in sequence to each other than to genes in the other cluster; thus each cluster is believed to have evolved by a series of sequential gene duplication events within the past 100 million years. The exon–intron patterns of the globin genes appear to have been remarkably conserved during evolution; each of the functional globin genes shown in Figure 3–10 has two introns at similar locations, although the sequences contained within the introns have accumulated far more nucleotide base changes over time than have the coding sequences of each gene, which have been under selection. The control of expression of the various globin genes, in the normal state as well as in the many inherited hemoglobinopathies, is considered in more detail both later in this chapter and in Chapters 6 and 11.

Several of the globin genes shown in Figure 3–10 do not produce any RNA or protein product; that is, they do not have any function. DNA sequences that closely resemble known genes but are nonfunctional are called **pseudogenes.** Pseu-

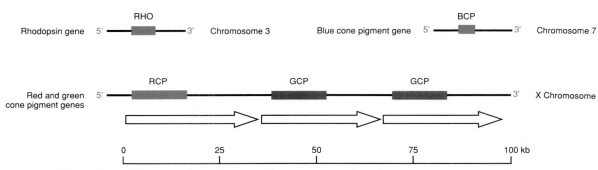

Figure 3-11. Chromosomal organization and gene structure of the human visual pigment gene family.

dogenes are widespread in the genome and are thought to be byproducts of evolution, representing genes that were once functional but are now vestigial, having been inactivated by mutations in coding or regulatory sequences. In some cases, as in the pseudo-α-globin and pseudo-β-globin genes, they presumably arose through the introduction of numerous mutations into extra copies of a once-functional gene generated by gene duplication. In other cases, pseudogenes have apparently been formed by a process involving transcription, generation of a DNA copy of the mRNA, and finally integration of such DNA copies back into the genome. This is the same process referred to previously for generation of copies of the dispersed repetitive elements, *Alu* and L1. Such pseudogenes lack introns and are often called "processed pseudogenes." They are not usually on the same chromosome (or chromosomal region) as their progenitor gene.

Another example of a gene family in the human genome includes genes encoding the various light-sensitive pigments required for color vision (Fig. 3–11). Biochemical evidence established that the different visual pigments are structurally homologous and probably arose from a common ancestral pigment gene. More recently, the isolation and characterization of these genes has confirmed the existence of a pigment gene family with members on at least three chromosomes (Fig. 3–11; Nathans et al., 1986). A single red pigment gene and a variable number of green pigment genes are located in a tandem array on the X chromosome. These X-linked genes show extraordinary homology to one another (about 98 percent nucleotide sequence identity) and appear to have evolved by gene duplications within the past 30 million years. Defects in the structure or the number, or both, of these genes are responsible for red-green color blindness, an X-linked condition (see Chapter 6). Two other members of this gene family, the blue pigment gene on chromosome 7 and the rhodopsin (rod photopigment) gene on chromosome 3, probably arose from the same ancestral pigment gene some 500 million years ago and, accordingly, are much more distantly related. Mutations at the rhodopsin locus are responsible for a significant proportion of cases of autosomal dominant retinitis pigmentosa, an ocular disorder involving photoreceptor degeneration.

Probably the largest gene family in the human genome is the so-called **immunoglobulin superfamily,** which includes many hundreds of genes involved in cell surface recognition events in the immune and nervous system, such as genes on chromosome 6 that make up the major histocompatibility (HLA) complex; genes on chromosomes 7 and 14 whose products make up the T cell receptor; genes that are involved primarily in neural tissues, such as genes for cell adhesion molecules or for myelin-associated glycoproteins; and, of course, genes on chromosomes 2, 14, and 22 that encode the immunoglobulin heavy and light chains themselves. The structure and function of many of these genes are examined in detail in Chapter 14.

FUNDAMENTALS OF GENE EXPRESSION

The flow of information from gene to polypeptide involves several steps (Fig. 3–12). Transcription of a gene is initiated at a site on chromosomal DNA just upstream from the coding sequences and continues along the chromosome, for anywhere from several hundred base pairs to more than 1 million base pairs, through both introns and exons and past the end of the coding sequences. After modification at both the 5' and 3' ends, the primary RNA transcript is then spliced so that the portions corresponding to introns are removed. After RNA splicing, the resulting mRNA (now colinear with only the coding portions of the gene) is transported from the nucleus to the cytoplasm, where it is translated into the amino acid sequence of the encoded polypeptide. Each of the steps in this complex pathway is prone to error, and mutations that interfere with the individual steps have been implicated in a number of inherited genetic disorders (see Chapters 6, 11, and 12).

Transcription

Transcription of protein-coding genes by RNA polymerase II (one of several classes of RNA polymerases) is initiated upstream from the first coding information at a point corresponding to the 5' end of the final RNA product, called the transcriptional "start site" (Figs. 3–9, 3–12). Synthesis of

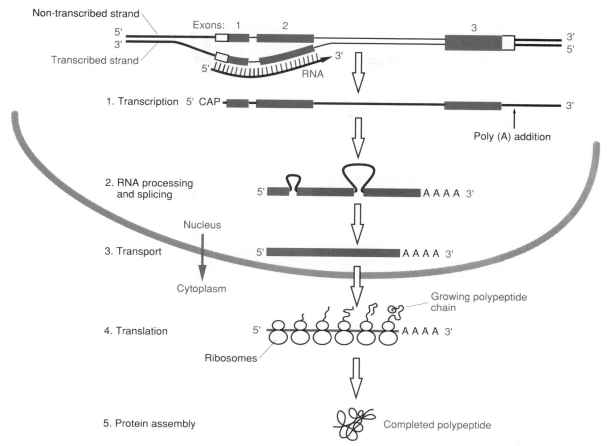

Figure 3–12. Flow of information from DNA to RNA to protein for a hypothetical gene with three exons and two introns. Steps include transcription, RNA processing and splicing, RNA transport from the nucleus to the cytoplasm, and translation.

the primary RNA transcript proceeds in a 5′-to-3′ direction, whereas the strand of the gene that is being transcribed is actually read in a 3′-to-5′ direction with respect to the direction of the deoxyribose phosphodiester backbone (Fig. 3–2). Because the RNA synthesized corresponds both in polarity and in base sequence (substituting U for T) to the 5′-to-3′ strand of DNA, this nontranscribed strand is sometimes called the "coding," or "sense," strand. The 3′-to-5′ transcribed strand is then called the "noncoding," or "antisense," strand. Transcription continues through both intron and exon portions of the gene, beyond the position on the chromosome that eventually corresponds to the 3′ end of the mature mRNA. Whether transcription ends at a predetermined 3′ termination point is unknown.

The primary transcript is processed by addition of a "CAP" structure to the 5′ end of the RNA and cleavage of the 3′ end at a specific point downstream from the end of the coding information. This cleavage is followed by addition of a polyA tail that marks the 3′ end and appears to increase the stability of the resulting mRNA. The location of the polyadenylation point is specified in part by the sequence AAUAAA (or a variant of this), usually found in the 3′ untranslated portion of the RNA transcript. These posttranscriptional modifications take place in the nucleus, as does the process of splicing the primary RNA transcript to excise the sequences corresponding to any introns. The fully processed, mature mRNA is then transported to the cytoplasm, where translation takes place (Fig. 3–12).

Translation and the Genetic Code

In the cytoplasm, mRNA is translated into protein by the action of a variety of tRNA molecules, each specific for a particular amino acid. These remarkable molecules, each only 70 to 100 nucleotides long, have the job of transferring the correct amino acids from the cytoplasm to their positions along the mRNA template, to be added to the growing polypeptide chain. Protein synthesis occurs on ribosomes, macromolecular complexes made up of rRNA (encoded by the 18S and 28S rRNA genes located on the short arms of the acrocentric chromosomes) and several dozen ribosomal proteins (Fig. 3–12).

The key to translation is the **genetic code**, which relates specific amino acids to combinations of three adjacent bases along the mRNA. Each set of three bases constitutes a **codon**, specific for a particular amino acid (Table 3–3). Almost infinite variations are theoretically possible in the arrangement of the bases along a polynucleotide chain. At any one position, there are four possibilities (A, T, C, or G); thus there are 4^n possible combinations in a sequence of n bases. For three bases, there are 4^3, or 64, possible triplet combinations. These 64 codons constitute the genetic code.

Table 3–3. The Genetic Code

First Base	Second Base								Third Base
	U		C		A		G		
U	UUU	phe	UCU	ser	UAU	tyr	UGU	cys	U
	UUC	phe	UCC	ser	UAC	tyr	UGC	cys	C
	UUA	leu	UCA	ser	UAA	stop	UGA	stop	A
	UUG	leu	UCG	ser	UAG	stop	UGG	trp	G
C	CUU	leu	CCU	pro	CAU	his	CGU	arg	U
	CUC	leu	CCC	pro	CAC	his	CGC	arg	C
	CUA	leu	CCA	pro	CAA	gln	CGA	arg	A
	CUG	leu	CCG	pro	CAG	gln	CGG	arg	G
A	AUU	ile	ACU	thr	AAU	asn	AGU	ser	U
	AUC	ile	ACC	thr	AAC	asn	AGC	ser	C
	AUA	ile	ACA	thr	AAA	lys	AGA	arg	A
	AUG	met	ACG	thr	AAG	lys	AGG	arg	G
G	GUU	val	GCU	ala	GAU	asp	GGU	gly	U
	GUC	val	GCC	ala	GAC	asp	GGC	gly	C
	GUA	val	GCA	ala	GAA	glu	GGA	gly	A
	GUG	val	GCG	ala	GAG	glu	GGG	gly	G

Abbreviations for amino acids:

ala (A)	alanine	leu (L)	leucine
arg (R)	arginine	lys (K)	lysine
asn (N)	asparagine	met (M)	methionine
asp (D)	aspartic acid	phe (F)	phenylalanine
cys (C)	cysteine	pro (P)	proline
gln (Q)	glutamine	ser (S)	serine
glu (E)	glutamic acid	thr (T)	threonine
gly (G)	glycine	trp (W)	tryptophan
his (H)	histidine	tyr (Y)	tyrosine
ile (I)	isoleucine	val (V)	valine

Other abbreviation:
stop   termination codon

Codons are shown in terms of messenger RNA, which are complementary to the corresponding DNA codons.

The genetic code was deciphered through experiments in which synthetic polynucleotides were used. The first synthetic mRNA used was polyuracil (polyU), a sequence of nucleotides in which all the bases are uracil. Upon translation, the polyU mRNA directed the synthesis of a polypeptide chain composed exclusively of phenylalanines, which thus established that the triplet code for phenylalanine is UUU. The other codons were then decoded in a similar manner. Because there are only 20 amino acids and 64 possible codons, most amino acids are specified by more than one codon; hence the code is said to be **degenerate.** For instance, the base in the third position of the triplet can often be either purine (A or G) or either pyrimidine (T or C) or, in some cases, any one of the four bases, without altering the coded message (Table 3–3). Leucine and arginine are each specified by six codons. Only methionine and tryptophan are each specified by a single, unique codon. Three of the codons are called **stop** (or **nonsense**) **codons** because they designate termination of translation of the mRNA at that point.

Translation of a processed mRNA is always initiated at a codon specifying methionine. Methionine is therefore the first (amino terminal) amino acid of each polypeptide chain, although it is usually removed before protein synthesis is completed. The codon for methionine (the initiator codon, AUG) establishes the **reading frame** of the mRNA; each subsequent codon is read in turn to yield a protein of the correct amino acid sequence.

The molecular links between codons and amino acids are the specific tRNA molecules. A particular site on each tRNA forms a three-base **anticodon** that is complementary to a specific codon on the mRNA. Bonding between the codon and anticodon brings the appropriate amino acid into the next position on the ribosome for attachment to the carboxyl end of the growing polypeptide chain by formation of a peptide bond. The ribosome then slides along the mRNA exactly three bases, bringing the next codon into line for recognition by another tRNA with the next amino acid. Thus proteins are synthesized from the amino terminus to the carboxyl terminus, which corresponds to translation of the mRNA in a 5'-to-3' direction.

As mentioned earlier, translation ends when a stop codon (UGA, UAA, or UAG) is encountered in the same reading frame as the initiator codon.

(Stop codons in either of the other two, unused reading frames are not read and have no effect on translation.) The completed polypeptide is then released from the ribosome, which becomes available to begin synthesis of another protein.

Posttranslational Processing

Many proteins undergo extensive posttranslational modifications. The polypeptide chain that is the primary translation product is folded and bonded into a specific three-dimensional structure that is determined by the amino acid sequence itself. Two or more polypeptide chains, products of the same gene or of different genes, may combine to form a single protein. For example, two α-globin chains and two β-globin chains combine to form a tetrameric $\alpha_2\beta_2$ hemoglobin molecule. The protein products may also be modified chemically by, for example, addition of carbohydrates at specific sites. Other modifications may involve cleavage of the protein, either to remove specific amino terminal sequences after they have functioned to direct a protein to its correct location within the cell (e.g., proteins that function within the nucleus or mitochondria) or to split the molecule into smaller polypeptide chains. For example, the two chains that make up insulin, one 21 and the other 30 amino acids long, are originally part of an 82 amino-acid primary translation product, proinsulin.

Example of Gene Expression: The Beta-Globin Gene

The flow of information outlined in the preceding sections can best be illustrated by reference to a particular well-studied gene, the β-globin gene. The β-globin chain is a 146 amino-acid polypeptide, encoded by a gene that occupies approximately 1.6 kb on the short arm of chromosome 11 (Fig. 3–13). The gene has three exons and two introns (see Fig. 3–9). The β-globin gene, as well as the other genes in the β-globin cluster (see Fig. 3–10), is transcribed in a centromere-to-telomere direction. This orientation, however, is not necessarily the same for other genes in the genome and depends on which strand of the chromosomal double helix is the coding strand for a particular gene.

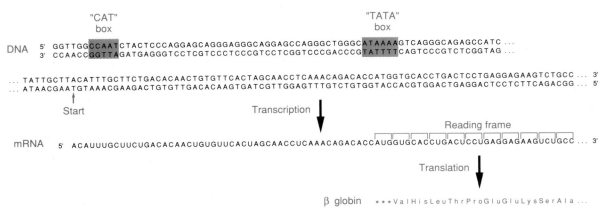

Figure 3–13. Structure and nucleotide sequence of the 5′ end of the human β-globin gene on the short arm of chromosome 11. Regulatory elements in the promoter are indicated in red. Transcription of the 3′- to-5′ (lower) strand begins at the indicated start site to produce β-globin mRNA. The translational reading frame is determined by the AUG initiator codon (***); subsequent codons specifying amino acids are indicated in red. The other two potential frames are not used.

DNA sequences required for accurate initiation of transcription of the β-globin gene are located in the promoter within approximately 200 base pairs upstream from the transcription start site. The double-stranded DNA sequence of this region of the β-globin gene, the corresponding RNA sequence, and the translated sequence of the first 10 amino acids are depicted in Figure 3–13 to illustrate the relationships among these three information levels. As mentioned previously, it is the 3′-to-5′ strand of the DNA that is actually transcribed, but the 5′-to-3′ sequence of the mRNA is most directly comparable with the 5′-to-3′ strand of DNA (and, in fact, is identical to it except that U is substituted for T). Because of this, it is the 5′-to-3′ strand of a gene (i.e., the strand that is *not* transcribed) that is generally reported in the scientific literature.

In accordance with this convention, the complete sequence of approximately 2.0 kb of chromosome 11 that includes the β-globin gene is given in Figure 3–14. (It is sobering to reflect that this page of nucleotides represents only 0.000067 percent of the sequence of the entire human genome!) Within these 2.0 kb are contained most,

but not all, of the sequence elements required to encode and regulate the expression of this gene. Indicated in Figure 3–14 are many of the important structural features of the β-globin gene, including conserved promoter sequence elements, intron and exon boundaries, RNA splice sites, the initiator and termination codons, and the polyadenylation signal.

Initiation of Transcription

The β-globin promoter, like many other gene promoters, consists of a series of relatively short functional elements that are thought to interact with specific proteins that regulate transcription, including, in the case of the globin genes, those proteins that control tissue-specific expression of these genes in erythroid cells, the tissue in which hemoglobin is produced. One important sequence is the "TATA box," a conserved region rich in adenines and thymines that is approximately 25 to 30 base pairs upstream to the start site of transcription (see Figs. 3–9, 3–13, and 3–14). The TATA box appears to be important for deter-

Figure 3–14. Nucleotide sequence of the complete human β-globin gene. The sequence of the 5′-to-3′ strand of the gene is shown. Capital letters represent sequences corresponding to mature mRNA. Lowercase letters indicate introns and flanking sequences. The CAT and TATA box sequences in the 5′ flanking region are boxed. The ATG initiator codon (AUG in mRNA) and the TAA stop codon (UAA in mRNA) are shown. The amino acid sequence of β globin is shown above the coding sequence; the three-letter abbreviations in Table 3–3 are used here. The GT and AG dinucleotides important for RNA splicing at the intron/exon junctions are boxed. (Based on Lawn RM, Efstratiadis A, O'Connell C, et al [1980] The nucleotide sequence of the human β-globin gene. Cell 21:647–651.)

```
5' ....agccacaccctagggttgg ccaat ctactcccaggagcagggagggcaggagccagggctgggc ataaaa
                                                                                    ***
gtcagggcagagccatctattgcttACATTTGCTTCTGACACAACTGTGTTCACTAGCAACCTCAAACAGACACCATG
```

Exon 1
```
ValHisLeuThrProGluGluLysSerAlaValThrAlaLeuTrpGlyLysValAsnValAspGluValGlyGlyGlu
GTGCACCTGACTCCTGAGGAGAAGTCTGCCGTTACTGCCCTGTGGGGCAAGGTGAACGTGGATGAAGTTGGTGGTGAG

AlaLeuGlyAr-
GCCCTGGGCAG gt tggtatcaaggttacaagacaggtttaaggagaccaatagaaactgggcatgtggagacagagaag
```

Intron 1
```
                                                                -gLeuLeuValValTyr
actcttgggtttctgataggcactgactctctctgcctattggtctatttttcccacccTT ag GCTGCTGGTGGTCTAC
```

Exon 2
```
ProTrpThrGlnArgPhePheGluSerPheGlyAspLeuSerThrProAspAlaValMetGlyAsnProLysValLys
CCTTGGACCCAGAGGTTCTTTGAGTCCTTTGGGGATCTGTCCACTCCTGATGCTGTTATGGGCAACCCTAAGGTGAAG

AlaHisGlyLysLysValLeuGlyAlaPheSerAspGlyLeuAlaHisLeuAspAsnLeuLysGlyThrPheAlaThr
GCTCATGGCAAGAAAGTGCTCGGTGCCTTTAGTGATGGCCTGGCTCACCTGGACAACCTCAAGGGCACCTTTGCCACA

LeuSerGluLeuHisCysAspLysLeuHisValAspProGluAsnPheArg
CTGAGTGAGCTGCACTGTGACAAGCTGCACGTGGATCCTGAGAACTTCAGG gt gagtctatgggacccttgatgtttt
```

```
ctttccccttctttctatggttaagttcatgtcataggaaggggagaagtaacagggtacagtttagaatgggaaac

agacgaatgattgcatcagtgtggaagtctcaggatcgtttttagtttcttttatttgctgttcataacaattgttttc

ttttgtttaattcttgctttctttttttttcttctccgcaatttttactattatacttaatgccttaacattgtgtat

aacaaaaggaaatatctctgagatacattaagtaacttaaaaaaaaaactttacacagtctgcctagtacattactatt
```

Intron 2
```
tggaatatatgtgtgcttatttgcatattcataatgtccctactttattttctttattttttaattgatacataatca

ttatacatatttatgggttaaagtgtaatgtttaatatgtgtacacatattgaccaaatcagggtaattttgcatt

tgtaattttaaaaaatgctttcttcttttaatatactttttgtttatcttatttctaatactttccctaatctcttt

ctttcagggcaataatgatacaatgtatcatgcctctttgcaccattctaaagaataacagtgataatttctgggtta

aggcaatagcaatatttctgcatataaatatttctgcatataaattgtaactgatgtaagaggtttcatattgctaa

tagcagctacaatccagctaccattctgcttttattttatggttgggataaggctggattattctgagtccaagctag
```

Exon 3
```
                                                    LeuLeuGlyAsnValLeuValCysValLeuAla
gcccttttgctaatcatgttcatacctcttatcttcctcccac ag CTCCTGGGCAACGTGCTGGTCTGTGTGCTGGCC

HisHisPheGlyLysGluPheThrProProValGlnAlaAlaTyrGlnLysValValAlaGlyValAlaAsnAlaLeu
CATCACTTTGGCAAAGAATTCACCCCACCAGTGCAGGCTGCCTATCAGAAAGTGGTGGCTGGTGTGGCTAATGCCCTG

AlaHisLysTyrHisTer
GCCCACAAGTATCAC TAAGCTCGCTTTCTTGCTGTCCAATTTCTATTAAAGGTTCCTTTGTTCCCTAAGTCCAACTAC

TAAACTGGGGGATATTATGAAGGGCCTTGAGCATCTGGATTCTGCCT AATAAA AAACATTTATTTTCATTGCaatgat

gtatttaaattatttctgaatatttttactaaaaagggaatgtgggaggtcagtgcatttaaaacataaagaaatgatg

agctgttcaaaccttgggaaaatacactatatcttaaactccatgaaagaaggtgaggctgcaaccagctaatgcaca

ttggcaacagcccctgatgcctatgccttattcatccctcagaaaaggattcttgtagaggcttga.... 3'
```

Figure 3–14. *See legend on opposite page*

mining the position of the start of transcription, which in the β-globin gene is approximately 50 base pairs upstream from the translation initiation site (see Fig. 3–13). Thus in this gene there are about 50 base pairs of sequence that are transcribed but do not get translated. In other genes, this 5' transcribed but untranslated region can be much longer and can, in fact, be interrupted by one or more introns. A second conserved region, the "CAT box," (actually CCAAT), is a few dozen base pairs farther upstream. Both experimentally induced and naturally occurring mutations in either of these sequence elements, as well as in the CACCC sequences even farther upstream (Fig. 3–14), lead to a sharp reduction in the level of transcription, thus establishing the importance of these sequences for normal gene expression. Several such promoter mutations in the TATA box and in the CACCC elements (but not as yet in the CAT box) have been characterized among patients with the disorder β-thalassemia (see Chapters 6 and 11).

Not all gene promoters contain these specific sequence elements. In particular, genes that are constitutively expressed in most or all tissues (sometimes called "housekeeping" genes) often lack the CAT and TATA boxes that are more typical of tissue-specific genes. Promoters of many housekeeping genes are often characterized by a high level of cytosines and guanines in relation to the surrounding DNA (see the promoter of the hypoxanthine phosphoribosyltransferase gene in Figure 3–9). These promoters are sometimes located in regions of the genome called **CG** (or **CpG**) **islands,** so named because of the unusually high concentration of the dinucleotide 5'-CG-3' that stands out from the more general AT-rich chromosomal landscape. Some of the GC-rich sequence elements found in these promoters are thought to serve as binding sites for specific transcription factors.

In addition to the sequences that constitute a promoter itself, there are other sequence elements that can markedly alter the efficiency of transcription. The best characterized of these "activating" sequences are called **enhancers.** Enhancers are sequence elements that can act at quite a distance (often several kilobases) from a gene to stimulate transcription. Specific enhancer elements function only in certain cell types and thus appear to be involved in establishing the tissue specificity of

many genes. In the case of the β-globin gene, there is some evidence for a tissue-specific enhancer in the 3' flanking region of the gene, downstream from the polyadenylation site. The interaction of enhancers with particular proteins leads to increased levels of transcription. A corollary of this, of course, is that mutations that disrupt or delete the enhancer sequence can affect the level of transcription, perhaps leading to genetic disease.

RNA Splicing

The primary RNA transcript of the β-globin gene contains two exons, approximately 100 and 850 base pairs in length, that need to be spliced out. The process is exact and highly efficient; 95 percent of β-globin transcripts are thought to be accurately spliced to yield functional globin mRNA. The splicing reactions are guided by specific DNA sequences at both the 5' and the 3' ends of introns. The 5' sequence consists of nine nucleotides, of which two (the dinucleotide GT located in the intron immediately adjacent to the splice site) are essentially invariant among splice sites in different genes (Fig. 3–14). The 3' sequence consists of about a dozen nucleotides, of which, again, two are obligatory for normal splicing, an AG located immediately 5' to the intron/exon boundary. The splice sites themselves are unrelated to the reading frame of the particular mRNA. In some instances, as in the case of intron 1 of the β-globin gene, the intron actually splits a particular codon.

The medical significance of RNA splicing is illustrated by the fact that mutations within the conserved sequences at the intron/exon boundaries commonly reduce or eliminate RNA splicing, with a concomitant reduction in the amount of normal, mature β-globin mRNA. A number of these splice site mutations, identified in patients with β-thalassemia, are discussed in detail in Chapter 11.

Polyadenylation

The mature β-globin mRNA contains approximately 130 base pairs of 3' untranslated material between the stop codon and the location of the polyA tail (Fig. 3–14). As in other genes, cleavage of the 3' end of the mRNA and addition of the polyA tail is controlled, at least in part, by an AAUAAA sequence approximately 20 base pairs before the polyadenylation site. Mutations in this polyadenylation signal in patients with β-thalassemia (as well as mutations in the corresponding polyadenylation signal in the α-globin gene in patients with α-thalassemia) document the importance of this signal for proper 3′ cleavage and polyadenylation. The 3′ untranslated region of some genes can be quite long, up to several kilobases. Other genes have a number of alternative polyadenylation sites, selection among which may influence the stability of the resulting mRNA and thus the steady-state level of the mRNA.

The Control of Gene Expression

The regulated expression of the 50,000 to 100,000 genes encoded in human chromosomes involves a set of complex interrelationships among different levels of control, including proper gene dosage (controlled by mechanisms of chromosome replication and segregation), gene structure, and finally transcription, translation, and protein processing. For some genes, fluctuations in the level of functional gene product, due either to inherited variation in the structure of a particular gene or to changes induced by nongenetic factors such as diet or the environment, are of relatively little importance. For other genes, even minor changes in the level of expression can have dire clinical consequences. The nature of inherited variation in the structure and function of chromosomes and genes, and the influence of this variation on the expression of specific traits, is the very essence of medical and molecular genetics and is dealt with in subsequent chapters.

General References

Alberts B, Bray D, Lewis J, et al. (1989) Molecular biology of the cell, 2nd ed. Garland, New York.

Lewin B (1990) Genes, 4th ed. Oxford University Press, Oxford, England.

Singer M, Berg P (1991) Genes and genomes. University Science Books, Mill Valley, CA.

Stamatoyannopoulos G, Nienhuis AW, Leder P, Majerus PW (1987) The molecular basis of blood diseases. WB Saunders, Philadelphia.

Watson JD, Hopkins NH, Roberts JW, et al. (1987) Molecular biology of the gene, 4th ed. Benjamin/Cummings, Menlo Park, CA.

Problems

1. The following amino acid sequence represents part of a protein. The normal sequence and four mutant forms are shown. By consulting Table 3–3, determine the double-stranded sequence of the corresponding section of the normal gene. Which strand is the strand that RNA polymerase "reads"? What would the sequence of the resulting mRNA be? What kind of mutation is each mutant protein most likely to represent?

   Normal   -lys-arg-his-his-tyr-leu-
   Mutant 1   -lys-arg-his-his-cys-leu-
   Mutant 2   -lys-arg-ile-ile-ile-
   Mutant 3   -lys-glu-thr-ser-leu-ser-
   Mutant 4   -asn-tyr-leu-

2. The following items are related to each other in a hierarchical fashion. What are these relationships? Chromosome, base pair, nucleosome, G-band, kilobase pair, intron, gene, exon, chromatin, codon, nucleotide.

3. The following schematic drawing illustrates a chromosome 5 in which the most distal band (band p15) on the short arm is deleted. This 5p− chromosome is associated with the cri du chat syndrome (see Chapter 9). Given what you know about the organization of chromosomes and the genome, approximately how much DNA is deleted? How many genes?

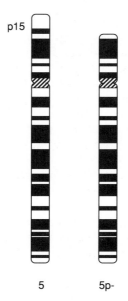

p15

5   5p−

CHAPTER 4

PATTERNS OF SINGLE-GENE INHERITANCE

In Chapter 1 the three main categories of genetic disorders — single-gene, chromosomal, and multifactorial — were named and briefly characterized. In this chapter the classical patterns of transmission of single-gene disorders are discussed in further detail, and some noteworthy exceptions to the usual patterns are described.

Single-gene traits are often called **Mendelian** because, like the characteristics of garden peas studied by Gregor Mendel, they segregate within families and, on the average, occur in fixed proportions among the offspring of specific types of matings. The single-gene phenotypes described so far are listed in Victor A. McKusick's classic reference, *Mendelian Inheritance in Man* (9th edition, 1990), which has been indispensable to medical geneticists for many years. The 1990 edition of this book lists more than 4500 loci, and at many of these there is at least one known mutant form that is associated with a clinically significant disorder. Thus of the estimated total of 50,000 to 100,000 human genes, approximately 5 percent to 10 percent have already been identified. The pace of new discovery is high, and it seems certain to accelerate because of international interest and activity in mapping and sequencing of the entire human genome.

Inherited variation in the genome is the cornerstone of human and medical genetics. Alternative forms of genetic information at a particular locus are called **alleles**. Many genes have only one normal version, which we call the "wild-type" allele. Other gene loci exhibit **polymorphism** (literally, "many forms"), meaning that in the population there are at least two relatively common normal alleles at the locus (see Chapter 6). In addition to the normal allele or alleles, most identified loci also have one or more rare alleles; in fact, many human loci were originally identified through a clinically significant disorder caused by a rare mutant allele.

The **genotype** of a person is his or her genetic constitution, either collectively at all loci or, more typically, at a single locus. The **phenotype** is the observable expression of a genotype as a morphological, biochemical, or molecular trait. A phenotype may, of course, be either normal or abnormal in a given individual, but in this book, which emphasizes disorders of medical significance, the focus is on abnormal phenotypes — that is, genetic disorders.

A single-gene disorder is one that is determined by a specific allele at a single locus on one or both members of a chromosome pair. The variant allele, which arose by mutation at some time in the recent or remote past and is usually relatively rare, replaces a normal wild-type allele on one or both chromosomes. When a person has a pair of identical alleles, he or she is said to be **homozygous** (a **homozygote**); when the alleles are different, he or she is **heterozygous** (a **heterozygote** or carrier). The term **compound**, or compound heterozygote, is used to describe a genotype in which two different mutant alleles are present, rather than one normal and one mutant. These terms (homozygous, heterozygous, and compound) can be applied either to a person or to a genotype. The term **mutation** is used in medical genetics in two senses: sometimes to indicate a new genetic change that has not been previously known in a kindred and sometimes merely to indicate an abnormal allele.

Single-gene disorders are characterized by their patterns of transmission in families. To establish the pattern of transmission, a usual first step is to obtain information about the family history of the patient and to summarize the details in the form of a **pedigree**, using standard symbols (Fig. 4–1). The patterns shown by single-gene disorders in pedigrees depend chiefly on two factors: (1) the chromosomal location of the gene locus, which may be **autosomal** (located on an autosome) or **X-linked** (located on the X chromosome) and (2) whether the phenotype is **dominant** (expressed even when only one chromosome of a pair carries the variant allele) or **recessive** (expressed only when both chromosomes of a pair carry a variant allele). Thus there are only four basic patterns of single-gene inheritance:

$$\text{Autosomal} \begin{cases} \text{dominant} \\ \text{recessive} \end{cases} \quad \text{X-linked} \begin{cases} \text{dominant} \\ \text{recessive} \end{cases}$$

Autosomal and X-Linked Inheritance

The distinction between autosomal and X-linked inheritance is obvious, as it depends solely on the chromosomal location of the gene. However, the clinical expression of an abnormal gene also depends on whether it is autosomal or X-linked. There are two considerations, which are discussed in more detail later: (1) Males have only a single X and are therefore said to be **hemizygous** with respect to X-linked genes, rather than homozygous or heterozygous; 46,XY males are *never* heterozygous for X-linked traits. (2) To compensate for the double complement of X-linked genes in females, as opposed to the single complement in males, alleles on only one of the two X chromosomes are expressed in any given cell of a female, whereas both alleles of any autosomal locus are active.

Dominant and Recessive Inheritance

By formal definition, a phenotype expressed in the same way in both homozygotes and heterozygotes is **dominant**, and a phenotype expressed only in homozygotes (or, for X-linked traits, hemizygotes) is **recessive**. In medical genetics, however, this definition does not strictly hold, and any phenotype expressed in heterozygotes is classified as dominant. Autosomal dominant disorders are typically more severe in homozygotes than in heterozygotes, and so far only one such disorder, Huntington disease, is known to be equally severe in both genotypes. When the expression of the heterozygous genotype is different from both homozygous types and intermediate between them, the phenotype may be described more precisely as incompletely dominant or incompletely recessive. If expression of each allele can be detected even in the presence of the other, the two alleles are termed **codominant**.

Each of the genetic disorders discussed in this book as an example of a genetic principle is described briefly from a clinical and genetic standpoint at an appropriate place in the text, often in a box. Refer to Table 1–1 and the index for information about where to find many of these clinical descriptions.

Strictly speaking, it is the phenotype rather than the allele that is dominant or recessive; however, genes are classified as dominant or recessive on the basis of their phenotypic expression, and the terms "dominant gene" and "recessive gene" are widely, if loosely, used.

The distinction between dominant and reces-

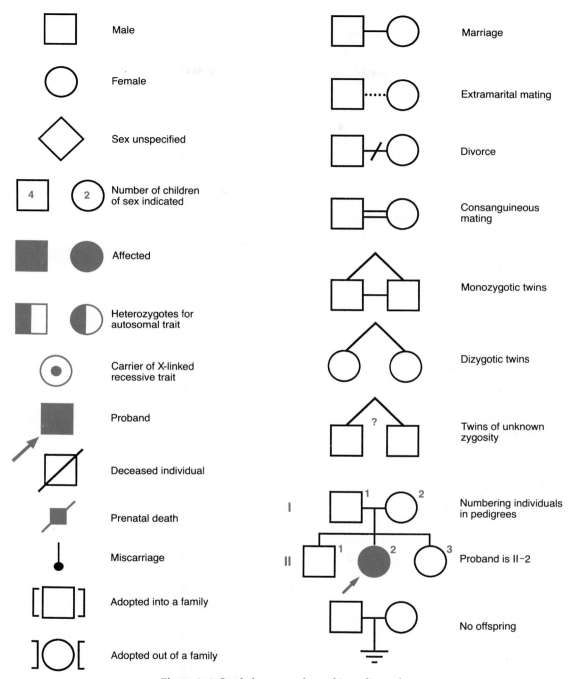

Figure 4–1. Symbols commonly used in pedigree charts.

sive inheritance is not absolute; rather, it is an arbitrary designation, based on clinical phenotypes, that may be without significance at the level of gene action. For autosomal loci, each allele is expressed as a gene product; in heterozygotes, one of

the alleles may be deleted, or its product may be defective and ultimately nonfunctional, but wherever it is biologically possible, both alleles are expressed, and the phenotype is the consequence of their combined expression. Although a recessive phenotype is defined as being clinically undetectable in heterozygotes, many traits classified as recessive do have heterozygous manifestations when examined at the cellular, biochemical, or molecular level.

For example, the well-known disorder of hemoglobin, **sickle cell disease** (or anemia), is inherited as an autosomal recessive disease (see Chapter 11 for further discussion). Patients with the disease are homozygous for a defective allele at the β-globin locus and consequently produce the abnormal hemoglobin S (Hb S) rather than normal adult hemoglobin (Hb A) in their red cells, which become sickle-shaped under conditions of low oxygen tension. Heterozygotes produce both Hb A and Hb S, a proportion of their red cells show the sickling phenomenon, and they have mild anemia. Thus at the level of hemoglobin synthesis, the normal β-globin allele and the defective allele are expressed as codominant alleles; at the level of physiological function, the normal allele is incompletely dominant (and the abnormal allele incompletely recessive); and at the clinical level, sickle cell disease behaves as a recessive trait.

In autosomal dominant disorders, the product of the normal allele is typically one that is required in a normal amount; a mutant gene that produces no protein, a reduced amount of protein, or protein in an abnormal form results in the abnormal phenotype. Broadly speaking, the normal gene product is often a nonenzymatic structural protein, such as collagen, or a protein component of a membrane or receptor; thus far, however, in the vast majority of autosomal dominant disorders, the nature of the defective or missing protein is still completely unknown. In contrast, many of the autosomal recessive disorders described to date are enzyme defects, in which there appears to be a margin of safety wide enough to allow normal function in heterozygotes even though only one of a pair of alleles is fully functional and the other (abnormal) allele is defective or nonfunctional. These considerations are discussed in detail in Chapter 12.

In summary, the distinction between a dominant and a recessive mutant allele is really a simple one: in the heterozygote, with one normal and one mutant allele, is the residual amount of gene product sufficient to perform its designed function? If the answer is yes, the mutant allele (and its associated disorder) is recessive. If the answer is no, the mutant allele (and its disorder) is dominant.

Other Factors Affecting Pedigree Patterns

Although as a general rule pedigrees of single-gene disorders can be readily classified as autosomal or X-linked and as dominant or recessive, the inheritance pattern of an individual pedigree is also determined by a number of other factors that may make the mode of inheritance difficult to interpret. Especially with the small family size typical of most developed countries today, the patient may be the only affected family member, and the genetic nature of the disorder may not be immediately apparent. Some other points to keep in mind are the chance segregation of genes from parents to children through the gametes; new mutation, which is not infrequent in some types of genetic disease; diagnostic difficulties due to absent or variable expression of the gene concerned; possible effects of other genes and of environment on gene expression; failure of persons of some genotypes to survive to the time of birth; and lack of accurate information about the presence of the disorder in relatives or about family relationships. As described in the section "Nonclassical Patterns of Single-Gene Expression," a number of rare and unusual biological mechanisms can lead to nonclassical pedigree patterns. Examples of some of the situations that can confound attempts to provide accurate genetic counseling are given in the problems at the end of this chapter.

Sometimes a pedigree pattern simulates a single-gene pattern even though the disorder does not have a single-gene basis. It is easy to be misled in this way by conditions that exhibit multifactorial inheritance, by certain types of familial chromosomal disorders, or by teratogenic effects. Inherited single-gene disorders can be distinguished from other types of familial disorders by their typical Mendelian segregation ratios within kindreds and by a number of other approaches, of which the most critical is the demonstration of a single defect at the level of the gene product or at the level of DNA that accounts for the phenotype.

Many patients with genetic disorders have no similarly affected relatives, but even if a genetic disorder occurs in only one member of a family group, it may still be possible to recognize that it is genetic. Because of the remarkable similarity of phenotype among different families with the same defect, well-established patterns of inheritance in other families with the same disorder can often be used as a basis for diagnosis and counseling (McKusick, 1990).

Heterogeneity

When a genetic disorder that appears to be a single entity is thoroughly analyzed, it is frequently found to be genetically heterogeneous; that is, it includes a number of phenotypes that are similar but are actually determined by different genotypes (see Table 4–1 for examples). Heterogeneity may be the result of different mutations at the same locus **(allelic heterogeneity)**, mutations at different loci **(nonallelic** or **locus heterogeneity)**, or both. Recognition of genetic heterogeneity is an important aspect of clinical diagnosis and genetic counseling.

For many phenotypes, pedigree analysis alone has been sufficient to demonstrate genetic heterogeneity. For example, **retinitis pigmentosa**, a common cause of visual impairment due to retinal degeneration associated with abnormal pigment distribution in the retina, has long been known to occur in autosomal dominant, autosomal recessive, and X-linked forms. In recent years the heterogeneity has been shown to be even more extensive; DNA analysis has demonstrated that there are at least two X-linked and three autosomal dominant forms. **Ehlers-Danlos syndrome**, in which there are numerous manifestations of an underlying defect of collagen structure, may also have autosomal dominant, autosomal recessive, or X-linked inheritance, and analysis at the clinical and molecular levels has shown that there are at least 10 distinct types of the disorder.

Allelic heterogeneity is an important cause of clinical variation. Many loci possess more than one mutant allele; in fact, at a given locus there may be several or many mutations, resulting in clinically indistinguishable or closely similar disorders. In other cases, different mutant alleles at the same locus result in very different clinical presentations. A classical example of allelic heterogeneity as the basis of clinical heterogeneity is the autosomal recessive disorder **Hurler syndrome**, a mucopolysaccharidosis resulting from deficiency of the enzyme α-L-iduronidase. A milder allelic disorder, **Scheie syndrome**, results from a different mutation at the same locus, and a phenotype of intermediate severity, **Hurler-Scheie syndrome**, is seen in patients with the compound genotype (see also Table 12–4).

Unless they have consanguineous parents, many people with autosomal recessive disorders probably have compound rather than truly homozygous genotypes, although for most purposes they are still usually referred to as homozygotes if they have a pair of abnormal alleles. Because different allelic combinations may have somewhat different clinical consequences, clinicians need to be aware of allelic heterogeneity as one possible explanation for variability among patients considered to have the same disease.

The Burden of Mendelian Disorders

The known Mendelian diseases exact a heavy cost in reproductive failure, premature death, and social handicap. They are primarily, but by no means

Table 4–1. **Heterogeneity in Selected Single-Gene Disorders**

Disorder	Type of Heterogeneity	Comments
Charcot-Marie-Tooth disease	Locus (nonallelic)	AD, XR forms
Cystic fibrosis	Allelic	Pancreatic insufficiency vs. sufficiency
Deafness, recessive congenital	Both allelic and locus	Numerous types described
Duchenne and Becker muscular dystrophy	Allelic	Clinically distinct
Ehlers-Danlos syndrome	Both allelic and locus	Many distinct variants
Homocystinuria	Both allelic and locus	Vitamin responsive vs. nonresponsive
Mucopolysaccharidoses	Both allelic and locus	Extensive heterogeneity
Myotonia congenita	Locus	AD, AR forms
Retinitis pigmentosa	Locus	AD, AR, and XR forms
Tay-Sachs disease	Allelic	Several forms
β-thalessemia	Allelic	Numerous different mutations in β-globin gene produce the phenotype

AD = autosomal dominant; AR = autosomal recessive; XR = X-linked recessive.

exclusively, disorders of the pediatric age range; fewer than 10 percent develop after puberty, and only 1 percent occur after the end of the reproductive period (Costa et al., 1985). Although individually rare, as a group they are responsible for a significant proportion of childhood diseases and deaths. In a population study of more than 1 million live births, the incidence of serious single-gene disorders was estimated to be 0.36 percent (Baird et al., 1988). In another study of liveborn and stillborn infants, 1 in 45 had some type of congenital anomaly; of the anomalies, about 1 in 30 appeared to be single-gene disorders, and about 1 in 4 of the single-gene disorders were thought to be new mutations (Nelson and Holmes, 1989). Among hospitalized children, 6 percent to 8 percent probably have single-gene disorders (Beaudet et al., 1989).

Terminology

Even though the principles of medical genetics are relatively easy to understand, the unfamiliar terminology may make the subject seem inaccessible at first. To help solve the language problem, some terms not previously defined are introduced here and illustrated by the pedigree in Figure 4–2.

The member through whom a family with a genetic disorder is first brought to attention (ascertained) is the **proband** (propositus), or if affected may be called the **index case**. The proband is usually a patient but may be some other member of the family. A family may have more than one proband, if it is ascertained through more than one source. Brothers and sisters are called **sibs** or siblings, and a family of sibs forms a **sibship**. The first-generation offspring of a mating constitute

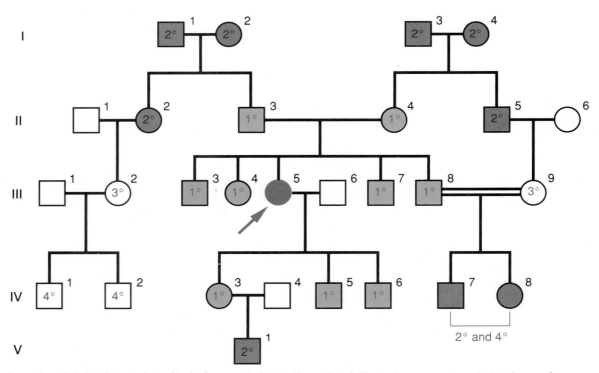

Figure 4–2. Relationships within a kindred. Arrow indicates the **proband**, III-5, who represents an **isolated case** of a genetic disorder. She has four **sibs**, III-3, III-4, III-7, and III-8. Her partner/spouse is III-6, and they have three children (their **F1** progeny). The proband has nine **first-degree** relatives (her parents, siblings, and offspring), nine **second-degree** relatives (grandparents, uncles/aunts, nieces/nephews, grandchildren), two **third-degree** relatives (first cousins), and four **fourth-degree** relatives (first cousins once removed). IV-3, IV-5, and IV-6 are **second cousins** of IV-1 and IV-2. IV-7 and IV-8, whose parents are **consanguineous**, are doubly related to the proband: second-degree relatives through their father and fourth-degree relatives through their mother.

the **F1** (first filial generation). Relatives are classified as **first-degree** (parents, sibs, and offspring of the proband), **second-degree** (grandparents and grandchildren, uncles and aunts, nephews and nieces, half-sibs), **third-degree** (first cousins, for example), and so forth, depending on the number of steps (in other words, the number of meioses) in the pedigree between the two relatives. The offspring of first cousins are second cousins, and a child is a "first cousin once removed" of his or her parents' first cousins. Couples who are related by descent are **consanguineous**. If there is only one affected member in a family, he or she is an "isolated" case or, if the disorder is determined to be due to new mutation, a "sporadic" case (Fig. 4–2).

AUTOSOMAL INHERITANCE

PATTERNS OF AUTOSOMAL DOMINANT INHERITANCE

Among the 4500 or so known Mendelian phenotypes, more than half are autosomal dominant traits. The incidence of some autosomal dominant disorders is quite high, at least in specific geographic areas: for example, 1 in 500 for familial hypercholesterolemia in populations of European or Japanese descent; more than 1 in 1000 for myotonic dystrophy in some parts of North America; and about 1 in 2500 to 3000 for several conditions such as Huntington disease (in populations of North European origin), von Recklinghausen neurofibromatosis, and polycystic kidney disease. Although many autosomal dominant disorders are much less common, they are so numerous that their total incidence is appreciable. The burden of autosomal dominant disorders is further increased because of their hereditary nature; they may be transmitted through families and become problems not only for individuals but for whole kindreds, often over many generations; and in some cases the burden is compounded by social difficulties resulting from physical or mental disability.

In classical autosomal dominant inheritance, every affected person in a pedigree has an affected parent, who also has an affected parent, and so on as far back as the disorder can be traced or until the occurrence of an original mutation. This is also true, as discussed later, of X-linked dominant pedigrees. However, autosomal dominant inheritance can readily be distinguished from X-linked dominant inheritance by **male-to-male transmission**, which is obviously impossible for X-linked inheritance since males transmit the Y chromosome, not the X, to their sons.

Most mutations that cause disease are rare in the population, in comparison with normal alleles; thus in matings that produce children with an autosomal dominant disease, one parent is usually heterozygous for the mutation, and the other parent is homozygous for the normal allele. The parents' genotypes can be written as

$A/a \times a/a$ A is dominant gene for abnormal phenotype; a is normal allele

Progeny of $A/a \times a/a$ Mating

Normal Parent

		a	a
Affected Parent	A	A/a Affected	A/a Affected
	a	a/a Normal	a/a Normal

Each child of this mating has a 50 percent chance of receiving the affected parent's abnormal allele A and thus being affected (A/a), and a 50 percent chance of receiving the normal allele a and thus being unaffected (a/a). (The unaffected parent can transmit only a normal a allele to each child.) Statistically speaking, each pregnancy is an "independent event," not governed by the outcome of previous pregnancies; thus within a family the distribution of affected and unaffected children may be quite different from the theoretical 1:1, although in the population as a whole the

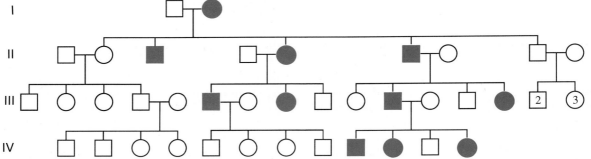

Figure 4–3. Pedigree of family with Huntington disease, an autosomal dominant disorder with relatively late age of onset.

offspring of $A/a \times a/a$ parents are approximately 50 percent A/a and 50 percent a/a.

Figure 4–3 is a hypothetical four-generation pedigree of a well-known autosomal dominant phenotype, **Huntington disease (HD)**, a disorder characterized by choreic movements and progressive dementia (see box). The onset age of HD is variable; only about half the people who have the HD gene show symptoms by the age of 40 years (Fig. 4–4). The disease was first described by the physician George Huntington in 1872 in an American kindred of English descent, but the original mutation is thought to have originated in northwestern Europe and to have spread from there around the world. New mutations, if they exist at all, are very rare; in other words, virtually all patients can be shown to have an affected parent, and a positive family history is one of the diagnostic criteria. Because HD does not usually make its

appearance until after the end of the reproductive years, it is likely to be passed on by persons who carry the mutant gene and who are unaware that they are at risk.

The largest HD group known lives in the region of Lake Maracaibo, Venezuela, to which the gene was introduced early in the 19th century (Gusella et al., 1983). About 100 living affected persons and another 900 each at 50 percent risk are currently known in the Lake Maracaibo community. High frequency of a disease in a local population descended from a small number of individuals, one of whom carried the gene responsible for the disease, is an example of **founder effect** (see Chapter 7).

HD was one of the first diseases in which molecular genetic methods led to the discovery of a DNA marker closely linked to the gene, which in suitable families allows presymptomatic and even

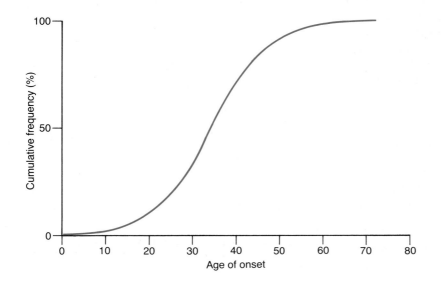

Figure 4–4. Onset age in Huntington disease. (From Conneally PM, Wallace MR, Gusella JF, Wexler NS [1984] Huntington disease: estimation of heterozygote status using linked genetic markers. Genet Epidemiol 1:81–88.)

HUNTINGTON DISEASE (HD)

Clinical features:	Progressive dementia, choreic movements; onset typically in 5th decade	Basic defect:	Unknown
		Pathophysiology:	Unknown
Incidence:	Variable (4 to 8 per 100,000), higher in some populations of Western European ancestry and in local populations	Prenatal diagnosis:	Possible with DNA techniques, but limited so far because ethical problems surrounding its use are still under study
Genetics:	Autosomal dominant	Treatment:	None available
	New mutation extremely rare (never documented)	Significance:	A classic autosomal dominant disorder associated with severe neurological and mental illness, particularly distressing because the onset age is typically in the postreproductive years. Also, the first Mendelian disorder mapped by linkage to DNA markers (in 1983)
	Similar expression in heterozygotes and homozygotes		
	Early-onset cases usually have paternal inheritance		
	Gene location 4p16		

prenatal diagnosis of individuals at risk (see Chapters 8 and 18). Because HD carries such a serious prognosis, there are major ethical implications associated with molecular analysis and genetic counseling for families with the disease. Does a person at risk have a right to know the result of the test? Does he or she have a duty to undergo testing and learn the result before reproducing? Is it ethical to allow children from HD families to be tested? Should a register of people at high risk of HD be kept, and if so, who should keep it? In view of these and related problems, approaches to presymptomatic testing in HD are being made with caution and with great concern for the family members who are found to be at risk.

In the idealized pedigree in Figure 4–3, each affected member has an affected parent, both males and females are affected, and both can pass on the phenotype to children of either sex. There are two examples of male-to-male transmission. Unaffected family members, who do not have the abnormal allele, have only unaffected descendants. About half the offspring of affected persons are affected. (Family members too young to express HD are omitted from this pedigree.)

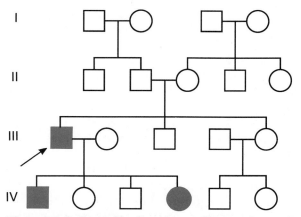

Figure 4–5. Pedigree of family with neurofibromatosis, type 1, apparently originating as a new mutation in the proband (arrow).

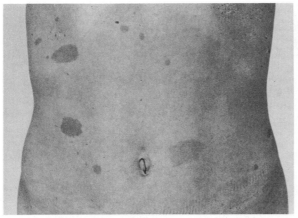

Figure 4–6. Neurofibromatosis, type 1: café-au-lait spots, hyperpigmented spots on the skin, a useful diagnostic sign in family members who otherwise may appear unaffected. Most patients have six or more spots at least 15 mm in diameter, usually on the trunk. (Photograph courtesy of Rosanna Weksberg, The Hospital for Sick Children, Toronto.)

Much more typical of the kind of autosomal dominant pedigree that comes to clinical attention is that shown in Figure 4–5, a pedigree of **neurofibromatosis** (NF1) (see box). NF1 is a common disorder of the nervous system, shown in one of its typical clinical presentations in Figure 4–6. The gene is clinically apparent in virtually everyone who carries it, and penetrance is therefore said to be 100 percent. However, there is great variability in its expression; even within a kindred, some individuals with NF1 are severely affected, whereas others show only mild symptoms (see discussion on "Penetrance and Expressivity"). Approximately half the cases of NF1 result from new mutation, and in the family shown in Figure 4–5, the proband (indicated by an arrow) appears to have a new mutant gene, since his parents and their parents are all unaffected. The chief genetic problem in counseling families of patients with NF1 is to

VON RECKLINGHAUSEN NEUROFIBROMATOSIS (NF1)

Clinical features:	Café-au-lait spots, fibromatous skin tumors, Lisch nodules in iris, risk of malignant tumors		none; secondary problems can be managed medically or surgically
Incidence:	~1 in 3000 to 1 in 5000	Significance:	A common autosomal dominant phenotype with extreme variation in expression from barely identifiable to dramatically abnormal. Gene cloned in 1990 by positional cloning approaches based initially on mapping gene by linkage to DNA polymorphisms. A very large gene (probably close to 400 kb) that includes several other genes within it encoded on the opposite DNA strand
Genetics:	Autosomal dominant Complete penetrance, highly variable expressivity ~50% of patients are new mutants Very high mutation rate ($\sim 1 \times 10^{-4}$), probably due to large gene Gene location 17q11.2		
Basic defect:	Mutations in gene proposed to be tumor suppressor gene		
Pathophysiology:	Unknown		
Prenatal diagnosis:	Possible in suitable families by DNA techniques		
Treatment:	For the primary defect,		

decide between two a priori, equally likely possibilities: Is the disease in this family due to new mutation, or has the patient inherited a clinically significant form of the disorder from a parent in whom the gene is present but only mildly expressed? If the patient has inherited the defect, the risk that any of his or her sibs will also inherit it is 50 percent, but if the child has a new mutant gene, there is almost no risk that any sib will be affected. In either case, the risk that the patient will pass the gene on to any one of his or her offspring is 50 percent. The unpredictability of the severity of the manifestations of NF1, a characteristic of many autosomal dominant disorders, is an added complication for genetic counseling. In view of these uncertainties, it is reassuring to families of NF1 patients to know that the NF1 gene has already been mapped (Barker et al., 1987) and cloned (Viskochil et al., 1990; Wallace et al., 1990). The disorder can now be detected presymptomatically and even prenatally by molecular genetic analysis. Unfortunately, there is no way to predict or detect the large proportion of cases that are due to new mutation.

Homozygotes for Autosomal Dominant Traits

In medical practice, homozygotes for rare dominant phenotypes are not often seen because matings that could produce homozygous offspring are rare. The parents of a homozygote might theoretically be $A/a \times A/a$, $A/A \times A/a$, or $A/A \times A/A$ (A representing the deleterious allele), or the patient might, in exceedingly rare instances, have received a new mutation from a genetically unaffected parent or even from both. Practically speaking, however, only the mating of two heterozygotes need be considered, and even that is an unusual event for most autosomal dominant conditions.

Parents: $A/a \times A/a$
                Affected $\times$ affected

Offspring: 1/4 A/A 1/2 A/a 1/4 a/a
           Homozygous   Heterozygous   Normal
           affected   affected

In human families, it is difficult to prove from a pedigree alone that a person affected by an autosomal dominant disorder is homozygous. The rule is that all the offspring of the homozygote are af-

fected and none are normal. This expectation can be proved statistically in experimental animals and plants, when the number of offspring is large, but human families are usually too small for such statistical verification. An A/a person with an a/a partner might by chance have only affected (A/a) children, even though the chance of an unaffected a/a child is 50 percent in each pregnancy. Thus when the phenotypes of A/A and A/a individuals are alike, an $A/A \times a/a$ mating cannot be distinguished from an $A/a \times a/a$ mating merely by the observation that all the offspring are affected. (The opposite, of course, is not true; the presence of even a single unaffected child from a mating involving an affected parent is sufficient to establish that the affected parent must be heterozygous and cannot be homozygous.)

Clinically, the distinction between affected heterozygotes and homozygotes can be made with considerable certainty in many cases because, as noted earlier, human autosomal dominant disorders are usually much more severe in homozygotes than in heterozygotes. Figure 4–7 shows a

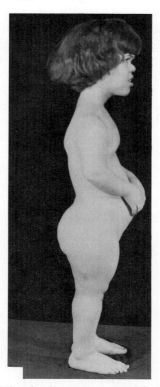

Figure 4–7. Achondroplasia, an autosomal dominant disorder that often occurs as a new mutation. Note small stature with short limbs, large head, low nasal bridge, prominent forehead, lumbar lordosis. (From Tachdjian MO [1972]. Pediatric orthopedics, Vol 1. WB Saunders, Philadelphia, p. 284.)

ACHONDROPLASIA

Clinical features:	Short-limbed dwarfism with characteristic facies and diagnostic radiological features of spine	Basic defect:	Unknown
		Pathophysiology:	Unknown
		Prenatal diagnosis:	Ultrasound examination
		Treatment:	None available
Incidence:	Probably ~ 1 in 10,000	Significance:	A major cause of short stature. Because the phenotype is so distinctive, it has been used to elucidate a number of principles of medical genetics (see text)
Genetics:	Autosomal dominant		
	Much more severe phenotype in homozygotes		
	~ 80% of patients are new mutants		
	Increased risk with late paternal age		

child with the typical heterozygous form of **achondroplasia**, a skeletal disorder of short-limbed dwarfism and large head size (see box). A homozygous child of two heterozygotes is often recognizable on clinical grounds alone; homozygous achondroplastics are much more severely abnormal than heterozygotes and commonly do not survive early infancy. Most achondroplastics have normal intelligence and lead normal lives within their physical capabilities. It is understandable that marriages between two achondroplastics are not uncommon.

Another example is **familial hypercholesterolemia**, an autosomal dominant disorder lead-

ing to premature coronary heart disease, in which the rare homozygous patients (Fig. 4–8) have a much more severe disease, with much shorter life expectancy, than do the relatively common heterozygotes (see box).

In fact, in virtually every reported example, homozygosity for a defective allele results in a more severely abnormal phenotype than does heterozygosity. As mentioned previously, HD is the sole exception; HD homozygotes can be distinguished from the far more common heterozygotes by molecular analysis with linked DNA markers, as described in Chapter 8. However, the clinical expression appears to be the same in both geno-

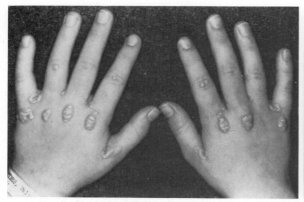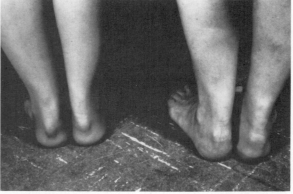

Figure 4–8. Comparison of severity of symptoms in familial hypercholesterolemia (FH): cutaneous xanthomas in an FH homozygote (left) and tendon xanthomas in FH heterozygotes (right). (Photographs courtesy of J. L. Goldstein, University of Texas Southwestern Medical Center, Dallas, Texas.)

FAMILIAL HYPERCHOLESTEROLEMIA (FH)

Clinical features:	In heterozygotes, elevated level of low-density lipoprotein (LDL) in plasma, deposition of cholesterol in tendons and skin (xanthomas) and arteries in adult life; coronary heart disease in early middle age In homozygotes, the clinical features are present earlier, and coronary heart disease is usually fatal in childhood		50% risk of myocardial infarction in heterozygous males by age 50 and in heterozygous females somewhat later
		Prenatal diagnosis:	Possible for homozygotes, by assay of LDL receptor activity in cultured amniotic fluid cells; possible by DNA techniques in suitable families
Incidence:	Heterozygotes very common, ~ 1 in 500 Homozygotes very rare, ~ 1 in 1,000,000	Treatment:	Lowering the plasma level of LDL by drugs and dietary restriction
Genetics:	Autosomal dominant Gene location 19p13 Multiple mutant alleles	Significance:	One of the most common genetic diseases and a leading cause of coronary heart disease. Joseph L. Goldstein and Michael S. Brown were awarded the 1985 Nobel prize in medicine for their discovery of the LDL receptor and their demonstration that FH is caused by mutation in the corresponding gene
Basic defect:	Mutations in the gene encoding the LDL receptor (see Chapter 12)		
Pathophysiology:	Excess cholesterol is deposited as xanthomas and arteriosclerotic plaques		

types (Wexler et al., 1987). This observation may provide clues to the nature of the long-sought primary defect in HD; it suggests that the basic defect is unlikely to be loss of function of an essential enzyme.

New Mutation in Autosomal Dominant Disorders

In any population, new alleles arise by mutation and are maintained or removed by selection. After a new mutation has arisen, its survival in the population depends on the **fitness** of persons carrying it, in comparison with that of persons carrying other alleles at the locus concerned.

The fitness of a condition is measured by the number of offspring of affected persons who survive to reproductive age, in comparison with an appropriate control group. Many autosomal dominant disorders are associated with reduced fitness. There is an inverse relation between the fitness of a given autosomal dominant disorder and the proportion of all patients with that disorder who have new mutant genes. When a disorder reduces the reproductive fitness of affected persons, a propor-

Criteria for Autosomal Dominant Inheritance

1. The phenotype appears in every generation, each affected person having an affected parent.

Exceptions or apparent exceptions to this rule in clinical genetics: (1) cases originating by fresh mutation in a gamete of a phenotypically normal parent; (2) apparent but not true exceptions in which the disorder is not expressed (nonpenetrant) or is expressed very mildly in a person who has inherited the responsible gene.

2. Any child of an affected parent has a 50% risk of inheriting the trait.

This is true for most families, in which the other parent is phenotypically normal. Because statistically each family member is the result of an "independent event," there may in a single family be wide deviation from the expected 1:1 ratio.

3. Phenotypically normal family members do not transmit the phenotype to their children.

Failure of penetrance or exceptionally mild expression of a condition may lead to apparent exceptions to this rule.

4. Males and females are equally likely to transmit the phenotype, to children of either sex. In particular, male-to-male transmission can occur, and males can have unaffected daughters.

tion of all those affected are likely to have received the defective gene as a new mutation in a gamete from a genotypically normal parent. Some disorders have a fitness of zero ($f = 0$); in other words, patients with such disorders never reproduce. Essentially all observed cases of the disorder are therefore due to new mutations. Other disorders, including some very serious conditions such as HD, have virtually normal reproductive fitness because of the late onset age in typical cases. If the fitness is normal ($f = 1$), the disorder is rarely seen as a result of fresh mutation; a patient is much more likely to have inherited the disorder than to have a new mutant gene. The measurement of mutation frequency and the relation of mutation frequency to fitness are discussed further in Chapter 7.

PATTERNS OF AUTOSOMAL RECESSIVE INHERITANCE

Autosomal recessive phenotypes are less common than autosomal dominants, accounting for about one third of the recognized Mendelian phenotypes. In contrast to autosomal dominant disorders, in which affected persons are usually heterozygous, autosomal recessive disorders are expressed only in homozygotes, who thus must have inherited a mutant allele from each parent. A classical pedigree illustrating autosomal recessive inheritance is shown in Figure 4–9. Both parents of an affected person are heterozygotes **(carriers)**, and their children's risk of receiving the recessive allele from each parent and therefore being affected is one in four. The proband may be the only affected family member, but if any others are affected, they are almost invariably in the same sibship, not elsewhere in the kindred. On occasion, other relatives may also be affected, especially in large inbred kindreds.

Although any mating in which each parent has at least one recessive allele can produce homozygous affected offspring, the most common one by far is the mating of two carriers. The three types, with the risk to the offspring in each case, are listed below. The mutant recessive allele is symbolized as r and its normal dominant allele as R.

Parents	Risk to offspring
Carrier × carrier: $R/r \times R/r$	$\frac{1}{4}$ R/R, $\frac{1}{2}$ R/r, $\frac{1}{4}$ r/r $\frac{3}{4}$ unaffected, $\frac{1}{4}$ affected
Carrier × affected: $R/r \times r/r$	$\frac{1}{2}$ R/r, $\frac{1}{2}$ r/r $\frac{1}{2}$ unaffected, $\frac{1}{2}$ affected
Affected × affected: $r/r \times r/r$	r/r only All affected

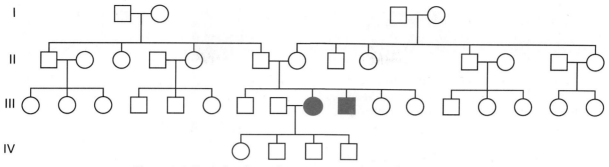

Figure 4–9. Typical pedigree showing autosomal recessive inheritance.

Gene Frequency and Carrier Frequency

Carriers of autosomal recessive genes are not usually clinically recognizable but, as the following discussion shows, they are far more common than homozygous affected individuals. Carrier frequency is clinically important for genetic counseling. Because an autosomal recessive disorder must be inherited *through both parents*, the risk that any carrier will have an affected child depends partly on the carrier frequency in the general population.

When the population frequency of the phenotype is known and when certain other idealized features of the population (described in Chapter 7) are met, the gene frequency and corresponding carrier frequency can be determined from the observed frequency of affected persons. The frequencies of the three possible genotypes (homozygous normal, heterozygous, and homozygous affected) depend on the relative frequencies of the alleles at that locus in the gene pool (i.e., all the genes at that locus in that population). For a typical locus, assuming only one normal allele and one mutant allele for a recessive disorder, one can think of the gene pool as a beanbag with beans of two colors, white representing the normal allele and blue representing the abnormal allele. Everyone has two "draws" from the beanbag, representing the pair of alleles at that locus, one on each of the homologous chromosomes. The chance that a person will draw two white beans (two normal alleles), one of each color (a normal and an abnormal allele), or two blue beans (two abnormal alleles) depends on the proportion of each color in the bag. If the proportion of white beans is p and the proportion of blue beans q (where $p + q = 1$, for a two-allele system), the relative proportions of the three combinations are p^2 (two white) : $2pq$ (one white, one blue) : q^2 (two blue). Because these are the only three possible genotypes, $p^2 + 2pq + q^2$ must equal 1. This is simply the expansion of the binomial $(p + q)^2$. A population in which the genotype frequencies for a given locus fit this prediction is said to be in **Hardy-Weinberg equilibrium**. Gene frequencies in populations are discussed further in Chapter 7; here our concern is with the clinical application of the rule.

The most common autosomal recessive disorder in Caucasian children is **cystic fibrosis (CF)** (see box). CF is virtually unknown in Asian populations and relatively rare in Black populations, but in Caucasian populations about 1 child in 2000 is homozygous for the CF allele and has the disease. In this population, therefore, q^2 (the frequency of the CF phenotype) is about 1 in 2000. Thus the frequency of the CF allele in this population, q, can be calculated as $\sqrt{1/2000}$, or about 1/45. The frequency of the normal allele, p, must therefore be $1 - q$, or 44/45. The proportion of carriers is $2pq$ ($2 \times 44/45 \times 1/45$) or approximately 1/22. In a population of 2000 Caucasians, then, one would expect 1 CF patient, 90 carriers of the CF mutation, and 1909 normal homozygotes. Because a patient has two CF alleles and a carrier has only one, 90/92 (about 98 percent) of all the CF genes in the population are hidden in carriers (who usually are unaware that they are carriers) and only 2 percent are in patients.

The chance that a carrier of CF might have an affected child depends on the chance that the other partner in the mating is a carrier. For the general Caucasian population, this chance is 1/22 or approximately 5 percent. Because the chance

CYSTIC FIBROSIS (CF)

Clinical features:	Chronic pulmonary disease, pancreatic exocrine insufficiency, increased concentration of sweat chloride		chronic lung infection and pancreatic insufficiency
Incidence:	Most common autosomal recessive disease in Caucasian children (1 in 2000); rare in other populations	Prenatal diagnosis:	Possible in suitable families by DNA techniques, usually only when there is already an affected child in the sibship. Assay of microvillar enzymes in amniotic fluid after detection of fetal meconium ileus by ultrasound screening is useful in detection of fetuses at unknown risk of CF. Widespread screening for CF carriers is under consideration
Genetics:	Autosomal recessive Gene location 7q31 Allelic heterogeneity associated with clinical heterogeneity A single mutation, a deletion of 3 bp, that results in the loss of a phenylalanine residue at position 508 in the predicted amino acid sequence, accounts for 70% of all mutations at the locus in populations of Northern European descent		
Basic defect:	Mutation in the gene encoding the cystic fibrosis transmembrane regulator (CFTR) protein, probably involved in the transport of anions across the cell membrane (see Chapter 12)	Treatment:	None as yet for the basic defect. Replacement of pancreatic enzymes, medical management of respiratory problems
Pathophysiology:	Defective ion transport in exocrine cells of the lungs, pancreas, and sweat glands results in	Significance:	The most common autosomal recessive disease in Caucasian children, requiring long-term medical treatment and generally fatal by the 4th decade. The first gene to be identified and cloned by positional cloning without prior knowledge of its map location or biochemical defect

that the child of two carriers would be homozygous for the mutant CF allele is 1/4, the chance that a carrier with an unrelated spouse would have an affected first child is the product of these probabilities, or 1/88 (about 1 percent). In this discussion it is assumed, of course, that there is no way to determine whether a person in the general population is a heterozygote at the locus in question; although this is true for most autosomal recessive conditions, many (though not yet all) carriers for cystic fibrosis can already be identified by DNA testing (see Chapters 6 and 12).

In clinical situations, the kind of calculation just outlined is most likely to arise when a parent of an affected child plans to have another child by a different partner. A more common problem in genetic counseling is the question of the risk that a sib or a more distant relative of a patient might have an affected child. Here the risk depends on the probability that the relative is a carrier, as well as on the probability that the partner is also a carrier. Some typical situations are described in the problems at the end of this chapter.

Consanguinity in Autosomal Recessive Inheritance

As discussed, most genes for autosomal recessive disorders are present in carriers rather than in homozygotes. They can be handed down in families for numerous generations without ever appearing in homozygous form; in fact, it is believed that everyone probably carries at least several genes for autosomal recessive disorders that would be severely damaging or even lethal if homozygous (see Chapter 6). The presence of such hidden recessive genes is not revealed unless the carrier happens to mate with someone who carries the same mutation, or a different mutation at the same locus, and the two deleterious alleles are both inherited by a child.

The chance that this will happen is increased by at least an order of magnitude if the parents are related by descent. Consanguinity of the parents of a patient with a genetic disorder is strong evidence (though not proof) for the autosomal recessive inheritance of that condition. (With rare exceptions, consanguinity in earlier generations is irrelevant.) For example, the disorder in the pedigree in Figure 4–10 is likely to be an autosomal recessive trait, even though other information in the pedigree may seem insufficient to establish this. Even if the parents consider themselves unrelated, they may have common ancestry within the past few generations, especially if they are of closely similar ethnic or geographic origin. Thus in taking a family history, it is important to ask about consanguinity and background.

The tendency for rare disorders to appear in the offspring of cousins was recognized long be-

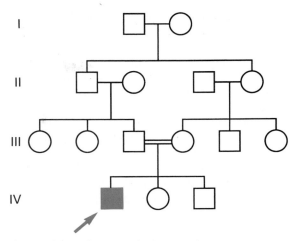

Figure 4–10. Pedigree in which parental consanguinity suggests autosomal recessive inheritance.

fore the underlying principle was understood, and it led to prohibition of cousin marriages in many societies. Early in the 20th century, when the physician Archibald Garrod first developed the concept of inborn errors of metabolism, he discussed with the biologist William Bateson two peculiarities that he had noticed in the family histories of his patients: if there was more than one affected family member, the affected members were always sibs, not other types of relatives, and the parents of the patients were often cousins or otherwise related by descent. At the time, Mendel's laws had recently been rediscovered, enabling Bateson to explain that the family histories of Garrod's patients were evidence that the inborn errors were inherited as Mendelian recessive traits.

Because the increased risk of birth defects in their offspring is well known though not widely understood, consanguineous couples sometimes request genetic counseling before they have children. There are two main points to be explained to such couples. First, the relative risk of abnormal offspring is higher for related than for unrelated parents, but still quite low: baseline risk figures for any abnormality are up to 3 percent for any child of any parents and about 4.5 percent to 5 percent for the offspring of first cousins (see Table 1–2). Second, any couple, consanguineous or not, who produces a child with an autosomal recessive disorder then faces a 25 percent recurrence risk in their future pregnancies, regardless of what their risk was before they had an affected child. This risk applies, of course, only to offspring of the same couple. Because both parents of affected children must be carriers, and because carriers are rare in comparison with normal homozygotes, a parent of a child with an autosomal recessive disorder is relatively unlikely to have another affected child with a different partner.

It is important to recognize that consanguinity is not the most common explanation for an autosomal recessive trait. The mating of unrelated persons, each of whom happens by chance to be a carrier, accounts for most cases of autosomal recessive disease. This is particularly true if a recessive trait has a high frequency in the population. Thus the overwhelming majority of cases of CF are *not* from consanguineous matings.

Rare Recessive Disorders in Genetic Isolates

There are many small groups in which the frequency of certain rare recessive genes is quite different from that in the general population. Such groups, genetic **isolates**, may have become separated from their neighbors by geographic, religious, or linguistic barriers (see Chapter 7). Although such populations are not, strictly speaking, consanguineous, the chance of mating with another carrier of a particular recessive condition may be as high as that observed in cousin marriages.

For example, among Ashkenazi Jews in North America, the gene for **Tay-Sachs disease** (G_{M2} gangliosidosis) is very common. Tay-Sachs disease is an autosomal recessive, neurological degenerative disorder that develops when a child is about 6 months old. Affected children develop blindness and regress mentally and physically (see box and Chapter 12). The disease is fatal in early childhood. The frequency of Tay-Sachs disease is 100 times as high in Ashkenazi Jews (1 in 3600) as in most other populations (1 in 360,000). Thus the Tay-Sachs carrier frequency among Ashkenazi Jews is approximately 3 percent.

TAY-SACHS DISEASE

Clinical features:	Severe mental and physical deterioration beginning in infancy; death occurs at age 2 to 3 years		cultured or uncultured amniotic fluid cells or cells of chorionic villi) for activity of the enzyme; also possible by DNA techniques in suitable families
Incidence:	About 1 in 3600 in Ashkenazi Jewish births; about 1 in 360,000 in most other populations	Treatment:	None available
		Significance:	Example of a lethal autosomal recessive disorder with high frequency in a specific, genetically isolated population. One of the first disorders for which heterozygote screening was carried out on a large scale, and one of the first metabolic disorders for which prenatal diagnosis was used
Genetics:	Autosomal recessive Gene location 15q23-q24		
Basic defect:	Mutations at the locus for the α subunit of hexosaminidase A		
Pathophysiology:	Deficiency or absence of the lysosomal enzyme hexosaminidase A leads to accumulation of ganglioside G_{M2}, mainly in neurons		
Prenatal diagnosis:	Possible by assay of fetal tissues (including		

When a recessive trait has a high frequency in a population, consanguinity is generally not a striking feature of pedigrees with the trait. Consequently, among Ashkenazi Jews the parents of affected children are usually not closely consanguineous, whereas in the other populations in which the frequency of carriers is very low, the consanguinity rate in the parents of Tay-Sachs patients is high.

The Offspring of Homozygous Recessives

Although many autosomal recessive disorders are so severe in homozygotes that they prohibit or greatly reduce reproduction, others are compatible with a normal life span and normal or only slightly reduced reproductive fitness. There are three mating types involving one homozygous recessive parent (genotype r/r), shown as follows:

Parents	Progeny	
	Genotypes	*Phenotypes*
$r/r \times R/R$	All R/r	All unaffected
$r/r \times R/r$	$\frac{1}{2}\,r/r$	$\frac{1}{2}$ affected
	$\frac{1}{2}R/r$	$\frac{1}{2}$ unaffected
$r/r \times r/r$	All r/r	All affected

In a mating of an affected homozygote with a heterozygote (the $r/r \times R/r$ mating just shown),

the offspring each have a 50 percent chance of being affected, just as in autosomal dominant inheritance. However, as Figure 4–11 illustrates, this **quasidominant** or pseudodominant pattern rarely persists over more than two generations because heterozygotes are so much less common than normal homozygotes that a sequence of matings of affected homozygotes with heterozygotes is statistically unlikely.

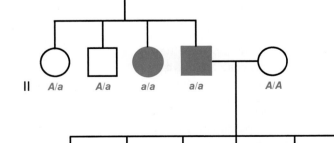

Figure 4-11. Pedigree showing "quasidominant" inheritance. See text for discussion.

X-LINKED INHERITANCE

The X and Y chromosomes, which are responsible for sex determination, are distributed unequally to males and females in families. For this reason, phenotypes determined by genes on the X have a characteristic sex distribution and a pattern of inheritance that is usually easy to identify. About 200 genes have already been mapped to the X chromosome.

Consider a mutant X-linked gene, X_h (representing the gene responsible for hemophilia A), in comparison with a normal allele, X_H. Because males have one X chromosome but females have two, there are two possible genotypes in males but three in females; males are hemizygous with respect to X-linked genes, whereas females may be homozygous for either allele or may be heterozygous.

	Genotypes	Phenotypes
Males	X_H	Unaffected
	X_h	Affected
Females	X_H/X_H	Homozygous unaffected
	X_H/X_h	Heterozygous
	X_h/X_h	Homozygous affected

X INACTIVATION AND THE EXPRESSION OF X-LINKED GENES

For many years the expression of X-linked genes was a puzzle to geneticists. Although males have only one "dose" of each X-linked gene, whereas females have two, the quantity of product formed by a single allele in the male or by a pair of alleles in the female was equivalent. The mechanism by which this "dosage compensation" was achieved was unknown. Another unexplained observation was that in female mice heterozygous for two X-linked coat-color alleles, the coat color was not uniform but mottled — that is, made up of patches of one or other of the two colors, random in arrangement and rarely crossing the midline (Fig. 4–12); males never had this patchy arrangement but had coats of a uniform color. A further observation was that the number of sex chromatin masses (Barr bodies) in a human's interphase cells was always one less than the number of X chromosomes seen at metaphase; thus, normal male cells have no Barr bodies, whereas normal female cells have one in every cell (see Chapter 10).

These observations were eventually explained by the formulation of the principle of X inactivation (Figure 4–13), which is often called the **Lyon hypothesis** because it was originally put forward in detail by Mary Lyon (1961, 1962). In brief, the principle has three points:

1. In the somatic cells of female mammals, only one X chromosome is active. The second X remains condensed and inactive and appears in interphase cells as the Barr body.

2. Inactivation occurs early in embryonic life, beginning in the morula stage about 3 days after fertilization, but is not complete in the inner cell mass, which forms the embryo, until about the end of the first week of development.

3. In any one female somatic cell the inactive

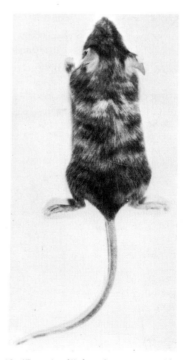

Figure 4–12. "Lyonized" female mouse, with mosaic coat-color phenotype illustrating the effects of random X chromosome inactivation. (From Thompson MW [1965] Genetic consequences of heteropyknosis of an X chromosome. Can J Genet Cytol 7:202–213.)

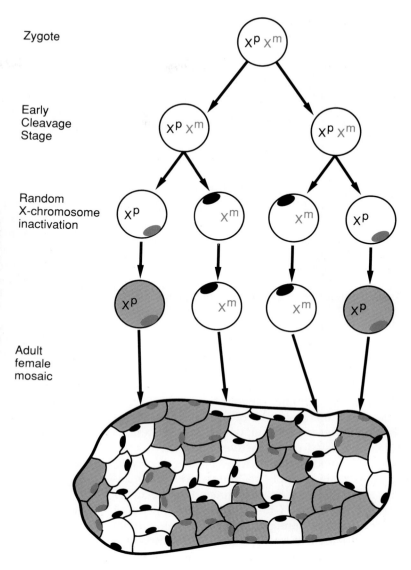

Figure 4–13. The Lyon hypothesis of random X chromosome inactivation in female somatic cells. X^p = paternally inherited X chromosome. X^m = maternally inherited X chromosome. Black or red ovals represent Barr bodies formed by the inactivated paternal or maternal X chromosome, respectively. Adult tissues (bottom) are a mosaic of clonal populations expressing alleles from either X^p or X^m. (Modified from Rosenberg LE [1980] Inborn errors of metabolism. *In* Bondy PK, Rosenberg LE [eds] Metabolic control and disease, 8th ed. WB Saunders, Philadelphia, pp. 73–102.)

X may be either the paternal or the maternal X (X^p or X^m); it is entirely a matter of chance which of the pair becomes inactivated in any one cell. However, after one X chromosome has become inactivated in a cell, all that cell's clonal descendants have the same inactive X. In other words, inactivation is randomly determined, but once made, the decision is permanent.

X inactivation has three consequences that are significant both genetically and clinically: dosage compensation, variability of expression in heterozygous females, and mosaicism.

Dosage Compensation

X inactivation provides an explanation for dosage compensation, since the inactive X chromosome is almost entirely condensed and, with a few exceptions, its genes appear not to be transcribed. Although the basic features of the Lyon hypothesis have been firmly established, the mechanism of X inactivation remains unknown.

Although much of the X is inactivated, several segments remain active. These segments include the distal region of the short arm, known as the

pseudoautosomal region because there are matching sequences on the Y chromosome by means of which the X and Y pair in meiosis. Among those genes known to escape inactivation is the locus for the enzyme steroid sulfatase, which when deficient causes the skin disorder X-linked ichthyosis. Steroid sulfatase escapes complete dosage compensation, although the total amount of gene product in normal female cells is somewhat less than double the amount in male cells. The possible role of noninactivated genes in determining phenotype in cases of abnormal X chromosome constitution is discussed in Chapter 10.

Variability of Expression in Heterozygotes

Because inactivation is random but is established at a stage of embryonic development when the developing embryo has only about 16 to 64 cells, carrier females have varying proportions of cells in which a particular allele is active and consequently exhibit variable phenotypes. The clinical variation in expression of X-linked disorders in heterozygotes can be extreme, ranging from entirely normal to full manifestation of the defect. A **manifesting heterozygote**, in whom the deleterious allele is located on the active X and the normal allele is located on the inactive X in all or most cells, is an extreme example of "unfavorable Lyonization." Manifesting heterozygotes have been described for many X-linked disorders, including color blindness, hemophilia A (classic hemophilia, factor VIII deficiency), hemophilia B (Christmas disease, factor IX deficiency), Duchenne muscular dystrophy (DMD), and several X-linked eye disorders.

Mosaicism

Females have two cell populations, in which one or the other X chromosome is the active one (Fig. 4–13); in other words, females are mosaics with respect to their X-linked genes. The mouse shown in Figure 4–12, with two coat-color genes and a mottled coat, is clearly mosaic. Mosaicism in human females is usually less obvious, though some X-linked disorders, such as Duchenne muscular dystrophy, exhibit typical mosaic expression,

allowing carriers to be identified by dystrophin immunostaining (Fig. 4–14). In addition, heterozygosity for a number of X-linked disorders can be demonstrated experimentally by culture of single cells to provide clones, which can then be analyzed to show that some clones have an active paternal X, whereas others have an active maternal X (Davidson et al., 1963).

X inactivation accounts for an important difference between autosomal and X-linked inheritance. In females, as in males, there is only one functional X in any cell. Consequently, although X-linked "dominant" and "recessive" patterns of inheritance are distinguished on the basis of the phenotype in heterozygous females, the distinction breaks down in practice. This is because in a female heterozygous for either a dominant or a recessive disorder, the mutant allele is the only functional allele in about half (but sometimes far more or less than half) of her somatic cells. In males, the inherited allele is inevitably expressed whether its expression in heterozygotes is dominant or recessive. Some medical geneticists prefer not to classify X-linked phenotypes as dominant or recessive, but others think that the distinction is useful because some X-linked phenotypes are consistently expressed in carriers (dominant), whereas others are usually not expressed in carriers (recessive). In the following discussion, X-linked dominance and recessiveness are examined separately.

PATTERNS OF X-LINKED RECESSIVE INHERITANCE

The inheritance of X-linked recessive phenotypes follows a well-defined and easily recognized pattern (Fig. 4–15). An X-linked mutation is typically expressed phenotypically in all males who receive it but only in those females who are homozygous for the mutation. Consequently, X-linked recessive disorders are generally restricted to males and, with the exception of rare manifesting heterozygotes (discussed earlier), are hardly ever seen among females.

Hemophilia A is a classic X-linked disorder in which the blood fails to clot normally because of a deficiency of factor VIII, an antihemophilic protein (see box). The hereditary nature of hemophilia and even its pattern of transmission have been recognized since ancient times, and the condition

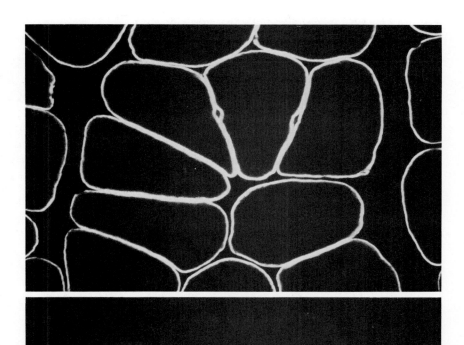

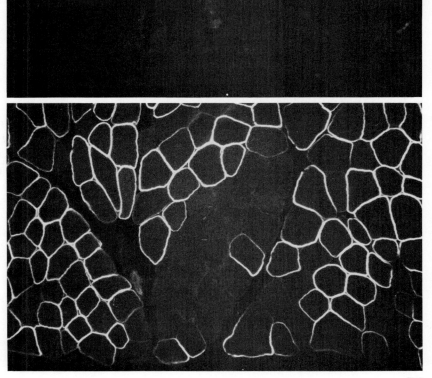

Figure 4-14. Immunostaining for dystrophin in muscle specimens from (top) a normal female (×480), (middle) a male with Duchenne muscular dystrophy (×480), and (bottom) a carrier female (×240). Muscle from DMD patients lack dystrophin staining. Muscle from DMD carriers exhibits both positive and negative patches of dystrophin immunostaining, reflecting X-inactivation. (Photographs courtesy of K. Arahata, National Institute of Neuroscience, Tokyo, Japan.)

HEMOPHILIA A (CLASSIC HEMOPHILIA)

Clinical features:	Coagulation disorder characterized by prolonged bleeding time, easy bruising, and hemorrhage into joints and muscles
Incidence:	About 1 in 10,000 males; rarely clinically evident in carrier females
Genetics:	X-linked recessive Gene location Xq28 Many different mutations reported
Basic defect:	Mutations in the gene that encodes factor VIII, a component of the coagulation cascade
Pathophysiology:	Deficiency of factor VIII eventually results in defective fibrin
	formation, impairing clotting ability
Prenatal diagnosis:	DNA-based diagnosis is possible
Treatment:	Replacement of factor VIII by means of factor VIII concentrate, prepared from blood or directly from cDNA by recombinant DNA technology
Significance:	A classic X-linked recessive disorder. Great Britain's Queen Victoria (1819–1901) was a carrier who, as the "grandmother of Europe," transmitted the gene to several other royal families

gained notoriety more recently as the "royal hemophilia" because of its occurrence among descendants of Queen Victoria, who was a carrier.

As in the earlier discussion, X_h represents the mutant factor VIII allele causing hemophilia A, and X_H represents the normal allele. If a hemophiliac mates with a normal female, all the sons receive their father's Y chromosome and a maternal X and are unaffected, but all the daughters receive the paternal X chromosome with its hemophilia allele and are obligate carriers.

Affected male x normal female: $X_h/Y \times X_H/X_H$

	X_H	X_H	
X_h	X_H/X_h	X_H/X_h	Daughters: all heterozygous (obligate carriers)
Y	X_H/Y	X_H/Y	Sons: all normal

Now assume that a daughter of the affected male mates with an unaffected male. Four genotypes are possible in the progeny, with equal probable abilities.

Normal male x carrier female: $X_H/Y \times X_H/X_h$

	X_H	X_h	
X_H	X_H/X_H	X_H/X_h	Daughters: $\frac{1}{2}$ normal, $\frac{1}{2}$ carriers
Y	X_H/Y	X_h/Y	Sons: $\frac{1}{2}$ normal, $\frac{1}{2}$ affected

The hemophilia of the affected grandfather, which did not appear in any of his own children, has a 50 percent chance of appearing in any son of any of his daughters. It will not reappear among the descendants of his sons.

A daughter of a carrier also has a 50 percent chance of being a carrier herself (Fig. 4–15). By chance, an X-linked recessive allele may be transmitted undetected through a series of carriers before it is expressed in a male descendant.

Genetic Counseling for Hemophilia

Because hemophilia A can be treated with considerable success with factor VIII concentrates and

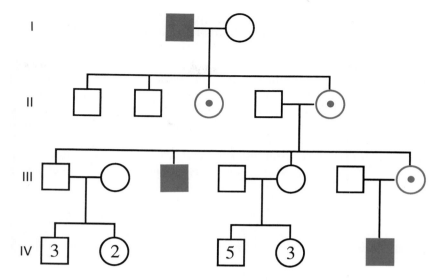

Figure 4-15. Pedigree pattern demonstrating an X-linked recessive disorder such as hemophilia A, transmitted from an affected male through females to an affected grandson and great-grandson.

blood transfusions, hemophilia families became for a time relatively unconcerned about the risk of an affected child, anticipating scientific progress to ensure a healthy life for their sons. However, the development of transfusion-associated acquired immunodeficiency syndrome (AIDS) in some hemophiliacs has changed the perception of the seriousness of hemophilia and has led to increased concern about the need for genetic counseling and prenatal diagnosis. A description of prenatal diagnosis for hemophilia A through DNA markers is given in Chapter 19.

Homozygous Affected Females

A gene for an X-linked disorder is occasionally present in both a father and a carrier mother, and female offspring can then be homozygous affected, as shown in the pedigree of X-linked color blindness, a relatively common X-linked disorder (Fig. 4-16). However, most X-linked diseases are so rare that it is very unusual for a female to be homozygous unless her parents are consanguineous.

Affected male x carrier female: $X_h/Y \times X_H/X_h$

	X_H	X_h	
X_h	X_H/X_h	X_h/X_h	Daughters: $\frac{1}{2}$ carriers, $\frac{1}{2}$ affected
Y	X_H/Y	X_h/Y	Sons: $\frac{1}{2}$ normal, $\frac{1}{2}$ affected

New Mutation for X-Linked Disorders

In males, genes for X-linked disorders are exposed to selection and tend to be lost. The selection is complete for some disorders and partial for others, depending on the fitness of the genotype. In heterozygous females, with some important excep-

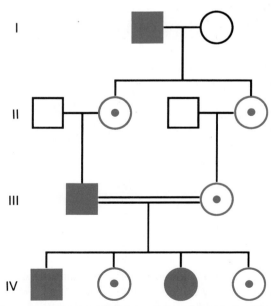

Figure 4-16. Consanguinity in an X-linked recessive pedigree, resulting in a homozygous affected female.

tions, the same genes confer little or no selective advantage or disadvantage. One third of the genes for hemophilia are carried in hemizygous males, with frequency q, whereas two thirds are found in carrier females, with frequency $2pq$ (very close to $2q$). Hemophiliacs have only about 70 percent as many offspring as unaffected males; that is, the fitness of affected males is about 0.70.

Selection against mutant alleles is even more dramatic for X-linked disorders such as DMD, a disease of muscle that affects young boys (see box and Chapter 12). The disorder is usually apparent by the time the child begins to walk and progresses inexorably, so that the child is confined to a wheelchair by about the age of 10 and is unlikely to survive his teens. Although the situation may change as a result of advances in research aimed at therapy for affected boys (see Chapter 13), DMD is said to be a **genetic lethal** because affected males usually fail to reproduce. It may, of course, be transmitted by carrier females, who themselves rarely show any clinical manifestation of the dis-

DUCHENNE MUSCULAR DYSTROPHY (DMD)

Clinical features:	Progressive muscle weakness, pseudohypertrophy of calf muscles; onset in early childhood, death by 3rd decade		structural gene for the protein dystrophin causes absent or grossly reduced levels of dystrophin in muscle
Incidence:	1 in 3000 to 1 in 3500 male births; carrier frequency ~1 in 2500 females	Pathophysiology:	Dystrophin is normally bound to the muscle membrane and helps to maintain the integrity of the muscle fiber; in its absence, the muscle fiber degenerates
Genetics:	X-linked recessive, lethal in males 1/3 of patients are new mutants; 2/3 have carrier mothers Gene location Xp21 Extremely large gene (more than 2000 kb) High mutation rate (1×10^{-4}), probably due to large size of gene 60% to 65% of the mutations are deletions, and about 6% are duplications Germline mosaicism in rare cases Allelic mutations in the same gene cause a milder disorder, Becker muscular dystrophy	Prenatal diagnosis: Significance:	Possible by DNA techniques in many families with a family history of the condition, especially if there is a deletion in the gene A classic X-linked recessive lethal disorder with a high mutation rate. The first gene to be cloned from knowledge of its chromosomal location, with the aid of chromosomal rearrangements that facilitated access to the appropriate region of the chromosome
Basic defect:	Abnormality of the		

Criteria for X-Linked Recessive Inheritance

1. The incidence of the trait is much higher in males than in females.

2. The gene responsible for the condition is transmitted from an affected man through all his daughters. Any of his daughters' sons has a 50 percent chance of inheriting it.

3. The gene is never transmitted directly from father to son, but it is transmitted by an affected male to all his daughters.

4. The gene may be transmitted through a series of carrier females; if so, the affected males in a kindred are related through females.

5. Heterozygous females are usually unaffected, but some may express the condition with variable severity.

PATTERNS OF X-LINKED DOMINANT INHERITANCE

An X-linked phenotype is described as dominant if it is regularly expressed in heterozygotes. The distinguishing feature of an X-linked dominant pedigree (Fig. 4–17) is that *all* the daughters and *none* of the sons of affected males are affected; if any daughter is unaffected or any son is affected, the inheritance must be autosomal, not X-linked. The pattern of inheritance through females is no different from the autosomal dominant pattern; because females have a pair of X chromosomes just as they have pairs of autosomes, each child of an affected female has a 50 percent chance of inheriting the trait, regardless of sex. As a general rule, rare X-linked dominant phenotypes are about twice as common in females as in males, although the expression is usually much milder in females, who are almost always heterozygotes.

Only a few genetic disorders are classified as X-linked dominants. One example is X-linked **hypophosphatemic rickets** (also called vitamin D–resistant rickets), in which the ability of the kidney tubules to reabsorb filtered phosphate is impaired. This disorder fits the criterion of an X-linked dominant disorder in that, although both sexes are affected, the serum phosphate level is less depressed and the rickets less severe in heterozygous females than in affected males. Another example of an X-linked condition that is usually classified as dominant is **ornithine transcarbamylase (OTC) deficiency**. Complete deficiency of OTC activity in the liver leads to lethal neonatal hyperammonemia in affected males. Heterozygous women ex-

ease. Because fully one third of all mutant alleles (the proportion being carried by affected males) are lost from the gene pool each generation, approximately one third of all cases of DMD (and other lethal X-linked recessive conditions) are expected to be due to new mutation, rather than being inherited from a carrier mother. The mathematics of the balance between new mutation and selection is discussed more fully in Chapters 7 and 18.

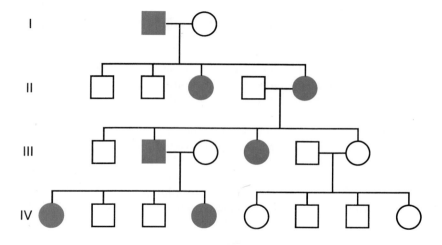

Figure 4–17. Pedigree pattern demonstrating X-linked dominant inheritance.

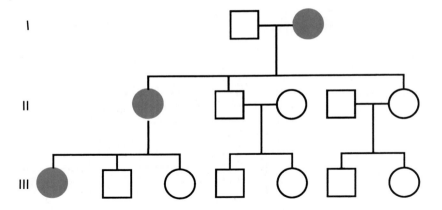

Figure 4-18. Pedigree pattern demonstrating an X-linked dominant disorder, lethal in males during the prenatal period.

hibit wide variation in clinical severity and in OTC levels in liver biopsies, as predicted by the Lyon hypothesis (Ricciuti et al., 1976). Symptomatic heterozygotes present as early as the first week of life or as late as adulthood with episodic lethargy and vomiting, protein avoidance, and, in extreme cases, seizures and coma. At least half of obligate carriers, however, appear to be asymptomatic; thus OTC deficiency might be better classified as an incompletely dominant X-linked disorder.

Some of the rare genetic defects expressed exclusively or almost exclusively in females appear to be X-linked dominant conditions that are lethal in males before birth. Typical pedigrees of these conditions show transmission by affected females, who produce affected daughters, normal daughters, and normal sons in equal proportions (Fig. 4–18). **Rett syndrome** (Fig. 4–19) is a striking mental retardation syndrome that has been hypothesized to be an X-linked dominant disorder, lethal in hemizygous males and precluding reproduction in heterozygous affected females. The disorder occurs exclusively in females, who are virtually always the only cases in their families and are considered to have genes that are new mutations. (Exceptions to this include two half-sisters with the same mother, who may have been a germline mosaic [see discussion later in this chapter] for the Rett syndrome gene, and an identical twin pair.) Rett syndrome is a reminder that although a family history usually points to a genetic basis for a disorder, the absence of a family history cannot be interpreted as evidence that the disorder does not have a genetic basis.

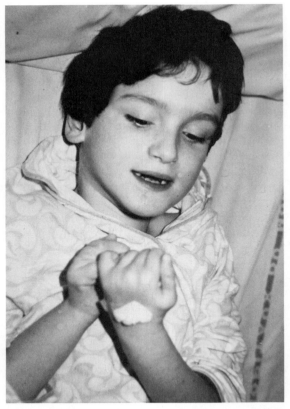

Figure 4-19. Rett syndrome, an X-linked dominant disorder that appears to be a prenatal lethal in hemizygous males and does not allow reproduction in affected females. (From Journel H, Melki J, Turleau C, et al. [1990] Rett phenotype with X/autosome translocation: possible mapping to the short arm of chromosome X. Am J Med Genet 35:142–147. Copyright © 1990, Wiley-Liss, Inc. Reprinted by permission of John Wiley and Sons, Inc.)

Criteria for X-Linked Dominant Inheritance

1. Affected males with normal mates have no affected sons and no normal daughters.

2. Both male and female offspring of carriers have a 50% risk of inheriting the phenotype. This is the same as the autosomal dominant pedigree pattern.

3. For rare phenotypes, affected females are about twice as common as affected males, but affected females typically have milder (though variable) expression of the phenotype.

THE FRAGILE X SYNDROME: A MUTATION WITH AN UNUSUAL PATTERN OF X-LINKED INHERITANCE

The fragile X syndrome (see box and Fig. 4 – 20) is the most common heritable form of moderate mental retardation and is second only to Down syndrome among all causes of moderate mental retardation in males. As mentioned in Chapter 2, the name refers to a cytogenetic marker, a ''fragile site'' in which the chromatin fails to condense during mitosis, on the X chromosome at Xq27.3 (Fig. 4 – 21). The fragile X syndrome, which has a frequency of at least 1 in 1500 male births, may account for much of the excess of males in the mentally retarded population. The basic defect responsible for the syndrome remains unknown. The combination of a single mutant gene and a specific cytogenetic abnormality is unique in medical genetics, and genetic analysis of the syndrome has revealed some unexpected and puzzling findings that are still not explained.

Although the fragile X syndrome is unquestionably X-linked, it cannot unequivocally be assigned to either the dominant or the recessive category, because carrier females may or may not be mentally retarded and may or may not reveal the fragile site in their cultured cells. Because of its characteristic cytogenetic marker, the syndrome is

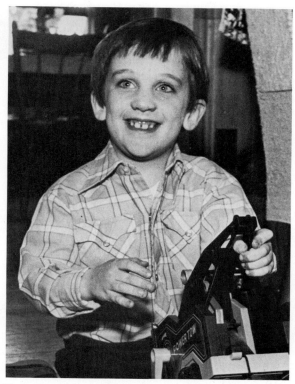

Figure 4 – 20. Characteristic facies of a patient with the fragile X syndrome. (Photograph courtesy of Michael Partington, Queen's University, Kingston, Ontario.)

regarded by some as a chromosomal rather than a single-gene disorder.

Demonstration of the fragile site requires special culture conditions, namely deprivation of folate and thymidine in the culture medium. Under these conditions, the fragile site in males who have

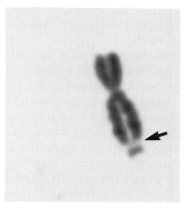

Figure 4 – 21. The fragile site at Xq27.3 associated with X-linked mental retardation.

FRAGILE X SYNDROME (X-LINKED MENTAL RETARDATION)

Clinical features:	Mental retardation, coarse facial features, and macroorchidism; carrier females are not dysmorphic, but about one third are mildly mentally retarded
Incidence:	Estimated to be 1 in 1100 to 1 in 1500 males; ~1 in 2000 to 1 in 3000 females show clinical signs
Genetics:	X-linked inheritance Associated with fragile site on the X chromosome at Xq27.3 Gene location Xq27.3 Unusual genetic transmission (see text) Highest mutation rate of any human gene, involves multistep changes in CGG repeat sequence
Basic defect:	Mutation in gene normally expressed in brain. Manifestation of mutation requires several sequential changes in unstable DNA sequences (Yu et al., 1991; Verkerk et al. 1991)
Pathophysiology:	Unknown
Prenatal diagnosis:	Possible in some cases by cytogenetic demonstration of the fragile site, though there are technical difficulties; DNA analysis possible in suitable families
Treatment:	None
Significance:	A major genetic cause of mental retardation in males. The only condition in which a heritable disorder is associated with a cytogenetic fragile site. Anomalies of pedigree pattern, as yet unexplained. Unusual multistep mutation. Gene cloned in 1991

the mutation is seen in up to 40 percent of the dividing cells. Carriers may not show the fragile site at all, and in those who do show it, the frequency is usually much lower than that observed in affected males.

A typical affected male is mentally retarded; heterozygous females have a 33 percent chance of being retarded. Surprisingly, whereas other X-linked disorders are virtually always expressed in hemizygotes, some males who by pedigree analysis can be shown to have the fragile X mutation are *not* retarded and do *not* show the cytogenetic marker. A nonexpressing but "transmitting" male of this type passes the gene to all his daughters, who usually are mentally normal themselves but have the expected proportion of retarded sons.

There are further complications. Molecular genetic analysis has shown different recombination frequencies between the mutation site and closely linked markers in different families (see Chapter 8). This X-linked locus has one of the highest mutation rates yet described for any human locus (see Chapter 6). Sequential mutations are required for phenotypic expression, an unstable "premutation" seen in heterozygous mothers and more severe full mutations in their affected sons. It is not surprising that difficulties arise both in diagnosis and in the provision of genetic counseling to relatives of affected males. Nevertheless, the syndrome is so common that it requires consideration in the differential diagnosis of mental retardation in both males and females. The fragile X syndrome is the subject of intensive molecular research activity and is among the most frequent reasons for requests for chromosome analysis, genetic counseling, and prenatal diagnosis.

ASPECTS OF PHENOTYPIC EXPRESSION

Many genetic conditions segregate sharply within families; that is, the abnormal phenotype can be distinguished clearly from the normal one. In clinical experience, however, some disorders are not expressed at all in genetically predisposed persons, and others have extremely variable expression in terms of clinical severity or onset age, or both. Expression of an abnormal genotype may be modified by other genetic loci or by environmental factors. These differences in expression, which are particularly characteristic of autosomal dominant disorders though by no means restricted to them, can often lead to difficulties in diagnosis and pedigree interpretation. Genetic heterogeneity has been mentioned earlier as a factor to be considered in pedigree analysis; here we consider failure of penetrance and variable expressivity, which are important characteristics of many autosomal dominant disorders; pleiotropy (multiple effects of a single basic defect); and examples of the effect of sex on phenotypic expression.

PENETRANCE AND EXPRESSIVITY

Penetrance and expressivity are characteristics of gene expression that are frequently confused but have quite distinct meanings. **Penetrance** is the probability that a gene will have any phenotypic expression at all; **expressivity** is the degree of expression of the phenotype.

Penetrance

When the frequency of expression of a phenotype is below 100 percent — that is, when some of those who have the appropriate genotype completely fail to express it — the gene is said to show **reduced penetrance**. Penetrance is an all-or-none concept. In statistical terms, it is the percentage of people with a particular genotype who are actually affected. For example, the fragile X mutation just discussed shows approximately 80 percent penetrance in males.

An example of an autosomal dominant mal-

formation with reduced penetrance is a type of ectrodactyly variously known as **split-hand deformity** or lobster-claw malformation (Fig. 4–22). Although the basic defect is not known, the malformation must originate in the 6th or 7th week of development, when the hands and feet are forming. Failure of penetrance in pedigrees of split-hand malformation can lead to apparent skipping of generations, and this complicates genetic counseling because an at-risk person with normal hands may nevertheless possess the gene for the condition and thus be capable of having children who are affected.

Figure 4–23 is a pedigree of split-hand deformity in which the person shown by the arrow is the consultand (the person who asks for genetic counseling). Her father is a nonpenetrant carrier of the split-hand mutation. Review of the literature on split-hand deformity suggests that the disorder has about 70 percent penetrance (i.e., only 70 percent of the people who have the gene exhibit the defect). Using this information in Bayesian analysis, a mathematical method for determining probabilities in pedigrees (see further discussion in Chapter 18), one can calculate the risk that the consultand might have a child with the abnormality.

Expressivity

When the manifestation of a phenotype differs in people who have the same genotype, the phenotype is said to have **variable expressivity**. Even within a kindred, a disorder may vary in its clinical expression, as discussed for neurofibromatosis earlier in this chapter. Many single-gene disorders are characterized by multiple phenotypic effects, and patients with one of these disorders may differ with respect both to the spectrum of abnormalities present and to the severity of any one manifestation.

A set of characteristics that occur together and thus are assumed to have a common basis constitutes a **syndrome**. The well-known autosomal dominant condition known as the **Marfan syndrome** (Fig. 4–24) is a disorder of fibrous connec-

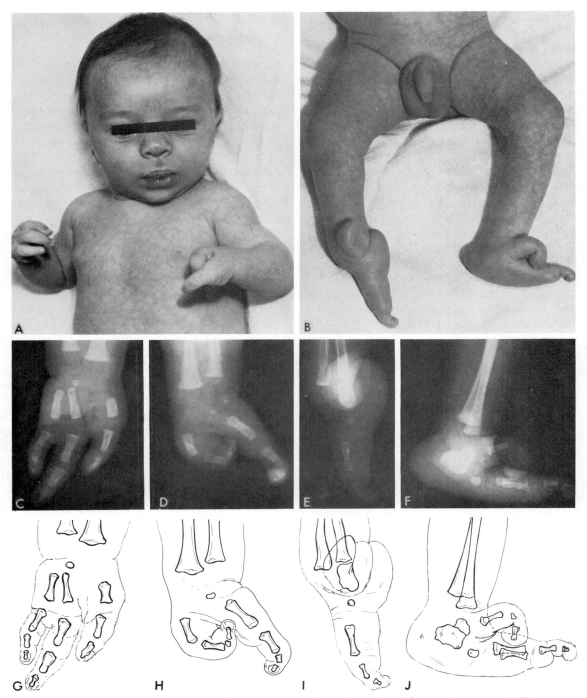

Figure 4-22. Split-hand deformity, an autosomal dominant trait involving the hands and feet, in a three-month-old boy. *A,* upper part of body; *B,* lower part of body; *C* to *F,* x-rays of the hands and feet; *G* to *J,* sketches illustrating the x-rays. (From Kelikian H [1974] Congenital deformities of the hand and forearm. WB Saunders, Philadelphia.)

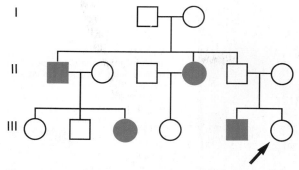

Figure 4-23. Pedigree of split-hand deformity demonstrating failure of penetrance in the father of the consultand. Consultand is indicated by the arrow. Reduced penetrance must be taken into account in genetic counseling.

tive tissue in which there are characteristic abnormalities of three systems (skeletal, ocular, and cardiovascular). Not only is there a wide range of clinical severity in this condition, but individual patients may show no clinical abnormality in at least one of the three systems that are typically affected. Diagnosis of a variable phenotype re-

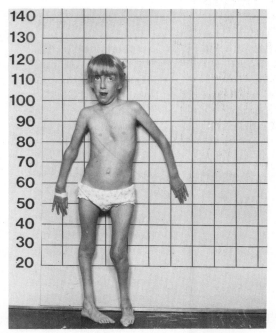

Figure 4-24. The Marfan syndrome, an autosomal dominant disorder with variable expressivity. The height of this patient, age 5.5 years, is above the 97th percentile for this age. She has long limbs with long extremities and arachnodactyly, genu valgum, long facies, and pectus excavatum. She also has a high narrow palate, bilateral ectopis lentis, and myopia. (Photograph courtesy of Victor McKusick, Johns Hopkins University, Baltimore.)

quires astute clinical observation, and a large part of clinical genetics is concerned with the diagnosis of disorders complicated by variable expressivity.

Myotonic dystrophy is an autosomal dominant myopathy that is notorious for its variable expression in both clinical severity and age of onset (Fig. 4-25). Pedigrees of myotonic dystrophy are said to show **anticipation**, the apparent worsening of the condition in successive generations. However, anticipation is probably simply a consequence of bias of ascertainment rather than a true biological phenomenon; patients with mild, late-onset expression are both less likely to be ascertained and more likely to transmit the disease to their offspring than are patients who have the disease in a severe form early in life. Until the advent of molecular genetic analysis, many members of myotonic dystrophy families who had inherited the gene for the disease actually remained undiagnosed.

One form of myotonic dystrophy, the congenital form, is particularly severe and may be associated with mental retardation or even be life-threatening. Virtually every child with the congenital form is the offspring of an affected mother, who herself may have only a mild expression of the disease and may not even know that she is affected. This particular feature, exclusively maternal transmission of the most severe cases, is unique to myotonic dystrophy and may be related to imprinting (see the section "Nonclassical Patterns of Single-Gene Inheritance"). Prenatal diagnosis of myotonic dystrophy by molecular genetic techniques is now possible for many families.

Onset Age

Not all genetic disorders are congenital; many are not expressed until later in life, some at a characteristic age and others (e.g., myotonic dystrophy) at variable ages. Because the terms *genetic* and *congenital* are frequently confused, it is important to keep in mind that a genetic disorder is one that is determined by genes, whereas a congenital disorder is merely one that is present at birth and may or may not have a genetic basis.

Many genetic disorders develop prenatally and thus are both genetic and congenital. Dysmorphic phenotypes of many kinds originate during development and are recognized at birth (or

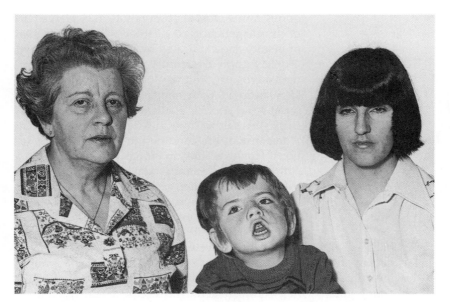

Figure 4–25. Myotonic dystrophy, an autosomal dominant condition with variable expression in clinical severity and age of onset. The grandmother in this family (left) has had bilateral cataracts but has no facial weakness or muscle symptoms; her daughter was thought to be unaffected until after the birth of her severely affected child, but she now has moderate facial weakness and ptosis, with myotonia, and has had cataract extraction. The child has congenital myotonic dystrophy. (From Harper PS [1989] Myotonic dystrophy, 2nd ed. WB Saunders, Philadelphia, p. 18.)

PHENYLKETONURIA (PKU)

Clinical features:	Developmental delay apparent in infancy, sometimes accompanied by other neurological manifestations such as seizures, hyperactivity, and behavioral disturbances; mental retardation if untreated
Incidence:	~ 1 in 5000 to 1 in 16,000 in Caucasian populations; less frequent in other ethnic groups (e.g., ~ 1 in 60,000 in Japan)
Genetics:	Autosomal recessive Gene location 12q22-q24 Four specific mutations account for most cases in Northern European populations
Basic defect:	Mutations in the gene for the liver enzyme phenylalanine hydroxylase, which converts phenylalanine to tyrosine (see Chapter 12)
Pathophysiology:	Phenylalanine or its derivatives damage the developing brain
Prenatal diagnosis:	Possible with DNA techniques
Treatment:	Dietary reduction of phenylalanine (see Chapter 13)
Significance:	The classic example of a treatable inborn error of metabolism. The first disease for which dietary restriction was successfully used to lower the level of a substrate, accumulation of which was responsible for the pathology. Also, the first genetic disease for which mass screening of newborns was successfully conducted

even prenatally, in some cases, by ultrasonography; see Chapter 19) as "birth defects." Some genetic disorders may be lethal in prenatal life. Others are expressed as soon as the infant begins its independent life; a well-known example is phenylketonuria (PKU; see box) discussed in Chapter 12. Still others appear even later or make their clinical appearance at a variety of ages extending from birth to the postreproductive years.

As previously mentioned, a classic example of a genetic disorder usually of late onset is Huntington disease (HD) (Fig. 4–4). Age of onset must be taken into account in genetic counseling for HD, and a method of doing this through Bayesian analysis is illustrated in Chapter 18.

Pleiotropy

Each gene has only one primary effect: it directs the synthesis of a polypeptide chain or an RNA molecule. From this primary effect, however, there may be multiple consequences. When a single abnormal gene or gene pair produces diverse phenotypic effects, its expression is said to be **pleiotropic**. The various characteristics seen in the Marfan syndrome are classical examples of pleiotropy.

Clinical syndromes offer many other examples of pleiotropy, and for most of these the connection between the various manifestations has not yet been established. In the Marfan syndrome, the underlying defect appears to be in the primary structure of fibrillin, a critical component of connective tissue. In contrast, in the rare autosomal recessive disorder known as the **Bardet-Biedl syndrome** (Fig. 4–26), the manifestations of hypogonadism, polydactyly, deafness, obesity, pigmentary retinopathy, and mental retardation have no obvious causative link.

There are a few rare **contiguous gene syndromes** (or **microdeletion syndromes**) in which

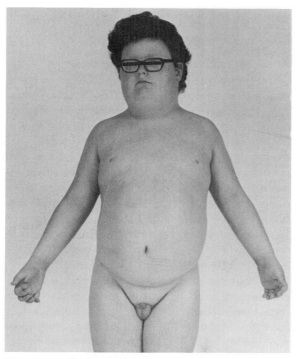

Figure 4-26. Bardet-Biedl syndrome, an autosomal recessive phenotype characterized by mental retardation, obesity, polydactyly, hypogenitalism, and retinitis pigmentosa.

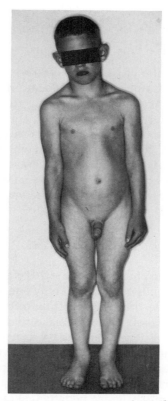

Figure 4-27. Male-limited precocious puberty (familial testotoxicosis), an autosomal dominant disorder expressed exclusively in males. This child, at 4.75 years, is 120 cm in height (above the 97th percentile for his age). Note the muscle bulk and precocious development of the external genitalia. Epiphyseal fusion occurs at an early age, and affected persons are relatively short as adults.

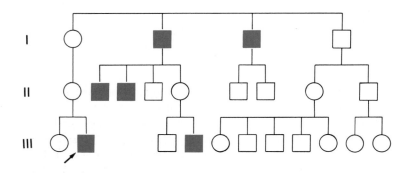

Figure 4-28. Pedigree pattern of male-limited precocious puberty in the family of the child shown in Figure 4-27. This autosomal dominant disorder can be transmitted by affected males or by unaffected carrier females. Male-to-male transmission shows that the inheritance is autosomal, not X-linked. Because the trait is transmitted through unaffected carrier females, it cannot be Y-linked.

deletion of multiple genes at closely linked loci results in diverse phenotypic effects (see Chapter 8). As a general rule, however, the presence of multiple phenotypic abnormalities is due to pleiotropy at a single locus rather than to loss of a sequence of several genes.

Sex-Limited and Sex-Influenced Phenotypes

If the sex ratio of persons who have a particular phenotype is not 1:1, there is a strong possibility that the phenotype is X-linked. However, for many phenotypes the sex ratio is abnormal even though the causative gene is autosomal. This is not unexpected, because the milieu in which any gene is expressed is conditioned partly by sexual constitution; moreover, differential prenatal and postnatal survival can distort the observed sex ratio.

Sex-Limited Phenotypes

A sex-limited phenotype is one that is autosomally transmitted but expressed in only one sex. An example is **male-limited precocious puberty** (familial testotoxicosis), an autosomal disorder in which affected boys develop secondary sexual characteristics and undergo an adolescent growth spurt at about 4 years of age (Fig. 4-27). There is no expression in heterozygous females. Figure 4-28, part of a much larger pedigree, shows that although the disease can be transmitted by unaffected females, it can also be transmitted directly from father to son, showing that it is autosomal, not X-linked.

Males with precocious puberty have normal fertility, and numerous multigeneration pedigrees are known. For disorders in which affected males do not reproduce, however, it is not always easy to distinguish sex-limited autosomal inheritance from X linkage because the critical evidence, absence of male-to-male transmission, cannot be provided. Other lines of evidence, especially gene mapping to learn whether the responsible gene maps to the X chromosome or to an autosome (see Chapter 8), can sometimes help to determine the pattern of inheritance and the consequent recurrence risk.

Sex-Influenced Phenotypes

A sex-influenced phenotype is one that is expressed in both sexes but with different frequencies. Among autosomal disorders, **hemochromatosis** is an example of a phenotype more common in males. In this autosomal recessive disorder of iron metabolism, there is enhanced absorption of dietary iron, which leads to iron overload with serious pathological consequences. The lower incidence (one tenth) of the clinical disorder in females is thought to be related to lower dietary intake of iron and menstruation.

Congenital adrenal hyperplasia occurs in several forms, one of which is autosomal recessive 21-hydroxylase deficiency (which itself has several variants representing combinations of different mutant alleles at the locus). This disorder is recognized at birth in female infants because they have ambiguous genitalia, but it may go unrecognized in males; however, without treatment, affected males develop consequences of excessive androgen production.

NONCLASSICAL PATTERNS OF SINGLE-GENE INHERITANCE

As a general rule, the patterns of inheritance and segregation ratios of single-gene disorders are in accord with the principles of Mendelian inheritance. Throughout the 20th century, since Garrod and Bateson first applied Mendel's laws to inborn errors of metabolism, few exceptions have been observed. However, close examination of certain unusual disorders and the analysis of mutations in molecular detail have shown that exceptions to Mendelian inheritance do occur in human genetics and must be taken into account in genetic medicine. In this section we briefly describe four nonclassical mechanisms that can affect the transmission or expression of single-gene disorders: mitochondrial inheritance, mosaicism, genomic imprinting, and uniparental disomy.

MITOCHONDRIAL INHERITANCE

It has been recognized for many years that a few pedigrees of inherited diseases cannot be explained by typical Mendelian inheritance of nuclear genes. A particular oddity has been **Leber's disease** (Leber's hereditary optic neuropathy, or LHON), which is expressed phenotypically as rapid, bilateral loss of central vision due to optic nerve death in young adults. Affected individuals may be male or female (there is a slight excess of males). The peculiarity of LHON pedigrees is that the patients are always related in the maternal line, and no affected male transmits the disease (Fig. 4–29).

Leber's disease and several other neuromuscular diseases (Table 4–2) are now known to be associated with mutations of mitochondrial DNA (mtDNA) (Wallace, 1989). The mtDNA is packaged into a circular chromosome, as described in Chapter 3. There are several copies of this chromosome per mitochondrion and thousands per cell. The mtDNA has been completely sequenced and is known to code for two types of ribosomal RNA, for 22 transfer RNAs, and for 13 polypeptides that are subunits of enzymes of oxidative phosphorylation; the other subunits of these enzymes are encoded in nuclear DNA. The mtDNA replicates within the mitochondrion, and the mitochondrion itself divides by simple fission. During cytokinesis, the mitochondria are randomly distributed to the two daughter cells. When a cell containing a mixture of normal and mutant mtDNAs divides, its daughter cells may contain

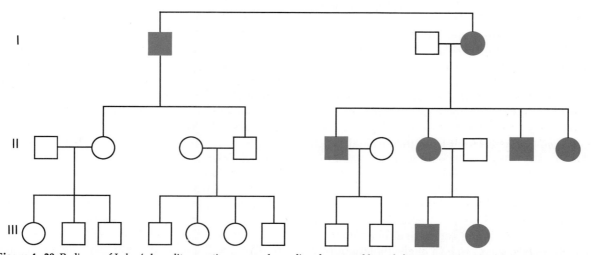

Figure 4–29. Pedigree of Leber's hereditary optic neuropathy, a disorder caused by a defect in mitochondrial DNA. Inheritance is only through the maternal lineage, in agreement with the known maternal inheritance of mitochondrial DNA. No affected male transmits the disease.

Table 4–2. Examples of Mitochondrial Disorders

Disease	Chief Distinguishing Features
Kearns-Sayre syndrome (KSS)	External ophthalmoplegia, retinal degeneration, heart block, high cerebrospinal fluid protein; usually sporadic; mitochondrial DNA deletions demonstrated
Leber's hereditary optic atrophy (LHON)	Rapid optic nerve death leading to blindness in young adult life; maternal inheritance; mutation in mitochondrial DNA demonstrated
Mitochondrial encephalomyopathy, lactic acidosis, and stroke-like episodes (MELAS)	As described in name, plus sensorineural hearing loss, dementia, short stature; sporadic mitochondrial DNA deletions demonstrated
Myoclonus epilepsy with ragged red fibers (MERRF)	As described in name; maternal inheritance

Based on Wallace DC (1989) Mitochondrial DNA mutations and neuromuscular disease. Trends Genet 5: 9–13.

only normal mtDNA, only mutant mtDNA, or a mixture. Because the phenotypic expression of a mutation in mitochondrial DNA depends on the relative proportions of normal and mutant mtDNA, variability of expression is a feature of the pedigrees of mitochondrial disorders.

A unique feature of mtDNA is its **maternal inheritance**. The ovum is well supplied with mitochondria, but sperm contain few, and even those few do not persist in the offspring. The mother transmits her mtDNA to all her offspring. Her daughters transmit it in their turn, but her sons do not.

MOSAICISM

Mosaicism is defined as the presence in an individual or a tissue of at least two cell lines, which differ genetically but are derived from a single zygote. Although we are used to thinking of ourselves as being composed of cells that all carry exactly the same complement of genes and chromosomes, this is in reality an oversimplified concept. Viable mutations arising in single cells in either prenatal or postnatal life can actually give rise to clones of cells genetically different from the original zygote (Fig. 4–30). Mosaicism is a clinically important phenomenon in chromosomal disorders (see Chapters 9 and 10), and somatic mutation is recognized as a major cause, if not the only cause, of many types of cancer (see Chapter 16). Mosaicism for mutations in single genes, in either somatic or germline cells, seems to be a likely explanation for a number of unusual clinical observations (Hall, 1988).

Somatic Mosaicism

A mutation affecting morphogenesis and occurring during embryonic development might be manifested as a segmental or patchy abnormality, depending on the stage at which the mutation occurred and the lineage of the somatic cell in which it originated. If it occurs at an early stage before the separation of germline cells from somatic cells, it is present in both somatic and germline cell lines and thus is transmissible to the offspring in its complete form, as well as being expressed somatically in mosaic form.

NF1 is sometimes segmental, affecting only one part of the body (Rawlings et al., 1987). In such cases, the patient has normal parents, but if he or she has an affected child, the child's phenotype is typical for NF1—that is, not segmental. The possible cause of segmental NF1 is mutation in a somatic cell ancestral to the affected segment. In cases in which NF1 is transmitted genetically by a patient who has the segmental form, however, the mutation must have occurred before separation of germline cells from the somatic cell line that carries the mutation.

Somatic mosaicism has been documented in a number of X-linked disorders in both males and females. A striking example is a case of mosaic OTC deficiency in a boy with an unusually mild form of the disorder (Maddalena et al., 1988). Molecular studies demonstrated that the boy had somatic mosaicism for a deletion mutation in the OTC gene. Somatic mosaicism has also been reported for hemophilia A and DMD in females who transmitted the mutation and therefore must have had germline, as well as somatic, mosaicism (Gitschier et al., 1989; Bakker et al., 1989).

Germline Mosaicism

Usually, a disorder due to a new autosomal dominant mutation does not recur within the sibship of the patient, but there are rare exceptions in which parents who are phenotypically normal have more than one affected child. There are a number of possible explanations, including variable expressivity or failure of penetrance. However, one potential cause of such unusual pedigrees is that during the early development of the parent, a somatic mutation has occurred in a germline cell or precursor, has persisted in all the clonal descendants of that cell, and has eventually reached a proportion of the gametes (Fig. 4–30). There are about 30 mitotic divisions in the cells of the germline before meiosis in the female and several hundred in the male, allowing ample opportunity for mutations to occur during the mitotic stages of germ cell development. Perhaps most mutations originate in diploid cells of the germline rather than at the stage of meiosis (see Chapter 6). Such mutations may in theory be relatively common in germ cell populations, although pedigrees in which more than one person receives the same new mutation are rare.

By chance, the same mutation could occur independently more than once in a sibship, and it used to be customary to advise parents of a child who apparently expressed a new mutation that the chance of the same defect in a subsequent child was equivalent to the population risk—a negligible risk, for example, for the autosomal dominant disorder **osteogenesis imperfecta** (Fig. 4–31). Now that the phenomenon of germline mosaicism has been recognized, geneticists are aware of the potential inaccuracy of predicting that a specific autosomal dominant phenotype that appears by every test to be a new mutation has an extremely low recurrence risk within the sibship. Although such exceptions are still considered quite unusual, pedigrees that could be explained by germline mosaicism have been reported for several well-known autosomal dominant (Fig. 4–31) and X-linked disorders. Phenotypically normal parents of a child with an autosomal dominant or X-linked disorder thought to be due to a new mutation should be informed that the recurrence risk is low, though not negligible (perhaps in the 1 percent to 7 percent range), and should be offered whatever prenatal diagnostic tests are appropriate.

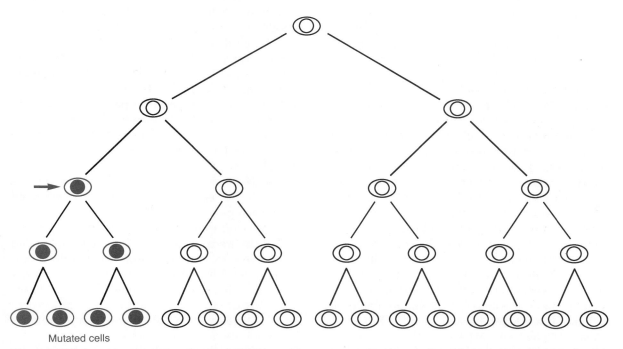

Figure 4–30. Schematic presentation of mitotic cell divisions. Mutations occurring during cell proliferation, in either somatic cells or during gametogenesis, lead to a proportion of cells carrying the mutation—that is, to either somatic or germline mosaicism.

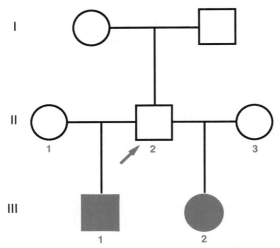

Figure 4–31. Pedigree demonstrating recurrence of the autosomal dominant disorder osteogenesis imperfecta. Both affected children have the same point mutation in a collagen gene. Their father (arrow) is unaffected and has no such mutation in DNA from examined somatic tissues. He must have been a mosaic for the mutation in his germline.

GENOMIC IMPRINTING

On the basis of Mendelian principles, we expect that an autosomal gene is equally likely to be transmitted from a parent of either sex and to an offspring of either sex; similarly, a female is equally likely to transmit either of her X chromosomes to a child of either sex. Little attention used to be paid to whether the sex of the transmitting parent had any effect on the expression of genes. We now know, however, that in a considerable number of genetic disorders, the expression of the disease phenotype depends on whether it has been inherited from the father or from the mother. Two examples have already been mentioned: the severe, early-onset form of myotonic dystrophy that occurs when the mutant gene has been inherited maternally, and the relatively early onset in HD when the mutant gene is inherited paternally. Other examples of differential effects on expression depending on the sex of the transmitting parent include the increased severity of NF1 with maternal transmission, and the earlier onset and more severe course of autosomal dominant spinocerebellar ataxia when inherited from the father. It is clear that maternal and paternal chromosomes can function differently and that differences in function that depend on parental origin, known as im-

printing, can influence the expression of human genetic disorders (Reik, 1989).

Perhaps the most unusual situations to come to light so far are those of **Prader-Willi syndrome** and **Angelman syndrome**. The Prader-Willi syndrome is a relatively common dysmorphic syndrome characterized by obesity, polyphagia, small hands and feet, short stature, hypogonadism, and mental retardation (Fig. 4–32). In many cases of the syndrome, there is a cytogenetic deletion (illustrated in Chapter 9) involving the proximal long arm of chromosome 15 (15q11q13), occurring on the chromosome 15 inherited from the patient's father (Butler and Palmer, 1983). Thus the genomes of these patients have genetic information in 15q11q13 that derives only from their mothers. In contrast, in many patients with the rare Angelman syndrome (also known as the "happy puppet" syndrome), which is phenotypically quite different from Prader-Willi syndrome (Fig. 4–33), there is a deficiency of the same chromosomal region but on the chromosome 15 inherited from the mother (Knoll et al., 1989). These patients, therefore, have genetic material in 15q11q13 only from their fathers. This unusual circumstance demonstrates strikingly that the parental origin of genetic material (in this case, on chromosome 15) can have a profound effect on the clinical expression of a defect.

In a further study of patients with Prader-Willi syndrome who did not have cytogenetic deletions, Nicholls and colleagues (1989) made the surprising discovery that two of their patients, each of whom had an intact pair of chromosome 15s, had inherited both members of the maternal chromosome pair but neither member of the paternal pair. This unusual situation, termed uniparental disomy (see next section), suggests that normal human development requires that a gene or genes in the region 15q11q13 must be inherited from each parent.

Differences in expression that depend on the sex of the transmitting parent have been studied extensively in transgenic mice (mice into which foreign genes have been implanted at an early developmental stage; see Chapter 17). The differences in expression are associated with differences in DNA methylation patterns, which in turn are related to transcriptional regulation of gene activity. Although there is little direct experimental evidence for genomic imprinting in humans, the pa-

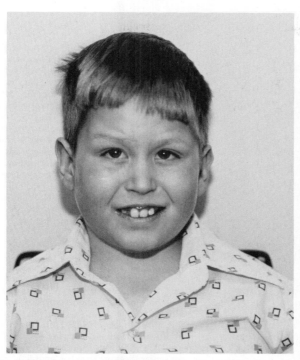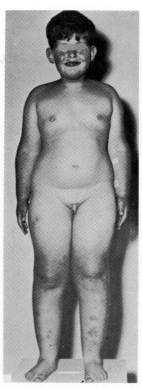

Figure 4–32. Prader-Willi syndrome. Left: Typical facies in a 9-year-old affected boy. (From Pettigrew AL, Gollin SM, Greenberg F, et al. [1987] Duplication of proximal 15q as a cause of Prader-Willi syndrome. Am J Med Genet 28:791–802. Copyright © 1990, Wiley-Liss, Inc. Reprinted by permission of John Wiley and Sons, Inc.) Right: Obesity, hypogonadism, and small hands and feet in a 9.5-year-old affected boy who also has short stature and developmental delay. (From Jones KL [1988] Smith's Recognizable patterns of human malformation, 4th ed. WB Saunders, Philadelphia, p. 173.)

rental effects on expression observed so far suggest that the process is important in gene expression and that there is much more to be learned about its extent and significance in human genetic disorders.

UNIPARENTAL DISOMY

Uniparental disomy is defined as the presence of a disomic cell line containing two chromosomes of a given kind, inherited from only one parent. If the same chromosome is present in duplicate, the situation is described as **isodisomy**; if both homologs from one parent are present, the situation is **heterodisomy**.

Until the late 1980s, uniparental disomy was unknown, but now that molecular genetic techniques allow the parental source of chromosomes to be identified, it has been documented in several clinical disorders. In the first such case to be reported (Spence et al., 1988), a female with CF and short stature was found to have two identical copies of most or all of her maternal chromosome 7. Homozygosity for the CF allele inherited from her carrier mother accounted for her cystic fibrosis; her growth failure was unexplained but might be related to genomic imprinting. A second example of uniparental disomy, also associated with CF and short stature, was described by Voss and associates (1989); this led to speculation that uniparental disomy may not be an uncommon phenomenon. As noted in the previous section, uniparental disomy (specifically, heterodisomy) has been recognized in some cases of Prader-Willi syndrome.

Uniparental disomy can also involve the sex chromosomes, as shown by a reported case of father-to-son transmission of hemophilia A, in which an affected boy inherited both his X and Y

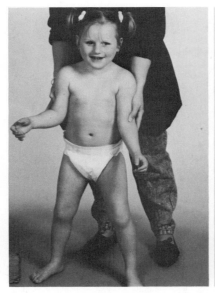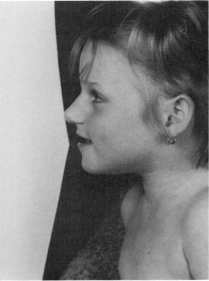

Figure 4–33. Angelman syndrome in a 4-year-old affected girl. Note wide stance and position of arms. Compare with phenotype of Prader-Willi syndrome in Figure 4–32. See text for discussion. (Photograph courtesy of Jan M. Friedman. From Magenis RE, Toth-Fejel S, Allen LJ, et al. [1990] Comparison of the 15q deletions in Prader-Willi and Angelman syndromes: specific regions, extent of deletions, parental origin, and clinical consequences. Am J Med Genet 35: 333–349. Copyright © 1990, Wiley-Liss, Inc. Reprinted by permission of John Wiley and Sons, Inc.)

chromosomes from his father with no sex chromosome contribution from his mother (Vidaud et al., 1989). Although it is too early to tell whether uniparental disomy is an interesting rarity or a relatively common phenomenon, the physician and the genetic counselor must keep it in mind as a possible cause of genetic disorders, especially in cases of autosomal recessive disorders in patients who have only one documented carrier parent, or in cases of X-linked disorders transmitted from father to son or expressed in homozygous form in females.

General References

Emery AEH, Rimoin DL (eds) (1990) Principles and practice of medical genetics, 2nd ed. Churchill Livingstone, Edinburgh.

Hall JG (1988) Somatic mosaicism: observations related to human genetics. Am J Hum Genet 43:355–363.

Hall JG (1990) Genomic imprinting: review and relevance to human diseases. Am J Hum Genet 46:857–873.

Harper PS (1989) Myotonic dystrophy, 2nd ed. WB Saunders, Philadelphia.

Hayden MR (1981) Huntington's chorea. Springer-Verlag, New York.

Jones KL (1988) Smith's Recognizable patterns of human malformation, 4th ed. WB Saunders, Philadelphia.

McKusick VA (1990) Mendelian inheritance in man: catalogs of autosomal dominant, autosomal recessive, and X-linked phenotypes, 9th ed. Johns Hopkins University Press, Baltimore.

Reik W (1989) Genomic imprinting and genetic disorders in man. Trends Genet 5:331–336.

Scriver CR, Beaudet AL, Sly WS, Valle D (eds) (1989) The metabolic basis of inherited disease, 6th ed. McGraw-Hill, New York.

Vogel F, Motulsky AG (1986) Human genetics: problems and approaches, 2nd ed. Springer-Verlag, New York.

Wallace DC (1989) Mitochondrial DNA mutations and neuromuscular disease. Trends Genet 5:9–13.

Problems

1. Cathy is pregnant for the second time. Her first child, Donald, has CF. Cathy has two brothers, Charles and Colin, and a sister, Cindy. Colin and Cindy are unmarried. Charles is married to an unrelated woman, Carolyn, and has a 2-year-old daughter, Debbie. Cathy's parents are Bob and Betty. Betty's sister Barbara is the mother of Cathy's husband, Calvin, who is 25. There is no previous family history of CF.
   a) Sketch the pedigree, using standard symbols.
   b) What is the pattern of transmission of CF, and what is the risk of CF for Cathy's next child?
   c) How does the risk of CF in Donald's first cousins compare with the population risk of 1/2000?
   d) Which people in this pedigree are obligate heterozygotes?

2. George and Grace, who have normal hearing, have 8 children. Two of their 5 daughters and 2 of their 3 sons are congenitally deaf. Another couple, Harry and Helen, both with normal hearing, also have 8 children; 2 of their 6 daughters and one of their 2 sons is deaf. A third couple, Gilbert and Gisele, who are congenitally deaf, have 4 children, also deaf. Their daughter Hedy marries Horace, a deaf son of

George and Grace, and Hedy and Horace in turn have 4 deaf children. Their eldest son Isaac marries Ingrid, a daughter of Harry and Helen; although both Isaac and Ingrid are deaf, their 6 sons all have *normal* hearing. Sketch the pedigree and answer the following questions. (Hint: how many different types of congenital deafness are segregating in this pedigree?)

a) State the probable genotypes of the children in the last generation.

b) Why are all the children of Gilbert and Gisele and of Hedy and Horace deaf?

3. Consider the following situations:

a) Retinitis pigmentosa occurs in X-linked and autosomal forms.

b) Two parents each have a typical case of familial hypercholesterolemia diagnosed on the basis of hypercholesterolemia, arcus corneae, tendinous xanthomas, and demonstrated deficiency of LDL receptors, together with a family history of the disorder; they have a child who has a very high plasma cholesterol level at birth and within a few years develops xanthomas and generalized atherosclerosis.

c) A couple with normal vision, from an isolated community, have a child with autosomal recessive gyrate atrophy of the retina. The child grows up, marries another member of the same community, and has a child with the same eye disorder.

d) A child has severe neurofibromatosis (NF1). Her father is phenotypically normal; her mother seems clinically normal but has several large café-au-lait spots and areas of hypopigmentation, and slit-lamp examination shows that she has a few Lisch nodules (hamartomatous growths on the iris that are common in persons with NF1).

e) Parents of normal stature have a child with achondroplasia.

f) An adult male with myotonic dystrophy has cataracts, frontal balding, and hypogonadism, in addition to myotonia.

g) A disorder chiefly affecting the muscles appears in all the offspring of an affected mother but is never transmitted by her sons.

h) A man with vitamin D–resistant rickets transmits the condition to all his daughters, who have a milder form of the disease than their father; none of his sons is affected. The daughters have approximately equal numbers of unaffected sons, affected sons, unaffected daughters, and affected daughters, the affected sons being more severely affected than their affected sisters.

i) A boy has progressive muscular dystrophy with onset in early childhood and is wheelchair bound by the age of 12 years. An unrelated man also has progressive muscular dystrophy but is still ambulant at age 30. Molecular analysis shows that both patients have a large deletion in the dystrophin gene, which is the abnormal gene in the Duchenne and Becker types of muscular dystrophy.

j) A patient with a recessive disorder is found to have inherited both copies of one chromosome from the same parent and no representative of that chromosome from the other parent.

Which of the concepts below are illustrated by the situations described above?
Variable expressivity
Uniparental disomy
X-linked dominant inheritance
New mutation
Allelic heterogeneity
Locus (nonallelic) heterogeneity
Homozygosity for an autosomal dominant trait
Pleiotropy
Quasidominant inheritance
Mitochondrial inheritance

4. Don and his maternal grandfather Barry both have hemophilia A. Don's partner Diane is his maternal aunt's daughter. Don and Diane have one son, Edward, and two daughters, Elise and Emily, all of whom have hemophilia A. They also have an unaffected daughter, Enid.

a) Draw the pedigree.

b) Why are Elise and Emily affected?

c) What is the probability that a son of Elise would be hemophilic? What is the probability that her daughter would be hemophilic?

d) What is the probability that a son of Enid would be hemophilic? A daughter?

5. A boy is born with a number of malformations but does not have a recognized syndrome. The parents are unrelated, and there is no family history of a similar condition. Which of the following conditions could explain this situation? Which are unlikely? Why?

a) Autosomal dominant inheritance with new mutation

b) Autosomal dominant inheritance with reduced penetrance

c) Autosomal dominant inheritance with variable expressivity

d) Autosomal recessive inheritance

e) X-linked recessive inheritance

f) Autosomal dominant inheritance, false paternity

g) Maternal ingestion of teratogenic drug at sensitive stage of embryonic development

6. A couple has a child with NF1. Both parents are clinically normal, and neither of their families shows a positive family history.

a) What is the probable explanation for NF1 in their child?

b) What is the risk of recurrence in other children of this couple?

c) If the husband has another child by a different mother, what would the risk of NF1 be?

d) What is the risk that any offspring of the affected child will also have NF1?

CHAPTER
5

TOOLS OF HUMAN MOLECULAR GENETICS

One of the foremost aims of modern medical and human genetics is to understand at a molecular level the basis for mutations that lead to genetic disease and to use that information to improve methods of diagnosis and potential treatment for those genetic diseases. These studies rely on the concepts of molecular genetics, which reflect a logical extension of concepts firmly rooted in cytogenetics, clinical genetics, and biochemical genetics. Like most advances in understanding, those in molecular genetics have been aided considerably by the development of key methodological and technological approaches that could hardly have been imagined even as late as the mid-1970s. The methods, if not the concepts, of molecular genetics have indeed been revolutionary. In the past 15 years, a number of techniques that permit the detailed analysis of both normal and abnormal genes were developed and used. The application of these techniques has both increased the understanding of molecular processes at all levels, from the gene to the whole organism, and provided the basis for a growing armamentarium of laboratory procedures for the detection and diagnosis of genetic diseases.

This chapter is not intended to be a "cookbook" of recipes for genetic experiments or of laboratory diagnostic methods. Rather, it serves only

as an introduction to the techniques that have been and continue to be largely responsible for advances in both basic and applied genetic research. The contents of this chapter both supplement the basic material presented in Chapters 2, 3, and 4 and provide a basis for understanding much of the molecular information contained in the chapters that follow. For readers who have had a course in molecular human genetics or who have had laboratory experience in molecular genetics, this chapter can be skimmed or even omitted altogether without interfering with the continuity of the text. For others who find the material in this chapter too brief, far more detailed accounts of modern techniques, along with complete references, can be found in the General References listed at the end of this chapter.

PRINCIPLES OF MOLECULAR CLONING

The process of molecular cloning involves isolating a DNA sequence of interest and obtaining multiple copies of it in an organism, usually a bacterium, that is capable of growth over extended periods. Large quantities of the DNA molecule can be then isolated in pure form for detailed molecular analysis (Fig. 5–1). The ability to generate virtually endless copies (clones) of a particular sequence is the basis of **recombinant DNA technology** and its application to human and medical genetics. The name "recombinant DNA" refers to novel combinations of DNA created between human (or other) DNA sequences of interest and bacterial (or other) DNA molecules capable of indefinite duplication in the laboratory. Like many technological advances, this one comes with its own jargon, the mastery of which may seem more imposing than the concepts involved (see box).

Restriction Enzymes

One of the key advances in the development of molecular cloning was the discovery in the early 1970s of bacterial **restriction endonucleases,** enzymes that recognize specific (usually short) double-stranded sequences in DNA and cleave the DNA at or near the recognition site. For example, the restriction enzyme *Eco*RI recognizes the specific six base-pair sequence

$$5'\ G A A T T C\ 3'$$
$$3'\ C T T A A G\ 5'$$

wherever it occurs in a double-stranded DNA molecule and cleaves the DNA at that site by introducing a nick on each strand between the G and the adjacent A. This generates two fragments, each with a four-base, single-stranded overhang at the end (Fig. 5–2). Such "sticky" ends are useful for subsequent joining reactions in the construction of recombinant DNA molecules. Other restriction enzymes recognize different sequences of nucleotides that are specific for each particular enzyme. Several hundred such enzymes are now known; some of the ones most commonly used are listed in Table 5–1. Most restriction enzymes have recognition sites that consist of four or six base pairs, although a few have longer sites. Usually, the sequences are **palindromes;** that is, they read the same 5' to 3' on both strands.

Cleavage of a DNA molecule with a particular restriction enzyme digests the DNA into a characteristic and reproducible collection of fragments, which reflect the frequency and the location of specific cleavage sites. This property of restriction enzymes has two important implications central to their role in recombinant DNA technology and its application to medical genetics. First, digestion of genomic DNA samples with, for example, the enzyme *Eco*RI generates a collection of approximately 1 million *Eco*RI fragments, each from a par-

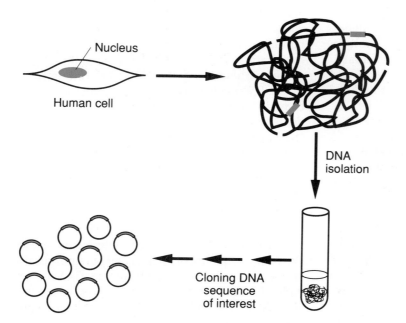

Figure 5–1. The rationale for molecular cloning to isolate infinite quantities of a particular desired DNA sequence in pure form.

The Language of Molecular Cloning

cDNA (complementary DNA): a synthetic DNA copied from messenger RNA (mRNA) by the enzyme reverse transcriptase. Used to refer to either a single-stranded copy or its double-stranded derivative. Usage: "a cDNA clone," "a cDNA library," or "to isolate a cDNA."

clone: a recombinant DNA molecule containing a gene or other DNA sequence of interest. Also, the act of generating such a molecule. Usage: "to isolate a clone" or "to clone a gene."

host: the organism used to isolate and propagate a recombinant DNA molecule. Usually a strain of the bacterium *Escherichia coli* or the yeast *Saccharomyces cerevisiae*. Usage: "What host did they use?"

hybridization: the act of two complementary single-stranded nucleic acid molecules forming bonds and becoming a double-stranded molecule. Usage: "The probe hybridized to a gene."

insert: a fragment of human DNA cloned into a particular vector. Usage: "They purified the insert."

library: a collection of recombinant clones from a source known to contain the gene, cDNA, or other DNA sequences of interest. In principle, a library may contain all the DNA sequences represented in the original cell, tissue, or chromosome. Usage: "a muscle cDNA library" or "a human genomic library."

ligation: the act of forming phosphodiester bonds to join two double-stranded DNA molecules with the enzyme DNA ligase. Ligation is the essential step in creating recombinant DNA molecules. Usage: "The fragments were ligated together."

probe: a cloned DNA or RNA molecule, labeled with radioactivity or another detectable tracer, used to identify its complementary sequences by molecular hybridization; also, the act of using such a molecule. Usage: "the β-globin probe" or "to probe a patient's DNA."

restriction endonucleases (restriction enzymes): enzymes that recognize specific double-stranded DNA sequences and cleave the DNA at or near the recognition site. Usage: "a restriction enzyme digest" (or just "a restriction digest") or "the restriction enzyme *Eco*RI."

Southern blot: a filter to which DNA has been transferred, usually after restriction enzyme digestion and gel electrophoresis to separate DNA molecules by size (named after the developer of the technique, Ed Southern); also, the act of generating such a filter and hybridizing it to a specific probe. Usage: "to probe a Southern blot" or "they did a Southern."

vector: the DNA molecule into which the gene or other DNA fragment of interest is cloned, capable of replicating in a particular host. Examples include plasmids, bacteriophage lambda, cosmids, and yeast artificial chromosomes. Usage: "a cloning vector" or "the cosmid vector."

ticular location in the genome. Because *Eco*RI cleaves double-stranded DNA specifically at each and every 5'-GAATTC-3' that it encounters, and because even a single base change in a potential cleavage site abolishes its recognition and cleavage by the enzyme, such digestion allows one to examine, in effect, this particular sequence of six nucleotides at approximately 1 million locations in the genome. (On average, an enzyme with a 6 base-pair recognition site should cleave human DNA every 4^6 base pairs, or once every 4 kb. However, in reality, such sites are located nonran-

domly, reflecting the particular base composition and sequence of different regions of the genome, and *Eco*RI fragments ranging in size from a few base pairs to well over 1 million base pairs are observed.)

Second, all DNA molecules digested with *Eco*RI, regardless of their origin, have identical single-stranded sticky ends, independent of the nature of the DNA sequences flanking a particular *Eco*RI site. Therefore, any two DNA molecules that have been generated by *Eco*RI digestion can be joined together by interaction of their complemen-

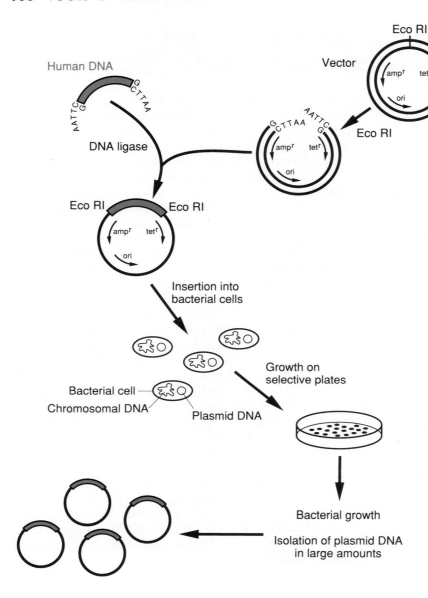

Figure 5–2. The process of cloning a segment of human DNA (between two *Eco*RI sites) into a plasmid cloning vector. "ori" denotes an origin of DNA replication for replicating the plasmid in bacterial cells. "amp^r" and "tet^r" denote bacterial genes conferring resistance to ampicillin and tetracycline. Growth of bacteria on plates containing antibiotics selects for those cells that contain copies of the plasmid, with its cloned human insert. (Modified from Fritsch EF, Maniatis T [1987] Methods of molecular genetics. *In* Stamatoyannopoulos G, Nienhuis AW, Leder P, Majerus PW (eds) The molecular basis of blood diseases. WB Saunders, Philadelphia, pp 1–27.)

tary four-base overhangs, which is followed by completion of the phosphodiester backbones on each strand by an enzyme called **DNA ligase.** This ligation step creates a "recombinant" DNA molecule, one end derived from one DNA source and the other end derived from a different source (Fig. 5–2). Many restriction enzymes, such as *Eco*RI, generate short overhangs; others, however, cut both strands at the same location, leaving blunt ends. DNA ligase can also join these molecules.

Vectors

A vector is a DNA molecule that can replicate autonomously in a host such as bacterial or yeast cells, from which it can be subsequently isolated in pure form for analysis. Cloning of human DNA fragments into a vector by means of restriction enzymes and DNA ligase, as just described, allows for the propagation of the cloned fragment along with the vector molecule. Because replicating vec-

Table 5–1. Examples of Restriction Enzymes and Their Recognition Sequences

Restriction Enzyme	Source	Recognition Sequence*
*Bam*HI	*Bacillus amyloliquefaciens* H	5'-G^GATC C-3' 3'-C CTAG^G-5'
*Eco*RI	*Escherichia coli* RY 13	G^AATT C C TTAA^G
*Hae*III	*Haemophilus aegyptius*	GG^CC CC^GG
*Hin*dIII	*Haemophilus influenzae* R_d	A^AGCT T T TCGA^A
*Not*I	*Nocardia otitidis-cavarium*	GC^GGCC GC CG CCGG^CG
*Sau*3A	*Staphylococcus aureus* 3A	^GATC CTAG^
*Sst*II	*Streptomyces stanford*	CC GC^GG GG^CG CC

* All recognition sequences are given in the 5'→3' polarity, as shown for *Bam*HI. Cleavage sites on each strand are indicated by the small circumflexes.

tors can achieve a high number of copies per cell and because the bacterial or yeast hosts can be grown indefinitely in the laboratory, vast quantities of the DNA sequences of interest can be obtained. A number of vectors are commonly used for this purpose, each with its own set of advantages and limitations (Table 5–2).

PLASMIDS

Plasmids are circular double-stranded DNA molecules that replicate extrachromosomally in bacteria or, less commonly, in yeast. Because they can be maintained in a moderate number of copies (Fig. 5–1), they are ideal for generating large quantities of a cloned DNA sequence. Plasmids specifically designed for molecular cloning are usually small (several kb in size) and contain an origin of replication (for replication either in *E. coli* or in yeast), one or more selectable markers (usually a gene that confers resistance to antibiotics), and one or more restriction sites for cloning foreign DNA molecules. A schematic drawing of the

important steps involved in cloning of foreign DNA into the *Eco*RI site of a plasmid is shown in Figure 5–2. Identification of colonies that contain the desired recombinant plasmid, followed by mass growth and isolation of pure plasmid DNA, allows the isolation of large amounts of the cloned insert. Cloning into plasmids is a standard procedure for the analysis of short DNA molecules (Table 5–2).

BACTERIOPHAGE LAMBDA

Another commonly used vector is bacteriophage lambda, a bacterial virus with a relatively large (approximately 45 kb) double-stranded DNA molecule. During growth in *E. coli,* lambda replicates to produce huge numbers of infectious viruses, eventually killing the bacterial cells thus infected and releasing 1 million or so bacteriophages. During this infectious phase of growth, approximately one third of the bacteriophage genome is nonessential (labeled "internal fragments" in Fig. 5–3) and can be replaced by other DNA sequences; thus

Table 5–2. Examples of Vectors Commonly Used in Molecular Cloning

Vector	Host	Type of Cloning	Insert Size Range
Plasmids	Bacterial, yeast	Genomic, cDNA	Usually < 5–10 kb
Bacteriophage lambda	Bacterial	Genomic, cDNA	Up to ~20 kb
Cosmids	Bacterial	Genomic	Up to ~50 kb
"Artificial chromosomes"	Yeast	Genomic	~100 to 1000 kb

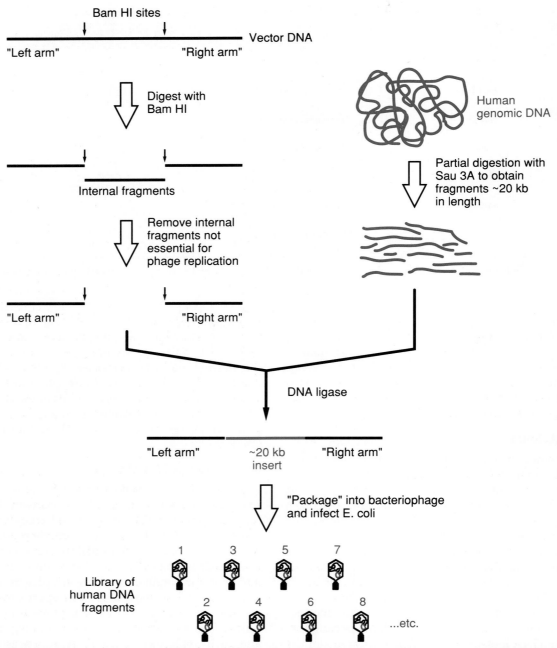

Figure 5–3. Construction of a "library" of DNA from the human genome in a bacteriophage vector. Each of the recombinant phage particles at the bottom contains a different fragment of human DNA. A collection of several hundred thousand such phages would represent all the DNA from the human genome.

it is highly suitable for cloning fairly large (up to about 20 kb) pieces of human DNA.

COSMIDS

Even larger fragments of foreign DNA (up to about 50 kb) can be cloned in cosmid vectors. Cos-

mids are basically plasmids that use the ability of bacteriophage lambda infectious particles to efficiently "package" large linear pieces of DNA and introduce them into bacterial cells. After infection of bacteria in a manner similar to that of a lambda virus, the cosmid recircularizes and replicates as a large plasmid.

YEAST "ARTIFICIAL CHROMOSOMES"

For many approaches to gene cloning and gene mapping, illustrated in Chapter 8, it is advantageous to isolate the largest piece of human chromosomal DNA possible. Until the mid-1980s, cosmid vectors represented the largest cloning vehicle available. In 1987, however, Olson and colleagues developed a technique to clone much larger pieces of DNA into vectors that replicate and segregate in the host *Saccharomyces cerevisiae* (common baker's yeast), as in normal linear yeast chromosomes (Burke et al., 1987). These yeast "artificial chromosomes" (YACs) have centromeres and telomeres, just like normal yeast chromosomes, and allow cloning and isolation of fragments of DNA up to 1000 kb in length, much smaller than a normal human chromosome but approximately the same size as a normal yeast chromosome.

Construction of Libraries

The purpose of molecular cloning, of course, is to isolate a particular gene or other DNA sequence in large quantities for further study. A common approach for achieving this is to construct a set of recombinant DNA clones from a source (genomic DNA or mRNA) that contains the gene or sequence of interest. Such a collection of clones is called a **library,** which at least theoretically contains all of the sequences found in the original source. Having a library, however, is only the first step. One then has to identify the clone or clones of interest from the library by using sensitive screening methods that are capable of finding, in some cases, even a single copy of the clone of interest in a collection of up to 10 million starting clones.

GENOMIC LIBRARIES

One approach to constructing a library of genomic DNA is shown in Figure 5–3. In this technique, first applied in the late 1970s, human genomic DNA is partially digested with a restriction enzyme like *Sau*3A in such a way that some of the sites are cleaved and others are not. In this way, if random cleavage of such sites is assumed, a collection of overlapping fragments of length suitable for cloning can be obtained and ligated into bacteriophage lambda "arms" prepared so that the *Sau*3A ends of human DNA fragments can be ligated into the vector (Fig. 5–3). After packaging of

the recombinant lambda chromosome into infectious bacteriophage particles, the library, containing 1 million or more fragments of genomic DNA, can be stored for the future isolation of many genes. One of the very first human genomic libraries, constructed by Maniatis and colleagues (Lawn et al., 1978), is still being used today in hundreds of laboratories around the world for the isolation of human genes.

One can greatly facilitate the process of screening for the sequence of interest by starting with a library that is already enriched for that sequence, thus considerably reducing the total number of recombinant clones that have to be screened. For genomic DNA, a particularly efficient way to achieve this is to use a library that contains only clones from a specific human chromosome. Thus if one wants to isolate a gene from, for example, chromosome 7, a **chromosome-specific library** representing clones only from chromosome 7 can be obtained. Such libraries are now available for all individual human chromosomes; these libraries are generated by the cloning of DNA from chromosomes separated on the basis of size from all of the other chromosomes by an approach called **fluorescence-activated chromosome sorting.** The applications of this particular approach are explained further in Chapter 8.

COMPLEMENTARY DNA LIBRARIES

Another common type of library used to isolate genes is a cDNA library, which represents **complementary DNA** (hence cDNA) copies of the mRNA population present within a particular tissue. Such cDNA libraries are often preferable to genomic libraries as a source of cloned genes (1) because the obtained clone is a direct representation of the coding sequences, without introns or other noncoding sequences found in genomic DNA, and (2) because the use of a particular mRNA source often enriches substantially for the sequences derived from a given gene known to be expressed selectively in that tissue. For example, the β-globin gene is represented at only one part per million in a human genomic library, but it is a major mRNA transcript in red blood cells. Thus a cDNA library prepared from red blood cells represents an excellent cloning source to isolate globin gene cDNAs. Similarly, a liver or muscle cDNA library is a good source of clones for genes known to be expressed preferentially or exclusively in those tissues.

A number of methods have been developed to clone cDNAs, all of which rely on the enzyme **reverse transcriptase,** an RNA-dependent DNA polymerase that can synthesize a cDNA strand from an RNA template (Fig. 5–4). Reverse transcriptase requires a primer to initiate DNA synthesis. Usually, a sequence of polythymine residues (oligo-dT) is used; this short homopolymer binds to the polyA tail at the 3'end of mRNA molecules and thus primes synthesis of a complementary copy. This single-stranded cDNA is then converted to a double-stranded molecule by one of several available methods, and the double-stranded cDNA can then be ligated into a suitable vector, usually a plasmid or a bacteriophage, to create a cDNA library representing all of the original mRNA transcripts found in the starting cell type or tissue (Fig. 5–4). Some cleverly engineered vectors contain transcription and translation signals adjacent to the cloning site to facilitate expression of the cloned cDNA in *E. coli* or in yeast. Such so-called expression vectors can then be screened with antibodies raised against, for example, the protein whose gene one is trying to isolate.

Representative cDNA libraries from different tissues or different times of development are valuable resources for gene cloning. Many such libraries are now widely available.

METHODS OF NUCLEIC ACID ANALYSIS

Many approaches to the analysis of RNA or DNA, or both, involve the detection of homologous sequences by using a "probe" to search out a particular DNA or RNA sequence among a collection of many other sequences and to mark that specific sequence in such a way that it can be readily observed and analyzed in a diagnostic or research laboratory. For genomic DNA, the problem is how to find and analyze the specific DNA fragment that one is interested in, among a genomic DNA sample that contains a total of several million DNA fragments. For RNA samples, the problem is how to detect and measure the amount and the quality of a particular mRNA in an RNA sample from a tissue in which the desired mRNA might

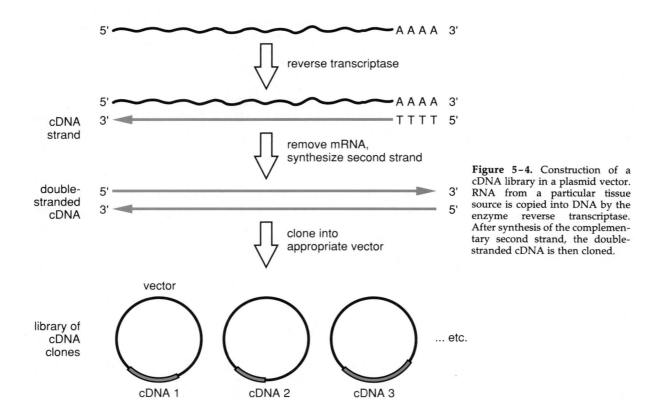

Figure 5–4. Construction of a cDNA library in a plasmid vector. RNA from a particular tissue source is copied into DNA by the enzyme reverse transcriptase. After synthesis of the complementary second strand, the double-stranded cDNA is then cloned.

account for only 1/1000 or less of the total RNA transcripts. The solution to both of these problems involves the method of **nucleic acid hybridization,** in which *single-stranded* nucleic acids (for example, genomic DNA isolated from a patient or RNA isolated from a tissue) are mixed with a specific probe and tagged in such a way as to allow its subsequent detection. Under appropriate conditions that favor formation of *double-stranded* nucleic acids, the probe hybridizes only to its complementary sequence, ignoring all of the other sequences in the mixture (Fig. 5–5). The desired sequence in the original DNA or RNA sample is now marked by the tag (usually a radioactive tracer or a histochemical compound) on the probe, which thus facilitates its subsequent detection and analysis.

What Are Probes and What Are They Good For?

Probes are either cloned or synthetic nucleic acid (usually DNA) molecules that are used in either DNA:DNA or DNA:RNA hybridization reactions (Fig. 5–5) to hybridize to a DNA or an RNA sequence of interest. For example, one might use a probe for the β-globin gene to analyze a sample of

patient DNA for a specific mutation thought to be responsible for sickle cell anemia. Or one might use a probe for the X-linked dystrophin gene to search a sample of muscle RNA obtained from a patient with X-linked Duchenne muscular dystrophy for dystrophin mRNA transcripts. Probes are absolutely critical for detecting mutations in clinical molecular diagnostic laboratories and for carrying out a variety of molecular genetics experiments in research laboratories. Without probes specific for different genes and for particular mutations in those genes, it would be impossible to examine DNA and RNA samples for the mutations underlying genetic diseases.

Many probes are cloned genes or cloned cDNA molecules obtained by use of the recombinant DNA technology described earlier in this chapter. In fact, one of the major reasons for wanting to clone a gene is to use it as a DNA probe for diagnostic purposes. Probes derived from cloned genes or cDNAs are usually several hundred to several thousand nucleotides in length and are typically labeled with a radioisotopic tracer such as phosphorus-32 (^{32}P) whose high energy exposes x-ray film. One can introduce ^{32}P into a probe by a variety of methods that substitute ^{32}P-labeled nucleotides for nonradioactive nucleotides in a double-stranded DNA molecule.

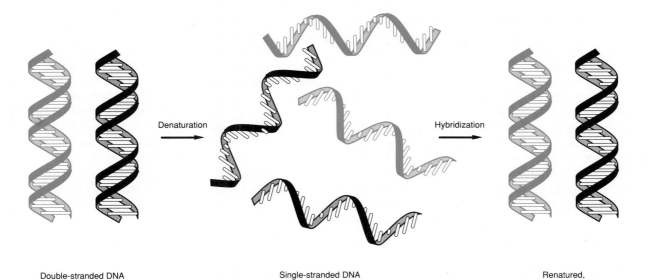

Double-stranded DNA   Single-stranded DNA   Renatured, double-stranded DNA

Figure 5–5. The principle of nucleic acid hybridization. The two complementary strands of a Watson-Crick double helix can be "denatured" by a variety of treatments (such as high temperature or very low salt conditions) to yield a collection of single-stranded DNA molecules. Under conditions that favor formation of renatured double-stranded DNA, complementary strands will "hybridize" to each other, but not to other fragments of DNA that have a different nucleotide sequence.

The Molecular Analysis of a Human Mutation

How does one proceed when one has a patient with a genetic disorder known or suspected to be due to a mutation in a particular gene? For example, consider a patient with a diagnosis of β-thalassemia, an autosomal recessive defect in the β-globin gene (see Chapter 11). The initial diagnosis is generally made on the basis of clinical and hematological findings alone. However, it is important to examine the gene itself, first to confirm the clinical diagnosis and second, to determine the specific mutation in the β-globin locus both for future use in carrier testing and possible prenatal diagnosis in the patient's family, and for increasing the understanding of the relationship between specific mutations in the gene and the resulting pathophysiology.

Several tests can be used initially to examine the gross integrity of the β-globin gene itself and its mRNA. Is the gene present in the patient in both normal amount (i.e., two copies) and structure? Or is one or both copies of the gene deleted or structurally rearranged, as has been described in some cases of β-thalassemia? If the gene is present, is it transcribed? The **Southern blotting** technique (see main text) is a now standard method for using a cloned gene probe (in this case, for the β-globin gene) to examine the integrity of a DNA sample. Southern blotting can address the question of whether a gene is present and whether it is grossly normal in structure. By this method one can detect large molecular defects that are well below the level of sensitivity of chromosome analysis. However, as currently used in diagnostic laboratories, it cannot reveal the presence of single mutations, such as base-pair changes or very small deletions of only a few base pairs. In order to examine whether mRNA is present, a technique called **Northern blotting** is used (see main text). This approach also enables one to detect major changes in mRNA levels or structure for a specific gene, but not to detect minor alterations.

Having asked whether there are gross changes in the gene or in its mRNA, one can proceed to a number of methods developed to examine gene structure and expression at increasingly finer levels of analysis. In β-thalassemia, as in many other genetic disorders, particular mutations responsible for the disease in other patients have been described previously. To determine whether one of these already known mutations is responsible for a particular case of β-thalassemia, one can apply particular direct molecular tests. Some of these entail the approach of **allele-specific oligonucleotides (ASOs)** that enable one to detect specific single base-pair mutations (see main text). In addition, it may be desirable to actually clone the mutant β-globin genes (or cDNAs) from the patient for comparison with a normal β-globin gene. Cloning of individual mutant genes (or portions of genes) from a patient's material is facilitated by use of the **polymerase chain reaction (PCR)** to specifically generate many millions of copies of a particular gene fragment (see main text). Once the mutant gene is isolated, one can then analyze it at the finest level possible by determining the **DNA sequence** of base pairs in the mutant gene for comparison with the normal gene. In this way, the specific mutation responsible for the genetic disorder in the patient can be determined and used to develop direct screening tests for that mutation in the patient's family.

Southern Blotting

The Southern blotting technique, developed in the mid-1970s, is the standard way of analyzing the structure of DNA cleaved by restriction enzymes.

In this procedure, diagrammed in Figure 5–6 for a genomic DNA sample, DNA is first isolated from an accessible source. Any cell in the body can be used as a DNA source, except for mature red blood cells, which have no nuclei. For analysis of patient

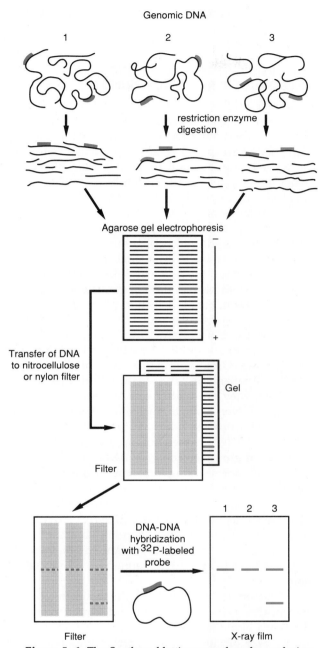

Figure 5-6. The Southern blotting procedure for analyzing specific DNA sequences in a complex mixture of different sequences, such as genomic DNA. In this example, sample 3 has a different restriction enzyme pattern for the DNA sequence detected by the probe. This variation might be due to a restriction fragment length polymorphism (see Chapter 6) or to a deletion of DNA near the detected sequence.

DNA samples, one typically prepares genomic DNA from lymphocytes obtained by routine venipuncture. A 10-cc sample of peripheral blood provides 50 to 100 μg of DNA, enough for 10 to 20 restriction enzyme digestions. However, genomic DNA can also be prepared from other tissue sources, including cultured skin fibroblasts, amniotic fluid or chorionic villus cells for prenatal diagnosis (see Chapter 19), or any organ biopsy (liver, kidney, placenta, etc.). The one million DNA fragments generated by restriction enzyme cleavage of a genomic DNA sample are separated on the basis of size by agarose gel electrophoresis, in which small fragments move more rapidly than larger ones. When digested DNA separated in this way is stained with a fluorescent DNA dye such as ethidium bromide, the genomic DNA fragments appear as a smear of fluorescing material because there are far too many DNA fragments for any one to stand out from the rest (Fig. 5–7, left). The Southern blotting technique allows one to find and examine at a gross level the one or two DNA fragments of interest in this seemingly uninformative collection of a million or so restriction enzyme fragments. Double-stranded DNA fragments are first denatured with a strong base to separate the two complementary DNA strands. The now single-stranded DNA molecules are then transferred from the gel to a piece of nitrocellulose or nylon filter paper by blotting and capillarity (hence, the name "Southern blot" or "Southern transfer").

To identify the one or more fragments of interest among the millions of fragments on the filter, a specific labeled probe is used. As described earlier, the probe is usually a piece of cloned DNA that has been radioactively labeled and itself denatured to the single-stranded state. The labeled probe and the filter are incubated together in solution under conditions that favor formation of double-stranded DNA molecules (as in Fig. 5–5). Because of the exquisite specificity of the DNA code, the probe anneals only to its complementary strand on the filter and ignores all of the other DNA fragments. If the probe is itself a piece of cloned genomic DNA, it usually hybridizes to one or two fragments on the filter, depending on how the gene or genes in the original DNA sample were cut by the specific restriction enzyme used. If the probe is a cloned cDNA, however, many fragments may hybridize because genomic DNA is usually not colinear with a gene's mRNA tran-

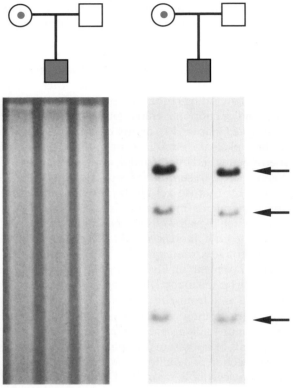

Figure 5–7. Detection of a gene deletion by Southern blotting. When genomic DNA from family members is digested with a restriction enzyme and the DNA stained with a fluorescent DNA dye (such as ethidium bromide) after electrophoresis, all samples appear the same (left). After Southern blotting and hybridization to a cDNA probe for the human X-linked androgen receptor gene, the individual with androgen insensitivity syndrome can be seen to be deleted for this gene (right, middle lane). (Figure courtesy of R. Lafreniere, Stanford University.)

script as a result of the presence of introns (see Chapter 3). After being washed to remove unbound probe, the filter (with its bound radioactive probe) is exposed to x-ray film to reveal the position of the one or more fragments to which the probe hybridized. Thus, as shown in Figure 5–7, specific radioactive bands show up on the x-ray film for each lane of human DNA on the original agarose gel. In this example, the Southern blotting technique shows that the gene for the X-linked androgen receptor, which is responsible for male secondary sex characteristics (see Chapter 10), is absent from a genomic DNA sample from a patient with X-linked **androgen-insensitivity syndrome** (also known as testicular feminization); it is present in normal males. Southern blotting is now a standard procedure in molecular diagnostic lab-

oratories in many medical centers around the world for the diagnosis of a growing number of genetic diseases.

ANALYSIS WITH ALLELE-SPECIFIC OLIGONUCLEOTIDE (ASO) PROBES

In some methods of nucleic acid analysis, probes are synthesized chemically from the individual nucleotide building blocks, following the known sequence corresponding to a particular gene, rather than by isolation of probes from cloned genes of cDNAs. Synthetic probes are usually much shorter (typically only a dozen or so bases in length) than cloned probes and are called **oligonucleotide probes** or, simply, **oligonucleotides.** The shorter length makes oligonucleotide probes much more sensitive to even single base-pair mismatches between the probe and the sample to be analyzed. Methods based on oligonucleotides are thus highly suitable for detection of specific mutations. When a particular mutation is known in at least some cases of a genetic disease, one can refine the analysis to ask specifically whether that mutation is present or absent in a DNA sample from a particular patient. Because oligonucleotide probes are short, they are highly sensitive to sequence changes at even a single nucleotide. Thus an oligonucleotide probe synthesized to match precisely the normal DNA sequence in a gene (an **allele-specific oligonucleotide,** or **ASO**) hybridizes only to the normal complementary sequence but not to an imperfect complementary sequence in which there are one or more mismatches as a result of a base change (Fig. 5–8). Similarly, an ASO made to the sequence corresponding to a mutant gene hybridizes only to the mutant complementary sequence but not to the sequence in a normal gene.

It is important to recognize the distinction between this type of analysis and conventional Southern blot analysis with cloned DNA probes. In the case of cloned DNA probes, the analysis cannot usually reveal a single base change. In the vast majority of cases, mutant genes due to single base changes or to similar small changes in the DNA (small deletions or insertions, for example) are indistinguishable from normal genes by Southern blot analysis with standard, cloned DNA probes. Only short ASO probes have this ability.

ASO analysis, then, allows for the precise genotyping of a DNA sample and can distinguish

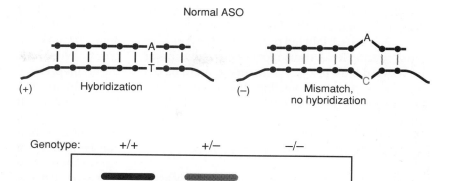

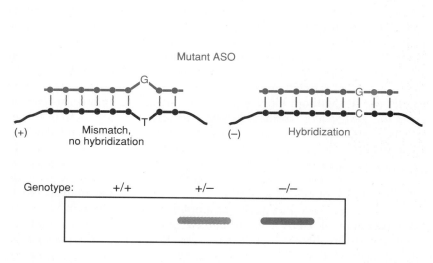

Figure 5-8. Detection of single base pair mutations using allele-specific oligonucleotide probes. The "normal" probe will bind only to DNA sequences that are identical to the probe (top). The "mutant" probe will bind only to DNA sequences that differ from the "normal" sequence by a specific single base pair mutation (bottom). Individuals of all three genotypes can be distinguished by this method.

people who are homozygous for the normal sequence (whose DNA hybridizes only with the normal ASO), heterozygous (whose DNA hybridizes with both ASO probes), or homozygous for the mutant sequence (whose DNA hybridizes only with the mutant gene ASO) (Fig. 5-8). Care must be taken, however, in interpreting results from ASO analysis because not all mutant genes at a given locus share exactly the same mutation. Thus failure to hybridize to the mutant gene ASO does not necessarily mean that the patient's DNA is normal at that gene; there may be a mutation elsewhere in that gene other than in the precise location examined by that particular ASO. ASO analysis is used primarily in cases for which there is a strong probability based on other lines of evidence that a family or an individual is at risk for a particular known mutation. The approach is usually feasible only for those genetic disorders that are char-

acterized by a finite and small number of different mutations. Specific examples of such diseases are considered in Chapters 6, 11, and 12.

Northern Blotting

The counterpart of the Southern blotting technique for analysis of RNA samples is called "Northern" blotting and is the standard approach for determining the size and abundance of the mRNA from a specific gene in a sample of RNA. RNA cannot be cleaved by the restriction enzymes used for DNA analysis. However, different RNA transcripts are of different lengths, depending on the size of the gene being transcribed. Thus cellular RNA (or purified mRNA) obtained from a particular cell type is separated according to size by agarose gel electrophoresis and transferred to nitrocellulose or nylon filters. As in the Southern blotting procedure, the filter is then incubated with a denatured, labeled probe, which hybridizes to the specific RNA transcripts. After exposure of the washed filter to x-ray film, one or more bands may be apparent, revealing the position and abundance of the specific transcript of interest.

The Polymerase Chain Reaction

Of all the techniques available for the analysis of DNA and RNA, none has had the impact or has the potential of a conceptually simple procedure developed in 1985, the polymerase chain reaction, or PCR (Saiki et al., 1985). PCR can selectively amplify a single molecule of DNA or RNA several millionfold in a few hours and has revolutionized both the molecular diagnosis and the molecular analysis of genetic disease. It allows the detection and analysis of specific gene sequences in a patient's sample without cloning and without the need for Southern or Northern blotting. Analyses can be performed on even a single cell obtained from a hair root, from the few cells present in mouth rinses, or from a drop of dried blood, thus eliminating the need to prepare large amounts of DNA or RNA from tissue samples.

PCR is based on the enzymatic amplification of a fragment of DNA that is flanked by two "primers," short oligonucleotides that hybridize to the opposite strands of the target sequence and prime synthesis of the complementary DNA sequence by the enzyme DNA polymerase. As diagrammed schematically in Figure 5–9, the primers are oriented in such a way that the two new strands of DNA are themselves complementary and effectively make up a second copy of the original target sequence. Repeated cycles of heat denaturation, hybridization of the primers, and enzymatic DNA synthesis result in the exponential amplification (2, 4, 8, 16, 32, . . . copies) of the target DNA sequence (Fig. 5–9). With the use of specifically designed "PCR machines," a round of amplification takes only about 10 minutes. In only a few hours, many millions of copies of a starting sequence can be created, an amount sufficient to easily detect a specific single-copy DNA sequence starting from less than 1 percent of the amount of genomic DNA required to perform a standard Southern blotting experiment!

The rapid amplification of specific sequences can also be used to facilitate cloning of specific genes from DNA samples for the analysis of mutation. What used to be a very laborious procedure, involving construction of a genomic or cDNA library from a patient's DNA or RNA followed by screening for the gene of interest, now can be carried out in less than a day. Particular portions of a gene (usually the exons) from DNA can be rapidly amplified through the use of specific primers known from the sequence of the normal gene. The mutant gene can then be either easily cloned for further analysis or analyzed directly as a PCR fragment (because it is now represented specifically and disproportionately in relation to the rest of the patient's genomic DNA).

PCR can also be applied to the analysis of small samples of RNA. A single-stranded cDNA is first synthesized from the mRNA of interest with the same reverse transcriptase enzyme that is used to prepare cDNA clone libraries (Fig. 5–4). PCR primers are then added along with DNA polymerase, as in the case of DNA PCR. One of the oligonucleotides primes synthesis of the second strand of the cDNA, which in its double-stranded form then serves as a target for PCR amplification.

PCR is rapidly becoming a standard method for analysis of DNA and RNA samples, both in research laboratories and, to an increasing extent, in clinical molecular diagnostic laboratories. PCR is faster, less expensive, more sensitive, and less demanding of patients' samples than any other method for nucleic acid analysis. Specific examples of its use for the detection of mutations in genetic disorders are presented in Chapter 6.

DNA Sequence Analysis

Methods for determining the nucleotide sequence of DNA fragments produced by DNA cloning were independently developed by Walter Gilbert and Fred Sanger, who shared the Nobel prize in 1980 for their work. (This was Sanger's second Nobel prize; he was also awarded one in 1958 for being the first to determine the amino acid sequence of a protein.) The sequence of virtually any purified DNA segment can now be determined, whether it comes from a cloned fragment or from a target sequence amplified by PCR. The most widely used approach for DNA sequence analysis

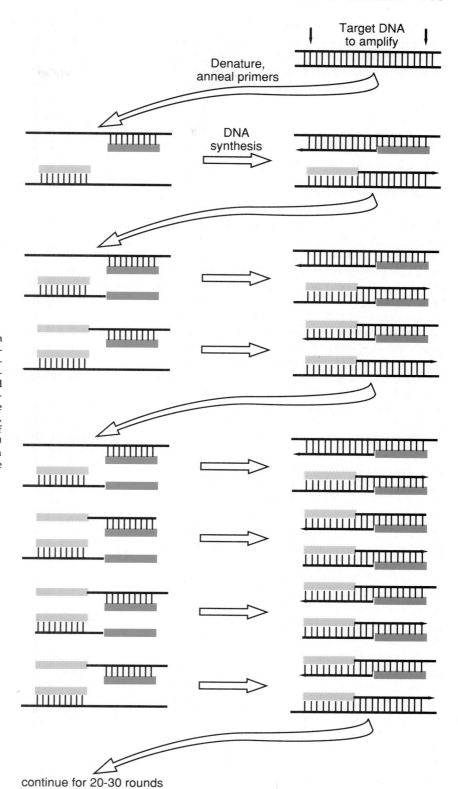

Figure 5–9. The polymerase chain reaction. By repeatedly synthesizing a region of DNA located between two DNA primers, this region of DNA is specifically and selectively amplified in an exponential fashion. Three successive rounds of amplification are shown, resulting in a total of eight copies of the targeted sequence. After 30 rounds of amplification, over a billion copies of the sequence are created.

is to utilize chemical analogs of nucleotides to inhibit the enzyme DNA polymerase as it synthesizes the complementary strand to the original template to be sequenced (Fig. 5–10). As with PCR, DNA synthesis is primed by a short oligonucleotide. DNA polymerase proceeds along the template sequence, incorporating either ^{32}P- or ^{35}S-labeled nucleotides into the newly synthesized sequence. One obtains sequence information by introducing one of the inhibitory analogs into each of four sequencing reactions. Thus in a reaction to define the location of G residues, a G analog is introduced, and DNA synthesis of a proportion of individual molecules stops at each G residue that the DNA polymerase encounters. Depending on the relative amounts of the normal G nucleotide and the G analog in this reaction, some newly synthesized strands are inhibited and stop at the first G, some at the second G, some at the third, and so forth. When this sample is then analyzed by gel electrophoresis, a series of radioactive bands is observed at lengths corresponding to the locations of each G residue. Similar reactions for the A, T, and C residues provide corresponding series of radioactive bands. The set of four reactions can then be read as a directional sequencing "ladder" to determine the nucleotide sequence of the DNA fragment being analyzed (Fig. 5–10).

Machines are now being developed to automate the procedure of DNA sequencing, which is routinely applied for analysis of both normal and mutant genes. In time, the nucleotide sequence of the entire human genome, including all of its genes, will be catalogued (see Chapter 8). DNA sequence information is critical for predicting the amino acid sequence of a newly isolated gene, for detecting individual mutations in genetic disease, and for designing either ASO probes or PCR primers used in molecular diagnostic procedures.

METHODS OF PROTEIN ANALYSIS

Many approaches to the analysis of both normal and abnormal gene function are based at the level of the protein. In most instances, one wants to know not only the molecular defect in the DNA, but also how that defect alters the encoded protein to produce the clinical phenotype.

Western Blotting

Shortly after development of Southern and Northern blotting for DNA and RNA, a conceptually related procedure for the detection of spe-

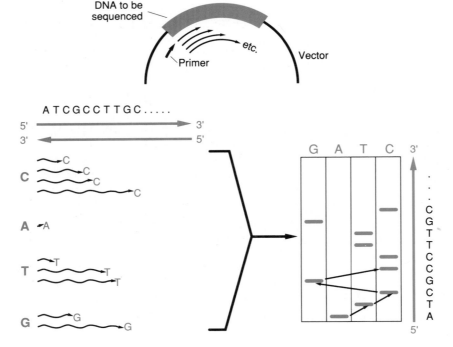

Figure 5–10. The Sanger method of determining the nucleotide sequence of a cloned DNA fragment. See text for description.

cific proteins was described and dubbed "Western" blotting. This technique can be used to obtain information on the size and amount of mutant protein in cell extracts from patients with genetic diseases. In this method, proteins isolated from a cell extract are separated according to size by polyacrylamide gel electrophoresis and then transferred to a nitrocellulose filter. The filter containing the separated proteins is then incubated with antisera that specifically recognize the protein to be analyzed. The specific interaction between the antibody and its antigen can then be detected by a second antibody against the first, tagged with a detectable histochemical, fluorescent, or radioactive substance. An example of a Western blot used to detect the presence or absence of the muscle protein dystrophin in patients with X-linked Duchenne muscular dystrophy is shown in Figure 5–11.

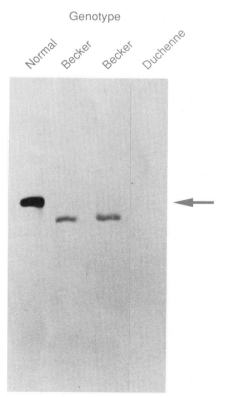

Figure 5–11. A "Western" blot demonstrating the presence or absence of the muscle protein dystrophin (arrow) in protein extracts from patients with the severe Duchenne or mild Becker form of X-linked muscular dystrophy. See Chapter 12 for further description. (Original photograph courtesy of R. Worton and D. Bulman, Hospital for Sick Children, Toronto.)

Amino Acid Sequencing

The techniques developed by Sanger in the late 1950s to determine the amino acid sequence of purified proteins continue to be used today. Typically, a purified protein is cleaved into a number of large peptide fragments with one or more chemical or enzymatic cleavage agents. Distinct peptide fragments are then isolated, and the sequence of 15 to 30 amino acids from the amino terminus of each fragment can be determined through the use of commercially available automated "sequenators." Amino acid sequencing is often the first important step in the attempt to isolate the gene for a particular protein, because knowledge of the amino acid sequence of even a small portion of a protein provides information about the underlying nucleotide sequence of the corresponding portion of the gene encoding that protein. Knowledge of the nucleotide sequence can then be used to synthesize oligonucleotide probes to screen genomic or cDNA libraries for the clone of interest.

Large-Scale Production of Proteins

One of the first applications of gene cloning was the ability to produce potentially unlimited quantities of the proteins encoded by the cloned genes. Cloned cDNAs can be propagated in either *E. coli* or yeast and expressed under the control of an appropriate promoter. Large quantities of such proteins can then be purified from the bacterial or yeast cultures more easily and less expensively than they could previously from human sources. This ability has led to the growth of a number of biotechnology firms that are interested in producing medically useful proteins. Proteins such as coagulation factor VIII (for treatment of hemophilia), insulin (for treatment of diabetes), and growth hormone (for treatment of growth disorders), among others, are now being produced by these methods. Large quantities of gene products can also be produced for structural and functional studies of the proteins themselves in efforts to understand the molecular mechanism of action of individual gene products.

General References

Caskey CT (1987) Disease diagnosis by recombinant DNA methods. Science 236:1223–1229.

Fritsch EF, Maniatis T (1987) Methods of molecular genetics. *In* Stamatoyannopoulos G, Nienhuis AW, Leder P, Majerus PW (eds) The molecular basis of blood diseases. WB Saunders, Philadelphia, pp 1–27.

Landegren U, Kaiser R, Caskey CT, Hood L (1988) DNA diagnostics—Molecular techniques and automation. Science 242:229–237.

Sambrook J, Fritsch EF, Maniatis T (1989) Molecular cloning: A laboratory manual, 2nd ed. Cold Spring Harbor Laboratory, Cold Spring Harbor, NY.

White TJ, Arnheim N, Erlich HA (1989) The polymerase chain reaction. Trends Genet 5:185–189.

Problems

1. Consider the following diagnostic situations. What laboratory method or methods would be most appropriate?
   a) Prenatal diagnosis of a male fetus at risk for Duchenne muscular dystrophy (DMD). Previous studies in this family have already documented a complete gene deletion.
   b) You want to estimate the amount of dystrophin mRNA present in a muscle specimen from a mildly affected obligate carrier of DMD.
   c) You want to determine the cellular localization of dystrophin in muscle biopsies from two unaffected sisters of a DMD boy in order to assess whether they are carriers.
   d) Prenatal diagnosis of a male fetus at risk for DMD. Previous studies have already documented a particular nucleotide base change that is responsible for the defect of this family.

2. What are some of the advantages or disadvantages of the polymerase chain reaction for diagnosis of genetic defects in comparison with Southern blotting? With biochemical assays of enzyme levels to diagnose enzyme deficiencies?

3. From which of the following tissues can DNA be obtained for diagnostic procedures: tissue biopsies, white blood cells, cultured amniotic fluid cells, and red blood cells?

4. Why is cloning of a gene considered such a significant advance for the field of medical genetics? What does the availability of a cloned gene allow one to do that one could not do before?

5. You want to clone a gene that is expressed in liver and is suspected to be involved in a genetic disease. Both a human genomic DNA library and a liver cDNA library are available to you. Which would you choose and why?

CHAPTER
6

GENETIC VARIATION, POLYMORPHISM, AND MUTATION

This chapter is one of several in which we explore the nature of genetically determined differences between individuals. Although the basis of phenotypic differences can be either genetic changes encoded in the DNA or nongenetic differences in the environment, we deal in this chapter with genetic variation that is due to permanent differences between individuals in the nucleotide sequence of their genomes. Not all such changes in the DNA are necessarily deleterious. One of the important concepts of human and medical genetics is that genetic disease is only the most obvious, and often the most extreme, manifestation of genetic change, superimposed on a background of entirely normal genetic variability.

Many different proteins are synthesized in each cell of the body. These proteins include enzymes and structural components responsible for all the developmental and metabolic processes of an organism. As demonstrated in Chapter 3, the fundamental relationship between genes and proteins is that the coding sequence of bases in the DNA of a given gene specifies the sequence of amino acids in the corresponding polypeptide

chain. Hence a nucleotide change, or **mutation,** in a gene may lead to the formation of a variant protein, which may have altered properties as a consequence of its changed structure. Other DNA changes, however, may have no phenotypic effect, either because the change does not alter the primary amino acid sequence of a polypeptide or because the resulting change in the encoded amino acid sequence occurs in a noncritical region of the polypeptide. Not all variant proteins, therefore, have clinical consequences. On the contrary, many proteins normally exist in two or more relatively common, genetically distinct, and structurally different forms. Such a situation is known as **polymorphism.**

The phenotypic changes produced by gene mutations are considered in detail in Chapters 11 and 12. In this chapter, we examine first the origins of genetic variation at both the protein and DNA level, and the nature of mutations that have produced different versions of the genetic material. We then discuss the molecular basis for different types of mutation and their detection in the context of inherited disease.

MUTATION

A mutation is defined as any permanent change in DNA: that is, a change in the nucleotide sequence or arrangement of DNA in the genome. In broad terms, mutations can be classified into three categories: **genome mutations, chromosome mutations,** and **gene mutations,** as outlined in Table 6–1. All three types of mutation occur at appreciable frequencies and underlie not only all genetic or heritable disease but also many instances of cancer and much of what is recognized as "normal" variation.

Mutations can occur in any cell, both in germline cells and in somatic cells. Only germline mutations, however, can be perpetuated from one generation to the next and are thus the ones responsible for inherited disease. This is not to say, however, that somatic cell mutations are not medically important. Indeed, the vast majority of cell divisions that produce an adult organism of an estimated 10^{13} cells from a single-cell zygote occur in somatic lineages, and thus most mutations occur there. Somatic mutations in a number of genes can give rise to a significant proportion of cancers, as a result of any of the three types of mutation described earlier. In this sense, cancer is fundamentally a "genetic" disease, and mutations are central to its etiology or progression, as is presented in Chapter 16. Moreover, somatic mutation at the level of the genome, the chromosome, or the gene, which results in somatic mosaicism, is a well-documented cause of phenotypic variation (see Chapters 4 and 9).

The Origin of Mutation

Genome mutations, responsible for conditions such as trisomy 21 (Down syndrome) (Chapter 9), involve the missegregation of a chromosome pair during cell division. They are the most common human mutations (Table 6–1). The estimated rate of one missegregation event per 25 to 50 meiotic cell divisions derives from the observed incidence of chromosomally abnormal fetuses and liveborn infants, as described in Chapter 9. This is clearly a minimal estimate because the consequences of many such events may be lethal and may be spontaneously aborted shortly after conception. Chromosome mutations are estimated to be much less frequent than genome mutations, occurring at a rate of approximately one rearrangement per 1700 cell divisions. Although these frequencies may seem high, genome and chromosome mutations are rarely perpetuated because they are usually incompatible with survival or normal reproduction (see Chapter 7). Most significant heritable mutations occur as relatively minor changes at the level of the gene.

Gene mutations, including base-pair substitutions, insertions, and deletions (Fig. 6–1), can originate by either of two basic mechanisms: errors introduced during the normal process of DNA replication or base changes induced by mutagens. DNA replication (see Fig. 3–4) is normally a remarkably accurate process. Even if mutations were introduced only once in every million base pairs, the burden of mutation on the organism would be intolerable, and our species would cease to exist. In fact, the DNA replication machinery does considerably better than this. Through a combination of nucleotide selection and molecular "proofreading," the enzyme DNA polymerase faithfully duplicates the double helix, introducing an incorrect nucleotide into one of the growing daughter strands only once every 10 million base pairs (all this while moving along a human chromosome at a rate of about 20 base pairs per second). The vast majority of these errors are rapidly removed from the DNA and corrected by a series of DNA repair enzymes that first recognize which

Table 6–1. Types of Mutation and Their Estimated Frequencies

Class of Mutation	Mechanism	Frequency (Approximate)	Examples
Genome mutation	Chromosome missegregation	10^{-2}/cell division	Aneuploidy
Chromosome mutation	Chromosome rearrangement	6×10^{-4}/cell division	Translocations
Gene mutation	Base pair mutation	10^{-10}/base pair/cell division	Point mutations
		10^{-5}–10^{-6}/locus/generation	

Based on Vogel F, Motulsky AG (1986) Human genetics (2nd ed). Springer-Verlag, Berlin.

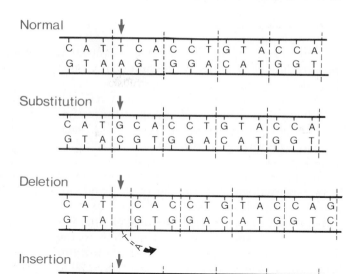

Figure 6–1. Examples of mutation. The first base of the second codon is mutated by a base substitution, deletion, or insertion. Both the single base-pair deletion and insertion lead to a frameshift mutation in which the translational reading frame is altered. See text for discussion.

strand in the newly synthesized double helix contains the incorrect base and then replace it with the proper complementary base. In all, more than 99.9 percent of errors of DNA replication are corrected in this manner. Thus the overall mutation rate as a result of replication errors is a remarkably low 10^{-10} per base pair per cell division. Because the human diploid genome contains approximately 6×10^9 base pairs of DNA, this mutation rate translates into less than one new base pair mutation introduced per cell division.

In addition to replication errors, DNA damage can be caused by spontaneous chemical processes such as depurination or deamination, by reaction with chemicals (natural or otherwise) in the environment, and by exposure to ultraviolet or ionizing radiation. In contrast to the proofreading and correction of replication-related DNA changes, many nucleotide changes introduced by mutagenesis remain as permanent mutations. One goal of current mutation research is to develop appropriate in vitro or in vivo tests to identify those substances that are the most significant in causing mutations responsible for both inherited disease and cancers.

As expected from the important role that DNA replication and repair enzymes play in mutation surveillance and prevention, inherited defects that alter the function of such enzymes can lead to a dramatic increase in the frequency of mutations of all types. Autosomal recessive disorders such as **xeroderma pigmentosum, ataxia telangiectasia, Fanconi anemia,** and **Bloom syndrome,** with documented or suspected defects in DNA repair or replication, are in fact characterized by a high frequency of both chromosome and gene mutations that are believed to underlie the predisposition of affected persons to cancer (see Chapters 9 and 16). There is some evidence that even people heterozygous for these disorders may have an increased chromosome or gene mutation rate.

The Frequency of New Mutations

The measurement of mutation rates at individual loci is presented later, but first it is worth considering the overall magnitude of the human mutational load. Given a frequency of 10^{-10} replication errors and an estimated 10^{15} cell divisions during the lifetime of an adult, replication errors result in thousands of new mutations at virtually every nucleotide position in the genome somewhere in the organism. Most mutations occur in somatic cells; depending on the nature of the mutation, its location in the genome, and the tissue involved, a given mutation may or may not lead to cancer or to phenotypic variation.

A small number of the new mutations occur in the germline, during any of the mitotic divisions that take place during spermatogenesis or oogenesis or during meiosis itself. As discussed in Chapter 2, both the number and timing of these divisions differ between the sexes. In oogenesis, each haploid ovum has gone through an estimated 22 mitotic divisions and one meiotic division; these occur only in fetal life and cease by the time of birth. Spermatogenesis, on the other hand, involves a continuous series of cell divisions throughout life, resulting in a total of approximately 1 billion spermatogonia. These cells are the result of about 30 mitotic divisions from the embryo stage to the time of puberty and about 20 to 25 division cycles per year thereafter. Thus each haploid sperm is the product of many hundreds of divisions, depending on age. Consequently, one might expect that the frequency of paternal new mutations is age-dependent and that certain kinds of new mutation in genetic disease are more often of paternal, rather than maternal, origin. In fact, this has been observed for some disorders, notably in neurofibromatosis (NF1), achondroplasia, and hemophilia A (when the maternal grandfather is the source of a new mutation). However, not all disorders appear to show this effect.

New germline mutations, although relatively rare, occur in what may seem like strikingly high numbers. Each sperm produced by a man 25 to 30 years old contains an estimated 100 new base pair combinations, as a result of DNA replication errors. Thus a normal ejaculate, containing approximately 100 million sperm, contains about 10 billion new mutations! Each base pair in the genome is mutated at least once in every ejaculate. According to calculated rates of deleterious mutations at individual loci (to be discussed), *approximately 1 in 10 sperm carries a new deleterious mutation.* Fortunately, most of these mutations are recessive (or lethal) and thus are not phenotypically apparent in a resulting conception and birth.

Estimates of Gene Mutation Rates

The mutation rate of a gene is usually expressed as the number of new mutations per locus per generation. The most direct way of estimating the rate is to measure the incidence of new, sporadic cases of an autosomal dominant or X-linked genetic disease that presents with a clearly recognizable phenotype at birth or shortly thereafter. **Achondroplasia** (see box, Chapter 4) is one such disease that meets most of the requirements for directly estimating a mutation rate. In one study, 10 achondroplastic children were born in a series of 94,075 consecutive births. Of the 10 affected children, 8 were born to parents of normal stature, and because achondroplasia is fully penetrant, these 8 cases were considered to represent new mutations. Assuming that the diagnoses were accurate and that a single locus is responsible for achondroplasia (a point that has not yet been firmly established), the new mutation rate can be calculated as eight new mutations of a total of $2 \times 94,073$ alleles, or approximately 4×10^{-5} mutations per locus per generation.

The mutation rate has been estimated for a number of inherited disorders, as shown in Table 6–2. The median gene mutation rate is approximately 1×10^{-6} mutations per locus per generation, but these mutation rates vary over a thou-

Table 6–2. Estimates of Mutation Rates for Selected Human Genes

Gene	Inheritance	Mutation Rate*	New Mutations per 10^6 Gametes
Achondroplasia	AD	$0.6–4 \times 10^{-5}$	6–40
Aniridia	AD	$2.5–5 \times 10^{-6}$	2.5–5
Duchenne muscular dystrophy	XR	$0.4–1 \times 10^{-4}$	43–105
Hemophilia A	XR	$3–6 \times 10^{-5}$	32–57
Hemophilia B	XR	$2–3 \times 10^{-6}$	2–3
Neurofibromatosis, type 1	AD	$0.4–1 \times 10^{-4}$	44–100
Polycystic kidney disease	AD	$0.6–1.2 \times 10^{-4}$	60–120
Retinoblastoma	AD	$5–12 \times 10^{-6}$	5–12

Based on data in Vogel F, Motulsky AG (1986) Human genetics (2nd ed). Springer-Verlag, Berlin.
AD = autosomal dominant; XR = X-linked recessive.
* Expressed as mutations/locus/generation.

sandfold range, from 10^{-4} to 10^{-7} mutations per locus per generation. The basis for these differences may be related to gene size or to the presence or absence of mutational "hot spots" in the genome. The Duchenne muscular dystrophy (DMD) locus is the largest yet described, estimated at over 2000 in in length; thus it is not surprising that the mutation rate measured at the DMD locus is quite high. The estimates in Table 6–2 reflect measurements made of very visible and deleterious mutations; less severe mutations or less phenotypically obvious mutations would have escaped detection, as would have more severe, lethal mutations. Thus the overall new mutation rate may be considerably higher.

New mutations have also been looked for by examining blood serum proteins by electrophoresis to separate polypeptides on the basis of charge and size. The appearance in a child of a new electrophoretic variant that is not present in either parent suggests a gene mutation that altered either the charge or the size of the encoded protein. Such variants are detected at a frequency of approximately 2×10^{-6} per locus per generation (Neel, 1983). Because only about one third of all amino acid changes would result in a charge change in the resulting polypeptide, the overall rate of new mutation determined by this approach, which is independent of the severity of the mutation, can be estimated to be as high as 6×10^{-6} per locus per generation.

Despite the limitations of these and other approaches for determining the average gene mutation rate, all methods yield essentially the same range of values for germline mutation rates: approximately 10^{-5} to 10^{-6} per locus per generation. Because there are about 50,000 to 100,000 genes in the genome, this suggests that *at least 1 in 10 people is likely to have received a newly mutated gene from one or the other parent.*

GENETIC DIVERSITY AMONG INDIVIDUALS

Most of the estimates of mutation rates just described involve detection of deleterious mutations with an obvious effect on phenotype. Many mutations, however, are not deleterious but are thought to be selectively neutral. On the basis of information presented earlier in this chapter, each new zygote would be expected to contain 100 or so new base pair combinations not present in the genome of either parent. Most of this variation is not confined to coding sequences but is found in extragenic sequences or in noncoding, heterochromatic regions of the chromosomes. Over the course of evolution, the steady influx of new nucleotide variation has ensured a high degree of genetic diversity and individuality. This theme extends through all fields in human and medical genetics; genetic diversity may manifest as changes in the staining pattern of chromosomes, as protein variation, or as nucleotide changes in DNA.

Chromosomal Heteromorphisms

In general, the karyotypes of normal persons of the same sex are quite similar. However, one can detect occasional variants in chromosome morphology or staining, called **heteromorphisms,** that reflect differences in the amount or type of DNA sequences at a particular location along a chromosome. Normal homologs can differ in size by many millions of base pairs (Trask et al., 1989), probably as a result of differences in the amount of heterochromatic DNA sequences. The most obvious examples of heteromorphism involve the heterochromatic regions of the Y chromosome long arm and the pericentromeric regions of chromosomes 1, 9, and 16. Such variants can be detected easily with many of the staining techniques discussed in Chapter 2, including C banding, G banding, and Q banding. Other heterochromatic regions also show variation, including the short arms of the acrocentric chromosomes and the centromeric region of many chromosomes (Fig. 6–2). Advances in molecular cytogenetics have increased the frequency with which heteromorphisms are detected, by using either specific DNA probes for heteromorphic satellite DNA sequences or restriction enzyme treatment of metaphase chromosomes (Miller et al., 1983) to reveal underlying differences in satellite sequences.

Protein Variation

Because of the degeneracy of the genetic code (see Table 3–3), not all nucleotide changes that occur

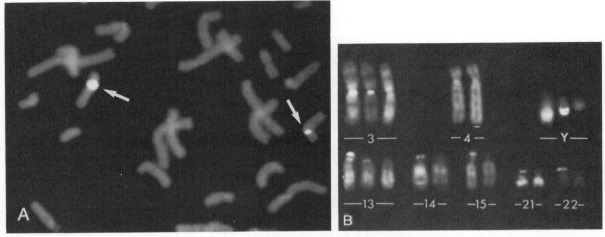

Figure 6-2. Examples of chromosomal heteromorphisms. *A,* Heteromorphism involving the centromeric region of chromosome 17, detected by a molecular cytogenetic assay. (Courtesy of V. E. Powers, Stanford University.) *B,* Chromosomes stained by Q banding, showing differences in intensity of fluorescent bands among homologs. (From Hirschhorn K [1987]. Chromosomes and their abnormalities. *In* Behrman RE, Vaughan VC [eds] Nelson Textbook of Pediatics, 13th ed. WB Saunders, Philadelphia, p. 250.)

in a gene lead to a structural change in the encoded polypeptide. About 25 percent of all mutations continue to encode the same amino acid and are thus called **"silent" mutations.** Other mutations that do alter the amino acid sequence may have only a subtle effect on the overall three-dimensional structure and function of a protein. These changes are unlikely to have a phenotypic effect. Furthermore, not all mutations that have demonstrable and recognizable effects on the protein necessarily influence the survival or fitness of the individual. Mutations of these latter two types result, therefore, in the occurrence of more than one version of a particular protein in a population.

The first instances of genetically determined protein variation were detected on antigens found in blood, the so-called **blood group antigens.** The now well-known variation at the ABO blood group locus on chromosome 9 was discovered by Landsteiner in 1900 through simple serological methods. Although for many years it was not clear whether examples such as this represented special and unusual forms of variation not typical of enzymes or proteins in general, subsequent studies clearly documented that protein variation in humans is a phenomenon that is much more common than had previously been suspected (Harris, 1980).

The Concept of Genetic Polymorphism

Many loci are characterized by a number of relatively common alleles that allow members of a naturally occurring population to be categorized into sharply distinct phenotypes. **Genetic polymorphism** is defined as the occurrence of multiple alleles at a locus, where at least two alleles appear with frequencies greater than 1 percent. By convention, then, **polymorphic loci** are those at which at least 2 percent of the population are heterozygous. However, because many polymorphic loci are characterized by a large number of different alleles, the proportion of heterozygotes at some loci is much greater. Again by convention, alleles with frequencies of less than 1 percent are called **rare variants.** As discussed further, most (but not all) deleterious mutations that lead to genetic disease are of this latter, rare class.

Over the years, a large number of different human enzymes and other proteins have been screened for electrophoretic variants in different populations. Of all loci tested, about one third have been found to exhibit detectable polymorphism in at least one major ethnic or racial group and often in all major population groups (Harris, 1980; Cavalli-Sforza and Bodmer, 1971).

USES OF POLYMORPHISMS IN MEDICAL GENETICS

The existence of different versions of the same genetic material in different people is more than a curiosity of interest only to the human geneticist. Polymorphisms are principally of value for their use as genetic "markers" to distinguish different inherited forms of a gene in family studies. As illustrated in subsequent chapters, genetic markers are of enormous practical use in medical genetics for:

• Mapping genes to individual chromosomes by linkage analysis.

• Presymptomatic and prenatal diagnosis of genetic disease.
• Detection of heterozygous carriers of genetic disease.
• Evaluation of high- and low-risk persons with a predisposition to common adult disorders, such as coronary heart disease, cancer, and diabetes.
• Paternity testing and forensic applications.
• Matching of donor-recipient pairs for tissue and organ transplantation.

The widespread occurrence of genetic polymorphism implies that any individual is likely to be heterozygous at many different gene loci. What is the proportion of loci in a given individual at which there will be two different alleles, each specifying a structurally distinct form of the gene product? It has been estimated from surveys of many enzymes that any individual is likely to be heterozygous at approximately 6 percent of enzyme-encoding loci. Correcting for the lack of detection of electrophoretically silent mutations, one can estimate that any individual is likely to be heterozygous for alleles determining structurally different polypeptides at approximately 12 to 18 percent of all loci. This figure is sometimes called the **average heterozygosity,** and it underscores the striking degree of biochemical individuality that exists within the human species.

Blood Groups and Their Polymorphisms

Numerous polymorphisms are known to exist in the components of human blood, especially in the antigens of red blood cells (Table 6–3). These markers illustrate many of the general principles of polymorphism. Red blood cell antigens have been useful genetic markers in family population studies and in linkage analyses because of their ready classification into different phenotypes,

their simple mode of inheritance, and their different frequencies in different populations. For many years, until the description and widespread use of DNA polymorphisms in the late 1970s, the blood group polymorphisms were, along with protein polymorphisms revealed by electrophoresis and cytogenetic heteromorphisms, among the few genetic markers available for genetic linkage analysis and family studies of inherited disease. Some human blood groups, particularly the ABO and Rh systems, are important in blood transfusion, tissue and organ transplantation, and the treatment of hemolytic disease of the newborn.

The ABO System

Landsteiner and colleagues found that human blood can be assigned to one of four types according to the presence of two antigens, A and B, on the

Table 6–3. Selected Examples of Polymorphic Antigens Identified on Red Blood Cells

Polymorphic System	Chromosomal Location	Common Alleles
ABO	9q34	*A, B,* and *O*
MNSs (glycophorin A, B)	4q28–31	*M* and *N; S* and *s*
Secretor (fucosyl-transferase)	19q	*Se* and *se*
Rh	1p34–36	See Table 6–4
Xg	Xp22.3	*Xg^a* and *Xg*

surface of red blood cells and the presence of the two corresponding antibodies, anti-A and anti-B, in the plasma.

There are four major phenotypes: O, A, B, and AB. Type A subjects have antigen A on their red blood cells, type B subjects have antigen B, type AB subjects have both antigens A and B, and type O subjects have neither. Thus the reaction of the red cells of each type with anti-A and anti-B is as follows:

Red Cell Phenotype	Reaction With		Antibodies in Serum
	Anti-A	*Anti-B*	
O	−	−	Anti-A, anti-B
A	+	−	Anti-B
B	−	+	Anti-A
AB	+	+	Neither

− represents no agglutination; + represents agglutination.

One feature of the ABO groups not shared by other blood group systems is the reciprocal relationship, in an individual, between the antigens present on the red blood cells and the antibodies in the serum. When the red blood cells lack antigen A, the serum contains anti-A; when the cells lack antigen B, the serum contains anti-B. The reason for this reciprocal relationship is uncertain, but formation of anti-A and anti-B is thought to be a response to the natural occurrence of A and B antigens in the environment (for example, in bacteria).

The primary importance of the ABO blood groups is in transfusion and transplantation. In the ABO blood group system, there are compatible and incompatible combinations, a compatible combination being one in which the red blood cells of a donor do not carry an A or a B antigen that corresponds to the antibodies in the recipient's serum. Although theoretically there are universal donors (group O) and universal recipients (group AB), a patient is given blood of his or her own ABO group, except in emergencies. The regular presence of anti-A and anti-B explains the failure of many of the early attempts to transfuse blood, because these antibodies can cause immediate destruction of ABO-incompatible cells. In tissue and organ transplantation, ABO compatibility of donor and recipient, as well as human leukocyte

antigen (HLA) compatibility (described in Chapter 14), is essential to graft survival.

Genetics of ABO. The ABO blood groups are determined by a locus on chromosome 9. The *A*, *B*, and *O* alleles at this locus are a classic example of multiallelism, in which three alleles, of which two are codominant and the third is recessive, determine four phenotypes. Because the relative proportions of the O, A, B, and AB types differ in different populations, frequency figures are valid only for the population from which they are derived, a point to which we shall return in Chapter 7. The following figures serve as an illustration:

Blood Type Genotype(s)	O *O/O*	A *A/A* or *A/O*	B *B/B* or *B/O*	AB *A/B*
Frequency				
W. European	.46	.42	.09	.03
African	.50	.29	.17	.04
Oriental	.30	.35	.23	.13

Genetic Pathways of A and B Antigen Synthesis. The A and B antigens are made by the action of the *A* and *B* alleles on a protein called H antigen (Watkins, 1980). In basic structure the A, B, and H antigens are complex glycosphingolipids embedded in the red blood cell membrane, with a core to which many sugar chains are attached (Fig. 6–3). The antigenic specificity is conferred by the terminal sugars. The enzymes (glycosyltransferases) that add the sugars to the core sphingolipids and glycoproteins are the direct products of the H and ABO genes. The relationship among the blood group genes, their products, and the red blood cell antigens is shown schematically in Figure 6–4.

The familiar genetically determined variation in ABO blood types is determined by allelic differences at the ABO locus. The *B* allele codes for a glycosyltransferase that preferentially recognizes the sugar D-galactose and adds it to the H substance. The *A* allele codes for a slightly different form of the enzyme that preferentially recognizes *N*-acetylgalactosamine instead of D-galactose and adds this to the precursor, thereby creating the A antigen. A third allele, *O*, codes for a version of the transferase that does not detectably affect H substance at all. The molecular differences in the glycosyltransferase gene that are responsible for the *A, B,* and *O* alleles have been determined (Yama-

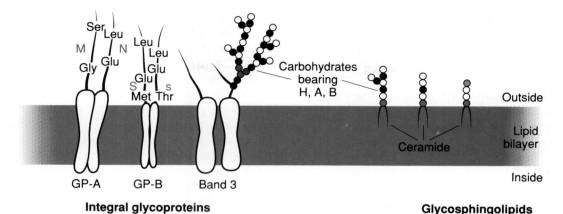

Integral glycoproteins   **Glycosphingolipids**

Figure 6-3. Diagram of the red cell membrane, showing the molecules that bear the antigens of the ABO and MNSs systems. The specificities H, A, and B are determined by different terminal sugars, not shown here. Amino acid differences that distinguish the *M* and *N* alleles or the *S* and *s* alleles at the GP-A and GP-B loci, respectively, are indicated. (Redrawn from Giblett ER [1983]. Erythrocyte antigens and antibodies. *In* Williams WJ, Beutler E, Erslev AJ, Lichtman MA: Hematology, 3rd ed. McGraw-Hill, New York, pp. 1491–1505.)

moto et al., 1990). Four nucleotide sequence differences are found between the *A* and *B* alleles. The *O* allele has a single base-pair deletion in the ABO gene coding region, which indicates that the lack of transferase activity in type O individuals is due to a frameshift mutation (to be described). Now that the DNA sequences are available, it is likely that ABO blood group typing will be performed directly at the genotype, rather than phenotype, level.

The Rh System

The Rh system ranks with the ABO system in clinical importance because of its role in hemolytic disease of the newborn and in transfusion incompatibilities. The name comes from Rhesus monkeys, which were used in the experiments that led to the discovery of the system. At the simplest level of explanation, the population is divided into Rh-positive individuals, who are either homozygous or heterozygous for a gene that specifies an antigen, and Rh-negative individuals who lack the antigen.

The Rh locus (or series of loci) is on chromosome 1. There is still controversy over the precise genetic interpretation of this system, which may be either a group of closely linked genes, each with a series of alleles, or a single locus with multiple alleles that determine the amino acid sequence of a

Figure 6-4. Diagram of the pathways of biosynthesis of the H, A, and B antigens. Alleles *h* and *O* have no detectable effect.

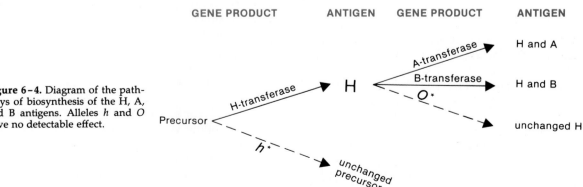

component of the red blood cell membrane. Each allele specifies a polypeptide with multiple antigenic sites, perhaps representing amino acid differences at more than one site in a single chain. The gene for one of the Rh polypeptides has been cloned (Cherif-Zahar et al., 1990), and the molecular elucidation of this complex polymorphic system should be forthcoming.

The Rh alleles determine at least eight antigenic combinations, shown in Table 6–4 with their frequencies in three selected populations. It is notable that each population has a different spectrum of common alleles. In addition, there are a number of instructive rare Rh variants. One is the Rh-null (Rh⁰) phenotype, in which the red blood cells lack all Rh antigens. Rh⁰ individuals have a form of autosomal recessive hemolytic anemia, a consequence that suggests that the Rh antigens are an essential part of the normal red blood cell membrane.

Clinically, the chief significance of the Rh system is that Rh-negative persons (genotype usually r/r) can readily form anti-Rh antibodies after exposure to Rh-positive red blood cells. When Rh-negative girls and women of childbearing age require transfusions, they must be given only Rh-negative blood. In pregnant Rh-negative women, the risk of immunization by Rh-positive fetal red blood cells can be minimized with injections of Rh immune globulin during and after pregnancy or after termination of pregnancy.

Hemolytic Disease of the Newborn. The discovery of the Rh system and its role in hemolytic disease of the newborn (HDN) has been a major contribution of genetics to medicine. At one time ranking as the most common human genetic disease, HDN is now relatively rare because Rh immune globulin usually prevents its development. In HDN, the life span of the fetal red blood cells is shortened by the action of antibodies formed by the mother against antigens of the fetus. Normally during pregnancy, small amounts of fetal blood cross the placental barrier and reach the maternal blood stream, where they may stimulate the mother to form antibodies, which return to the fetal circulation, damaging the fetal red blood cells, with consequences that can be severe if not treated.

There are two main types of HDN: one due to Rh incompatibility, when the mother is Rh-negative and the fetus is Rh-positive, and the other due to ABO incompatibility, when the mother is type O and the fetus is type A or B. Most cases of HDN recognized clinically are due to Rh incompatibility; ABO incompatibility is difficult to diagnose but tends to be mild and to require no treatment.

The MNSs System: Polymorphism of the Glycophorin Genes

The A and B glycophorins are two major glycoproteins of the red cell membrane. Polymorphisms at the glycophorin A and B loci determine the MN and Ss blood group systems, respectively. The MN system (unrelated to the ABO blood group system) was discovered when Landsteiner and Levine injected human blood into rabbits and found that the immune serum formed by the rabbits could be used to distinguish between human red cell samples. This polymorphism involves a pair of codominant alleles, M and N, which produce three genotypes, M/M, M/N, and N/N, and three corresponding phenotypes, M, MN, and N. The different antigenic specificities in the MN system result, not from terminal sugars as in the ABO system, but from differences in the amino acid sequence of the encoded glycophorin A molecules (Fig. 6–3). The products of the M and N alleles at the glycophorin A locus differ in two amino acids.

The Ss subdivisions of the MN groups are also based on the response of different red blood cell samples to an antiserum, in this case one that detects allelic differences in glycophorin B molecules

Table 6–4. Major Alleles of the Rh Blood Group System

	Allele Frequencies		
Allele	*W. Europe*	*Africa*	*Asia*
R^1	.45	.10	.55
r	.37	.15	.10
R^2	.14	.10	.35
R^0	.02	.60	<.01
r''	.01	<.01	<.01
r'	.01	<.01	<.01
R^z and r^V	<.01	<.01	<.01

Data from Giblett ER (1983). Erythrocyte antigens and antibodies. *In* Williams WJ, Beutter E, Erslev AJ, Lichtman MA (eds) Hematology, 3rd ed. McGraw-Hill, New York, pp. 1491–1505.

on the red blood cell surface (Fig. 6–3). There is a single amino acid difference between the products of the two alleles, *S* and *s*, at the glycophorin B locus. The combinations of alleles at the glycophorin A and B loci are called **haplotypes,** defined as the genotypes from two or more separate loci, close together on a chromosome. In this case, the four haplotypes—*MS, NS, Ms,* and *Ns*—are inherited as units because the genes for glycophorins A and B are very closely linked on chromosome 4. The significance and application of haplotypes for genetic analysis in families segregating for genetic diseases are discussed further in Chapter 8.

The major significance of the MNSs blood group polymorphism in medical genetics is that the relative frequencies of the alleles and the codominant pattern of their inheritance make them useful genetic markers. Because of the simple relationships between genotype and phenotype, the MNSs system is often used to illustrate basic genetic principles, and it is used for this purpose in determining gene frequencies in Chapter 7.

Genetic Polymorphism as a Universal Concept

Although first discovered in blood groups, polymorphism is a widespread and universal phenomenon that has been documented at many loci, encoding many different types of protein products. Mutant alleles that lead to severe genetic disease are often only the most obvious form of genetic diversity; on examination, many proteins have been found to exist in different populations in several relatively common, distinguishable forms. Some of these polymorphic alleles are clinically significant, either individually or in combination with a rare deleterious allele.

Genetic Variation at the Galactosemia Locus

Galactosemia results from the inability to metabolize galactose, a monosaccharide that is a component of lactose (milk sugar). People with this autosomal recessive disease completely lack the enzyme galactose-1-phosphate uridyltransferase (GALT), which normally catalyzes the conversion of galactose-1-phosphate to uridine diphospho-

galactose. Infants with galactosemia are usually normal at birth but begin to develop gastrointestinal problems, cirrhosis of the liver, and cataracts in the weeks after they are given milk. If not recognized, galactosemia causes severe mental retardation and is often fatal. Complete removal of milk from the diet, however, can protect against most of the harmful consequences of GALT deficiency.

Affected infants are homozygous at the GALT locus for a rare mutant allele (*g*) with a frequency of approximately 0.5 percent. (Actually, at the molecular level, alleles that cause galactosemia are heterogeneous, although the exact number and frequency of *g* alleles remains to be determined [Reichardt and Woo, 1991].) There are also a number of other variant alleles, identified either electrophoretically or by reduced GALT activity, that alone or in combination with a galactosemia allele can also have clinical consequences. At least two of these variant alleles are polymorphic: the Duarte allele (*D*), a variant with only about 50 percent normal activity that has an allele frequency of about 5 percent; and the Los Angeles allele (*LA*), with an allele frequency of about 1 to 2 percent, which actually encodes a gene product with greater than usual enzyme activity (approximately 140 percent). A number of other allelic variants, whose frequencies have been less well established, have also been described; their GALT activities range from approximately 5 to 45 percent of normal. With regard to the three most readily identifiable variant alleles and the "normal" (*G*) allele, the approximate frequencies, enzyme activities, and phenotypes of various genotypes are listed in Table 6–5. An important concept to emerge from the data in the table is that clinically

Table 6–5. Selected Genotypes and Phenotypes at the Galactose-1-Phosphate Uridyltransferase Locus

Genotype	Frequency (%)	Enzyme Activity (%)	Phenotype
G/G	87.4	100	Normal
G/D	7.5	75	Normal
G/LA	3.7	120	Normal
G/g	0.9	50	Normal
D/D	0.16	50	Normal
D/LA	0.16	95	Normal
LA/LA	0.04	140	Normal
D/g	0.04	25	Borderline
LA/g	0.02	70	Normal
g/g	0.0025	<5	Galactosemia

For abbreviations, see text.

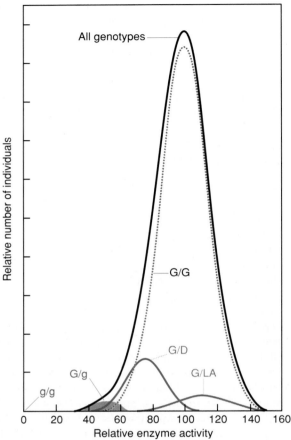

Figure 6-5. Population distribution of "normal" GALT activity. Major subgroups of individuals with different genotypes are indicated by separate curves. Total population distribution for GALT activity is indicated by the solid black curve, with a population average of 100 percent activity. Distributions based on data in Table 6-5.

normal persons do not necessarily have exactly the same "normal" level of GALT activity. Depending on their genotype at this locus, their enzyme levels may vary over a two- to threefold range (Fig. 6-5).

Genetic Variation of Alpha$_1$-Antitrypsin

Alpha$_1$-antitrypsin (α_1-AT) is a major serum protein that inhibits the activity of a number of specific proteolytic enzymes, such as trypsin, chymotrypsin, and pancreatic elastase. Its major target is leukocyte elastase, an enzyme that, if not inactivated by α_1-AT, destroys lung connective tissue proteins, particularly elastin, leading to alveolar wall damage in the lung. The gene for α_1-AT, known as the PI (protease inhibitor) locus, is on chromosome 14 and is highly polymorphic: there are several relatively common alleles (frequencies of 10 to 75 percent in different populations) and 25 or so rare alleles (Table 6-6). The three most common alleles (*M1*, *M2*, and *M3*) each encode a structurally different version of a functionally normal protein, as do at least some of the rare alleles. Other alleles give rise to α_1-AT molecules with significantly reduced protease inhibitor activity, several of which are clinically significant.

The principal medical significance of α_1-AT polymorphisms lies in alleles whose product is deficient in α_1-AT activity. The most common and important of these is the Z allele, which has a frequency of 1 to 2 percent in Caucasian populations. People with the Z/Z genotype have less than 15 percent of the normal plasma concentration of

Table 6-6. Selected Alleles at the Alpha$_1$-Antitrypsin Locus in Different Populations

Population	Allele Frequencies					
	M1	*M2*	*M3*	*S**	*Z**	*Other*
U.S. Caucasians	.724	.137	.095	.023	.014	.007
U.S. Blacks	.982	—	—	.015	.004	—
Denmark	.728	.136	.082	.022	.023	.009
Portugal	.510	.260	.053	.150	.009	.018
Japan	.786	.153	.062	—	—	—

Based on electrophoretic studies summarized by Cox DW (1989) α_1-Antitrypsin deficiency. In Scriver CR, Beaudet AL, Sly WS, Valle D (eds) The metabolic basis of inherited disease, 6th ed. McGraw-Hill, New York, pp. 2409-2437.
* The *S* and *Z* alleles encode products with reduced activity, ~60% and ~15% of normal, respectively.

SIGNIFICANCE OF PROTEIN POLYMORPHISM

An important concept to emerge from the many examples of genetic variation and polymorphism is the considerable degree of individual diversity that must exist among the members of a population in their makeup of enzymes and other gene products. Because the distinct genotypes that reflect each of the thousands of polymorphisms that exist are inherited more or less independently of each other, it should be clear that a nearly infinite combination of genotypes (and thus phenotypes) must exist. Because the products of many of the encoded metabolic pathways interact, one may plausibly conclude that each individual, regardless of his or her state of health, has a unique, genetically determined chemical makeup and thus responds in a unique manner to environmental, dietary, and pharmacological influences. Awareness of this individuality is a cornerstone of the genetic approach to medicine.

α_1-AT and have a high risk of obstructive lung disease in early adult life, as discussed in detail in Chapter 12. α_1-AT deficiency is seen at a frequency of 1/2000 to 1/8000 in Caucasian populations, but only rarely in Black or Asian populations.

As seen also with respect to variation at the GALT locus, genetic polymorphism at the PI locus leads to a severalfold variation in α_1-AT activity among apparently "normal" persons. Some of this variation may be highly significant from a public health standpoint because there is a suggestion of predisposition to a number of disorders, such as lung disease (particularly in smokers), asthma, and rheumatoid arthritis (as well as other immune disorders) among people heterozygous for either the Z or the S allele (estimated at approximately 3 to 5 percent of Caucasian populations).

INHERITED VARIATION AND POLYMORPHISM AT THE DNA LEVEL

The previous sections concentrated on mutations and polymorphism in portions of the genome encoding proteins, an estimated 5 percent of the total genomic DNA. What about genetic diversity in the remaining 95 percent of DNA? Estimates are that any two copies of the human genome differ at 1/100 to 1/500 of all nucleotide positions. Thus if one could directly compare the nucleotide sequence of an individual's paternally and maternally derived haploid genomes, there would be more than 10 million differences, the accumulation of mutations over the course of human evolution.

From a number of large surveys in which cloned DNA probes (described in the previous chapter) were used, the total proportion of polymorphic base positions (also called the **DNA heterozygosity index**) has been estimated to be about 1 in 270 base pairs for any randomly chosen piece of DNA in the genome (Cooper et al., 1985). This figure is about ten times higher than the proportion of heterozygous nucleotides estimated for protein-coding regions of the genome (about 1 in 2500 base pairs). The difference is not altogether surprising, for it seems intuitively likely that protein-coding regions are under more rigid selective pressure, and thus the incidence of mutations in those regions throughout evolution should be lower.

We have presented the remarkable degree of DNA variation in the genome among different individuals in a population without considering how these estimates were derived or how this variation is detected. In practice, the most commonly used approach to screen for DNA variation is to use the Southern blotting procedure to examine restriction enzyme sites in a particular region of DNA, with cloned DNA probes. The major virtue of this technique, which has revolutionized human and medical genetics in a way not seen since the original application of electrophoresis to protein analysis in the late 1940s and the 1950s, is to allow visualization of a single small fragment of genomic DNA among the millions of other fragments in the genome (see Chapter 5).

Restriction Fragment Length Polymorphisms

Soon after the application of Southern blotting to genome analysis in the late 1970s, it was discovered that not all people have exactly the same distribution of restriction enzyme sites (Lawn et al., 1978; Jeffreys, 1979; Kan and Dozy, 1978). Although the existence of some nucleotide variation could be predicted by what was known about mutation and protein polymorphisms, the degree of variation as detected by Southern blotting came as a surprise.

Because restriction enzymes have specific recognition sequences in DNA, sequence changes in genomic DNA that are due to either inherited or new mutation will lead to the creation or abolition of particular cleavage sites, thereby altering the size of one or more DNA fragments apparent after Southern blotting and hybridization to a cloned

DNA probe (Fig. 6–6). Because several hundred restriction enzymes are available for detecting a wide variety of four to eight base-pair recognition sequences, this method allows extensive examination of the nucleotide sequence in the immediate vicinity of a given cloned DNA probe. DNA-based variations at restriction sites detected in this manner are called **restriction fragment length polymorphisms** (RFLPs; Botstein et al., 1980). The different fragment lengths constitute codominant alleles at a DNA locus. Thus one can easily examine a Southern blot and read off the different fragment lengths directly as a reflection of the genotype (the DNA sequence) at a particular restriction site (Fig. 6–7). RFLPs may also arise from deletion or insertion of DNA, rather than from single nucleotide changes. If a segment of DNA between two restriction sites is deleted or inserted, the size of the resulting restriction fragment is different (Fig. 6–6).

The discovery of DNA polymorphisms has greatly increased the extent to which individual copies of particular genes are recognized as being truly unique. However, conceptually, DNA polymorphisms are nothing new; they are simply the molecular manifestation of variation in the ge-

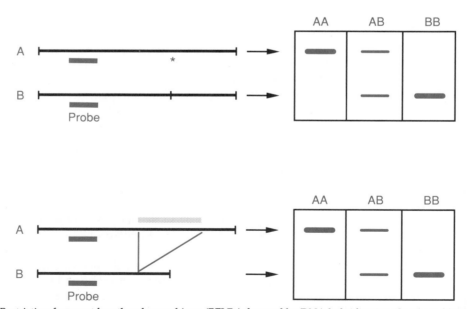

Figure 6–6. Restriction fragment length polymorphisms (RFLPs) detected by DNA hybridization (Southern blotting). At the top, polymorphism is due to variation at a specific cleavage site for a restriction enzyme; in the *A* allele, the site is absent (asterisk), and the resulting restriction fragment detected by the probe is larger than in the *B* allele. At the bottom, polymorphism is due to insertion or deletion of a DNA segment (grey bar) within a particular restriction fragment detected by the probe. For both types of polymorphism, Southern blotting patterns observed in DNA from persons with the three possible genotypes at this locus are indicated.

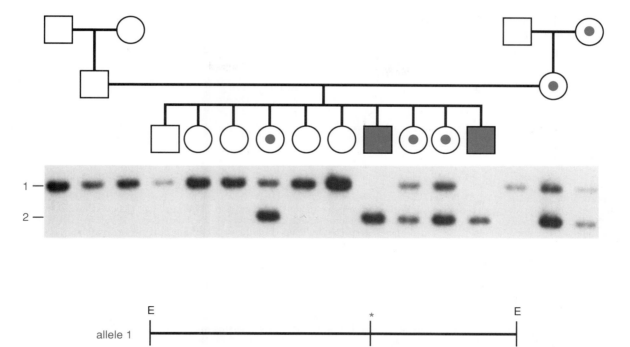

Figure 6–7. Codominant inheritance of an X-linked RFLP. Alleles 1 and 2 differ by variation at a recognition site for the restriction enzyme EcoRI (E). Red symbols indicate inheritance of allele 2.

nome that has long been apparent from the study of protein polymorphisms.

As an illustration, consider again variation at the α_1-AT locus. As discussed earlier and presented in Table 6–6, extensive polymorphism has been documented at the protein level in population studies and in studies of patients with inherited α_1-AT deficiency. A similar degree of sequence variation is indicated from analysis of DNA at the α_1-AT locus. Figure 6–8 depicts the structure of the α_1-AT gene, including the positions and frequencies of some of the most common sites of DNA variation, some first identified as RFLPs, some as pathological mutations, and some as benign protein polymorphisms. It is worth noting in Figure 6–8 that the mutations responsible for RFLPs are conceptually identical to those responsible for the pathological Z and S alleles seen in cases of α_1-AT deficiency or to that responsible for the M3 allele detected by protein electrophore-

sis in 10 to 20 percent of people. The only differences among the three types of polymorphism lie in their allelic frequencies, the methods of ascertaining and detecting them, and their pathological consequences, if any.

VNTR Polymorphisms

As mentioned earlier, some DNA polymorphisms are based on the insertion or deletion of DNA, rather than on nucleotide changes. A special class of insertion/deletion polymorphism, first described by Wyman and White (1980), consists of a series of allelic fragment lengths, related to each other by a variable number of tandem repeated DNA sequences (VNTRs) in the interval between two restriction sites. This class of RFLPs has been called "hypervariable," because such loci are characterized by many alleles (Fig. 6–9). The most in-

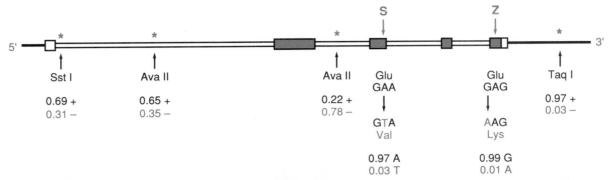

Figure 6–8. Schematic of the α_1-AT gene, its mutations and its DNA polymorphisms. Exons are boxed. Asterisks indicate sites of selected DNA polymorphisms detected with the indicated restriction enzymes (*Sst*I, *Ava*II, or *Taq*I). Frequencies below each polymorphic site indicate frequencies of Caucasian chromosomes that are cleaved (+) or not cleaved (−) at that site. Red S and Z indicate sites of mutations in the S and Z alleles, respectively. DNA mutations and amino acid substitutions are indicated. Frequencies of bases at these polymorphic sites are also indicated.

formative markers have up to several dozen or more alleles, and so no two unrelated individuals are likely to share the same alleles. VNTR markers are highly informative for genetic linkage analyses (see Chapter 8), as well as for individual identification (forensics and paternity testing).

RFLPs of both the two-allele and the VNTR classes have greatly increased the number of polymorphic markers available to examine genetic diversity among individuals and to follow the segregation of different portions of the genome through

families. Several thousand such DNA polymorphisms located thoughout all of the different chromosomes have now been described (Kidd et al., 1989; Williamson et al., 1990).

DNA Fingerprinting

The DNA polymorphisms just described are found through the use of a particular single-copy DNA probe to examine a *unique locus* in the genome.

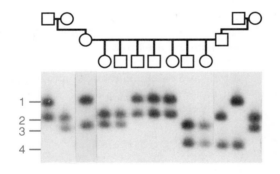

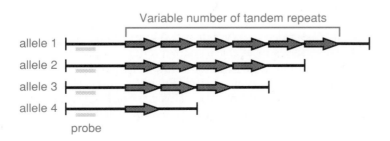

Figure 6–9. Codominant inheritance of a hypervariable autosomal DNA polymorphism caused by a variable number of tandem repeats (VNTR). Alleles 1 to 4 are related to each other by a variable number of identical (or nearly so), short DNA sequences (arrows). Size variation can be detected after restriction enzyme digestion and hybridization with a unique probe that lies outside of the VNTR sequences themselves but inside the restriction sites used to define the allelic fragments. (Original photograph courtesy of A. Bowcock, Stanford University.)

However, Jeffreys discovered in 1985 that the repeated sequences found in many different VNTR-type polymorphisms were sufficiently similar to permit detection of *many loci* simultaneously (Jeffreys et al., 1985). By using as a probe a repeated sequence shared by different VNTR polymorphisms, one can show that each individual's pattern of hybridization is unique and serves as a DNA "fingerprint." Only identical twins show an indistinguishable pattern (Fig. 6–10). DNA fingerprinting has extensive applications in forensic medicine and identification.

THE MOLECULAR BASIS OF MUTATIONS AND THEIR DETECTION

Many types of mutation are represented among the diverse alleles detected at individual loci. Underlying both normal variation in the population and examples of inherited disease, mutations ranging from single base pair changes to deletion of many millions of base pairs have been documented. With the now seemingly routine application of molecular techniques to mutation detection and elucidation, a large number of specific mutations are being discovered in scores of different genetic disorders. The description of different mutations not only increases awareness of human genetic diversity and of the fragility of human genetic heritage but also, more significantly, contributes diagnostic tools for the detection and screening of genetic disease in particular families at risk, as well as, for some diseases, in the population at large.

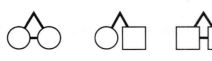

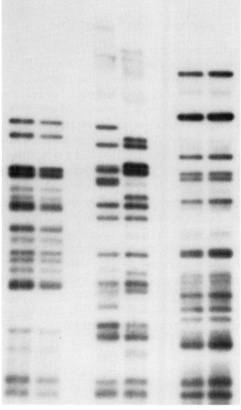

Figure 6–10. DNA fingerprinting of twins by means of a probe that detects VNTR polymorphisms at many loci around the genome. Each pair of lanes contains DNA from a set of twins. The twins of the first set (as well as the twins of the third set) have identical DNA fingerprints, indicating that they are identical (monozygotic) twins. The set in the middle have clearly distinguishable DNA fingerprints, indicating that they are fraternal twins. The figure also demonstrates the degree of variation detectable between nonidentical siblings and between unrelated people by comparing pairs of twins. (Southern blot provided courtesy of Alec Jeffreys, University of Leicester, United Kingdom.)

TYPES OF MUTATION IN HUMAN GENETIC DISEASE

Nucleotide substitutions (point mutations)
  Missense mutations (amino acid substitutions)
  Nonsense mutations (premature "stop" codons)
  RNA splicing mutations (intron/exon splice sites or cryptic sites)
Deletions and insertions
  Frameshift mutations (number of bases involved is not a multiple of 3)
  Codon deletions and insertions (number of bases involved is a multiple of 3)
  Gene deletions and duplications (often mediated by unequal crossing over)
  Insertion of repeated elements (interrupts coding sequence)

Here we consider the nature of different mutations, their underlying mechanisms, and their effect on the genes involved. In Chapters 11 and 12, we turn to the ways in which mutations cause disease. Each type of mutation discussed here is illustrated by one or more disease examples; however, it should be remembered that mutations in most genetic diseases are quite heterogeneous. Different cases of a particular disorder will therefore usually be caused by different underlying mutations.

Nucleotide Substitutions

A single nucleotide substitution (or **point mutation**) in a DNA sequence can alter the code in a triplet of bases and cause the replacement of one amino acid by another in the gene product. Point mutations leading to amino acid substitutions in the α_1-AT gene were illustrated in Figure 6–8. Such mutations are called **missense mutations** because they alter the "sense" of the coding strand of the gene by specifying a different amino acid. In many disorders, such as the hemoglobinopathies described in Chapter 11, the vast majority of detected mutations are missense mutations.

Other base substitutions occurring either within or outside the coding sequences of a gene can also have extensive effects on the gene product or interfere directly with the transcription process itself. As discussed in detail in Chapter 11, a number of mutations in the 5' promoter region or the 3' untranslated region of the β-globin gene lead to a sharp decrease in the amount of mature, processed β-globin mRNA produced. Indeed, such mutations have been critical for elucidating the importance of particular nucleotides in these regions for gene expression. As another example, the mutation shown in Figure 6–11 was detected in the 5' untranslated region of the factor IX gene from two unrelated patients with **hemophilia B,** an X-linked clotting disorder. The affected boys showed only about one third the normal amount of anti-clotting activity, which suggests that the base pair affected by the mutation is important for expression of the factor IX gene at normal levels. Indeed, studies have demonstrated that this mutation prevents the binding of a key transcription factor that normally activates the factor IX promoter (Crossley and Brownlee, 1990).

Chain Termination Mutations

Normally, translation of mRNA ceases when a termination codon is reached (see Chapter 3). A mutation that creates a termination codon can cause premature cessation of translation, whereas a mutation that destroys a termination codon allows translation to continue until the next termination codon is reached. A mutation that generates one of the three "stop" codons is called a **nonsense mutation.** In general, such mutations have no effect on transcription. However, the truncated translation product may be either grossly abnormal in shape and function or so unstable that it is rapidly degraded within the cell. An example of a nonsense mutation in the NF1 gene (see box, Chapter 4) is shown in Figure 6–12. Detection and elucidation of this particular NF1 mutation by White and colleagues in 1990 was instrumental in establishing the causative role of this possible tumor suppressor gene in NF1 (Cawthon et al., 1990).

Factor IX gene promoter

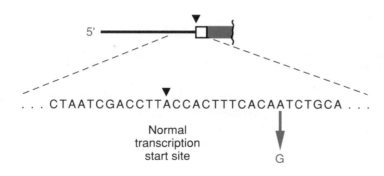

Figure 6–11. A single base mutation in the 5' untranslated region of the factor IX gene. This A→G mutation affects the level of factor IX gene expression, leading to hemophilia.

. . . CTAATCGACCTTACCACTTTCACAATCTGCA . . .

Normal
transcription
start site

G

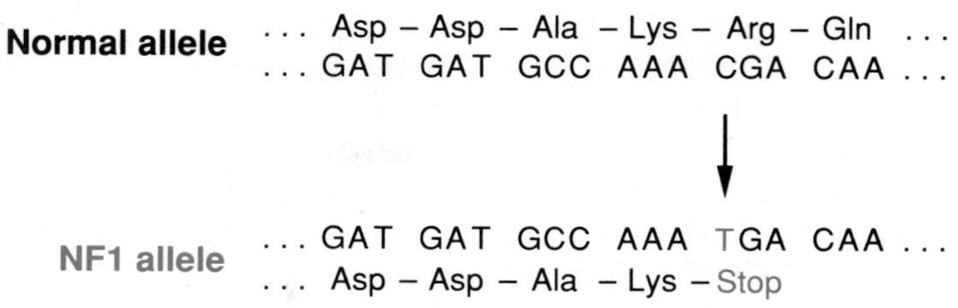

Normal allele   . . . Asp – Asp – Ala – Lys – Arg – Gln . . .
                     . . . GAT GAT GCC AAA CGA CAA . . .

NF1 allele   . . . GAT GAT GCC AAA TGA CAA . . .
                     . . . Asp – Asp – Ala – Lys – Stop

Figure 6–12. Nonsense mutation in the coding sequence of the neurofibromatosis, type 1 (NF1) gene, resulting in premature termination of translation.

RNA Splicing Mutations

As described in Chapter 3, the normal mechanism by which introns are excised from unprocessed RNA and exons spliced together to form a mature mRNA is dependent on particular nucleotide sequences located at intron/exon (acceptor site) and exon/intron (donor site) boundaries. Two general classes of splicing mutations have been described. Mutations that affect the required bases at either the splice donor or acceptor site interfere with (and in some cases abolish) normal RNA splicing at that site. An example of such a mutation is a single base-pair substitution at the donor site in the hexosaminidase A gene found in a proportion of Ashkenazi Jewish patients with Tay-Sachs disease (see box, Chapter 4). As shown in Figure 6–13, the G→C mutation occurs in the normally invariant GT dinucleotide required for proper splicing. Hexosaminidase A mRNA detected in these patients contains an unspliced intron between exon 12 and exon 13, consistent with the mutation abolishing normal splicing at this site (see Chapter 12). Similar splice site mutations have been documented in other genetic disorders, including phenylketonuria, hemophilia B, and, as described in detail in Chapter 11, β-thalassemia.

A second class of splicing mutations involves intron base substitutions that do not affect the donor or acceptor site sequences themselves. Such mutations may create alternative donor or acceptor sites that compete with the normal sites during RNA processing. Thus at least a proportion of the mature mRNA in such cases may contain improperly spliced intron sequences. Examples of this mechanism of mutation are also presented in Chapter 11.

"Hotspots" of Mutation

Nucleotide changes that involve the substitution of one purine for the other (A↔G) or one pyrimidine for the other (T↔C) are called **transitions.** In contrast, the replacement of a purine for a pyrimidine (or vice versa) is called a **transversion.** If nucleotide substitutions were random, there should be twice as many transversions as transitions, because every base can undergo two transversions, but only one transition. However, different mutagenic processes may preferentially cause one or the other type of substitution. Thus the finding of a higher frequency of transitions than expected among a collection of mutant alleles has been taken as evidence of a favored mechanism of mutation, rather than spontaneous or random base substitution.

Insight into the excess of transitions among

Figure 6–13. RNA splicing mutation at the splice site between exon 12 and intron 12 in the hexosaminidase A gene in Tay-Sachs disease. Normal splicing does not occur in RNA transcribed from the mutant allele; thus generation of mature mRNA and normal hexosaminidase product is prevented.

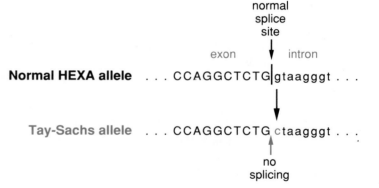

normal
splice
site

exon   intron

Normal HEXA allele   . . . CCAGGCTCTG|gtaagggt . . .

Tay-Sachs allele   . . . CCAGGCTCTG ctaagggt . . .

no
splicing

single base-pair substitutions causing genetic disease has come with the finding that the major form of DNA modification in the human genome involves methylation of cytosine residues (to form 5-methylcytosine), specifically when they are located immediately 5′ to a guanine (i.e., as the dinucleotide 5′-CG-3′). Spontaneous deamination of 5-methylcytosine to thymidine (compare the structures of cytosine and thymine in Fig. 3–1) in the CG doublet gives rise to C→T or G→A transitions (depending on in which strand of DNA the 5-methylcytosine is mutated). More than 30 percent of all single nucleotide substitutions detected in many inherited disorders are of this type, including most notably hemophilia A and B (Youssoufian et al., 1986; Antonarakis, 1988). Similar data have been reported for mutations leading to RFLPs. In all, 5-methylcytosine mutations both in mutant genes and in polymorphic DNA sequences are found at a tenfold to fortyfold higher frequency than that of any other base mutation (Cooper and Krawczak, 1990). Thus the CG doublet represents a true "hotspot" for mutation in the human genome. This finding has implications for developing strategies for the detection of new mutations in diagnostic settings.

Deletions and Insertions

Mutations can also be caused by the insertion or deletion of one or more base pairs. Some deletions and insertions involve only a few nucleotides and can generally be detected only through molecular analysis involving nucleotide sequencing. In other cases, a substantial segment of a gene or an entire gene is deleted. Such mutations are usually detected at the level of Southern blotting of a patient's DNA; large insertions or duplications can also be detected in this manner. In rare instances, deletions are large enough to be visible at the cytogenetic level. To be detected even with high-resolution prometaphase banding, these mutations generally must delete at least 3 to 5 million base pairs of DNA. In many instances, such deletions remove more than a single gene and are associated with a **microdeletion syndrome** or **contiguous gene syndrome** (see Chapter 9).

In the case of deletions or insertions involving only a few base pairs, when the number of bases involved is not a multiple of three (i.e., is not an integral number of codons), such a mutation in a coding sequence alters the reading frame of translation from the point of the mutation on, which results in a different amino acid sequence at the carboxyl terminus of the encoded protein. These mutations are called **frameshift mutations.** One example mentioned briefly earlier is a single base-pair deletion at the ABO blood group locus, a mutation that distinguishes the nonfunctional *O* allele from the *A* allele (Fig. 6–14). The deletion alters the translational reading frame at codon 86 until a premature termination codon (normally out of frame and therefore not read in the *A* allele) is reached 30 amino acids later. The resulting truncated protein (only about one third as large as either the type A or type B glycosyltransferase) would be expected to be very different from the normal gene product.

An example of an insertion that causes a frameshift is the most common mutation found in Ashkenazi Jewish patients with Tay-Sachs disease (Fig. 6–15). A four base-pair insertion creates a translational frameshift that leads, as in the ABO *O* allele example, to a premature stop codon. In this case, no detectable hexosaminidase A protein

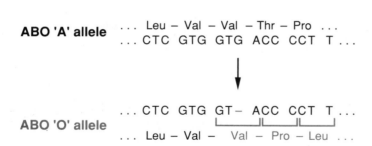

ABO 'A' allele

```
... Leu – Val – Val – Thr – Pro ...
... CTC  GTG  GTG  ACC  CCT  T ...
```

ABO 'O' allele

```
... CTC  GTG  GT–  ACC  CCT  T ...
... Leu – Val –  Val – Pro – Leu ...
```

altered reading frame ⟶

Figure 6–14. Single-base deletion at the ABO (glycosyltransferase) locus, leading to a frameshift mutation responsible for the *O* allele.

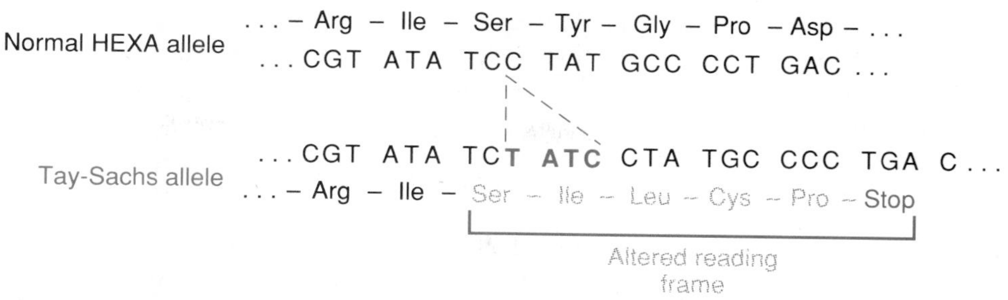

Normal HEXA allele

... – Arg – Ile – Ser – Tyr – Gly – Pro – Asp – ...
...CGT ATA TCC TAT GCC CCT GAC...

Tay-Sachs allele

...CGT ATA TCT ATC CTA TGC CCC TGA C...
... – Arg – Ile – Ser – Ile – Leu – Cys – Pro – Stop

Altered reading frame

Figure 6–15. Four-base insertion in the hexosaminidase A gene in Tay-Sachs disease, leading to a frameshift mutation. This mutation is the major cause of Tay-Sachs disease in Ashkenazi Jews.

is made, and this accounts for the complete enzyme deficiency and the severe phenotype classically observed in the infantile form of the disease.

Other small insertions or deletions do not cause a frameshift because the number of base pairs involved is a multiple of three. A notable example is a three base-pair deletion observed in the most common mutant allele that causes cystic fibrosis (CF; see box, Chapter 4). This mutation, found in nearly 70 percent of all mutant CF alleles examined to date (see Chapter 12), causes synthe-

sis of an abnormal gene product that is missing a single amino acid, the phenylalanine at amino acid position 508 (Fig. 6–16).

Large Deletions and Insertions

Alterations of gene structure large enough to be detected by Southern blotting have been described in numerous inherited disorders (see Fig. 5–7). The observed frequency of such mutations differs markedly among different genetic diseases; some

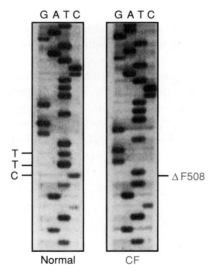

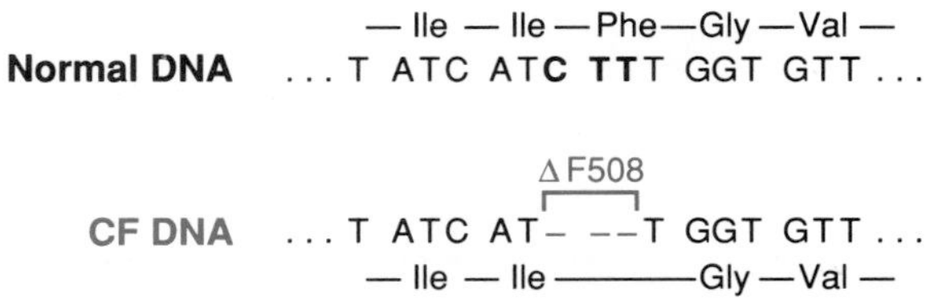

Figure 6–16. Three-base deletion in the common cystic fibrosis (CF) allele results in synthesis of a protein that is missing amino acid 508 (phenylalanine). Because the deletion is a multiple of three, this is not a frameshift mutation. This depiction of a portion of a DNA sequencing gel (see Fig. 5–10) shows the relevant portion of the CF gene in a normal person and in an affected person. (Based on a photograph provided by L.-C. Tsui, Hospital for Sick Children, Toronto.)

Normal DNA

— Ile — Ile — Phe — Gly — Val —
... T ATC ATC TTT GGT GTT ...

CF DNA

ΔF508
... T ATC AT– ––T GGT GTT ...
— Ile — Ile ———— Gly — Val —

disorders are characterized by a high frequency of detectable deletions, whereas in others deletion is a very rare cause of mutation. Total deletion of the steroid sulfatase locus, for example, is observed in more than 90 percent of cases of X-linked ichthyosis, whereas deletion is observed in less than 10 percent of cases of X-linked ornithine transcarbamylase deficiency. Deletions within the large dystrophin gene on the X chromosome in DMD are present in more than 60 percent of cases (see Chapter 12). Many cases of α-thalassemia are due to deletion of one of the two α-globin loci on chromosome 16, whereas β-thalassemia is only rarely due to deletion of the β-globin gene (see Chapter 11). In some cases, the basis for gene deletion is well understood and is probably mediated by aberrant recombination between multiple copies of similar or identical DNA sequences (see the next section). In other cases, the basis for deletion is unknown.

Insertion of large amounts of DNA is a less frequent cause of mutation than is deletion. A novel mechanism of mutation, however, has been described in two unrelated, sporadic cases of hemophilia A. As discussed in Chapter 3, the L1 family of interspersed repetitive sequences probably represents a class of repeated DNA that is capable of moving to different sites in the genome through an RNA-mediated process. In 2 of about 200 patients with hemophilia A, L1 sequences several kb long were found to be inserted into an exon in the factor VIII gene, interrupting the coding sequence and inactivating the gene. This finding suggests that at least some of the estimated 10,000 copies of the L1 family in the human genome are capable of causing disease by insertional mutagenesis (Kazazian et al., 1988).

Deletions and Duplications Caused by Recombination

A frequent cause of mutation involves deletion or duplication mediated by recombination between highly similar or identical DNA sequences. Many genes exist as members of multigene families (see Chapter 3). When the members of such a gene family are located in a head-to-tail tandem fashion in the same chromosomal region, they sometimes misalign and pair out of register either in meiosis (when two homologs pair) or in mitosis after replication (when the two sister chromatids often exchange DNA). Recombination occurring between mispaired chromosomes or sister chromatids can lead to gene deletion or duplication (Fig. 6–17). The mechanism of **unequal crossing over** is thought to be responsible for gene deletions in the growth hormone gene family in cases of familial isolated growth hormone deficiency, for deletion of one of the α-globin genes in α-thalassemia (see Chapter 11), and for variation in the copy number of green visual pigment genes in the red and green visual pigment gene cluster on the X chromosome, both in people with normal color vision and in males with X-linked defects in green or red color perception (Fig. 6–18).

Recombination between homologous non-coding DNA sequences can also cause genetic disease. Recombination between different members of the *Alu* family class of interspersed repeated

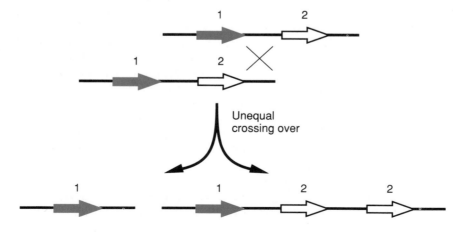

Figure 6–17. Unequal crossing over between misaligned sister chromatids or homologous chromosomes containing two highly homologous copies of a DNA sequence (either members of a gene family or copies of a repetitive DNA family) leads to two products, one with only a single copy and one with three copies of the sequence. See text for discussion.

Unequal
crossing over

Normal Vision

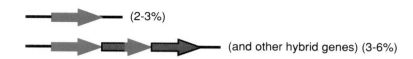

(20-47%)

(29-46%)

(8-17%)

(3-5%)

(1-2%)

Figure 6–18. Variation in the number and structure of the X-linked red and green visual pigment genes in normal persons and in males with red or green vision defects. Variation is thought to be due to unequal crossing over. Red arrow = red visual pigment gene. Grey arrow = green visual pigment gene, present in 1 to 5 copies per X chromosome. (Based on data in Nathans et al., 1989; Drummond-Borg et al., 1989; and Jorgensen et al., 1990.)

Deuteranopia/Deuteranomaly (green vision defects)

(2-3%)

(and other hybrid genes) (3-6%)

Protanopia/Protanomaly (red vision defects)

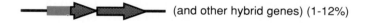

(and other hybrid genes) (1-12%)

DNA (see Chapter 3) has been documented (Lehrman et al., 1987) as the cause of a duplication of several exons in the low-density lipoprotein receptor gene in familial hypercholesterolemia (see box, Chapter 4, and Chapter 12). As a second example, the mutational event in a case of XX maleness (phenotypically male individuals with a 46,XX karyotype; see Chapter 10) resulted from aberrant exchange between an *Alu* repeat on the short arm of the X chromosome and one on the Y chromosome (Rouyer et al., 1987). Other classes of repetitive DNA have been implicated in deletion events causing somatic mutations in retinoblastoma, a dominantly transmitted disorder characterized by malignant tumors in the eyes of affected children (Chapter 16). Because the retinoblastoma gene serves as a model for the study of recessively acting oncogenes, the results suggest that aberrant recombination between short repeated DNA elements may play a role in the genesis of other human cancers.

One of the most striking examples of recombination between misaligned copies of a repeated sequence explains the unusually high frequency of gene deletion in X-linked ichthyosis, mentioned earlier; the steroid sulfatase (STS) gene on the short arm of the X chromosome is completely deleted in the vast majority of cases of X-linked ichthyosis. Shapiro and colleagues documented that in 24 of 26 cases examined, the deletion is apparently due to recombination between two copies of a short, tandemly repeated DNA sequence located nearly 2 million base pairs apart, one on either side of the STS gene locus (Yen et al., 1990). Because the opposite by-product of a proposed unequal crossing over event, a duplication of the STS gene, has not been documented, this recurring mutation might involve an *intrachromosomal* recombination event (Fig. 6–19). An estimated 0.01 per cent of the population have an X chromosome in which the STS locus has been deleted by this mechanism.

Intermolecular model:

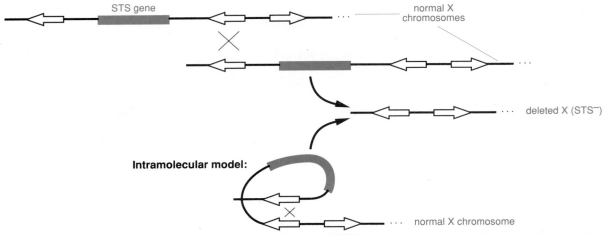

Figure 6-19. Two models to explain deletion of the steroid sulfatase (STS) gene in patients with X-linked ichthyosis, based on unequal crossing over between two copies of a repetitive DNA sequence, three of which (open arrows) are found near the STS gene in band Xp22.3.

The Detection of Mutations Causing Genetic Disease

One approach to the diagnosis of genetic disease involves identification of the precise mutation underlying a particular disorder. Depending on the nature of the mutation, a variety of diagnostic tools are used (Table 6-7). As an increasing number of specific mutations are being analyzed at the molecular level, the use of these methods in diagnostic laboratories will constitute an important part of the clinical management of families with genetic disease. This is particularly so for the com-

mon alleles that account for a significant proportion of all the cases of a particular genetic disease in a population.

Many of these approaches have already been mentioned in the preceding discussion. Southern blotting is, of course, useful for detecting gene rearrangements or deletions (see Figs. 5-7 and 12-12). In addition, Southern blotting in combination with digestion of a patient's DNA with particular restriction enzymes can reveal specific mutations that create or abolish that restriction site. Thus particular mutations can be detected directly by this approach and can be tracked through fami-

Table 6-7. **Diagnostic Approaches for the Detection of Mutations**

Method	Material	Mutations Detected	Examples*
Southern blotting	Genomic DNA	Large deletions, insertions, rearrangements	DMD (Chap. 12), androgen insensitivity (Chap. 5)
Restriction enzymes	Genomic DNA	Point mutations in a restriction site	Sickle cell disease (Chap. 11), hemophilia A
PCR	Genomic DNA	Deletions	Lesch-Nyhan syndrome
PCR, restriction enzyme	Genomic DNA, cDNA	Point mutations in a restriction site	Tay-Sachs disease, hemophilia A
Denaturing gels	Genomic DNA, RNA	Point mutations, deletions, insertions	NF1, OTC deficiency, hemophilia A
Single-strand gels	Genomic DNA, cDNA	Point mutations	Many
RNAse A cleavage	RNA	Point mutations	Lesch-Nyhan syndrome
PCR, direct sequence	Genomic DNA, cDNA	Point mutations (all)	Many
Allele-specific oligonucleotides	Genomic DNA	Any known mutation	CF, retinitis pigmentosa (Chap. 8)

*When presented in the book, example is in this chapter, unless otherwise specified.

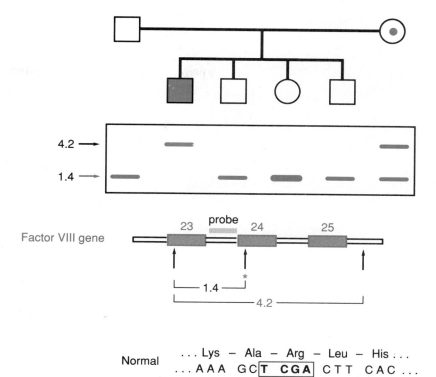

Figure 6–20. Detection of a single-base substitution that alters the recognition sequence for the restriction enzyme *Taq*I in exon 24 of the factor VIII gene in a family with hemophilia A. A factor VIII gene probe detects a 1.4-kb *Taq*I fragment on normal X chromosomes but a 4.2-kb fragment on X chromosomes carrying the mutation. In this family, the sister of the proband can clearly be shown not to be a carrier of the mutation.

lies (Fig. 6–20). In many instances, the polymerase chain reaction (PCR) is replacing Southern blotting for routine diagnostic purposes because it is easier and faster and requires considerably less of a patient's DNA. For example, PCR can be used to detect large gene deletions (Fig. 6–21), specific point mutations, or small insertions or deletions. Such analyses require only a few cells from any accessible source and can provide a specific diagnosis within a few hours.

Another approach for the direct detection of mutations is the application of allele-specific oligonucleotides (ASOs), as described in Chapter 5. Figure 6–22 illustrates the detection of the three base-pair deletion causing CF with the use of PCR and ASOs. Such an assay is of considerable use in clinical laboratories for the detection of CF carriers and for the prenatal diagnosis of CF (Lemna et al., 1990).

In addition to their use in routine diagnosis,

many of the approaches described in Table 6–7 are being used to efficiently analyze new mutations in order to establish the exact nature of a mutation or to confirm that a candidate gene is, in fact, responsible for a particular genetic condition. With PCR, specific regions of genes can be rapidly isolated from a patient's DNA and then directly sequenced in order to identify a mutation. Electrophoresis of denatured or single-stranded DNA samples can be used to efficiently identify "mismatches" between a patient's sample and a normal copy of the gene sequence or its mRNA (denaturing gradient gel electrophoresis and single-strand conformation analysis; see Table 6–7). Such mismatches may indicate a potential site of a mutation responsible for the genetic disease under study. Of course, once a particular mutation is identified and confirmed, direct tests can be developed for use in diagnosing future cases of that disease.

Lesch-Nyhan syndrome

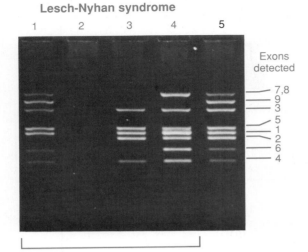

HPRT gene deletions

Figure 6–21. Detection of HPRT gene deletions in Lesch-Nyhan syndrome by the polymerase chain reaction (PCR; Gibbs et al., 1990). PCR amplification of the normal HPRT gene detects all nine exons, as shown in normal DNA in lane 5. PCR analysis of DNA samples from four males with Lesch-Nyhan syndrome reveals a deletion of exon 2 (lane 1), a total gene deletion (lane 2), deletion of exons 6 to 9 (lane 3), and deletion of exon 9 (lane 4). (Based on a photograph provided courtesy of R. A. Gibbs and C. T. Caskey, Baylor College of Medicine, Houston.)

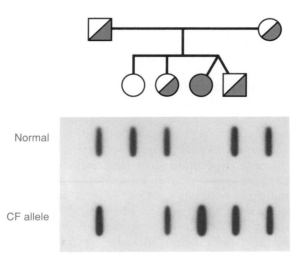

Figure 6–22. Detection of the three base-pair deletion in cystic fibrosis, by means of allele-specific oligonucleotides for the normal allele (top) and the ΔF508 CF allele (bottom). Assay allows genotyping of unaffected siblings of a CF child and allows detection of CF carriers and prenatal diagnosis (Lemna et al., 1990). (Based on a photograph provided courtesy of A. Beaudet, Baylor College of Medicine, Houston.)

General References

Antonarakis SE (1989) Diagnosis of genetic disorders at the DNA level. N Engl J Med 320:153–163.
Caskey CT (1987) Disease diagnosis by recombinant DNA methods. Science 236:1223–1229.
Crow JF, Denniston C (1985) Mutation in human populations. Adv Hum Genet 14:59–124.
Harris H (1980) The principles of human biochemical genetics (3rd ed). Elsevier-North Holland, Amsterdam.
Vogel F, Motulsky AG (1986) Human genetics (2nd ed). Springer-Verlag, Berlin.

Problems

1. Suggest possible explanations for the following observed phenotypes at the galactose-1-phosphate uridyltransferase (GALT) locus:
   a) A normal amount of GALT protein, but with no enzymatic activity.
   b) A normal amount of mRNA, but no observable GALT protein.
   c) Absent mRNA and absent GALT protein.
   d) A protein product with normal activity, but with variant electrophoretic charge.
   e) Reduced (but measurable) levels of GALT protein.
   f) Altered restriction enzyme pattern in the GALT gene, but with normal GALT enzymatic activity.

2. Among 4.5 million births in one population over a period of 40 years, 41 children diagnosed with the autosomal dominant condition aniridia were born to normal parents. Assuming that these cases were due to new mutations, what is the estimated mutation rate at the aniridia locus? On what assumptions is this estimate based, and why might this estimate be either too high or too low?

3. The following patterns are observed for a DNA polymorphism, after digestion of genomic DNA with a particular restriction enzyme: in males, a fragment at either 9 or 11 kb; in females, a fragment at 9 or 11 kb, or both.
   a) What is the likely origin of these patterns?
   b) What would you predict if the DNA samples were digested with a different restriction enzyme?

4. A VNTR-type DNA polymorphism detects five different alleles, each with a frequency of 0.20. What proportion of individuals would be expected to be heterozygous at this locus?

5. There are several common polymorphic alleles at the autosomal apolipoprotein(a) locus that determine plasma levels of the macromolecular complex, lipoprotein(a). Consider three alleles, Lp^B, Lp^S, and a null

allele, Lp^0, with estimated frequencies of .01, .61, and .38, that contribute additively plasma lipoprotein(a) levels of 25 mg/dl, 10 mg/dl, and 0 mg/dl. (Persons homozygous for the Lp^B allele, in other words, have lipoprotein(a) plasma concentrations of approximately 50 mg/dl.) Determine the possible genotypes and their frequencies. What will the distribution of lipoprotein(a) plasma levels be? High concentrations (> 30 mg/dl) are associated with an increased risk of premature coronary heart disease. What proportion of individuals have a genetically determined increased risk of premature coronary heart disease?

CHAPTER 7

GENES IN POPULATIONS

Genetics is unique among the various disciplines in medicine because of its focus on a family rather than on an individual patient. Medical genetics is concerned not only with making the correct diagnosis in a particular case but with determining the genotypes of other family members and estimating recurrence risks both for the parents of an affected person and for his or her sibs, as well as for more distant relatives. Furthermore, because such risks are usually affected not only by the genotypes of directly related family members but also by the genotypes of persons from the general population who have married into the family, genetic counseling must take into account the likelihood of specific genotypes in different populations. Thus in order both to make a genetically correct clinical diagnosis and to determine recurrence risks as part of effective genetic counseling, it often matters, for example, whether a family has its origins in the British Isles or in the Mediterranean or in Finland, whether there is a family history of consanguinity, or whether the family is Caucasian, Black, or Asian. In genetics more than in any other medical specialty, the patient is a reflection of the population to which he or she belongs.

Population genetics is the study of the distribution of genes in populations and of how the frequencies of genes and genotypes are maintained or changed. The theme of this chapter is that knowledge about the different disease genes that are common in different populations, and

their effect or lack of effect on reproductive fitness, can be a valuable asset in clinical diagnosis and in genetic counseling. Population genetics has much in common with epidemiology, the study of the interrelationships of the various genetic and environmental factors that determine the frequency and distribution of diseases in human communities. The two areas fuse in the field of genetic epidemiology, which is chiefly concerned with diseases that have complex patterns of inheritance or are caused by a combination of heritable and environmental factors. As described further in Chapter 15, this approach has already improved our understanding of the genetics of many diseases, especially the common disorders of adult life.

In this chapter we describe the underlying principle of population genetics, Hardy-Weinberg equilibrium; we consider its assumptions and the factors that may cause true or apparent deviation from equilibrium in real as opposed to idealized populations; and we consider how to determine the frequencies and mutation rates of certain genes of clinical importance, both autosomal and X-linked.

HUMAN POPULATIONS

The human species of close to 5 billion members is divided into many distinguishable subpopulations, the largest of which are commonly called

races. Races are defined as major population groups whose gene pools differ from each other. There are three major racial divisions, Caucasians, Blacks, and Asians, each of which has numerous genetically different subgroups. Although the human chromosomes and the loci that they contain are identical in all members of the species, allele frequencies at many loci vary widely among population groups. As discussed in the previous chapter, some variants are virtually restricted to members of a single group, although they are not necessarily present in all members of the group. More often, variant alleles have different frequencies in different populations. Within each population there is extensive variation, greater on the average than the mean differences between groups.

The basis of the genetic differences among races and among their subpopulations is mutation. The selection of favorable mutations in response to environmental conditions or the chance survival of specific neutral or even harmful mutations, together with a degree of reproductive isolation between the groups, allowed genetic differences between population groups to become established. In the most recent glacial period, 100,000 years or so ago, the Eurasian land mass, where small and scattered human settlements were developing, was divided into three distinct regions, separated by mountainous glaciated areas that were physical barriers to communication and interbreeding. Within these regions, geographi-

cally and thus genetically isolated from one another, the three major racial groups are believed to have developed. Subsequently, each group subdivided further into numerous distinct subpopulations, often called **ethnic groups,** with their own characteristic sets of gene frequencies. There are often dramatic differences in allele frequencies between population groups, both for alleles that cause genetic disease and for presumably selectively neutral genetic markers, such as certain blood group and protein polymorphisms and

Table 7–1. **Selected Examples of Disease Alleles With Different Frequencies in Different Populations**

Allele/Disease	Population Variation
β^s allele of β-globin gene (sickle cell anemia)	High in Africa, less common elsewhere
β^c allele of β-globin gene	High in West Africa specifically
Cystic fibrosis	High in European and U.S. Caucasian populations; low in Asian and African populations; low in Finland
Tay-Sachs disease	High frequency of several alleles in Ashkenazi Jews; low in most non-Ashkenazi populations
Choroideremia	Common in Finland; very rare elsewhere
Myotonic dystrophy	About 1 in 10,000–20,000 in most populations, but >1 in 1000 in parts of Quebec

Table 7–2. **Examples of Polymorphic Loci with Different Allele Frequencies in Different Populations**

Locus	Allelic Variation
ABO blood group system	Wide variation; e.g., *B* allele common in Asians but absent in American aboriginal populations (see Chapter 6)
Other blood group systems	Wide variation in frequency of common alleles; some rare alleles show restricted distribution (Rh allele R^0 found only in Africa; see Chapter 6)
Alpha$_1$-antitrypsin	Frequencies of three major *M* alleles vary between populations (e.g., *M1* from 0.51 to 0.98; *M2* from 0.00 to 0.20)
Alcohol dehydrogenase	Three loci: ADH1, ADH2, ADH3. Variant of ADH2 much more common in Japanese (90%) than in Europeans (15%)
Aldehyde dehydrogenase	Deficiency of ALDH1 in 50% of Asians, <5% of North American Indians
HLA system	Numerous alleles at each sublocus, wide variation in frequency (see Chapter 14)
Lactase activity	Two major alleles, for high and low activity. Low activity after early childhood common in Africans and Asians (allele frequency 0.8–0.95), less common in Northern Europeans and U.S. Caucasians (allele frequency 0.17–0.48)
Apolipoprotein A-I levels	Plasma concentration varies from <10 to >100 mg/dl and is correlated with risk of coronary heart disease; allele for low apoA-I level is common in Chinese, but less common in other populations.

some DNA polymorphisms (Tables 7–1 and 7–2). Although the former are highly significant for determining recurrence risks for genetic diseases in specific population groups, the latter are important as markers of recent human evolution.

PHENOTYPES, GENOTYPES, AND GENE FREQUENCIES

Although one requires knowledge of a person's genotype to accurately determine recurrence risks, in most instances it is only the phenotype that one can observe and directly measure. Thus there is a need to be able to use incidence figures for an inherited disease or other genetic trait to calculate individual allele frequencies. To do this requires knowledge of genes in populations and their transmission from generation to generation.

Single-gene phenotypes, such as those introduced in Chapter 4, segregate sharply in families and, on average, tend to occur in fixed and predictable proportions. A simple example of a common autosomal hereditary trait governed by a single pair of alleles can be used to illustrate the basic principles that underlie the inheritance of genes in populations. Consider the MN blood group system (the glycophorins), in which a pair of codominantly expressed alleles, M and N, give rise to three genotypes, M/M, M/N, and N/N, and the three corresponding phenotypes, M, MN, and N (see Chapter 6). As is clear from the principles of single-gene inheritance discussed in Chapter 4, a specific mating of an MN female and an MN male would result in three types of distinguishable offspring (M, MN, and N), in the expected proportions 1/4 M, 1/2 MN, and 1/4 N.

These same principles can be extended to matings within the population in general. A sampling of individuals from a population provides absolute numbers of MN phenotypes (and thus genotypes) that can be converted into relative frequencies by dividing them all by the total number of observations. Thus for a British population studied by Race and Sanger (1975):

Phenotype	Genotype	Number of people	Relative frequency
M	M/M	392	0.276
N	N/N	320	0.226
MN	M/N	707	0.498
Total		1419	1.000

We use the observed relative frequencies to estimate the frequencies of the M and N alleles in this population because it is this estimate that is needed to make predictions about matings and their likely outcome. On the basis of the observed phenotype and genotype frequencies, we can directly determine the gene frequencies, remembering that each autosomal genotype consists of two alleles. In this example, then, the observed frequency of the M allele is

$$\frac{(2 \times 392) + 707}{1419 \times 2} = 0.53.$$

Similarly, one can calculate the frequency of N as 0.47, either by adding up the number of N alleles directly (1347 of a total of 2838 alleles) or simply by subtracting the frequency of M from 1 (therefore, the frequency of $N = 1 - 0.53 = 0.47$), since the relative frequencies of the two alleles must add up to 1.

We have used this small sampling of individuals in a population to derive estimates of the relative frequency of the two alleles in the population as a whole. In this context, when we refer to the population frequency of a gene (allele), we are considering a **gene pool**, which contains all of the alleles at a particular locus for the entire population. The likelihood of an individual's being of a particular genotype at the MN locus thus depends on the frequency of the M and N alleles in the gene pool. If the relative frequencies of the two alleles in the gene pool are 0.53 (for M) and 0.47 (for N), then for the population from which this sampling of 1419 people was tested, the relative proportions of the three combinations of alleles (genotypes) are $0.53 \times 0.53 = 0.281$ (for drawing two M alleles from the pool), $0.47 \times 0.47 = 0.221$ (for two N alleles), and $(0.53 \times 0.47) + (0.47 \times 0.53) = 0.498$ (for one M and one N allele).

THE HARDY-WEINBERG LAW

Putting the above example in more general terms, if p is the frequency of one allele and q is the frequency of the other allele, then the frequencies of the three combinations of alleles will be:

$$\begin{array}{ccc} p^2 & +\ 2pq\ + & q^2 \\ M/M & M/N & N/N \end{array}$$

An important consequence of the relation-

Table 7–3. Frequencies of Mating Types and Offspring for a Population in Hardy-Weinberg Equilibrium with Parental Genotypes in the Proportion $p^2 : 2pq : q^2$

Mating Types			Offspring		
Mother	Father	Frequency	M/M	M/N	N/N
M/M	M/M	$p^2 \times p^2 = p^4$	$1(p^4)$		
M/M	M/N	$p^2 \times 2pq = 2p^3q$	$1/2(2p^3q)$	$1/2(2p^3q)$	
M/N	M/M	$2pq \times p^2 = 2p^3q$	$1/2(2p^3q)$	$1/2(2p^3q)$	
M/M	N/N	$p^2 \times q^2 = p^2q^2$		$1(p^2q^2)$	
N/N	M/M	$p^2 \times q^2 = p^2q^2$		$1(p^2q^2)$	
M/N	M/N	$2pq \times 2pq = 4p^2q^2$	$1/4(4p^2q^2)$	$1/2(4p^2q^2)$	$1/4(4p^2q^2)$
M/N	N/N	$2pq \times q^2 = 2pq^3$		$1/2(2pq^3)$	$1/2(2pq^3)$
N/N	M/N	$2pq \times q^2 = 2pq^3$		$1/2(2pq^3)$	$1/2(2pq^3)$
N/N	N/N	$q^2 \times q^2 = q^4$			$1(q^4)$

Sum of M/M offspring $= p^4 + 2p^3q + p^2q^2 = p^2 (p^2 + 2pq + q^2) = p^2$.
Sum of M/N offspring $= 2p^3q + 4p^2q^2 + 2pq^3 = 2pq (p^2 + 2pq + q^2) = 2pq$.
Sum of N/N offspring $= p^2q^2 + 2pq^3 + q^4 = q^2 (p^2 + 2pq + q^2) = q^2$.
The proportion of genotypes in the offspring is $p^2 : 2pq : q^2$, as in the parental generation.

ships among phenotype, genotype, and allele frequencies is that the proportions of the genotypes do not change from generation to generation. In the generation that follows random mating of a population in which the genotypes M/M, M/N, and N/N are present in the proportions $p^2 : 2pq : q^2$, the genotypes appear in the same relative proportions (Table 7–3).

That genotypes are distributed in proportion to the frequencies of individual alleles in a population and remain constant from generation to generation is the basic tenet of the cornerstone of population genetics, the **Hardy-Weinberg law.** This law was named for George Hardy, an English mathematician, and Wilhelm Weinberg, a German physician, who independently formulated this thesis in 1908. It seemed surprising to some at that time that a dominant allele does not automatically increase in frequency until it replaces its recessive counterpart, or a deleterious recessive allele, such as that responsible for cystic fibrosis in Caucasian children (Chapter 4), does not automatically fall in frequency until it is eliminated altogether from a population. The Hardy-Weinberg law explained the basis for the constant gene frequencies as an application of the binomial theorem.

The Binomial Distribution

The binomial distribution, originally discovered by Sir Isaac Newton, was given its first rigorous proof by Jakob Bernoulli, a mathematician. In gen-

eral terms, when there are two alternative events, one with probability p and the other with probability $1 - p = q$, the frequencies of the possible combinations of p and q in a series of n trials are given by the expansion of $(p + q)^n$. We now examine a simple example that has some clinical relevance: the distribution of boys and girls in successive births.

We assume that both male and female births have a probability of $1/2$, even though the true probability of human male birth (p) is actually a little higher than $1/2$. Then the distribution of sibships with 2 boys, 1 boy and 1 girl, and 2 girls in 2-child families is given by the expansion of the binomial $(p + q)^2$; in 3-child families, by the expansion of $(p + q)^3$; and so forth, where $p = q = 1/2$.

Thus among 2-child sibships,

$(p + q)^2 = p^2 + 2pq + q^2$;
$p^2 = 1/4$ of sibships contain 2 boys;
$2pq = 1/2$ contain 1 boy and 1 girl;
$q^2 = 1/4$ contain 2 girls.

In 3-child sibships,

$(p + q)^3 = p^3 + 3p^2q + 3pq^2 + q^3$;
$p^3 = 1/8$ of sibships contain 3 boys;
$3p^2q = 3/8$ contain 2 boys and 1 girl;
$3pq^2 = 3/8$ contain 1 boy and 2 girls;
$q^3 = 1/8$ contain 3 girls.

Of course, regardless of the sex distribution of the preceding children in a sibship, each new sib has equal probabilities of being male or female.

Mathematicians may prefer to use the general term of the binomial expansion, which is

$$\frac{n!}{m!(n-m)!}\, p^m q^{n-m},$$

where n = number in series, p = probability of a specified event, q = probability of the alternative event, m = number of times p occurs (i.e., the exponent of p), and $n!$ (n factorial) is $n(n-1)(n-2)\ldots1$.

In this example, the values of p and q are each 1/2, but the binomial distribution can be used for other values as well. The same method is applied, for example, to give the distribution of a known autosomal recessive trait among the progeny of two heterozygous parents. Here, the probability of one event (that a child is affected) is 1/4, and the probability of the other event (that a child is unaffected) is 3/4. Thus the probability of having 1 affected child in a 5-child sibship is

$$\frac{5\times4\times3\times2\times1}{(1)(4\times3\times2\times1)}\,(1/4)^1(3/4)^4 = 405/1024 = 0.40.$$

Similarly, the probability of having 3 affected children can be calculated to be 90/1024, or approximately 9 percent.

Genetic Ratios

One of the important uses of the binomial distribution in population genetics is to determine whether a particular disorder whose pattern of inheritance has not been previously established is autosomal recessive, by examining whether its distribution in sibships fits the 25 percent expectation for autosomal recessive inheritance. For example, assuming recessive inheritance, what proportion of 3-child families would have 0, 1, 2, and 3 affected children? According to the approach used earlier, p (chance of clinically normal child) = 3/4, q (chance of affected child) = 1/4, $n = 3$, and $(p+q)^3 = p^3 + 3p^2q + 3pq^2 + q^3$. Thus the theoretical expectation, based on autosomal recessive inheritance, is that

27/64 of all such families have no affected child;
27/64 have 1 affected child;
9/64 have 2 affected children;
1/64 have 3 affected children.

Bias of Ascertainment

We have determined the expected proportions of affected children in 3-child families of parents who are carriers for an autosomal recessive disorder. As shown, if we ascertain a family only when it has at least 1 affected child, and if we ascertain all such families, then 27 of the 64 families at risk (42 percent) will be missed. Of the 37 ascertained families,

27 (73 percent) have 1 affected child;
9 (24 percent) have 2 affected children;
1 (3 percent) have 3 affected children.

In the ascertained group, then, the total number of affected children among 111 children in 37 families is $27 + (9 \times 2) + (1 \times 3) = 48$ or 43 percent, far above the theoretical 25 percent expected for autosomal recessive inheritance. Where did we go wrong?

This is an example of **bias of ascertainment,** a bias to avoid in medical research, especially in medical genetics. In tests for autosomal recessive inheritance, sibships with no affected members are inevitably missed, and depending on the mode of ascertainment, a sibship's chance of being ascertained may be higher when it has 2 or more affected members than when it has only 1. A number of statistical methods to correct for bias under different conditions of ascertainment are known and are described in many statistics texts. Bias of ascertainment is mentioned here chiefly because failure to recognize its importance can lead to serious errors.

Frequency of Autosomal Genes and Genotypes

As we have seen, Hardy-Weinberg distributions of genotypes in populations are simply binomial distributions. Symbols p and q represent the frequencies of two alternative alleles at a locus (where $p + q = 1$), and $n = 2$, representing the pair of alleles at any autosomal locus or any X-linked locus in females. (Because males are unique in having only a single X chromosome, frequencies of X-linked genes in males are considered separately later.) If a locus has three alleles, p, q, and r, the genotypic distribution can be determined from $(p + q + r)^2$. In general terms, the genotypic fre-

Table 7–4. Incidence, Gene Frequency, and Heterozygote Frequency for Selected Autosomal Recessive Disorders in Different Populations

Disorder	Population	Incidence (q^2)	Gene Frequency (q)	Heterozygote Frequency $(2pq)$	Heterozygotes / Homozygotes $(2pq/q^2)$
Alpha$_1$-antitrypsin deficiency (genotype Z/Z)	Denmark	1 in 2000	.023	1 in 22	90
	U.S. Blacks	1 in 100,000	.004	1 in 125	800
Congenital adrenal hyperplasia, nonclassic type	Ashkenazi Jews	1 in 28	.19	1 in 3	9
	Non-Ashkenazi Europeans	1 in 1000	.036	1 in 14	70
Cystic fibrosis	U.S. Caucasians	1 in 2000	.023	1 in 22	90
Phenylketonuria	Scotland	1 in 5300	.014	1 in 30	175
	Finland, Japan, Ashkenazi Jews	1 in 200,000	.002	1 in 250	800
Tay-Sachs disease	U.S. Ashkenazi	1 in 3900	.016	1 in 30	130
	U.S. non-Ashkenazi Caucasians	1 in 112,000	.003	1 in 170	660

Data from Cox (1989); New et al. (1989); Scriver et al. (1989); and Sandhoff et al. (1989).
Figures are approximate.

quencies for any known number of alleles can be calculated binomially.

In clinical genetics, by far the chief use of the Hardy-Weinberg law is for calculating gene and heterozygote frequencies when the frequency of a genetic trait is known, as was illustrated earlier in the case of a codominantly expressed trait for the MN locus. A related application for determining the frequency of carriers of an autosomal recessive condition was demonstrated in Chapter 4 with reference to cystic fibrosis; further examples of the application of these calculations are given in Table 7–4, in which the gene frequencies and heterozygote frequencies of several disorders in high-incidence and low-incidence populations are compared.

Frequencies of autosomal dominant genes can also be estimated from incidence data. Usu-

ally, homozygotes for autosomal dominant conditions are so rare that for purposes of calculation they can be ignored (Table 7–5). Because almost every patient is therefore a heterozygote with one normal and one abnormal allele, the frequency of the mutant allele (q) is approximately half the disease incidence ($2pq$, or about $2q$, since p is very nearly 1). The observed incidence of familial hypercholesterolemia (FH), for example, is approximately 1/500. Therefore, we can calculate that the frequency of the mutant FH gene is half of this, or about 0.001 (Table 7–5).

Hardy-Weinberg Equilibrium

A population that demonstrates the basic features of the Hardy-Weinberg law is said to be in **Hardy-**

Table 7–5. Incidence and Gene Frequency for Selected Autosomal Dominant Disorders

Disorder	Incidence $(2pq + q^2)$	Gene Frequency (q)	Heterozygotes / Homozygotes $(2pq/q^2)$
Achondroplasia	1/20,000	.000025	80,000
Familial hypercholesterolemia	1/500	.001	2000
Huntington disease	1/10,000	.00005	40,000
Neurofibromatosis, type 1	1/3000	.00017	12,000

Incidence figures are estimates. Other figures rounded off.

Weinberg equilibrium. In the example of the MN blood group locus considered earlier, if we now compare the observed and expected proportions of the M, MN, and N phenotypes, we can test whether the distribution in this population is in Hardy-Weinberg equilibrium.

Phenotype	Observed	Expected
M	392	$p^2 \times 1419 = 399$
MN	707	$2pq \times 1419 = 707$
N	320	$q^2 \times 1419 = 313$
Total	1419	1419

In this example, the agreement between the observed and expected values is so close that even without statistical analysis it is obvious that the population is in Hardy-Weinberg equilibrium. However, this is not always the case. Suppose there had been 543 people with the M phenotype, 419 with the MN phenotype, and 457 with the N phenotype in the population. Even though the allele frequencies in this population sample are the same as in the original sample (0.53 for M and 0.47 for N), is this population in Hardy-Weinberg equilibrium? An appropriate statistical test used to answer this question is the chi-square (χ^2) test, described in Appendix II, where this example is worked out as an illustration. This test is a comparison of the observed and expected frequencies of the different genotypes. As illustrated in the Appendix, the observed frequencies in this example differ significantly from expectations based on assumptions of Hardy-Weinberg equilibrium.

Another example involves the autosomal recessive disorder sickle cell disease, caused by a mutation in the β-globin gene (see Chapter 11). Consider two alleles, the normal A allele and the mutant S allele, which give rise to three genotypes: A/A (normal), A/S (heterozygous carriers), and S/S (sickle cell disease). In a sample of 12,387 individuals from an adult West African population (Cavalli-Sforza and Bodmer, 1971), the three genotypes were detected in the following proportions: 9365 A/A : 2993 A/S : 29 S/S. By applying the binomial theorem, one can calculate the allele frequencies to be 0.877 for the A allele and 0.123 for the S allele. Is this population in Hardy-Weinberg equilibrium? According to the chi-square test, the observed frequencies in this population also differ from expectations; there are significantly more heterozygotes and fewer affected persons than expected. Some of the factors affecting frequencies of genes in populations that might account for these deviations from Hardy-Weinberg equilibrium are discussed later in this chapter.

Frequency of X-Linked Genes and Genotypes

Recall that for X-linked genes, there are only two possible male genotypes but three female genotypes. To illustrate gene frequencies and genotype frequencies when the gene of interest is X-linked, we use the trait known as red–green color blindness, which is caused by mutations in the series of red and green visual pigment genes on the X chromosome (see Chapter 6). The advantage of using color blindness as an example is that, as far as we know, it is not a deleterious trait (except for possible difficulties with traffic lights), and color-blind persons are not subject to selection. As discussed later, allowing for the effect of selection complicates estimates of gene frequencies.

We use the symbol cb for the mutant color-blindness allele and the symbol $+$ for the normal allele, with frequencies q and p respectively, as shown in the box below.

Sex	Genotype	Phenotype	Incidence (Approximate)
Male	X^+	Normal color vision	$p = 0.92$
	X^{cb}	Color blind	$q = 0.08$
Female	X^+/X^+	Normal (homozygote)	$p^2 = (0.92)^2 = 0.846$
	X^+/X^{cb}	Normal (heterozygote)	$2pq = 2(0.92)(0.08) = 0.147$
		Normal (total)	$p^2 + 2pq = 0.993$
	X^{cb}/X^{cb}	Color blind	$q^2 = (0.08)^2 = 0.0064$

The frequencies of the normal and mutant alleles can be determined directly from the incidence of the corresponding phenotypes in *males*. Because females have two X chromosomes, their genotypes are distributed binomially, exactly like autosomal genotypes, but because color-blindness alleles are recessive, the normal homozygotes and heterozygotes are not distinguishable. As shown in the box, the frequency of color blindness in females is much lower than that in males, even though the allele frequencies are of course the same in both sexes. Less than 1 percent of females are color blind, but nearly 15 percent are carriers of the mutant color-blindness allele and are therefore at risk of having color-blind sons.

FACTORS AFFECTING HARDY-WEINBERG EQUILIBRIUM

The Hardy-Weinberg law makes several fundamental assumptions that are not always true of actual human populations:

1. The population is characterized by **random mating,** with little if any stratification, assortative mating, or inbreeding.
2. The locus under consideration exhibits a **constant mutation rate,** and mutant alleles lost by death are replaced by new mutations.
3. There is **no selection** for or against a particular phenotype; all genotypes at a locus are equally viable.
4. The population is sufficiently large that there has been **no random fluctuation** of frequencies resulting from transmission of any one genotype simply by chance.
5. There has been no change in the population structure by **migration,** which can gradually change gene frequencies by increasing or decreasing the number of individuals with a particular genotype.

If in a given population one or more of these assumptions does not hold true, the genotypes in that population may not be in Hardy-Weinberg equilibrium. In the next sections we consider the genetic consequences of nonrandom mating, alteration in mutation rate, selection, genetic drift, and gene flow.

Exceptions to Random Mating

The principle of random mating is that, for any locus, each genotype has a purely random probability of combining with any other, the proportions being determined only by the relative frequencies of the different genotypes in the population. However, simple observation shows that a number of factors, some genetically significant and others probably genetically neutral, enter into mate selection. These factors include **stratification, assortative mating,** and **consanguinity.**

Stratification

A stratified population is one that contains a number of subgroups that have remained largely distinct genetically during modern evolution. Worldwide there are numerous stratified populations; for example, the U.S. population is stratified into two major subgroups, Caucasians and Blacks, and several smaller subgroups, including Native Americans, Asians, and Hispanics. Similarly, gene frequencies vary significantly between countries across Europe. When mate selection in a mixed population is restricted to members of the same subgroup, the result is an excess of homozygotes and a corresponding deficiency of heterozygotes in the population as a whole for any locus with more than one allele.

Because the subgroups are likely to have different frequencies of a number of autosomal recessive disease genes, their characteristic diseases are likely to differ. Classic examples include Tay-Sachs disease in people of Ashkenazi Jewish ancestry, characteristic types of thalassemia in people of Mediterranean or East Asian descent, sickle cell anemia in Blacks, and cystic fibrosis and phenylketonuria (PKU) in Caucasians (Tables 7–1 and 7–4). Each subgroup seems to have its own profile of disorders that are more common, and others that are less common, than in the species as a whole.

Awareness of stratification can be relevant in some clinical situations. Thus not only the frequency but the specific mutant alleles in different genetic disorders vary between population groups. For example, studies of β-thalassemia have led to the identification of specific molecular defects in the β-globin gene and recognition of their population distributions. Even though there are dozens of different alleles that can cause β-thalassemia, these alleles tend to be highly specific to individual populations, so that each population has only a few common alleles (see box). Furthermore, the alleles that are common in one population are rare in other populations. For example,

Population	Number of mutant alleles
Mediterranean	15 (6 account for 92 percent of the total)
Chinese/Southeast Asian	9 (4 account for 91 percent of the total)
Asian Indian	10 (5 account for 90 percent of the total)

This information is of great practical value in prenatal diagnosis. For example, in North America, when a couple of Mediterranean descent are at risk of having a child with β-thalassemia, testing of parental DNA for just six mutant alleles has over a 90 percent probability of providing the information needed for prenatal diagnosis (Kazazian and Boehm, 1988).

Assortative Mating

Assortative mating is the choice of a mate because the mate possesses some particular trait. Assortative mating is usually positive; that is, people tend to choose mates who resemble themselves (e.g., in native language, intelligence, stature, skin color, musical talent, or athletic ability). Negative assortative mating, the selection of a mate with characteristics different from those of oneself, is less common. To the extent that the characteristic shared by the partners is genetically determined, the overall genetic effect is an increase in the proportion of the homozygous genotypes at the expense of the heterozygous genotype.

A clinically important aspect of assortative mating is the tendency to choose partners with similar medical problems, such as congenital deafness or blindness or exceptionally short stature (dwarfism). In such a case, the expectations of Hardy-Weinberg equilibrium do not apply because the probable genotype of the mate cannot be determined by the allele frequencies found in the general population. Of course, not all blindness, deafness, or short stature has the same genetic

Ethnicity of Genetic Disease

Many genetic disorders are characterized by specific allelic mutations that vary among different population groups. Although not all allelic heterogeneity can be explained in terms of population genetics, much of it can, suggesting in those cases that there were a small number of ancestral mutations that became prevalent in particular populations. The existence of population-specific mutant alleles has significance for understanding the origins of genetic disease and also provides opportunities for diagnosis of specific alleles in an at-risk population. Examples include the following disorders.

β-**Thalassemia.** Several different common mutations are found in each high incidence population, not present or present on different haplotypes in other populations. In West Africa: two alleles; in Northern Africa and Mediterranean: three alleles; in India: one deletion allele accounting for 30 percent; in Southeast Asia: five alleles.

α^0-**Thalassemia.** Different deletion mutations in the Mediterranean and Southeast Asia.

Gyrate Atrophy. A single predominant mutation in the ornithine aminotransferase gene in Finland; different mutations in other populations.

Familial Hypercholesterolemia. Mutational heterogeneity in most populations, but French Canadians have two predominant mutations; the Lebanese have one largely specific mutant allele.

Tay-Sachs disease. Two common mutations in Ashkenazi Jews; different alleles in other populations. French Canadians have different but specific mutant alleles.

basis, but when mates have disorders caused by the same mutation or allelic mutations, there are likely to be severe consequences for their offspring. Although the long-term population effects are trivial, the family immediately concerned may find itself at very high genetic risk.

Consanguinity

Consanguineous mating (inbreeding), like stratification and positive assortative mating, brings about an increase in the frequency of both homozygous genotypes and a decrease in the corresponding heterozygous form. Unlike the disorders in stratified populations, where each subgroup is likely to have a high frequency of a few alleles, consanguineous mating allows less common alleles to become homozygous, and the kinds of recessive disorders seen in the offspring of related parents may be very rare and unusual.

As mentioned in Chapter 4, an important feature of some rare recessive disorders is that they often appear among the progeny of consanguineous matings. This tendency is stronger the rarer the disorder is. Thus most affected persons with a relatively common disorder, such as cystic fibrosis, are *not* the result of consanguinity because the mutant allele is so common in the general population. However, consanguinity is more frequently found in the background of patients with very rare conditions. In xeroderma pigmentosum, a rare autosomal recessive condition of DNA repair (see Table 9-8), for example, more than 20 percent of cases are reported to result from marriages between first cousins.

Although in most populations in Western societies today the incidence of cousin marriage is low, in some groups it is relatively common. For that matter, all matings are at least remotely consanguineous, in that any two persons are likely to have at least one ancient ancestor in common. If there have been about three generations per century, the young adults of today each have 64 (2^6) ancestors (great-great-great-grandparents) who were young adults at the time of the French Revolution (1789), and these may well have been 64 different people; but each person has about 2^{24}, or almost 17 million, ancestors who were living at the time of the Magna Carta (1215). It is very unlikely if not impossible that 17 million different individuals were involved. Thus a child of virtually any mating today is likely to be homozygous by descent at one or more loci, having inherited the identical copy of a gene through both parental lineages.

Although genealogical research casts light on the history of the human species as a single family, the genetic risk to the offspring of marriages between related people is not as great as is sometimes imagined. The absolute risks of abnormal offspring for marriages between first cousins is less than double the overall population risk for marriages between unrelated persons (see Table 1-2). Consanguinity at the level of third cousins or more remote relationships is not considered to be genetically significant, and the increased risk of abnormal offspring is negligible in such cases. Even so, probably many people who are homozygous for a rare allele have inherited it through both parents from a remote common ancestor who was heterozygous.

The Measurement of Consanguinity

The measurement of consanguinity is relevant in medical genetics because the risk of a child's being homozygous for some rare recessive allele is proportional to the closeness of the parents' relationship. Some types of consanguineous mating that carry an increased risk are shown in Figure 7–1.

The **coefficient of inbreeding** (F) is the probability that a homozygote has received both alleles of a pair from an identical ancestral source; it is also the proportion of loci at which a person is homozygous by descent. In Figure 7–2, person IV-1 is the offspring of a first-cousin mating. For any specific allele that his father possesses, the chance that his mother has also inherited that same allele *from the same source* is 1/8. Thus for any gene the father passes to his child, the chance that the mother transmits the same one is 1/8 (the chance that she carries that allele) $\times$ 1/2 (the chance that she will transmit it) = 1/16. This is the coefficient of inbreeding for the child of first cousins. It means that a child of a first-cousin mating has a 1/16 chance of being homozygous by descent ("autozygous") at any one locus or, alternatively, that the child is autozygous at 1/16 (about 6 percent) of his or her loci. An alternative way of reaching the same conclusion (and the same F coefficient) is to consider that each of the

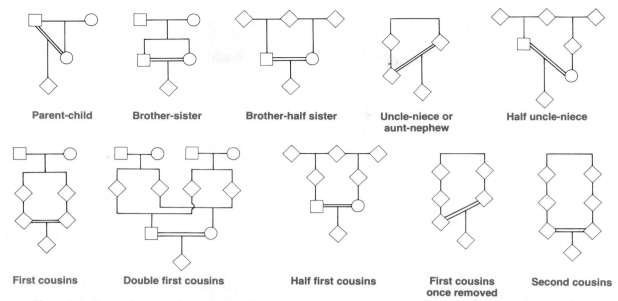

Figure 7–1. Types of consanguineous mating. Incestuous matings are those in which marriage of the partners is illegal.

four alleles at locus A in generation I has a 1/64 chance of being homozygous in IV-1; thus the probability that IV-1 is homozygous for any one of the four alleles is $4 \times 1/64 = 1/16$. Table 7–6 shows the coefficients of inbreeding for the offspring of a number of consanguineous matings. If a person is inbred through more than one line of descent, the separate coefficients are summed to find his or her total coefficient of inbreeding.

Average coefficients of inbreeding can be measured for populations as well as for individuals, and some examples are given in Table 7–7. Thus individuals from a fairly restricted population may have a significant F coefficient, even though they may not think of themselves as consanguineous. For some highly inbred populations, the average value is as high as or higher than the value for children of second cousins; for example, F = 0.04 for Samaritans, a group numbering only about 500 people that has been genetically isolated for more than 3000 years, in comparison with 0.016 for offspring of second cousins. In Japan, F is about 0.005 (0.5 percent), meaning that on the average, a Japanese person is homozygous by descent at some 500 loci.

Mutation and Selection

The molecular basis for mutation has been considered in detail in the previous chapter. In the present context, we consider mutation from the point of view of **fitness,** the chief factor (and in some views, the only factor) that determines whether a mutation is lost immediately, survives

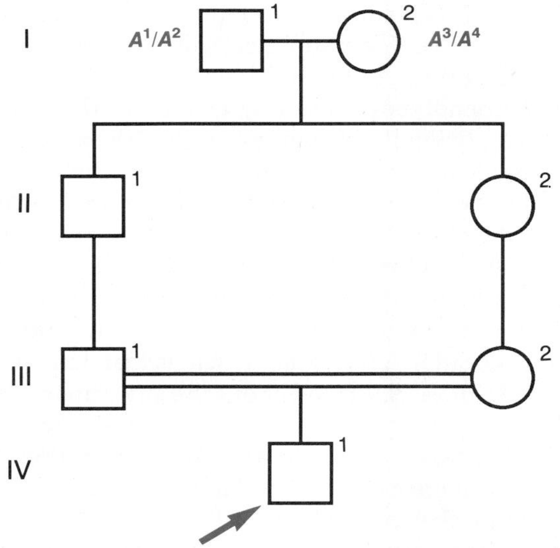

Figure 7–2. A cousin marriage, used in the text to demonstrate how to calculate the coefficient of inbreeding, F, of the child IV-1.

Table 7–6. Consanguineous Matings

Type	Degree of Relationship	Proportion of Genes in Common	Coefficient of Inbreeding of Child (F)
MZ twins	—	1	—
Parent-child	1st	1/2	1/4
Brother-sister (including DZ twins)	1st	1/2	1/4
Brother-half sister	2nd	1/4	1/8
Uncle-niece or aunt-nephew	2nd	1/4	1/8
Half uncle-niece	3rd	1/8	1/16
First cousins	3rd	1/8	1/16
Double first cousins	2nd	1/4	1/8
Half first cousins	4th	1/16	1/32
First cousins once removed	4th	1/16	1/32
Second cousins	5th	1/32	1/64

for a few generations, or eventually becomes the predominant allele at the locus concerned.

Mutation sometimes leads to loss or change of function of a gene. Because a random change is unlikely to lead to an improvement, the vast majority of detected mutations are either deleterious or selectively "neutral." The frequency of an allele in a population represents a balance between the mutation rate of that gene and the effects of selection. If either the mutation rate or the effectiveness of selection is altered, the allele frequency is expected to change.

Many mutations are lethal to the persons who receive them. In the genetic sense, a mutation that prevents reproduction by an adult is just as lethal as one that causes early abortion of an embryo, because in neither case is the mutation transmitted to the next generation. Mutations that allow survival are likely to be identified, however, whereas the ones that cause early prenatal loss may never be known. Other mutations are sublethal or neutral in their effects, and a small proportion are actually favorable. The number of generations during which a mutation persists before failing to be passed on (undergoing "genetic death") is closely related to the selection rate against it. For example, a mutation that causes a reduction in reproductive fitness of 20 percent survives, on the average, for five (1/0.20) generations.

Charles Darwin postulated **natural selection** as the crucial factor in evolution, with the idea that the fittest individuals in a given environment were the ones who survived to reproduce. In modern terms, Darwinian natural selection is interpreted as taking place through the action of selection on new phenotypes caused by genotypes that have arisen originally through mutation. There is considerable controversy at present over the reason for the persistence of mutations. According to one view (the "selectionist" view), it is due to Darwinian selection for the fittest genotypes. The opposing view (the non-Darwinian or "neutralist" view) is that it is largely a matter of chance whether a new mutation, once it has arisen, is maintained or lost. As more is learned about the structure of the human genetic material, it is becoming increasingly apparent that the amount of variation in DNA sequence in the population is very high, and it seems likely that much of the variation is random and selectively neutral. There is no question, however, that numerous deleterious alleles are

Table 7–7. Examples of Coefficient of Inbreeding (F) for Some Human Populations

Population	F
Canada	
Roman Catholic	.00004–.0007
United States	
Roman Catholic	0–.0008
Hutterites	.02
Dunkers (Pennsylvania)	.03
Latin America	0–.003
Southern Europe	.001–.002
Japan	.005
India (Andhra Pradesh)	.02
Samaritans	.04

subject to selection and that in some cases the selection can be very effective. The relative roles of selection and random chance in the long-term evolution of the genome cannot be determined at this time.

Individuals who are more fit have, by definition, a greater probability of surviving to maturity and having offspring than do less well adapted individuals. Over time, the proportion of more fit individuals tends to increase in a population, as they have proportionately more progeny. Similarly, the frequency of whatever alleles contribute to their increased fitness increases. Fitness is thus the outcome of the joint effects of survival and fertility. It is most meaningful in comparisons of different genotypes in a population and is valid only in the context of a particular environment within which there is a fitness difference. Factors such as diet (which may increase or decrease the fitness of a particular genotype), medical treatment (which increases the fitness of a particular genotype), and prenatal diagnosis and selective termination of pregnancy (which decreases the fitness of a particular genotype) alter the process of natural selection for a gene. In the biological sense, fitness has no connotation of superior endowment except in a single respect: comparative ability to contribute to the gene pool of the next generation.

Selection thus distorts Hardy-Weinberg equilibrium, which, as mentioned earlier, depends on the assumption that no selection favors one genotype over another. Dominant mutant alleles are openly exposed to selection, in contrast to recessive mutant alleles, most of which are "hidden" in heterozygotes. Consequently, the effects of selection are more obvious and can be more readily measured for dominant traits.

Selection Against Autosomal Dominant Mutations

A harmful dominant gene, if fully penetrant, is exposed to selection in heterozygotes as well as in homozygotes. Whether it is transmitted to the succeeding generation depends on how deleterious it is. If it is just as likely as the normal allele to be represented in the next generation, its fitness is 1. If it causes death or sterility (in other words, if its fitness is zero), selection acts against it very effectively, removing all the genes responsible for the disorder in a single generation. There are several human diseases that are thought to be autosomal dominants with zero or near-zero fitness and thus always to result from new autosomal dominant mutations (Table 7–8).

If a mutation is deleterious but not lethal, affected persons may nevertheless contribute fewer than the average number of offspring to the next generation; that is, their fitness, f, may be reduced. Such a mutation is lost through selection at a rate proportional to the loss of fitness of heterozygotes. The coefficient of selection, s, is a measure of the loss of fitness. Fitness is measured as $f = 1 - s$. An example mentioned in Chapter 4 was that achondroplastic dwarfs have only about one fifth as many children as do people of normal stature in the population. Thus their average fitness is 0.20, and the coefficient of selection is 0.80. In the sub-

Table 7–8. Examples of Disorders Occurring as Sporadic Conditions, Possibly Determined by Autosomal Dominant Genes with Zero Fitness

Disorder	Features
Acrodysostosis	Multiple congenital abnormalities, especially short hands with peripheral dysostosis, small nose, mental deficiency
Apert syndrome (acrocephalosyndactyly)	Very rarely, a person with this dysmorphic syndrome has offspring; if so, about 50% of the offspring are affected
Atelosteogenesis	Early lethal form of short-limbed dwarfism
Cornelia de Lange syndrome	Mental retardation, micromelia, synophrys, and other abnormalities
Lenz-Majewski hyperostosis syndrome	Dense, thick bone; symphalangism; cutis laxa
Osteogenesis imperfecta, Type 2	The perinatal lethal type, with a defect in Type 1 collagen (see Chapter 12)
Thanatophoric dysplasia	Early lethal form of short-limbed dwarfism, sometimes misdiagnosed as achondroplasia

Data from Jones KL (1988) Smith's Recognizable patterns of human malformation, 4th ed. WB Saunders, Philadelphia.

sequent generation, the frequency of achondro-plasia alleles passed on from the current generation falls to 20 percent. The remaining 80 percent of mutant genes required to maintain the constant frequency of achondroplasia in the population are added through new mutation.

Thus the observed gene frequency in any one generation represents a balance between loss of alleles through the effects of selection and gain of mutant alleles through recurrent mutation. This does not mean that a gene "knows" when it must mutate. Rather, it means that an equilibrium gene frequency is reached at whatever level balances the two opposing forces: one (selection) that removes mutant alleles from the gene pool and one (new mutation) that adds new ones back. Thus if the fitness of affected persons suddenly improved, the observed incidence of achondroplasia in the population would increase and reach a new equilibrium. Retinoblastoma and certain other dominant embryonic tumors with childhood onset are examples of conditions that now have a greatly improved prognosis, with a theoretical risk of increased frequency. On the other hand, if affected persons elected to have no children at all (thus effectively reducing the fitness of the mutant allele to zero), the disease incidence would immediately fall, not to zero, but to a level maintained by the introduction of new mutations to the gene pool in each generation.

Selection Against Autosomal Recessive Mutations

Selection against harmful recessive mutations is less effective than selection against dominant mutations because, as discussed earlier, only a small proportion of the genes are present in homozygotes and are therefore exposed to selective forces. Even if there were complete selection against homozygous recessive persons ($f = 0$), as in many lethal autosomal recessive conditions, it would take many generations to reduce the gene frequency appreciably because there are many copies of the mutant allele in the heterozygous state (with normal fitness) for every copy of the mutant allele removed from the gene pool by selection (Table 7–4). Removing selection against an autosomal recessive disorder such as CF or PKU by successful medical treatment would have just as slow an effect on increasing the gene frequency over many

generations. Thus in contrast to the situation for autosomal dominant mutations, the rate of increase would be so slow as to be of little if any clinical significance.

Selection Against X-Linked Recessive Mutations

Almost all X-linked phenotypes of medical interest are recessive, and therefore, as a general rule, selection occurs in hemizygous males, not in asymptomatic heterozygous females. This statement is, in fact, an oversimplification of the real-life situation because, as a consequence of X inactivation (Chapters 4 and 10), a small proportion of females are manifesting heterozygotes with low fitness; examples include rare carriers of Duchenne muscular dystrophy (DMD) who are physically handicapped by the disease and about one third of carriers of the fragile X syndrome (Chapter 4) who are moderately retarded. In this brief discussion, however, we assume that heterozygous females have normal fitness.

If an X-linked phenotype is benign and if affected males have normal fitness, one third of the corresponding genes are in males and two thirds in females, as shown in the example used earlier in this chapter of gene frequencies in color blindness. For such phenotypes, the ratio of affected males to carrier females is 1:2. However, if the phenotype has reduced fitness and affected males are selected against, a higher proportion of the *mutant genes capable of being transmitted* are found in heterozygous (but asymptomatic) females. Since affected males (who can transmit only to carrier daughters) are less fit, the relative proportion of heterozygous females in the next generation will *decrease*, and the proportion of affected males will *increase*. In DMD, for example, the ratio of affected males to carrier females is 3:4, and in classic hemophilia, with an estimated reduced fitness of 0.7 in affected males, there are less than 2 carrier females for each affected male (Emery, 1986).

In X-linked disorders such as DMD in which affected males do not reproduce, only the genes present in carrier females are transmitted to the next generation. Such diseases are called X-linked **genetic lethals.** Thus one third of all copies of such a mutant gene are lost each generation. As we saw in the case of autosomal dominant mutations, these mutant genes must be replaced by recurrent new mutations to maintain the observed disease incidence. Therefore, one third of all cases of such disorders are new mutants, born to genetically normal mothers who have no risk of having subsequent children with the same disorder. In a later section in this chapter, we return to the relation between mutation rate and fitness for DMD and for other genetic lethals.

In less severe disorders such as hemophilia A, the proportion of affected individuals with new mutant genes is less than one third (currently about 15 percent). Because the treatment of hemophilia is improving rapidly, the total mutant gene frequency can be expected to rise relatively rapidly and to reach a new equilibrium, as we saw in the case of autosomal dominant conditions. Assuming that the mutation rate at this locus stays the same, the *proportion* of hemophiliacs who result from a new mutation decreases, even though the incidence of the disease increases. Such a change would have significant implications for genetic counseling for this disorder (see Chapter 18).

Selection Against Heterozygotes

Selection may act against heterozygous genotypes as well as against homozygotes. Most of the blood group systems, especially the Rh system, tend to select against heterozygotes through maternal–fetal incompatibility. As recently as 1970, Rh hemolytic disease of the newborn was ranked as one of the most common genetic diseases, but it is no longer a serious threat to children's health because the sensitization of an Rh-negative mother (homozygous for a recessive allele) to the antigens of an Rh-positive fetus (who must of course be heterozygous) is now preventable by the administration of Rh immune globulin. Removal of selection against the heterozygotes would be expected, over time, to raise the incidence of the recessive Rh-negative allele.

As a second example, heterozygotes for sickle cell disease (see Chapter 11), although they are at an advantage in malarial areas (see next section), may be less fit than normal homozygotes in other environments. U.S. military recruits in basic training who were heterozygous for the sickle cell mutation have been reported to have a substantially increased risk of exercise-related sudden death unexplained by any known pre-existing disease (Kark et al., 1987).

Selection for Heterozygotes (Heterozygote Advantage)

The considerations in the preceding sections explain the present-day frequencies of rare mutant alleles as a balance between loss by selection and gain by new mutation. However, how then can we explain disorders such as CF and sickle cell anemia in which the mutant allele achieves quite high frequencies? Given the substantial selection against homozygotes for these mutant alleles, the only possible explanations are either that these genes have an extraordinarily high mutation rate or that heterozygous carriers are more fit in particular environments than even the normal homozygotes. Either explanation could ensure the constant replenishment of mutant alleles lost to selection against homozygous recessive persons. There is no evidence of high mutation rates in these disorders. However, it is known that there are environmental situations in which heterozygotes for some diseases are at a selective advantage in comparison with both homozygous genotypes. Even a slight **heterozygote advantage** can lead to an increase in frequency of a gene that is severely detrimental in homozygotes. If heterozygote advantage of a particular genotype is present but unrecognized, the mutation rate of the gene may be grossly overestimated.

The classic example of heterozygote advantage, though not the only one, is resistance to malaria by heterozygotes for sickle cell anemia. The sickle cell gene has reached its highest frequency in certain regions of West Africa, where heterozygotes are more fit than either type of homozygote. Heterozygotes are resistant to the malarial organism *Plasmodium vivax*, a parasitic protozoan that spends part of its life cycle in the red cells of vertebrates, to which it is introduced by the bite of the *Anopheles* mosquito. In regions where malaria is endemic, normal homozygotes are susceptible to malaria and probably almost all are infected and become relatively unfit; sickle cell homozygotes are even more seriously disadvantaged, with a fitness approaching zero. Heterozygotes, whose red cells are inhospitable to the malaria organism although their hemoglobin is quite adequate for normal environmental conditions, are relatively more fit than either homozygote and reproduce at a higher rate (Table 7–9). Thus over time the sickle cell gene has reached a frequency as high as 0.15 in

Table 7–9. Example of Heterozygote Advantage: The Sickle Cell Gene

Genotype	Observed Frequency Among Adults	Expected Frequency if in Hardy-Weinberg Equilibrium*	Ratio of Observed: Expected	Normalized Fitness
S/S	29	187	0.155	0.155/1.12 = 0.14
S/A	2993	2673	1.12	1.12/1.12 = 1.00
A/A	9365	9527	0.983	0.983/1.12 = 0.88
Total	12,387	12,387		

Data from Cavalli-Sforza LL, Bodmer W (1971) The genetics of human populations. WH Freeman, San Francisco.
* Sample calculation: Frequency of S allele = $[(29 \times 2) + 2993]/(2 \times 12,387)$ alleles = 0.123; Expected frequency of S/S persons = $q^2 = 0.123^2 = {\sim}187/12,387$.

some areas, far higher than could be accounted for by recurrent mutation. Earlier in this chapter we used this example of the sickle cell allele to illustrate deviations from Hardy-Weinberg equilibrium in a population of West African adults. It can now be seen that this deviation can be explained by the forces of selection on different genotypes.

When selective forces operate in both directions, toward the maintenance of a deleterious allele and toward its removal, the situation is described as a **balanced polymorphism.** Change in the selective pressures would be expected to lead to a rapid change in the relative frequency of the allele. Today many sickle cell heterozygotes live in nonmalarial regions, and even in malarial areas, major efforts are being made to eradicate the mosquito responsible for transmitting it. There is evidence that in the Black population in the United States, the frequency of the sickle cell gene may already be falling from its high level in the original immigrant African population of several generations ago.

Some other deleterious genes, including genes for hemoglobin C, the thalassemias, and glucose-6-phosphate dehydrogenase (G6PD) deficiency (see Chapter 12), as well as the benign *Fy* allele of the Duffy blood group system, are also thought to be maintained at their present high frequencies in certain populations because of the protection that they provide against malaria. The high frequencies of CF in Caucasians and of Tay-Sachs disease and other disorders affecting sphingolipid metabolism in the Ashkenazi Jewish population may, therefore, be due to heterozygote advantage. In fact, there is some evidence that heterozygotes for CF might have more children (i.e., be more fit) than normal homozygotes. However, genetic drift (to be discussed below), is a

powerful mechanism for the alteration of gene frequencies and may adequately account for the unusually high frequencies that some deleterious genes achieve in some environments. For CF and Tay-Sachs disease, the question may be resolved as methods of DNA analysis that allow unequivocal identification of heterozygotes are applied widely to population studies.

Genetic Drift

New alleles arise from mutation. When a mutation occurs, its frequency is represented by only one copy among all the copies of that gene in the population. The likelihood that such a new mutation will survive from one generation to the next is determined both by chance and by natural selection. Depending on chance, the allele frequency fluctuates from generation to generation, particularly if the population size is small. This phenomenon is called **genetic drift** and applies both to the establishment of new mutant alleles in a population and to the formation of a small subpopulation by isolation from a larger population from which it originated. In the new population, the gene frequencies may be rather different from those of the parent population because the new group represents only a small sample of the parent group and, by chance, may not truly reflect the gene frequencies of the parent group. Over the next few generations, while the population size remains small, there may be considerable fluctuation in gene frequency, although these changes are likely to smooth out as the population increases in size.

If one of the original founders of the new group happens to carry a relatively rare allele, that allele may become fixed in the new group at a relatively high frequency. This is the basis of the **founder effect.** One example cited earlier is the high incidence of Huntington disease in the region of Lake Maracaibo, Venezuela (see Chapter 4), but there are numerous other examples in genetic isolates throughout the world.

The Old Order Amish, a religious isolate of European descent that settled in Pennsylvania, gave rise to a number of small, genetically isolated subpopulations throughout the United States and Canada, with large families and a high frequency of consanguineous marriage. The incidence of specific rare syndromes such as Ellis – van Creveld syndrome (Fig. 7 – 3) in some Amish communities but not in others is an illustration of the founder effect.

One of the most striking examples of founder effect is provided by the Afrikaner population of South Africa (Diamond and Rotter, 1987). The population was established by a small number of immigrants, mainly from Holland, over a few decades beginning in 1652, and underwent explosive growth in its early years. Today, nearly 1 million of the 2,500,000 living Afrikaners bear the names of only 20 original settlers. One early settler brought the gene for **variegate porphyria** (VP), an autosomal dominant disorder of relatively late onset. VP results from deficiency of the enzyme protoporphyrinogen oxidase, which is in the heme synthesis pathway. Heterozygotes develop photosensitivity and neurovisceral symptoms, induced by barbiturates and other factors. Homozygotes have a more severe disorder, with earlier onset and retardation of growth and mental development. Today the incidence of VP in South Africa is 3/1000, far higher than in the population of Holland or anywhere else in the world.

The French-Canadian population of Canada also has high frequencies of certain disorders that are rare elsewhere. One disease characteristic of the relatively isolated Lac Saint Jean region of Quebec is tyrosinemia; this autosomal recessive condition has an overall frequency of about 1/100,000 in other parts of Quebec and in Norway and Sweden, but 1/685 in Lac Saint Jean, where the founder effect has been demonstrated (Laberge, 1969).

The population of Finland, long isolated genetically by geography, language, and culture, has expanded in the last 300 years from 400,000 to about 5 million. The isolation and population expansion have allowed Finland to develop a distinctive pattern of single-gene disorders. There is a high frequency of at least 20 disorders that are rare elsewhere. For example, choroideremia, an X-linked degenerative eye disease, is very rare worldwide; only about 400 cases have been described. However, fully one third of these are from a small region in Finland, populated by a large extended family descended from a founding couple born in the 1640s (Fig. 7 – 4). Conversely, disorders that are common in other European populations, such as PKU, are quite rare in Finland.

One of the Finnish genetic diseases is hyperornithinemia with gyrate atrophy (GA) of the choroid and retina, an autosomal recessive condition

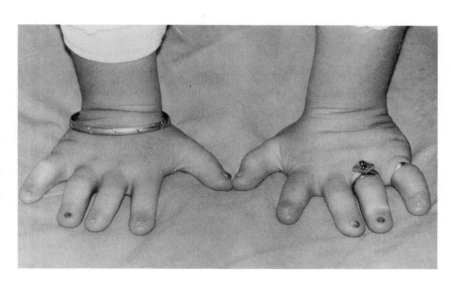

Figure 7 – 3. The hands of a patient with Ellis – van Creveld syndrome, a disorder seen in some Amish groups. Note the characteristic short fingers and hypoplastic nails, (Photograph courtesy of David Rimoin, Cedars-Sinai Medical Center, Los Angeles.)

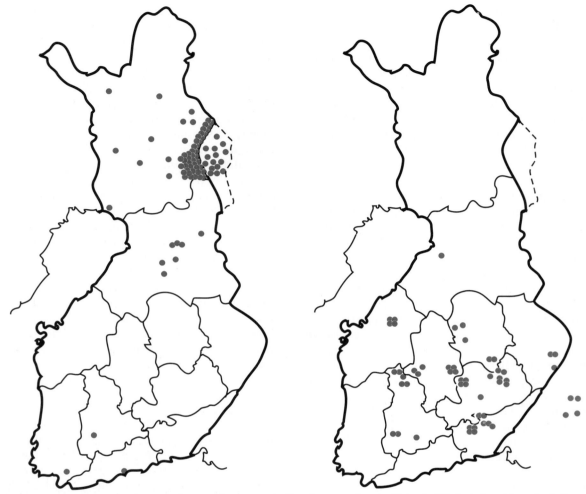

Figure 7–4. The geographical origin of cases of two genetic disorders prevalent in Finland: X-linked choroideremia (left) and hyperornithinemia with gyrate atrophy of the choroid and retina (right). Most cases of each disease originate from particular communities in Finland, but the distributions of the diseases differ. (Based on Mitchell et al., 1989, and Norio et al., 1973.)

caused by deficiency of ornithine aminotransferase (OAT) and leading to loss of vision in young adulthood. The structural gene for OAT has been characterized, and several different mutations have been identified. One mutation was found in homozygous form in the vast majority of apparently unrelated cases of GA in Finland, but it was not observed at all in non-Finnish cases (Mitchell et al., 1989).

Thus one of the outcomes of genetic drift is that each population may be characterized by its own particular molecular mutations. This type of ethnic and racial specificity of mutation has considerable implications for the application of DNA

techniques to the diagnosis of inherited disease (see box on p. 151 in this chapter). DNA-based screening and diagnostic tests designed to detect a specific mutation (such as tests based on allele-specific oligonucleotides; see Chapter 5) may have to be uniquely targeted to individual population groups.

As these examples show, genetic drift can favor the establishment at high incidence of genes that are not favorable or even neutral but are actually harmful. The relative mobility of most present-day populations, in comparison with their ancestors of only a few generations ago, may reduce the effect of genetic drift in the future.

Gene Flow

In contrast to genetic drift, which leads to random gene variation in small populations, **gene flow** is defined as the slow diffusion of genes across a racial barrier (Cavalli-Sforza and Bodmer, 1971), a process that involves a large population and a gradual change in gene frequencies. The genes of migrant populations with their own characteristic gene frequencies are gradually merged into the gene pool of the population into which they have migrated. (The term "migrant" is used here in the broad sense of crossing a racial division, not necessarily requiring physical movement to a different region.) Whereas the mechanism of genetic drift is chance, the mechanism of gene flow is population migration.

The frequencies of the different alleles of the ABO blood group system, which have been studied in many populations all over the world, provide convincing evidence for gene flow. The frequency of the B allele of the ABO system declines from about 0.30 in Eastern Asia to 0.06 in Western Europe, suggesting that the mutation originated in the Orient and gradually diffused into the more westerly populations (Fig. 7–5).

The transfer of genes between racial groups is a classic example of gene flow. By several measures, such as comparison of the frequency of the strictly African R^0 allele in African and American Blacks (Table 7–1), the percentage of alleles of one racial group carried by members of another can be determined. In one study the proportion of Caucasian genes in American Blacks ranged from 0.04 to 0.28 (Reed, 1969). Another example of gene flow between population groups is reflected in the frequency of specific mutant alleles causing PKU (see box in Chapter 4). There is strong evidence that the most common mutations were of Celtic origin (Woolf et al., 1975). These same mutations have now turned up in many populations around the world. The presence of the same PKU alleles in different populations reflects the geographical migration of the Celts. Thus the frequency of PKU is approximately 1/4500 in Ireland, but the disorder is progressively less prevalent across Northern and Southern Europe. There has been considerably less gene flow to East Asia. The incidence of PKU

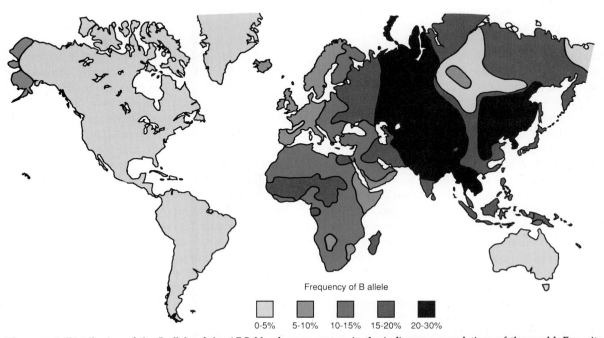

Frequency of B allele

0-5%   5-10%   10-15%   15-20%   20-30%

Figure 7-5. Distribution of the B allele of the ABO blood group system in the indigenous populations of the world. From its supposed origin in eastern Asia, the frequency of B declines fairly steadily across Asia and Europe. (Redrawn from Mourant AE [1983] Blood relations: Blood groups and anthropology. Oxford University Press, Oxford.)

in Japan is only about 1/50,000 (Scriver et al., 1989).

MEASUREMENT OF HUMAN MUTATION RATES

As described in Chapter 6, the mutation rate of a gene is defined as the rate of mutation per locus per generation, or, equivalently, the rate per locus per gamete. It must be distinguished from another clinically important concept, the proportion of all cases of the disorder that are due to new mutation; in a balanced population, the latter is equivalent to the proportion of alleles lost as a result of reduced fitness. A gene's frequency, mutation rate, and fitness are related; thus if any two of these three characteristics are known, the third can be estimated.

Mutation Rate of Autosomal Dominant Genes

The mutation rate of autosomal dominant disorders can be measured either directly or indirectly. Direct measurement is accurate only when all cases of a disorder in the population are correctly diagnosed and ascertained and those patients with unaffected parents are identified. This is easier said than done, but estimates have been made for a number of conditions. As described in Chapter 6, the highest mutation rate known for any autosomal dominant disease is that of neurofibromatosis (NF1), which is about 1×10^{-4}. At the other extreme, there is no convincing report of a new mutation at the Huntington disease locus.

One can also measure the incidence of new mutation indirectly by taking fitness into account. Achondroplasia, like many other autosomal dominant disorders of early onset, is associated with reduced fitness. As mentioned earlier, fitness in achondroplasia is about 0.20. The mutation rate at this locus therefore must be sufficient to account for the proportion of mutant alleles lost by selection (in this case, 80 percent). Thus the mutation rate will be equal to 80 percent of the allele frequency. Because the observed incidence of achondroplasia ($q^2 + 2pq$) is about 1/20,000, the frequency of the mutant allele (q) is about 1/40,000.

The mutation rate estimated by this method is therefore $(0.8)(1/40,000) = 2 \times 10^{-5}$. To state this generally,

$$\mu = s \times q,$$

where μ = mutation rate, s = selective disadvantage, and q = mutant allele frequency. This indirect estimate is only slightly less than that estimated by the direct method in Chapter 6. The difference probably reflects diagnostic difficulties or erroneous estimates of fitness.

Mutation Rate of Autosomal Recessive Genes

Although one can measure mutation rates for autosomal recessive mutations by equating the rate of new mutation to the number of genes lost through selection, those rates are of little medical significance. When a disorder shows autosomal recessive inheritance, the probability that a parent is a carrier is far greater than the probability that one or both parents could have transmitted a fresh mutation to the child. For most autosomal recessive genes of medical interest, the population frequency of the abnormal allele (q) is about 0.02 to 0.003 (see Table 7–4 for examples). Thus the calculated probability that both parents of an affected child are carriers ($2pq \times 2pq$) is far greater than the chance that one is a carrier and one not ($2pq \times \mu$) or that neither is a carrier (μ^2).

Does this mean that recessive mutant alleles are never generated by new mutation? No. In fact, it seems reasonable to assume that the rate of new mutation at, for example, the CF or PKU locus is approximately the same as that at loci for autosomal dominant disorders. However, given the relatively high frequency of pre-existing mutant alleles already present in the population (in the form of heterozygous carriers), it is *a priori* unlikely that a new mutation will come to attention. For example, even assuming a probably unreasonably high mutation rate of 1×10^{-4} at the CF locus, one can calculate that more than 99 percent of all patients with CF will be born to carrier parents. For general purposes, then, the parents of a child with an autosomal recessive condition are considered obligate heterozygotes, and the possibility of a new mutation is discounted.

Mutation Rate of X-Linked Genes

For X-linked genes, the method of calculation of mutation rate must take into account the fact that males, being hemizygous, inevitably express X-linked mutations, whereas females, being heterozygous, usually do not. In disorders due to X-linked recessive genes that are genetic lethals, with a fitness of zero, *all* the alleles in affected males are lost in each generation. These represent one third of the alleles for that disorder in the population. In a population at equilibrium, the number of new mutations at the locus should equal the number lost in affected males; thus one third of the alleles responsible for the disease in males are new mutations. The general formula for the mutation rate for such an X-linked disorder is

$$\mu = \frac{s \times q}{3},$$

where μ = mutation rate, s = selective disadvantage, and q = mutant allele frequency.

The proportion (m) of all patients with an X-linked recessive disease who are new mutants can be measured by the following formula, often referred to as Haldane's rule because it was first shown by J.B.S. Haldane, in 1935:

$$m = \frac{s \times \mu}{2\mu + v},$$

where s = selective disadvantage, v = mutation rate in males, and μ = mutation rate in females.

The question of whether μ and v are equal has been examined for a number of X-linked loci but remains unsettled. There is no strong reason to expect that ova and sperm, with their very different histories, should have the same mutation rate. However, for most of the few loci tested so far, there seems to be little if any difference in the male and female mutation rates. For practical purposes, therefore, it seems acceptable at present to assume that $\mu = v$ for most X-linked disorders. If so, the Haldane equation becomes

$$m = 1/3(s),$$

and if $s = 1$ (for a genetic lethal with $f = 0$), as it does for many X-linked lethal disorders, then

$$m = 1/3.$$

In other words, for X-linked lethal disorders, one third of all the affected males have new mutant alleles. In Chapter 18, Haldane's rule is used to demonstrate how to determine carrier risk in X-linked pedigrees.

EUGENIC AND DYSGENIC EFFECTS ON GENE FREQUENCIES

The term **eugenics,** introduced by Darwin's cousin Francis Galton in 1883, refers to the improvement of a population by selection of only its best specimens for breeding. Plant and animal breeders have followed this practice since ancient times. In the late 19th century, Galton and others began to promote the idea of using selective breeding to improve the human species, thus initiating the so-called eugenics movement, which was widely supported for the next half century. Eventually, a strong reaction developed against eugenics, partly because it was used in Nazi Germany as a false justification for racism and prejudice, but also because of a growing appreciation of the theoretical and practical difficulties of carrying out eugenics programs.

Ethical considerations aside, the major theoretical difficulty in planning eugenics programs is that there is little agreement about what hereditary characters are desirable. A second problem, which is a source of increasing concern to plant and animal breeders today, is that selective breeding reduces genetic diversity and thus limits the capacity of a species to adapt to changes in environmental conditions.

Medical treatment can have a dysgenic effect by reducing selection against a particular genotype and thus allowing the incidence of harmful genes to rise. The effect of relaxed selection is more striking for autosomal dominant and X-linked disorders than for autosomal recessive disorders, as discussed earlier. Research workers have begun to be optimistic that successful treatment of DMD and CF will be achieved (see Chapter 13). Successful therapy for DMD could cause the incidence of the disease to rise sharply because the DMD genes of the affected males would then be transmitted to all their daughters, which would greatly increase the proportion of carriers in the population. In contrast, if all persons affected with CF could survive and reproduce at a normal rate, the incidence of the disease would rise from 1 in 2000 to only about 1 in 1550 over 200 years.

Genetic disorders with complex inheritance, discussed in Chapter 15, could also become more common if selection is removed. Congenital heart malformations and pyloric stenosis are multifactorial traits that are now treated successfully by surgery in many cases. To the extent that such disorders are caused by genetic factors, they will rise in incidence. Similarly, the discovery of insulin, a major medical advance, could conceivably lead to an increase in the incidence of insulin-dependent diabetes mellitus (IDDM) by allowing juvenile diabetics to survive and reproduce.

On the other hand, genetic counseling and parental decisions to limit reproduction can have the effect of greatly reducing the incidence of some diseases. As we have mentioned, if no one at risk of Huntington disease reproduced, there could be a large effect on the incidence of the responsible gene. Other late-onset autosomal dominant diseases such as myotonic dystrophy would also become less common if at-risk family members were identified and chose not to reproduce or chose to have prenatal diagnosis to ensure that the disease gene was not passed on. In contrast, restriction of reproduction would have no appreciable effect on the incidence of most autosomal recessive diseases.

The long-term impact of activities in medical genetics that can affect gene frequencies may be difficult to predict. As prenatal diagnosis (Chapter 19) becomes widespread, significant numbers of pregnancies in which the fetus has a genetic defect are terminated, with the potential effect of reducing the frequency of the disorders and of the genes responsible for them. At present, however, no one has measured to what extent pregnancy termination for genetic reasons is followed by **reproductive compensation** — that is, by the birth of additional, unaffected children, many of whom are carriers of the deleterious gene. Some families with X-linked disorders have chosen to terminate pregnancies in which the fetus was male, but of course daughters in such families, though unaffected, may be carriers. Thus reproductive compensation has the potential long-term effect of raising the frequency of the genetic disorder that led to loss of an affected child.

CONCLUSION: DISEASE GENES IN PATIENT POPULATIONS

The purpose of this chapter has been to provide some insight into the population aspects of medical genetics, especially into the differences that exist between members of different, more or less genetically isolated groups, and to show the medical significance of this kind of information. Some understanding of this aspect of genetics is important, especially in a region such as North America with its mixed population of diverse origins, where a single genetics clinic may have patients of several ethnic backgrounds, each at high risk of one or more different genetic disorders.

Practically speaking, regardless of the effect of medical treatment or genetic counseling on the gene pool of the population, the true focus of concern is not the general population, but the individual patient and family. We need to be aware of the population aspects of a disease gene because the knowledge can help in diagnosis, treatment, and genetic counseling. Broader considerations, such as the risk of increasing the load of deleterious genes in the population, are beside the point, and this is just as well because it is rare for genetic advice in a single case to have any significant effect on the gene pool of the population, though it may have profound effects on the individual patient and family.

General References*

Bodmer WF, Cavalli-Sforza LL (1976) Genetics, evolution, and man. WH Freeman, San Francisco.

Cavalli-Sforza LL, Bodmer WF (1971) The genetics of human populations. WH Freeman, San Francisco.

Emery AEH (1986) Methodology in medical genetics, 2nd ed. Churchill Livingstone, Edinburgh.

Eriksson AW, Forsius HR, Nevanlinna HR, et al. (1980) Population structure and genetic disorders. Academic Press, London.

Hartl DL (1987) A primer of population genetics, 2nd ed. Sinauer Associates, Sunderland, England.

Kevles DJ (1985) In the name of eugenics. Knopf, New York.

Morton NE (1982) Outline of genetic epidemiology. Karger, Basel.

---

*See also the General References listed at the end of Chapter 1.

Problems

1. In a population at equilibrium, three genotypes are present in the following proportions: A/A, 0.81; A/a, 0.18; a/a 0.01.
   a) What are the frequencies of A and a?
   b) What will their frequencies be in the next generation?
   c) What proportion of all matings in this population are $A/a \times A/a$?

2. In a screening program to detect carriers of β-thalassemia in an Italian population, the incidence was found to be about 4%. Calculate
   a) the frequency of the β-thalassemia allele (assuming that there is only one common β-thalassemia mutation in this population);
   b) the proportion of matings in this population that could produce an affected child;
   c) the incidence of affected fetuses or newborns in this population;
   d) the incidence of β-thalassemia among the offspring of couples both found to be heterozygous.

3. Which of the following populations is in Hardy-Weinberg equilibrium?
   a) A/A, 0.70; A/a, 0.21; a/a, 0.09.
   b) MN blood groups: (i) M, 0.33; MN, 0.34; N, 0.33. (ii) 100% MN.
   c) A/A, 0.32; A/a, 0.64; a/a, 0.04.
   d) A/A, 0.64; A/a, 0.32; a/a, 0.04.
   What explanations could you offer to explain the frequencies in those populations that are *not* in equilibrium?

4. You are consulted by a couple, Abby and Andrew, who tell you that Abby's sister Anna has Hurler syndrome (a mucopolysaccharidosis) and that they are concerned that they themselves might have a child with the same disorder. Hurler syndrome is an autosomal recessive condition with a population incidence of about 1 in 90,000 in your community.
   a) If Abby and Andrew are not consanguineous, what is the risk that Abby and Andrew's first child will have Hurler syndrome?
   b) If they are first cousins, what is the risk?
   c) How would your answers to the above questions differ if the disease in question were cystic fibrosis, instead of Hurler syndrome?

5. In a certain population three disorders — autosomal dominant retinoblastoma, autosomal recessive Friedreich's ataxia (a neuromuscular disorder), and X-linked choroideremia (a cause of loss of vision in males at an early age) — each have a population frequency of ~1/25,000.
   a) What are the gene frequency and the heterozygote frequency for each of these?
   b) Suppose that each one could be successfully treated, so that all selection against it was removed. What would be the effect on the gene frequency in each case? Why?

6. As discussed in this chapter, the autosomal recessive condition tyrosinemia has an observed incidence of 1/685 individuals in one population in the province of Quebec but an incidence of about 1/100,000 elsewhere. What is the frequency of the mutant tyrosinemia allele in these two groups?

7. For the population in question 6, would you expect the mutant tyrosinemia alleles to be homogeneous or heterogeneous? How about for cases of autosomal dominant achondroplasia in the same French-Canadian population? X-linked Duchenne muscular dystrophy? X-linked color blindness?

THE HUMAN GENE MAP: GENE MAPPING AND LINKAGE ANALYSIS

Geneticists working in many different organisms depend on the mapping of genes to establish the identity of genes controlling different traits. Gene mapping in human and medical genetics has proven to be no exception to this pattern and has, in addition, paid a rich dividend in providing information of enormous practical value for biology and medicine. As alluded to in earlier chapters, human gene mapping is one of the most rapidly expanding areas of study in medical genetics today. This is largely due to the realization that gene mapping can provide a direct route for identifying genes responsible for genetic diseases. As applications of gene mapping information to disease diagnosis, gene isolation, and genetic counseling have become more widely appreciated, the impetus behind achievement of a complete human gene map — an encyclopedia of all of our genes and their associated genetic disorders — has gained strength. Today, medical journals are full of reports assigning genetic diseases to particular chromosomes, and medical charts are full of laboratory reports in which genetic markers have been used to assist in providing accurate genetic counseling or diagnoses.

There are two fundamentally different approaches for assembling gene maps of human chromosomes: physical mapping and genetic mapping. **Physical mapping** uses a variety of methods to assign genes to particular locations along a chromosome. With these methods, map positions are described in units that are a reflection of some physical measurement performed with somatic cells in the laboratory. **Genetic mapping,** on the other hand, is the measurement of the tendency of two genes to segregate together through meiosis in family studies and thus is a description of a gene's meiotic behavior rather than its physical location. In this chapter, we discuss both types of mapping and examine several of their applications for identifying and isolating particular human genes and for providing diagnostic information in medical genetics.

PHYSICAL MAPPING OF HUMAN GENES

The assignment of genes to particular human chromosomes initially relied exclusively on family

The Growth of Human Cells in Culture

Techniques for cell culture took a long time to develop and to become widely used, partly because of the strict nutritional requirements of cultured cells and partly because successful maintenance of a culture for long periods requires exacting precautions to avoid contamination by microorganisms, yeasts, or other cultured cell lines. The nutritional requirements include the use of a semidefined medium with 5 to 15 percent fetal or newborn calf serum (containing largely unidentified growth factors), as well as glucose, amino acids, vitamins, minerals, salt, and a buffering system.

The kinds of cultures most frequently used in human and medical genetics, including gene mapping studies, include the following:

Peripheral Lymphocytes in Short-Term Cultures. These cells do not meet the requirement of long-term survival, persisting in culture for only about 72 hours. Such short-term cultures are used extensively for chromosome analysis, as discussed in Chapter 2.

Fibroblasts. Fibroblasts are among the most useful cell types for somatic cell genetic studies, including physical gene mapping. They are cultured from small explants of skin or other tissue. The cells, which have a characteristic spindle shape, grow in monolayers attached to a plastic or glass substratum and must be subcultured at frequent intervals because overcrowding leads to contact inhibition of growth. Fibroblast cultures usually maintain the karyotype of the original cells (normal or abnormal), although clones of cells with somatically altered karyotypes arise in culture rarely. Fibroblast cultures senesce after about 30 to 100 generations in culture; the duration of survival in culture is longer for cell lines set up from young persons than for cell lines from older persons. Fibroblasts cultured from patients with a suspected genetic disorder are a common source of metaphase chromosomes for cytogenetic analysis, of cell extracts for biochemical studies, and of DNA for molecular studies. In addition, human fibroblasts are often used in somatic cell hybridization experiments for gene mapping.

Permanent Lines of Transformed Cells. Some cell lines undergo transformation in culture and become capable of unlimited growth, either spontaneously or experimentally by viral infection; other permanent cell lines are established directly from tumors. Such lines do not exhibit contact inhibition, do not senesce, and do not maintain a stable karyotype, but often exhibit characteristics of the type of transformed cell from which they were derived. As such, they are quite useful for analysis of the genetic basis of transformation and malignancy.

Lymphoblast Cell Lines. Although cultures of peripheral blood lymphocytes do not ordinarily persist in culture, they can be induced to do so when transformed by the Epstein-Barr virus. Lymphoblast cultures, derived from B-cell lineages, grow in suspension, rather than as an attached monolayer of cells, and do not senesce. Thus they are an essentially permanent source of material from patients with genetic disorders.

Fetal Cell Lines. Fetal cells can be obtained prenatally either by sampling amniotic fluid by amniocentesis or by chorionic villus sampling from a pregnant woman (see Chapter 19). A proportion of fetal cells so obtained retain at least some growth potential in culture, although such cultures tend not to grow as well (or for as long) as skin fibroblasts. Amniotic fluid cell or chorionic villus cultures are used for determining the fetal karyotype, for analysis of enzyme levels, and for DNA analysis to provide prenatal diagnosis.

studies in large pedigrees to ascertain the mode of inheritance. X-linked traits could be assigned to the X chromosome because of their unique pattern of transmission. In addition, as discussed later in this chapter, a few autosomal traits could be assigned to individual chromosomes because of the fortuitous discovery of their cotransmission through many meioses with other well-known autosomal genes. This was a generally slow and painstaking business, however, until the discovery in the 1960s that mammalian chromosomes, and particularly human chromosomes, could be made to "segregate" in somatic cells in culture, not just in germ cells in family studies, thus establishing a so-called "parasexual" alternative for gene mapping. Because of its central importance to the field of gene mapping, we first discuss the establishment and growth of cells in culture and then describe the specific applications of this approach to physical gene mapping.

Somatic Cell Genetics

Somatic cell genetics, in broad terms, is the study of gene organization, expression, and regulation in cultured cells of somatic origin. As an approach to many problems in human and medical genetics, it has been remarkably successful since the 1960s. Somatic cell genetics was originally seen as a way of investigating single-gene and chromosomal disorders in long-term culture in the laboratory rather than in living patients. The approach has many obvious advantages. If a cell line from a patient with a rare disorder or an unusual karyotype can be established when the patient is available, it can be frozen more or less permanently in liquid nitrogen and studied later by different groups of investigators at any convenient time, even decades after the demise of the patient.

The field of gene mapping has taken advantage of the ability of a number of different cell types to grow, sometimes indefinitely, in cell culture (see the box on p. 168). Indeed, it is doubtful that many of the advances in gene mapping could have come about so quickly without the capability of culturing somatic cells.

Physical mapping of genes encompasses a variety of different methods, designed to provide mapping information of different types and different levels of resolution, ranging from an entire chromosome to the single base pair (Table 8–1).

Somatic Cell Hybrids and Gene Mapping

One of the principal applications of somatic cell genetics to gene mapping involves the transfer of genetic material from a human cell to another type of cell in culture, a procedure called **gene transfer.** The amount of transferred DNA may range from a short segment of chromosomal DNA to much of an entire genome. Gene transfer is a well-known mechanism in bacterial, viral, and fungal genetics, and geneticists have long recognized that the frequency with which two genetic markers are transferred together can be used as a measure of their physical proximity in the donor genome. Thus, not long after it became clear that human and other mammalian cells could be maintained in culture, human geneticists searched for ways to transfer human genes from one cell to another in the laboratory as a parasexual means of segregating different genes and their alleles.

The most widely used approach, developed in the 1960s, involves fusion of cells from different species to make interspecific **somatic cell hybrids.** Cultured somatic cells growing as monolayers or in suspension, as well as living cells obtained di-

Table 8–1. Approaches for Physical Gene Mapping

Method	Goal	Typical Mapping Resolution (in base pairs)
Rodent/human somatic cell hybrids	Chromosome assignment	50 to 250 $\times 10^6$
Translocations, deletions	Regional localization	5 to 20 $\times 10^6$
Gene dosage analysis	Regional localization	5 to 20 $\times 10^6$
In situ hybridization	Within a chromosome band	1 to 2 $\times 10^6$
Long-range restriction mapping	Fine mapping of gene region	$10^5 - 10^6$
Cloning in yeast artificial chromosomes	Gene cloning (large scale)	$10^5 - 10^6$
Cloning in *Escherichia coli*	Gene cloning	10^3 to 5×10^4
DNA sequencing	Nucleotide sequence	1

rectly from patients, can be fused by using either inactivated Sendai virus or polyethylene glycol. These agents promote fusion of membranes from two types of cell, thus forming homokaryons (if two cells of the same type fuse) or heterokaryons (if two cells of different type fuse), in which two nuclei are maintained separately in the same cytoplasm (Fig. 8–1). After mitosis and cell division, the two nuclear contents are mixed in a single "hybrid" nucleus. Under appropriate selective culture conditions, the two parental cell types, as well as hybrids derived from homokaryons, are incapable of survival, thus selecting for growth of intercell hybrids. Although a number of selective schemes have been developed, one of the first and most commonly used involves selection in medium containing hypoxanthine, aminopterin, and thymidine (the so-called HAT medium). Cells can grow in HAT medium only if they possess the enzyme hypoxanthine guanine phosphoribosyl-

transferase (HPRT), which utilizes hypoxanthine and guanine in DNA synthesis (see Fig. 12–2). Cells deficient in HPRT activity (HPRT⁻) require de novo synthesis of purines for survival and cannot survive in HAT medium because aminopterin inhibits purine (as well as pyrimidine) biosynthesis.

When HPRT⁻ rodent cell lines (usually either mouse or hamster) are fused with HPRT⁺ human cells, only rodent/human somatic cell hybrids are capable of prolonged growth in HAT medium: the parental mouse or hamster line dies in HAT, and the parental human cells (depending on their source) are selected against by virtue of their lack of long-term growth potential (if peripheral leukocytes are used), their generally slow growth (if primary skin fibroblasts are used), or their fortuitous and characteristic sensitivity (in comparison with rodent cells) to the compound ouabain (Fig. 8–1).

Somatic Cell Hybridization

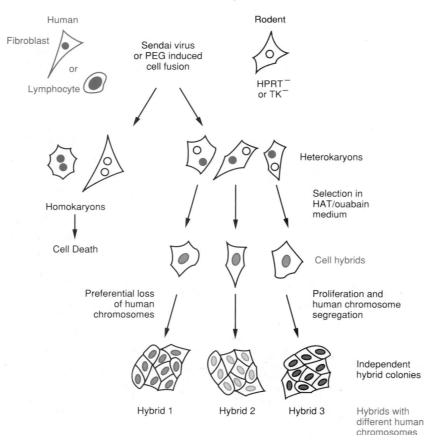

Figure 8–1. Interspecific somatic cell hybridization scheme. After cell fusion, human/rodent somatic cell hybrid clones are selected in a selection system, such as HAT medium. These cell hybrids preferentially lose human chromosomes, which makes it possible to isolate hybrid clones containing different combinations of human chromosomes. These clones can then be analyzed for the presence or absence of a particular human gene, thus allowing assignment of the gene to a specific human chromosome.

Somatic cell hybrids are originally polyploid, containing the full chromosome complement of both the rodent and human parental cells. In time, however, many of the chromosomes of one of the species are lost because their continued presence is not required for hybrid survival. Only the chromosome carrying the gene for a marker being selected (for example, the X chromosome, carrying the HPRT gene) is necessarily present in all cells, although, in general, at least a few other donor chromosomes also persist. The basis for chromosome loss or retention is still unknown; the important characteristic of rodent/human somatic cell hybrids is that it is the human, not rodent, chromosomes that are preferentially lost, resulting in hybrid cells retaining different numbers and combinations of human chromosomes, as determined by a number of karyotyping techniques that distinguish between rodent and human chromosomes (Figs. 8–1, 8–2).

This parasexual system of human chromosome segregation makes it possible to map any gene or DNA segment that can be distinguished between the species to a particular human chromosome. When the residual human chromosomes present in a panel of independent somatic cell hybrids are compared to the presence or absence of a particular human gene in the same series of hybrids, that human gene can be seen to correlate completely with the presence or absence of a specific chromosome. In this way, for example, the presence or absence of the gene for hexosaminidase A (HEXA), mutations at which cause Tay-Sachs disease (see Chapters 4 and 12), could be shown to correlate with human chromosome 15 (Table 8–2). All hybrids that retained a human chromosome 15 contained the human HEXA gene; all those that no longer had chromosome 15 did not contain human HEXA. This perfect concordance was observed only for chromosome 15 and not for any other human chromosome, thus allowing assignment of the HEXA gene to chromosome 15. In this type of analysis, the presence of a human gene can be monitored either by activity measurements (if the gene is expressed in somatic cell hybrids), by using electrophoresis to distinguish human from rodent cell activity, or, more commonly now, by DNA hybridization methods with the Southern blotting technique and restriction enzyme differences to distinguish the human gene from the rodent gene (Fig. 8–3). By using this type of concordance analysis in a panel of interspecific somatic cell hybrids, many hundreds of genes have been assigned to individual human chromosomes. Genes that have been mapped to the same chromosome are said to be **syntenic** (lit-

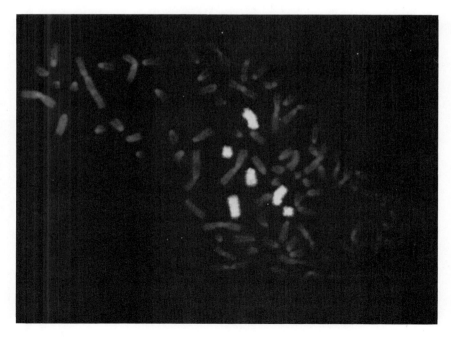

Figure 8–2. Metaphase chromosome spread from a mouse/human somatic cell hybrid. Human chromosomes can be identified by a detection method that specifically labels human but not mouse DNA. This hybrid contains six human chromosomes, identified as chromosomes 13, 20 (two copies), and the X (three copies). (Courtesy of V. E. Powers, Stanford University.)

Table 8–2. **Mapping a Human Gene by Using Somatic Cell Hybrids**

Hybrid	HEXA Gene	1	2	3	4	5	6	7	8	9	10	11	12	13	14	15	16	17	18	19	20	21	22	X	Y
																Human Chromosomes									
I	+	+	−	−	−	−	−	−	−	−	+	+	−	−	+	+	−	+	−	−	+	−	+	+	−
II	−	+	+	−	−	+	−	−	+	+	−	−	−	+	−	−	+	−	−	+	+	−	+	+	−
III	+	−	−	−	+	−	−	+	+	−	−	+	−	+	+	+	−	−	−	+	−	−	+	+	+
IV	−	−	−	−	−	−	−	+	+	−	+	−	+	+	+	−	−	−	+	+	−	+	−	+	−
V	−	−	+	+	−	+	−	−	+	+	−	−	+	−	+	−	−	+	−	−	+	+	+	+	+
VI	+	+	+	−	−	−	−	−	−	−	−	−	−	−	+	+	−	−	+	+	−	+	−	+	−
VII	+	+	−	+	−	−	−	+	+	−	+	+	+	−	+	+	+	−	−	+	+	−	−	+	−
VIII	+	−	−	−	−	−	−	−	−	−	−	−	−	−	−	+	−	−	−	−	−	−	−	+	−

Note: A panel of mouse/human somatic cell hybrids, each containing 2 to 13 human chromosomes, was used to test for the presence or absence of the human hexosaminidase A gene (HEXA) by means of Southern blotting of DNA prepared from the hybrids (see Fig. 8–3). There is a perfect correlation between the presence or absence of HEXA and the presence or absence of human chromosome 15. For all other human chromosomes, there are hybrids that contain HEXA but are missing the chromosome, and there are hybrids that contain the chromosome but are missing HEXA. Thus these results indicate that the HEXA gene must be on human chromosome 15.

erally, "on the same thread"), regardless of how close together or how far apart they lie on that chromosome.

Studies such as this using human/rodent hybrids allow assignment of a gene to a particular chromosome. Additional resolution can be gained by the segregation in hybrids of structurally abnormal human chromosomes, of which many examples are described in Chapters 9 and 10. If a particular gene cosegregates in a panel of rodent/human somatic cell hybrids with a deleted or translocated chromosome, then the gene can be localized to the portion of the chromosome retained in the hybrids. Alternatively, if a gene is known to map to a particular chromosome but is absent from a hybrid containing a deleted or translocated copy of that chromosome, then the gene can be assigned to the portion of the chromosome that is missing. Figure 8–4 depicts two structurally abnormal X chromosomes used in gene mapping to localize X-linked genes and DNA sequences to particular regions of the X chromo-

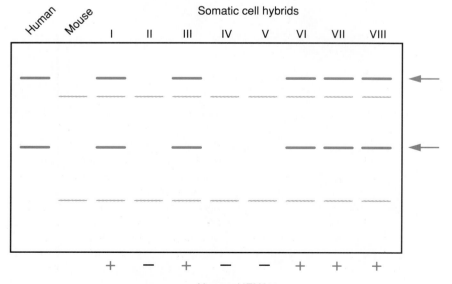

Figure 8–3. Southern blot experiment to map the human HEXA gene to chromosome 15, in a series of mouse/human somatic cell hybrids. Only hybrids I, III, VI, VII, and VIII contain human HEXA sequences, which can be distinguished from the mouse gene sequences by different restriction sites in the gene in the two species.

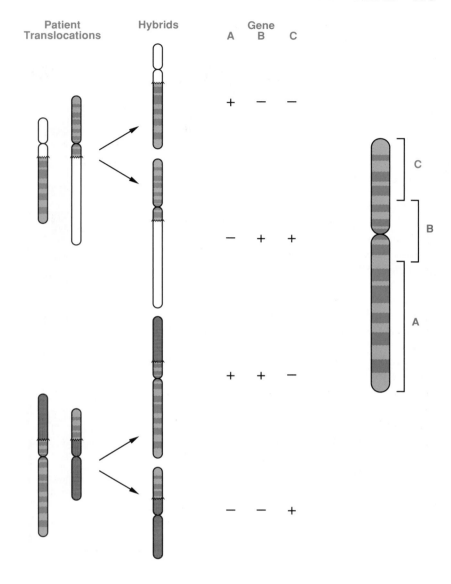

Figure 8–4. Regional mapping of X-linked genes by analysis of X;autosome translocation chromosomes in somatic cell hybrids. The reciprocal products of two different X;autosome translocations are segregated in somatic cell hybrid clones and can be analyzed for the presence or absence of genes from the human X chromosome. The combined results allow regional localization of the three genes to different portions of the X, as indicated at the right.

some. By examination of hybrids containing portions of these translocation chromosomes, the X chromosome could be divided into three intervals and different genes assigned to each. Extension of this strategy and examination of increasingly smaller regions of the chromosome of interest in hybrids has made it possible to localize genes to even smaller regions. Although this approach significantly improves the level of resolution of gene mapping, the chromosome regions defined are still quite large in comparison with the size of an average gene.

Mapping by Gene Dosage

A conceptually related approach also takes advantage of structurally rearranged chromosomes for gene mapping but does not rely on having to first segregate the abnormal chromosomes into somatic cell hybrids. This approach depends on detection of dosage differences in either gene products or the gene sequences themselves between patients' cell lines containing different numbers of copies of a particular gene. Although this method requires very careful analysis and interpretation, it has been used to assign genes to or exclude them from a region involved in a duplication or deletion (see Chapter 9). It was originally used to assign genes to chromosome 21 by detecting levels of enzyme activity in cell lines from patients with Down syndrome (three doses of chromosome 21) that were higher than levels in cell lines from chromosomally normal persons (two doses). At the DNA level, the dosage approach has been used increasingly to assign DNA markers to the X chromosome (by comparing DNA dosage in persons with one [i.e., a normal male karyotype] to five [i.e., a 49,XXXXX karyotype] X chromosomes) (Fig. 8–5) or to small regions of a particular chromosome (by examining collections of patients with partial trisomies [three copies] or monosomies [one copy]; see Chapter 9).

One of the most direct applications of mapping by gene dosage is the regional assignment of X-linked disease genes by examining males with cytogenetically detectable deletions of part of the X chromosome. In one well-studied case, a boy (B. B.) with no known history of any genetic disease presented with four normally distinct X-linked conditions: Duchenne muscular dystrophy (DMD), chronic granulomatous disease (CGD), retinitis pigmentosa (RP), and a rare red blood cell phenotype. Careful cytogenetic analysis revealed a small but detectable deletion in band Xp21 (Fig. 8–6). The coexistence of four single-gene disorders with the small chromosome deletion led to the conclusion that the genes for these four X-linked traits mapped to the deleted interval. Ex-

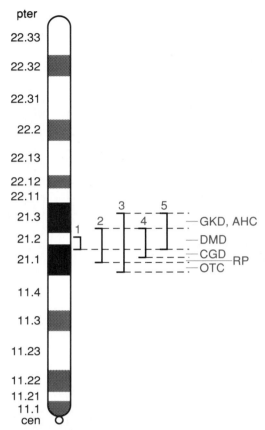

Figure 8–6. Regional localization of X-linked genes in patients with X chromosome deletions. Correlation of the extent of the cytogenetic deletion with the particular disorders present in each case allows fine mapping of the individual disease genes to particular regions on the X chromosome. DMD = Duchenne muscular dystrophy, OTC = ornithine transcarbamylase deficiency, CGD = chronic granulomatous disease, RP = retinitis pigmentosa, GKD = glycerol kinase deficiency, AHC = congenital adrenal hypoplasia. (Courtesy of U. Francke, Stanford University.)

tension of this type of analysis to other individuals simultaneously affected with multiple X-linked diseases has allowed the regional assignment of a number of genes in this region of the X chromosome (Fig. 8–6). The case of B. B. turned out to be even more significant for medical genetics because (as described more fully later in this chapter) his deleted X chromosome was used directly to allow cloning of the genes for both DMD and CGD. This provides yet another example of how recognition of the unusual in medicine—in this case, the occurrence of multiple genetic diseases in a single individual—can provide important new information about normal genes, their organization, and their function.

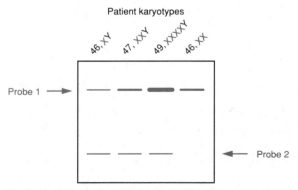

Figure 8–5. Examples of mapping by dosage analysis. DNA probe 1 used at the left can be mapped to the X chromosome because the intensity of hybridization appears to be a function of the number of Xs present in each DNA sample. DNA probe 2 shows the same intensity hybridization in lanes 1 to 3, but is missing from lane 4. This locus maps to the Y chromosome.

Gene Mapping by In Situ Hybridization

The mapping methods just discussed are indirect in that they provide information on the physical location of a gene on a particular chromosome but without actually visualizing the gene's map position. A more direct approach is **in situ hybridization**, which involves hybridizing DNA (or RNA) probes directly to metaphase chromosomes spread on a slide as described in Chapter 2 and visualizing the hybridization signal (and thus the location of the gene to which the probe hybridizes) under a microscope. The DNA in metaphase chromosomes is denatured in place (hence, in situ) on the slide, and hybridization of a labeled probe is allowed to proceed.

Methods for mapping single-copy gene sequences by in situ hybridization originally were laborious and slow, requiring long exposures of the slides under photographic emulsion to detect the location of hybridized probe that had been labeled with low-level isotopes, such as tritium. Mapping with confidence required analysis of many metaphase spreads to distinguish the real hybridization signal from background radioactivity. However, more sensitive techniques have now been developed that enable rapid detection of hybridized probes labeled nonradioactively with compounds that can be visualized by fluorescence microscopy (Fig. 8–7). Even in a single metaphase spread, one can easily see the position of the gene being mapped. In combination with banding methods for chromosome identification (see Chapter 2), fluorescence in situ hybridization can be used to map genes to within 1 to 2 million base pairs (1000 to 2000 kb) along a metaphase chromosome. Although this degree of resolution is a considerable improvement over other methods, it is still substantially larger than the size of most individual genes.

Chromosome Sorting

Fluorescence-activated chromosome sorting is a method that allows separation and purification of individual chromosomes on the basis of their in-

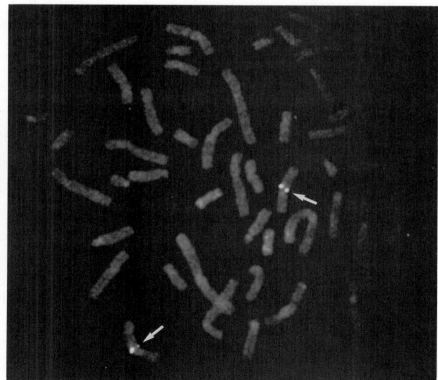
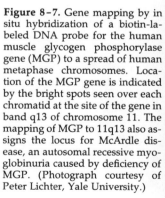

Figure 8–7. Gene mapping by in situ hybridization of a biotin-labeled DNA probe for the human muscle glycogen phosphorylase gene (MGP) to a spread of human metaphase chromosomes. Location of the MGP gene is indicated by the bright spots seen over each chromatid at the site of the gene in band q13 of chromosome 11. The mapping of MGP to 11q13 also assigns the locus for McArdle disease, an autosomal recessive myoglobinuria caused by deficiency of MGP. (Photograph courtesy of Peter Lichter, Yale University.)

tensity after being stained with one or more fluorescent DNA dyes. Metaphase chromosomes are isolated from a population of mitotic cells in culture, stained in solution, and allowed to flow past one or more laser beams set to deflect particles (chromosomes) of a particular fluorescence intensity into collection vessels. Each of the different types of human chromosomes can be separated from the others for karyotype analysis (Fig. 8–8). Millions of copies of a particular human chromosome can thus be purified from other chromosomes and used for gene mapping or DNA cloning. Flow-sorted chromosomes have been used to generate highly enriched clone libraries for individual chromosomes, which, as mentioned in Chapter 5, are often the source of choice for attempting to clone a particular gene whose chromosomal localization is already known, because the use of such libraries gives a ten- to thirtyfold enrichment for the clones of interest over the use of a total human genomic library. Flow-sorted chromosomes have also been used for rapid gene mapping by Southern blotting or polymerase chain reaction amplification of DNA isolated from the different fractions.

High-Resolution Mapping Approaches

All these cytogenetically based methods are designed to localize genes and other DNA sequences to regions of individual chromosomes covering anywhere from approximately a million base pairs (about 0.5 to 2 percent of the linear length of a typical chromosome) to nearly entire chromosomes. However, fine mapping of genes, as needed for cloning and detailed characterization of disease genes, requires a number of additional physical mapping approaches to map and clone regions of DNA in the range between the nucleotide sequence (single base pairs) and about 1000 kb. These methods include long-range restriction mapping, using restriction enzymes (see Chapter 5) whose recognition sites are very rare and that therefore cleave genomic DNA only once in several hundred to thousands of kilobases. Such restriction maps, which require a special type of electrophoresis of very long DNA molecules, called **pulsed-field gel electrophoresis**, are useful for establishing the order and distance between loci that map to the same small region of a chromosome, as determined by the mapping methods described earlier.

From the standpoint of medical genetics, the ultimate purpose of physical mapping with ever-increasing levels of resolution is, of course, to isolate genes responsible for genetic disease. Cloning of large DNA fragments, to facilitate moving along a chromosome toward a gene that one wants to identify and isolate, can be achieved through a number of cloning methods introduced in Chapter 5. One of the most useful approaches involves isolating human DNA fragments cloned as yeast

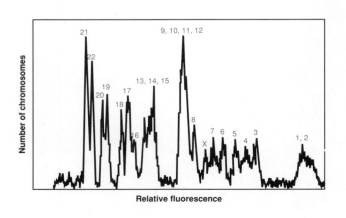
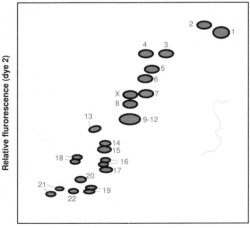

Figure 8–8. Flow karyotype measured for chromosomes isolated from a peripheral blood sample from a normal female, with either one (left) or two (right) DNA stains. Most of the human chromosomes can be separated from each other into specific peaks. Chromosomes can be analyzed for karyotype analysis, or DNA can be isolated from purified fractions for DNA cloning and gene mapping. (Data from Young et al., 1981, and Trask et al., 1989.)

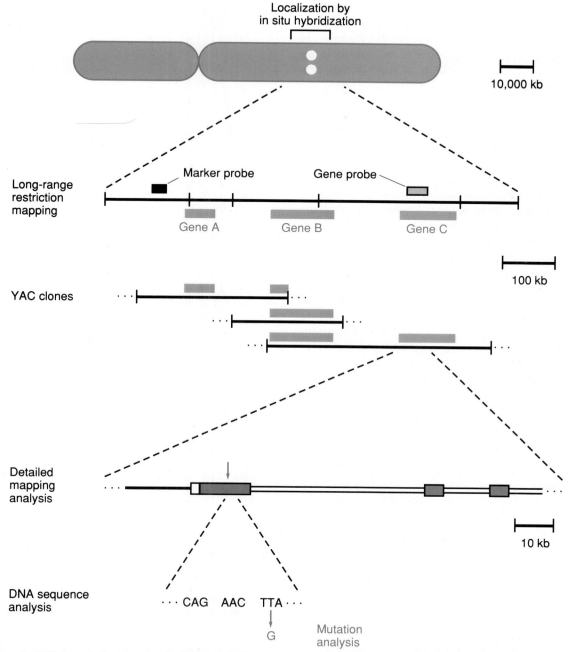

Figure 8–9. High-resolution mapping for cloning and analysis of a hypothetical disease gene. Resolution of analysis increases from in situ hybridization to metaphase chromosomes, to long-range restriction mapping, to cloning in yeast artificial chromosomes, to gene isolation and characterization, and finally to identification of a molecular defect by DNA sequence determination. Initial localization may be achieved through a DNA probe for a particular gene or a DNA probe for a "marker" locus that is known, by means discussed in the text, to map very near the disease gene of interest.

artificial chromosomes (YACs). YAC libraries can contain fragments up to 1000 kb long, and screening such libraries with a DNA probe of interest is therefore a rapid way to isolate considerable stretches of genomic DNA in a cloned form suitable for further detailed analysis (Fig. 8–9).

GENETIC MAPPING OF HUMAN GENES

In contrast to physical mapping methods, which rely on the parasexual segregation of homologous chromosomes in somatic cell hybrids or on measurements of gene position that are directly related to the linear scale of a chromosome (and thus its DNA), genetic mapping methods are based on the observed segregation of homologous chromosomes (and thus the alleles they carry) in meiosis in family studies. Although **genetic linkage analysis**, the method of mapping genes by virtue of their cosegregation (i.e., their "linkage") on a chromosome through meiosis, is laborious and computationally more complex than direct mapping of a gene by physical means, it is a tremendously important and powerful approach in medical genetics because it is the only method that allows mapping of genes, such as some disease genes, that are detectable only as phenotypic traits. The vast majority of genes that underlie genetic disease fall into this category because neither their biochemical nor their molecular basis has yet been elucidated. It is often the successful mapping of a disease gene by linkage analysis that provides the first real evidence that a collection of clinical abnormalities observed in family members actually is due to mutations at a particular, identifiable gene.

Genetic Linkage Analysis

In order to understand fully the concepts underlying genetic linkage analysis, it is necessary to review briefly the behavior of chromosomes and genes during meiosis I. As discussed in Chapter 2, each set of homologs pairs during meiosis I and undergoes a number of recombination events, exchanging homologous sections by crossing over and creating new combinations of alleles in the products of meiosis (Fig. 8–10). Crossing over

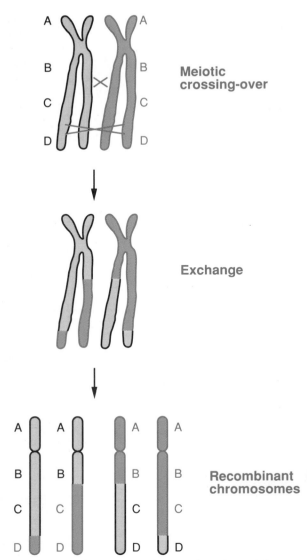

Figure 8–10. Crossing over between homologous chromosomes in meiosis, resulting in a new combination of maternally and paternally derived genes in the recombinant chromosomes. Two crossovers are diagrammed; as discussed in the text, a pair of large chromosomes will usually have several crossovers per meiosis.

takes place at the four-strand stage of meiosis, when there are four chromatids per chromosome pair. However, each crossing over event involves only two of the four chromatids. Thus for each recombination event, there are four products, two of which are **recombinant** and two **nonrecombinant.** One genetic crossover, then, is equivalent to 50 percent recombination between loci on opposite sides of the crossover.

We previously considered the chromosome as a unit of heredity; at this extreme, there are 23 pairs of homologous chromosomes that segregate in meiosis I, and one member of each pair is transmitted to each gamete and each child. At the other extreme, there are an estimated 50,000 to 100,000 genes, each in two copies, and one copy of each must be transmitted to each gamete and each child.

Considering both chromosomes and genes together, then, there are three possible ways for pairs of alleles to segregate in meiosis (Fig. 8–11):

1. Alleles at loci on different chromosomes assort independently in meiosis; thus for two loci D and M, with alleles *D* and *d* and *M* and *m*, one observes four types of offspring (i.e., four types of gametes) in equal proportions: *DM, Dm, dM,* and *dm* (Fig. 8–11A). (Within a single family, of course, these proportions may deviate significantly because of the relatively small numbers of offspring that are typical of human populations. However, by combining data obtained with different families, one can verify this expected result.)

2. At the opposite extreme, genes extremely close together on the same chromosome are transmitted together essentially all of the time; thus only two of the possible allele combinations will be observed in offspring; which two will depend on the particular combinations in the parental chromosomes (*DM* and *dm* in Fig. 8–11B). Assortment will *not* be independent, and no recombination will be observed.

3. Finally, in between these two extremes, alleles at two loci that are located on the same chromosome but some distance apart tend to be transmitted together unless a recombination event in meiosis creates a new combination (Fig. 8–11C). In this case, we observe all four combinations of alleles in offspring, the relative proportions of which will depend on the frequency of recombination between the two loci.

Genetic linkage can be defined as the tendency for alleles close together on the same chromosome to be transmitted together, as an intact unit, through meiosis. The strength of linkage can then be used as a unit of measurement to distinguish how close genetically different loci are to each other. This unit of map distance will, as said earlier, be a reflection of physical distance. However, the frequency of recombination is not constant along the length of a chromosome or throughout the genome. Thus genetic distance (measured as percentage recombination) and physical distance (measured in base pairs or chro-

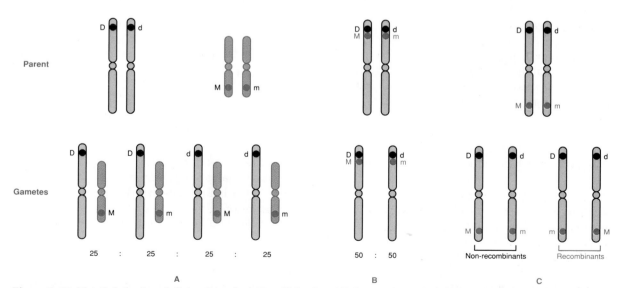

Figure 8–11. Meiotic behavior of alleles at two loci, D and M, when (A) they are located on separate chromosomes, (B) they are located very close together on the same chromosome, and (C) when they are located on the same chromosome but sufficiently far apart for meiotic crossovers to occur.

mosome bands) are different map parameters that should not be confused.

The unit of measurement for genetic linkage is the genetic length of a chromosome over which, on average, one recombination event is observed per meiosis. This unit is called a **Morgan** (named after Thomas Hunt Morgan, who first observed genetic crossing over, in the fruit fly *Drosophila*). Thus a **centiMorgan** (cM) is the genetic length over which one observes recombination 1 percent of the time. The total genetic length of the human genome was originally estimated to be 3000 cM, on the basis of the observed number of chiasmata seen in meiosis I in spermatogenesis (see Chapter 2). Thus because the genome corresponds to a haploid physical length of approximately 3×10^9 base pairs, 1 cM translates roughly into one million base pairs. This estimate suggests that individual chromosomes will each be approximately 100 to 300 cM long. One expects, then, on average, about 1 to 3 recombination events per chromosome per meiosis. This fact emphasizes the concept that a chromosome inherited by a child from, for example, the mother is essentially never exactly the same as either of the two copies of that chromosome in the mother's genome. Rather the child's chromosome is a patchwork, consisting of alternating portions of the maternal grandmother's chromosome and the maternal grandfather's chromosome (Fig. 8–12). Extending this concept over the entire karyotype reinforces the notion of human genetic individuality.

Linkage Analysis in Medical Genetics. The principal value of genetic linkage analysis in human and medical genetics is to aid in identifying, mapping, and diagnosing the genes responsible for inherited disease. Localization of genes by linkage analysis provides an opportunity to identify medically relevant genes that have not yet yielded to biochemical or molecular analyses. In suitable families, then, one can detect genetically the inheritance of a particular disease gene, whose phenotypic detection may be made difficult or impossible by lack of penetrance, late onset of symptoms, or uncertain clinical findings, by following the transmission of other, closely linked loci, called "marker loci."

Consider the family shown in Figure 8–13. The mother has neurofibromatosis, type 1 (NF1), an autosomal dominant condition with variable expressivity, the gene for which is on chromosome 17 (see box in Chapter 4). She is also heterozygous for two other loci on chromosome 17, one close to the NF1 gene and one not. One can see that transmission of the NF1 mutant allele "follows" that of one of the marker loci, locus 1. All the offspring who inherited their mother's *NF1* allele also inherited the *A* allele at marker locus 1, whereas all the offspring who inherited their mother's normal allele inherited the *a* allele. However, the NF1 gene shows no tendency to cosegregate with marker locus 2. Thus one would say that the NF1 gene and marker locus 1 are linked, but NF1 and locus 2 are not linked (even though they are still syntenic). In this family, even without any clinical examination, one could have predicted the presence or absence of NF1 by following the inheritance of alleles at the linked marker locus. However, marker locus 1 is *not* the NF1 gene itself; it is another fragment of DNA from chromosome 17, mapping close enough to the NF1 locus to track its inheritance through a family. This analysis would yield an incorrect diagnosis only in the event of a meiotic crossover between NF1 and marker locus 1 in the mother. The chance of an incorrect diagnosis is the chance that a crossover has occurred and is therefore equivalent to the genetic distance between the disease locus and the marker locus. This chance has to be taken into account in genetic counseling, especially for a disease such as NF1 in which the clinical symptoms are so variable, because an apparently unaffected person may have inherited the mutant gene but may show only very mild symptoms that might escape clinical attention.

Detection and Measurement of Linkage

There are two major requirements for carrying out a linkage analysis: a family must be **informative** for the loci being considered and the particular alignment of alleles in the parent (known as the **phase**) must be known or able to be determined. Detection of linkage requires that a parent be heterozygous (and thus informative) both at a disease locus and at marker loci. If the mother in the family shown in Figure 8–13 had been homozygous at the marker loci, evaluation of linkage would have been impossible. The loci most informative for

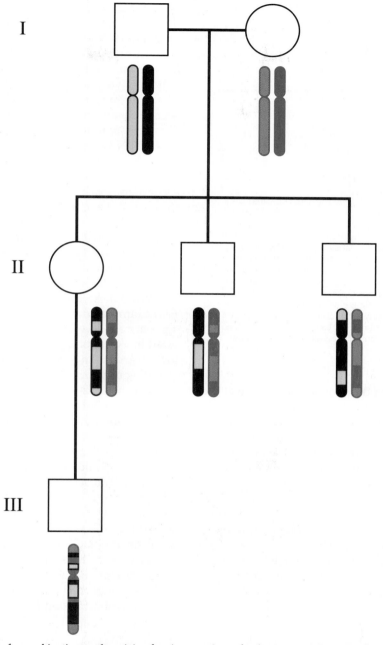

Figure 8–12. The effect of recombination on the origin of various portions of a chromosome. Because of meiotic crossing over, the copy of a chromosome inherited by the boy in generation III is actually a mosaic of parts of all four of the grandparental copies of that chromosome.

linkage analysis, therefore, are the ones that are highly polymorphic and are heterozygous in a large proportion of individuals; today, most of the loci used in linkage analysis are detected by restriction fragment length polymorphisms (RFLPs) with DNA probes. Especially valuable are the multiallelic variable number of tandem repeat (VNTR) loci introduced in Chapter 6, because most people are heterozygous at these loci. The second requirement for linkage analysis is knowl-

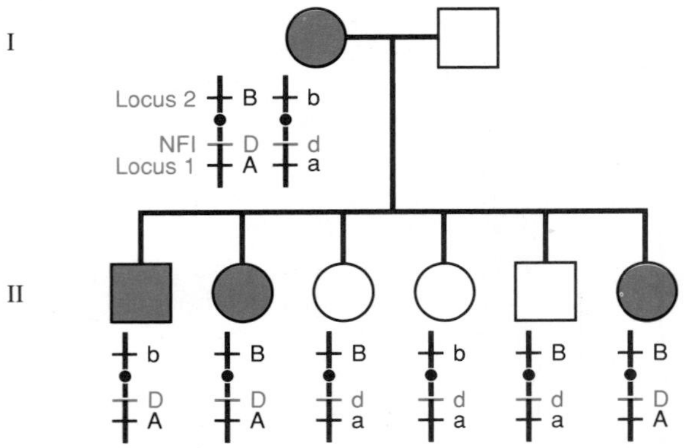

Figure 8–13. Linkage of the gene for neurofibromatosis 1 to a marker locus. The mother (I-1) is affected with this dominant disease and is heterozygous at the NF1 locus (*Dd*), as well as at two other loci, 1 and 2, on chromosome 17. She carries the *A* and *B* alleles on the same chromosome as the mutant NF1 allele (*D*). The unaffected father is homozygous normal (*dd*) at the NF1 locus, as well as at the two marker loci (*AA* and *BB*). All three affected offspring have inherited the *A* allele at marker 1, whereas the three unaffected offspring have inherited the *a* allele. Thus all six offspring are nonrecombinant for NF1 and marker locus 1. However, individuals II-1, II-3, and II-5 are recombinant for NF1 and marker locus 2, indicating that meiotic crossing over has occurred between these two loci.

reason, three-generation families are more useful than two-generation families. There are two related and parallel approaches to linkage in human genetics today. One is to develop a detailed genetic linkage map of the entire human genome, with a battery of very useful, large three-generation families. The purpose of this effort is to measure as accurately and finely as possible the linkage relationships among hundreds of informative loci, mostly DNA markers. The families are normal and do not manifest any known genetic diseases. The value of these families, however, is related to the second approach to genetic mapping, which is to measure linkage to disease loci. Because families that segregate genetic diseases tend to be small and not optimal for detecting linkage, the detection of linkage in such families is aided immeasurably by having a detailed normal map for comparison (White and Lalouel, 1988).

With these introductory comments, we can now examine how one detects and measures linkage between two loci. Suppose that one is interested in evaluating possible linkage between two loci, A and B, in a series of families. Among the offspring of informative meioses (those in which a parent is heterozygous at both loci), 80 percent are nonrecombinant and 20 percent are recombinant. The recombination frequency, therefore, is 20 percent, and loci A and B are estimated to lie approximately 20 cM apart genetically. This estimate, however, is valid only if the number of offspring has been sufficient to be confident that the observed 80:20 ratio of nonrecombinants to recombinants is really different from the 50:50 ratio expected for independently assorting loci, either far apart on the same chromosome or on different chromosomes. To evaluate this, one must determine the relative likelihood (odds) of obtaining the observed data when the two loci are linked at some recombination fraction θ, in comparison with the

edge of the phase of the genetic information at the two loci under consideration. When a person is heterozygous at a marker locus (as in Fig. 8–13), it must be determined which of the two alleles is on the chromosome with the mutant disease gene allele. Alleles on the same chromosome are said to be **in coupling** (or *cis*), whereas alleles on homologous chromosomes are said to be **in repulsion** (or *trans*) (Fig. 8–14). The importance of both of these requirements for genetic mapping is illustrated in sections below.

For the detection of linkage, large families are of greater value than small ones, but, particularly in studies of linkage with a genetic disease, large families are not always available. For the same

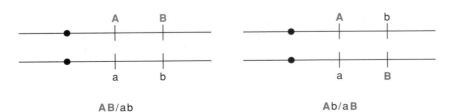

Figure 8–14. Possible linkage phases of alleles at two loci.

AB/ab

A and B in **coupling**
A and b in repulsion

Ab/aB

A and b in coupling
A and B in **repulsion**

situation in which they are not. Thus if of five children four were nonrecombinant and one was recombinant, this ratio would not be considered significantly different from the result expected for randomly assorting loci. However, if one observes the same 80:20 ratio after scoring several dozen children from several families, it would certainly be considered different from 50:50.

Lod Scores

In linkage analysis, one calculates a series of likelihood ratios (relative odds) at various possible values of θ, ranging from $\theta = 0.0$ (no recombination) to $\theta = 0.50$ (random assortment). Thus, the likelihood at a given value of θ

$$= \frac{\text{likelihood of data if loci linked at } \theta}{\text{likelihood of data if loci unlinked}}$$

The computed likelihoods are usually expressed as the $\log_{10}$ of this ratio and called a "lod score" (Z) for "logarithm of the odds." The use of logarithms allows data collected from different families to be combined by simple addition. Positive values of Z suggest that the two loci are linked, whereas negative values suggest that linkage is less likely (at that value of θ) than the possibility that the two loci are unlinked. By convention, a combined lod score of

+3 or greater (equivalent to greater than 1000:1 odds in favor of linkage) is considered definitive evidence that two loci are linked. The value of θ at which Z is greatest is accepted as the best estimate of the recombination fraction. This is often called the **maximum likelihood estimate.**

To illustrate the approach, we consider two examples that also demonstrate the importance of knowing phase information in linkage analysis. Figure 8–15 shows pedigrees of two families with neurofibromatosis, type 1 (NF1). In the two-generation family, the affected mother is heterozygous at both the NF1 locus (D/d) and a marker locus ($1/2$), but we do not know whether the NF1 allele is in coupling with the 1 or 2 allele at the marker locus. The father in this analysis is uninformative; he transmits to his offspring a chromosome that has the normal allele (d) and the 1 allele, regardless of how far apart the loci are or whether recombination has occurred. By inspection, then, we can infer which alleles in each child have come from the mother. Two children have inherited the D and 2 alleles, and one has received d and 1. Depending on the actual phase of these alleles in the mother, either all three offspring are recombinants or all three are nonrecombinants (Fig. 8–15, left).

Which is correct? There is no way to know for certain, and thus we must compare the likelihoods

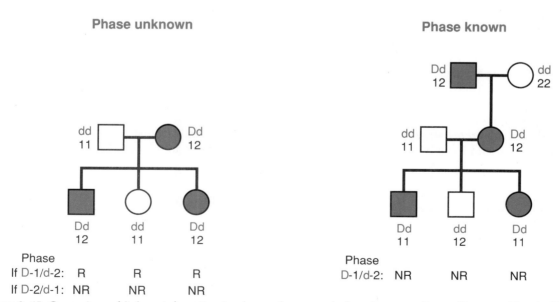

Figure 8–15. Comparison of linkage information in phase-unknown and phase-known pedigrees. R = recombinants; NR = nonrecombinants. See text for discussion.

of the two possible results. We can illustrate this for the situation in which we assume that the loci are completely linked ($\theta = 0.0$). If the correct phase is *D2* and *d1*, only two types of gametes would be produced; each child would have a 1/2 chance of receiving each combination. Thus the probability of having three children with the observed genotypes is $(1/2)^3$, or 1/8. However, there is an equally likely chance a priori that the correct phase is *D1* and *d2*. Thus the combined likelihood of these data, assuming linkage at $\theta = 0.0$, is $1/2 \times 1/8$, or 1/16.

On the other hand, if there is no linkage between these loci (phase, therefore, being irrelevant), one expects independent segregation of the two loci. Each child, then, has an equal probability of receiving *D1*, *D2*, *d1*, or *d2*. The probability of three children with the observed genotypes is $(1/4)^3$, or 1/64. The relative odds for this pedigree, then, are 1/16 : 1/64, or 4 : 1, in favor of linkage. The maximum lod score Z is the $\log_{10}$ of 4, or 0.602 (Table 8–3). Because this is far short of a lod score greater than 3, we would need at least five equivalent families to establish linkage (at $\theta = 0.0$) between this marker locus and NF1. With slightly more complex calculations (usually requiring computer programs written to facilitate linkage analysis), one can calculate the lod scores for other values of θ (Table 8–3). (Examples of lod scores for a range of recombination values and for families with up to seven offspring are given in a table in Appendix III.)

The second family in Figure 8–15 is similar, except that the mother's parents are available for analysis. By inspection, it is clear that the maternal grandfather must have transmitted both the NF1 allele (*D*) and the *1* allele. (This finding does not require any assumption about whether a crossover occurred in the grandfather's germline. Such an assumption would have been unwarranted.) The

phase in the mother must, therefore, be *D1* on one chromosome and *d2* on the other. The availability of a third generation makes this a **phase-known pedigree.** The three children can now be scored definitively as nonrecombinant. Comparing the likelihoods of linkage and nonlinkage is now simplified because we do not have to consider the opposite phase. The probability of having three children with the observed genotypes is now 1/8, not 1/16. As in the previous, phase-unknown pedigree, the probability of the observed data if there is no linkage between the loci is 1/64. Overall, the relative odds for this pedigree are 1/8 : 1/64, or 8 : 1 (instead of 4 : 1), in favor of linkage, and the lod score Z at $\theta = 0.0$ is 0.903 (Table 8–3). Thus the strength of the evidence supporting linkage is twice as great in the phase-known situation as in the phase-unknown situation.

The two families in Figure 8–15 illustrate another very important concept. In one family, the NF1 mutant allele was associated with the *1* allele at the closely linked marker locus; in the other family, NF1 was associated with the *2* allele. In general, there is no association between disease alleles and particular alleles at a linked polymorphic locus. The linkage phase has to be established for each family independently of any unrelated families. The allelic frequencies at the two loci are said to be in **linkage equilibrium**; the relative proportions of the possible allelic combinations can be predicted by the product of the population frequencies of the alleles at the individual loci. Thus, if a disease is linked to a polymorphic marker with two alleles of equal frequency, the disease allele will be associated with one of the marker alleles in half of affected families and with the other allele in half of the families. Exceptions to this are unusual and extremely valuable for genetic analysis, as illustrated later in this chapter with reference to the cystic fibrosis gene.

Table 8–3. Maximum Likelihood Analysis for Linkage Between NF1 and Marker Locus in Pedigrees in Figure 8–15

Type of Pedigree	Lod scores (Z) at various values of θ							Z_{max}	θ_{max}
	0.00	0.01	0.05	0.10	0.20	0.30	0.40		
Phase unknown	.602	.589	.533	.465	.318	.170	.049	.602	.00
Phase known	.903	.890	.837	.765	.612	.438	.237	.903	.00

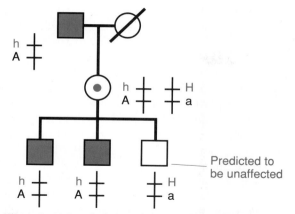

Figure 8–16. In X-linkage, the maternal grandfather's phenotype can reveal the linkage phase in his daughter. In this pedigree, the affected maternal grandfather's X chromosome carries allele *A* at a marker locus closely linked to the gene for hemophilia A (*h*). Thus his daughter carries these alleles on one of her X chromosomes and alleles *a* and *H* on the other, even though there is no direct information on her mother's genotypes. Knowledge of this phase can be used to predict the genotypes of her male offspring, including a male fetus diagnosed prenatally.

$\theta = 0.12$ and linked to B with a maximum lod score at $\theta = 0.05$. With only these two-point data, order can be established by inspection: the likely order would be A-B-C, with the following map.

|====0.10==== | ==0.05==|

---- A -------------------- B ----------- C ----

|=======0.12=======|

Note that the A-C distance as measured by recombination frequency is less than the sum of the A-B and B-C distances. This is due to the fact that double crossovers (one in the A-B interval and one in the B-C interval) do not result in recombination between A and C and, therefore, lead to an underestimate of the distance between them.

An alternative method for determining order among three loci is to consider all the data together, rather than the individual two-point

DETERMINING PHASE IN X-LINKED PEDIGREES

For linkage analysis in X-linked pedigrees, the mother's father's genotype is particularly important because, as illustrated in Figure 8–16, it provides direct information on linkage phase in the mother. Because there can be no recombination between X-linked genes in a male and because the mother always receives her father's only X, any X-linked marker in her genotype, but not in her father's, must have been inherited from her mother. This direct demonstration of phase is important for genetic counseling in X-linked disorders.

Genetic Linkage Maps

The previous section began with the observation that two loci, A and B, were linked. Let us assume that they are linked at a distance of approximately 10 cM. We can now begin to construct a genetic map for the chromosome on which the A and B loci map. Additional loci can be added to the linkage map if their distances from the A and B loci can be measured. Consider a third locus C, which we find is linked to A with a maximum lod score at

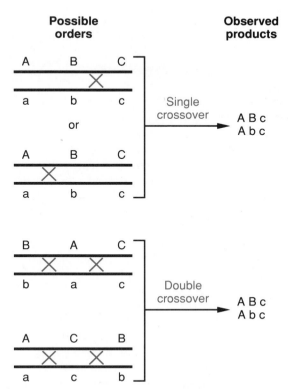

Figure 8–17. Determination of marker order by using multifactor crosses. Orders other than A-B-C require double crossovers to produce the observed patterns of recombination and nonrecombination among the three markers.

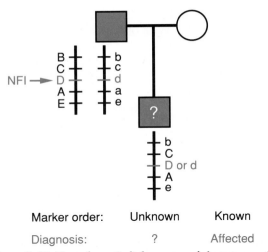

Marker order: Unknown   Known

Diagnosis: ?   Affected

Figure 8–18. Normal genetic linkage map of chromosome 17 and its application to genetic counseling for NF1. Knowing the order of markers on the chromosome 17 map allows interpretation of linkage data in the family. Without the normal map for comparison, the family would have been uninformative because the position of the observed crossovers with respect to the NF1 locus would have been unknown.

crosses separately. The principle of multipoint analysis is to establish marker order by minimizing the number of apparent multiple crossovers (Fig. 8–17). Particularly in very complex mapping studies, involving dozens of marker loci, multipoint analysis can provide strong statistical support that a particular order of markers is correct. These maps can then be used as frameworks to provide diagnostic information for use in genetic counseling (Fig. 8–18).

With increased attention focused on gene mapping as part of the Human Genome Project (see box), detailed genetic maps of all human chromosomes are becoming available, as a result of the thousands of RFLPs (and other forms of DNA polymorphism) detected in the genome (Williamson et al., 1990; Stephens et al., 1990). There is no longer any genetically "uncharted territory," and new genes, including many medically relevant ones, are being placed on the map weekly.

The Human Genome Project

Human and medical geneticists have been identifying and mapping genes for decades. However, a radical departure to the "map-as-map-can" approach was proposed in 1986 by Dulbecco, who suggested that if scientists really wanted to understand the role of genes in cancer—not to mention in genetic disorders in general—all they had to do was sequence the entire 3 billion base pairs and find all the genes! After much discussion and debate (some of which still rages), the Human Genome Project, an international effort to first map and eventually sequence all of the estimated 50,000 to 100,000 genes, was born. The initial emphasis of the project is on building both physical and genetic linkage maps of all 22 autosomes and the sex chromosomes and on assembling overlapping and contiguous collections of clones (called "contigs") covering each chromosome from telomere to telomere, in order to facilitate gene identification and isolation (Fig. 8–9). In the United States, the project is headed by James D. Watson, who, along with Francis Crick, discovered the structure of the double helix in 1953. The international effort is monitored by the Human Genome Organization (HUGO), which organizes a series of annual Human Gene Mapping Workshops to formally assemble and compare maps and to compile a list of all mapped human genes. An updated catalog is published annually (see General References) and maintained in a continually edited computer data base that tracks all of the current mapping data and makes it available electronically, together with information on human genetic disorders (*On-Line Mendelian Inheritance in Man; OMIM;* accessible through the Genome Data Base at Johns Hopkins University, Baltimore, Maryland; McKusick, 1990; Pearson, 1991).

APPLICATIONS OF HUMAN GENE MAPPING

There are three major applications of gene mapping to medical genetics: providing diagnostic information for genetic counseling, guiding efforts to clone genes responsible for genetic disease, and raising and testing hypotheses about the basis of particular genetic diseases. In all three instances, the building of both physical and genetic maps is interdependent. Genetic mapping is aided by the knowledge of the physical map position of polymorphic markers being used in linkage analysis. Physical mapping efforts to finely localize a gene can be guided by the existence of specific meiotic crossovers, detected as part of linkage analyses.

Detection of Mutant Genes by Linkage Analysis

That a genetic linkage map could be used to diagnose genetic diseases even in the absence of any concrete information about the biochemical or molecular nature of the disorder is a classic genetic concept that has been appreciated for decades (Haldane and Smith, 1947; Edwards, 1956). Despite the importance of this concept, however, linkage mapping has been widely accepted as being medically relevant only since the formulation of the idea that RFLPs could form the basis of a human genetic map (Botstein et al., 1980).

As discussed in Chapter 11, Kan and Dozy (1978) were the first to apply a DNA polymorphism to clinical diagnosis; they used a polymorphism 3' of the β-globin gene to diagnose cases of sickle cell disease by linkage analysis. Although the frequency of recombination between the polymorphic site and the site of the sickle cell mutation in the β-globin gene was negligible, it is important to recognize that the linkage approach to mutation detection, even when one is using informative polymorphisms in the cloned gene that is responsible for a genetic defect, is indirect and carries a risk of recombination between the genetic marker and the actual mutation. In most instances, this risk is probably very low. Very large genes, such as the DMD gene, provide exceptions to this generalization because crossing over within the gene occurs at a detectable frequency. In Figure 8–19

we illustrate the use of cloned genes as polymorphic markers for disease diagnosis, using as an example another defect at the β-globin locus, β-thalassemia, a common autosomal recessive condition that is described in detail in Chapter 11. The examples illustrate, once again, the requirements that a genetic marker must be informative and that it must be possible to assign phase in order to perform linkage analysis.

The value of a genetic map for disease diagnosis is most apparent when a gene has been localized on a chromosome, but not yet cloned. In this case, one has to rely on using one or more genetic markers that show detectable recombination with a disease locus. We have already alluded to this approach in discussing the detection of linkage earlier in this chapter. Diagnosis in this case is complicated by having to take into consideration

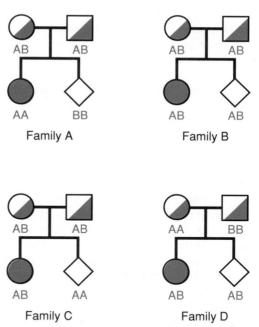

Figure 8–19. Examples of molecular diagnosis in β-thalassemia, with polymorphisms in the β-globin locus. The chance of recombination between the polymorphic marker and the mutation is assumed to be negligible. In family A, phase can be determined from the affected sibling, and a diagnosis of unaffected is possible. In family B, phase cannot be determined completely; no diagnosis is possible, because the second child could be either affected (50 percent chance) or unaffected (50 percent chance). In family C, phase cannot be determined completely, but it is possible to provide a diagnosis that the second child will be a heterozygous carrier. In family D, no diagnosis is possible; the family is uninformative.

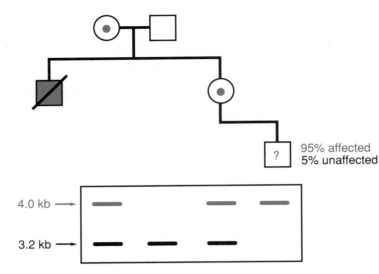

95% affected
5% unaffected

Figure 8–20. Example of molecular diagnosis by using genetic linkage with a polymorphic marker known to map a distance of about 5 cM from an X-linked disease locus. Pedigree is phase-known. The mutant allele must be located on the X chromosome with the 4.0-kb allele at the marker locus.

the possibility of crossing over in meiosis; thus for a genetic marker that shows 5 percent recombination with a disease locus, the diagnosis carries a 5 percent chance of error, even when the marker is completely informative and the phase is known (Fig. 8–20). The possibility of recombination can also complicate the determination of the phase, when the phase is inferred from a child rather than from the grandparental generation. For example, in the family shown in Figure 8–21, a diagnosis of myotonic dystrophy (DM), a variable autosomal dominant condition, is possible with only 82 percent certainty in individual III-2 (see legend to Fig. 8–21), despite the fact that the linked genetic marker being used shows only 10 percent recombination with the DM mutation. This is because phase information is provided by only the genotype of the affected child (III-1) in this family.

The accuracy of diagnosis by using genetically linked markers with an appreciable recombination frequency between the marker and the disease locus can be increased markedly by using two informative genetic markers that flank the disease gene. In this instance, the chance of a misdiagnosis is reduced significantly, since misdiagnosis will result only if *two* crossovers occur, one on each side of the disease gene. For example, for flanking markers that each show 10 percent recombination with a disease gene, diagnosis by genetic linkage will be 99 percent accurate (instead of 90 percent for a single marker). The benefit of using flanking markers reinforces the value of an accurate genetic

linkage map, with well-mapped markers of known order and distance.

Additional examples of the use of genetic linkage analysis for diagnosis of inherited disease are discussed in Chapters 18 and 19.

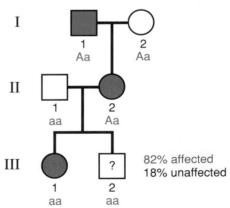

82% affected
18% unaffected

Figure 8–21. Example of molecular diagnosis by using genetic linkage in a phase-unknown pedigree with a polymorphic marker known to map a distance of about 10 cM from the myotonic dystrophy (DM) locus. Phase in individual II-2 cannot be determined from her parents because her affected father could have transmitted the mutant DM allele along with either the *A* or *a* allele at the marker locus. The genotype of the affected child, III-1, suggests that the mother's phase is DM-*a*, but this conclusion is only 90 percent certain because there is a 10 percent chance that her phase is DM-*A* and that a crossover occurred in the meiosis when her daughter was conceived. Thus the overall chance that III-2 will be affected is 82 percent, calculated as $(0.9 \times 0.9) + (0.1 \times 0.1)$.

Mapping of Disease Genes by Linkage Analysis

The preceding section focused on the use of a genetic linkage map for providing diagnostic information when a disease gene is already known to be genetically linked to one or more markers. However, how were these linkage relationships discovered?

The two essential requirements for mapping disease genes are, first, sufficient numbers of families to establish linkage and, second, adequate informative DNA markers. As mentioned earlier, the second requirement can be met relatively easily now. Finding suitable families can, however, be a challenge, particularly for rare disorders or for disorders in which affected persons die at a young age (and are thus unavailable for analysis). Two general approaches have been used (Fig. 8–22). In one, a small number of very large families is ascer-

tained and DNA is obtained from family members to be typed for DNA polymorphisms. The advantage of this approach is that all affected members of the pedigree are known to have the same genetic disease, caused by a mutation at a single locus. The alternative approach is to collect a large number of somewhat smaller families. This is easier to do for relatively common diseases, such as cystic fibrosis (Fig. 8–22), but it carries the risk that not all families may have the genetically identical disorder. **Genetic heterogeneity,** exemplified by the situation in which identical clinical symptoms are caused by defects at two or more genetic loci, can confound genetic linkage analysis and give the impression that a marker is unlinked to a disease locus when in fact it may be linked, but only in a subset of the families analyzed. This situation is illustrated later in the case of linkage in autosomal dominant retinitis pigmentosa.

In practice in human genetics, one can hope to

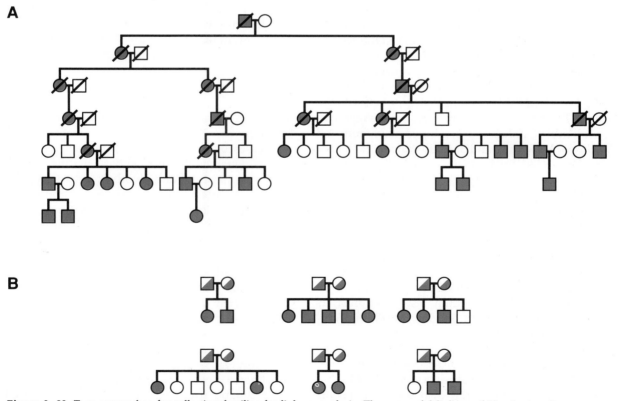

Figure 8-22. Two approaches for collecting families for linkage analysis. The successful linkage of Huntington disease to a polymorphic marker on chromosome 4 relied in large part on a single large Venezuelan pedigree, a small part of which is shown in A. The successful linkage of cystic fibrosis to a polymorphic marker on chromosome 7, however, relied on a collection of many smaller families, some of which are shown in B. (Adapted from Gusella et al., 1983, and Tsui et al., 1986.)

find linkage only at a distance of approximately 20 cM or less because at longer distances one usually cannot find sufficient family material to establish significant evidence for linkage (a lod score >3) compared to nonlinkage. Thus a polymorphic marker generally has to be within roughly 20 million base pairs of the disease gene of interest in order for linkage to be detected. For an autosomal trait, this is less than 1 percent of the genome, and so one would predict that, on average, 100 or so well-spaced autosomal polymorphic markers would have to be scored in the family collection before a positive linkage result is found. In fact, among the several dozen successful applications of this approach, the range is 12 RFLPs (for the most fortunate search) to over 200 (for the most difficult). It should be clear that the situation is considerably easier for X-linked diseases because one already knows the chromosomal location of the gene. Consequently, only polymorphic markers from the X chromosome need to be tested for linkage to the disease.

When one begins a search for linkage, the expectation for any given polymorphic marker is that, by chance, it will *not* be linked to the disease gene (in fact, by chance, it is not even likely to be on the same chromosome as the disease gene). Thus it may take only a few informative meioses to establish that the polymorphism is not close to the gene of interest. When a marker shows suggestive evidence of linkage (a combined maximum lod score of between 2 and 3, for instance), the search can be aided by knowing where the potential marker locus maps physically. If, for example, the marker maps to a position on the long arm of chromosome 7, then one can focus attention on other polymorphic markers in that region to efficiently confirm or reject the suggested linkage result. It is at this point that the extensive physical and genetic maps of each human chromosome become extremely valuable. Once a suspected linkage result is confirmed, one can then test other markers known to map close to the one found, in an attempt to move closer and closer to the gene of interest. Once one or more markers are found within about 5 cM of the disease gene, they can be used for diagnostic purposes, as illustrated in previous sections. They can also serve as starting points for fine mapping studies, to attempt to isolate the disease gene.

Human Gene Mapping and "Positional Cloning"

The application of gene mapping to medical genetics has met with spectacular success in some instances. The overall strategy — mapping the location of a disease gene by linkage analysis to define markers for use in disease diagnosis and genetic counseling, followed by attempts to clone the gene based on its map position — can best be illustrated by specific examples. The examples to be discussed illustrate several approaches; the one that is ultimately successful for a given disease depends on the unique characteristics and circumstances of that disease.

The approach of cloning a gene on the basis of its map position can be called **positional cloning,** to distinguish it from the more typical strategy for gene cloning, in which one begins with a known protein, determines its amino acid sequence, and uses that information to isolate the gene (see Chapter 5). Positional cloning relies only on the chromosomal location of the gene. This strategy has in the past been called "reverse genetics." However, in fact, this approach is firmly rooted in the traditions of classical genetics (Botstein, 1990).

Huntington Disease

Although linkage between an inherited disease and a marker locus had been demonstrated in a few cases by means of serum protein polymorphisms (such as the linkage between the "secretor" polymorphism and myotonic dystrophy), the first successful application of the RFLP strategy for linkage detection was carried out by Gusella and colleagues in 1983 for Huntington disease (HD). As described in Chapter 4, HD is an autosomal dominant disorder with late onset. A number of attempts had been made previously to find linkage with serum protein markers, but without success.

The family in which linkage was first demonstrated was from a large Venezuelan community in which there are numerous cases of HD; all patients had inherited the disease from a common ancestor (Fig. 8–22), thus eliminating the possibility of genetic heterogeneity from the initial analysis. A collaborative team of investigators collected DNA samples from thousands of members of this extended Venezuelan family and began what was

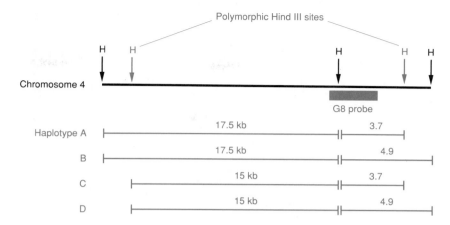

Figure 8-23. Four haplotypes at the D4S10 locus detected with the probe G8. All four haplotypes have been associated with the HD mutation in different families.

originally anticipated as a long search for a linked DNA marker. By a stroke of enormous good luck, particularly considering the fact that there were relatively few polymorphic DNA markers available in the early 1980s (in contrast to the thousands available today), close linkage to HD was found with only the 12th probe tested! The probe, called G8, detected two polymorphisms with the restriction enzyme *Hind*III, which led to a total of four different combinations of alleles, or **haplotypes** (Fig. 8-23). These polymorphisms were linked to HD with a peak lod score of 8.53 at $\theta = 0.0$, representing odds of greater than 100 million to one in favor of linkage. Subsequent studies in additional families have demonstrated crossovers between HD and this marker locus and have established that the G8 marker maps about 3 to 5 cM from the HD gene.

By analysis of somatic cell hybrids and by in situ hybridization, the locus detected by G8 was mapped physically to the most distal band on the short arm of chromosome 4, thereby demonstrating that the HD gene maps to this region on chromosome 4. Intensive investigations on the part of a large number of laboratories have isolated a number of additional DNA markers from band 4p16

that are also linked to HD (Fig. 8-24). Consideration of specific meiotic crossover events detected in family studies has permitted localization of the HD locus to a position extremely close to the telomere of the chromosome 4 short arm, within a region of 1000 kb or so.

In parallel with efforts to clone the gene and understand its function and to elucidate the basic defect in HD, the available markers are being used to offer presymptomatic detection of the HD gene in suitable families. Predictive testing of whether a clinically unaffected person carries the HD mutant allele requires extreme care with respect to confidentiality and to the psychological effects of a positive diagnosis made perhaps decades before the onset of symptoms. Such testing raises a number of important legal and ethical issues (Huggins et al., 1990).

The discovery of linkage of HD to a DNA polymorphism provided striking verification of the RFLP approach for disease gene mapping and provided impetus to the entire field of human gene mapping. In the years since the HD discovery, many of the major single-gene disorders have been mapped to regions of chromosomes by this approach (Table 8-4), and new disorders are

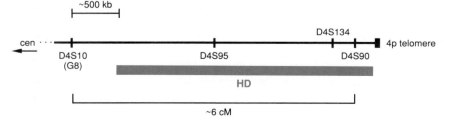

Figure 8-24. A map of the HD region near the telomere of the chromosome 4 short arm. Markers indicated are DNA probes that detect polymorphisms linked to HD.

Table 8–4. Selected Examples of Single-Gene Disorders
Mapped by Linkage Analysis

Disorder	Inheritance	Map Location
Alport syndrome	XR	Xq22
Ataxia telangiectasia	AR	11q22–23
Cystic fibrosis	AR	7q31–32
Duchenne muscular dystrophy	XR	Xp21
Fragile X syndrome	XR	Xq27
Friedreich ataxia	AR	9q13–21.1
Huntington disease	AD	4p16.3
Marfan syndrome	AD	15q
Multiple endocrine neoplasia, type 1	AD	11q
Multiple endocrine neoplasia, type 2A	AD	10cen
Multiple endocrine neoplasia, type 2B	AD	10cen
Myotonic dystrophy	AD	19q
Neurofibromatosis, type 1	AD	17q11.2
Neurofibromatosis, type 2 (acoustic)	AD	22q
Polycystic kidney disease	AD	16p13
Polyposis of colon, familial	AD	5q21–22
Retinitis pigmentosa	XR*	Xp11, Xp21
Retinitis pigmentosa (some families)	AD	3q21–24
Retinoblastoma	AD	13q14

AD = autosomal dominant; AR = autosomal recessive; XR = X-linked recessive.
    * Two loci.

being added to the list at a rapid pace. For many of these, establishing linkage provided the possibility of prenatal or presymptomatic detection for the first time, by using the approaches discussed earlier.

Cystic Fibrosis

Because of its relatively high frequency, particularly in Caucasian populations, cystic fibrosis (CF) represented another obvious target for the linkage strategy. Many families were studied and samples collected for DNA analysis (Fig. 8–22). Hundreds of DNA markers were tested for linkage without success before, quite ironically, linkage was demonstrated in 1985 between CF and an "old-fashioned" serum protein polymorphism, paraoxonase (PON; Eiberg et al., 1985). However, PON

activity is not expressed in somatic cell hybrids, and thus, despite the linkage, the chromosomal localization of PON (and thus of CF) remained unknown. Shortly thereafter, Tsui and colleagues (1985) demonstrated linkage of both CF and PON to a DNA polymorphism from the long arm of chromosome 7, using a collection of nearly 50 CF families. This linkage was quickly confirmed, and additional DNA markers were also shown to be linked to CF in the 7q31–q32 region. Because of the large number of meioses available for study, it was possible to use multipoint mapping analyses to pinpoint the location of the CF locus among a series of ordered and finely mapped DNA markers (Fig. 8–25). Long-range physical mapping techniques demonstrated that the distance between the MET and D7S8 loci was about 1.5 million base pairs. Because these two markers could be shown by inspection of crossover events to clearly flank

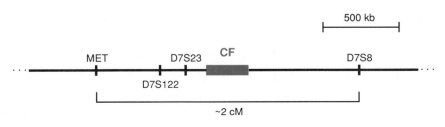

Figure 8–25. A map of the CF region in band q31 of chromosome 7, determined by long-range restriction mapping, extensive DNA cloning, and analysis of genetic linkage data. Markers indicated are DNA probes that detect polymorphisms linked to CF.

the CF locus, this meant that the CF gene must lie within this region.

The CF gene was isolated in 1989 after an intensive series of investigations that illustrate the importance of both physical and genetic mapping (Rommens et al., 1989). By examining the location of individual crossovers in CF families, the possible location of the gene could be further reduced. Eventually all such recombination points were identified, and a region of some 500,000 base pairs still remained. At this point, however, an unusual feature of CF genetics emerged. Despite the fact that the closest markers were still some distance from the CF gene, it became clear that almost all chromosomes carrying the CF mutation, in many unrelated families, had the same genotype at the linked polymorphic loci. Approximately 90 percent of CF chromosomes have a particular genotype that is found in only about 25 percent of normal (non-CF) chromosomes. This situation is called **linkage disequilibrium,** which can be defined as the preferential association of a disease gene with specific alleles at closely linked markers. This is in contrast, for example, to what was observed in HD, in which the mutation in different families can be linked to any of the haplotypes detected by the linked G8 marker (Fig. 8–23). The usual interpretation of linkage disequilibrium is that most chromosomes carrying the disease mutation are descended from a common ancestor who had the haplotype most often associated with the mutant allele, as illustrated in Figure 8–26. This model predicts that the highest degree of disequilibrium should be found closest to the disease mutation, as has indeed been observed across the region near the CF gene, inasmuch as markers at the extreme limits of the region (MET and D7S8) show relatively little disequilibrium (Kerem et al., 1989). In terms of a strategy for positional cloning, the existence of linkage disequilibrium suggests that one should focus attention on regions with the highest degree of disequilibrium because these should be closest to the site of the ancestral mutation.

Guided by these genetic considerations, Tsui and Collins and their colleagues searched for genes in the remaining ~500 kb by concentrating on two features usually associated with coding sequences, but not with noncoding sequences: the presence of mRNA transcripts and DNA sequences that are conserved through evolution.

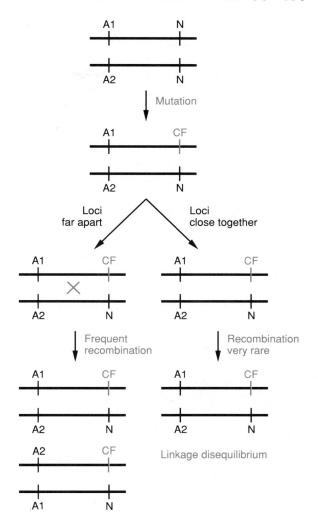

Figure 8-26. An explanation for linkage disequilibrium between a disease locus, such as cystic fibrosis, and a closely linked marker locus. Frequencies of haplotypes reach equilibrium if the marker locus is far enough away from the disease locus for many crossovers to have occurred during evolution, since the time of the original mutation. For markers very closely linked to the disease locus, little recombination has occurred, and thus the distribution of alleles observed in chromosomes with the CF mutation will be different from that observed in normal chromosomes.

Among the four genes identified and studied from within this region, one showed additional features expected of a candidate for the CF defect in that its transcripts were present in tissues affected in CF (lung, pancreas, and sweat glands; Rommens et al., 1989). Proof of its being the CF gene, however, required demonstration of a molecular defect, a 3 base-pair deletion in the coding sequence found in approximately 70 percent of all CF chromosomes in Northern European populations but never in normal alleles at this locus (Riordan et al., 1989; Kerem et al., 1989). Details of the CF gene and its molecular genetics are discussed further in Chapter 12.

Duchenne Muscular Dystrophy

Positional cloning of the X-linked DMD gene (see box in Chapter 4) illustrates a different strategy from that just discussed: the use of rare chromosome rearrangements to identify the gene responsible for a genetic disease. DMD (and the less severe Becker allelic form, BMD) was one of the first genetic diseases localized by genetic linkage analysis, to band Xp21.

Successful cloning of the gene relied on two different approaches, both of which involved rare chromosome defects. First, as mentioned earlier in this chapter, a small proportion of DMD boys have cytologically detectable deletions within Xp21. Second, DMD, being an X-linked recessive disorder, is only rarely observed in females. Cytogenetic investigations of some such affected girls have shown X;autosome translocations. The autosome involved differed in each case, but the site of the translocation on the X was always the same: Xp21.

In the first approach, Kunkel and colleagues (1985) cloned the DMD gene by using DNA from the patient B.B., referred to earlier, who had a deletion of Xp21 (Fig. 8–6). By enriching for X-linked DNA sequences that were missing from B.B.'s X chromosome, they isolated cloned fragments that were present in band Xp21 on normal X chromosomes but were deleted in B.B. These sequences

represented candidates for DMD. Indeed, one of the clones was also shown to be deleted in a proportion of affected boys with *no* apparent cytogenetic deletion. A number of such sequences were isolated from the X chromosome in this region; some of these turned out to correspond to DMD coding sequences.

The second approach relied on one of the rare affected females with an X;autosome translocation, in which the autosomal breakpoint happened to go through an already known sequence, the ribosomal RNA genes on the short arm of chromosome 21. The portion of the DMD gene translocated to chromosome 21 was identified and isolated by cloning X chromosome DNA joined to the ribosomal RNA genes. Although the site of the translocation break on the X chromosome turned out to be in the middle of a very large intron, eventually portions of the DMD coding sequence were identified (Ray et al., 1985).

The cloning of the DMD gene and its cDNA by relying on cytogenetic defects has allowed intensive study of this disorder and its basic defect. Unlike the situation in CF, the majority of mutations in DMD are due to complete or partial gene deletions. The molecular genetics of DMD (and BMD) and the nature of the encoded protein, dystrophin, are discussed in Chapter 12.

X;Autosome Translocations in X-Linked Disease. The existence of translocation breakpoints through the gene, although rare among all affected persons with a particular X-linked disease, is in fact a relatively common observation among X-linked recessive disorders present in females (Table 8–5). The basis for expression of the defect in females with balanced X;autosome translocations is nonrandom X inactivation of the normal X chromosome in most or all cells (see Chap-

Table 8–5. Examples of X;Autosome Translocations Observed in Females Affected With X-Linked Disorders

Disorder	X Chromosome Breakpoint	Site of Gene Confirmed by Linkage
Choroideremia	Xq21	Yes
Duchenne muscular dystrophy	Xp21	Yes
Hunter syndrome	Xq27	Yes
Hypohidrotic ectodermal dysplasia	Xq12	Yes
Lowe syndrome	Xq25	Yes
Menkes syndrome	Xq13	Yes
Norrie disease	Xp11	Yes

Based on Harper et al. (1989)

ters 4 and 10). Because the allele on the normal X is inactivated, only the allele on the translocated X is potentially active, and its disruption by the translocation precludes normal expression. According to this model, the site of the translocation should reveal the site of the gene involved in the X-linked disorder (Jacobs et al., 1981). In general, this appears to be the case (Table 8–5).

Retinitis Pigmentosa

Retinitis pigmentosa (RP) is a group of inherited retinopathies involving photoreceptor degeneration. Clinical features typically include reduced night and peripheral vision, as well as retinal degeneration. RP is a major cause of blindness in humans, with an estimated prevalence of about 1 in 4000. Genetically, RP is clearly heterogeneous on the basis of its mode of inheritance. Among familial cases, about 25 percent of pedigrees are classified as autosomal dominant, 30 percent as X-linked, and 45 percent as autosomal recessive.

Linkage analysis has revealed even more heterogeneity. There are at least two distinct forms of X-linked RP: one mapping in Xp11 and one in Xp21. The latter X-linked locus was the one deleted in patient B.B., who had the Xp21 deletion. Extensive computational analyses of X-linked RP families have suggested that 60 to 80 percent of X-linked cases involve the Xp21 locus, whereas 20 to 40 percent are due to mutations at the Xp11 RP locus.

Autosomal dominant RP has been subclassified clinically into two groups on the basis of age of onset and differential patterns of rod and cone degeneration. Because this clinical heterogeneity raised the possibility of multiple responsible loci, linkage studies concentrated on single large pedigrees, rather than on a collection of smaller ones. Extensive analyses excluded the defect from about half of the autosomes. Finally, very close linkage of RP to a marker locus on the long arm of chromosome 3 was demonstrated in one large Irish pedigree (McWilliam et al., 1989).

This finding led directly to identification of the responsible gene and illustrates another strategy used in positional cloning. In CF and DMD, the successful isolation of the responsible genes was not based on any features of the gene other than its known chromosomal location. An alternative strategy is called the **candidate gene approach.** In this approach, one selects already cloned genes that are known to map to the same chromosomal region or that are known to have a role in the physiology of the tissue affected in the disease. A variety of methods for finding mutations (see Chapter 6) are then used to screen the candidate gene for defects in a group of patients.

The mapping of autosomal dominant RP to the long arm of chromosome 3 immediately raised the hypothesis that the gene for rhodopsin, a rod photoreceptor gene that had previously also been assigned to the long arm of chromosome 3, might be responsible for RP in this family. Indeed, a single base mutation was identified in the rhodopsin gene in about 15 percent of unrelated patients with autosomal dominant RP (Dryja et al., 1990) (Fig. 8–27). Although some of the remaining patients have other defects in the rhodopsin gene, this is not the case for all such patients. In at least some families with autosomal dominant RP, the inherited defect does *not* cosegregate with polymorphisms at the rhodopsin locus. Thus in these families, some other autosomal locus must be responsible. For both the autosomal dominant and the X-linked forms of RP, recognition of genetic heterogeneity is an important aspect of linkage studies because misclassification of a case could lead to erroneous prenatal or preclinical diagnoses based on using polymorphic DNA markers that are, in fact, not linked (or not as closely linked) to the disease locus in question.

Other Applications of the Candidate Gene Approach. The success of the candidate gene approach illustrates nicely the value of gene mapping. Rhodopsin was originally cloned and mapped for reasons unrelated to RP. However, if it were not on the chromosome 3 gene map, it is unlikely that the defect in autosomal dominant RP would have been uncovered so quickly. The candidate gene approach allows the raising and testing of hypotheses about the cause of an inherited disease on the basis of its clinical and cellular phenotype and the role of candidate proteins in the relevant tissue.

One other inherited disorder illustrates further the value of this approach. X-linked Alport syndrome is a relatively common hereditary nephritis in which progressive loss of kidney function is accompanied by ultrastructural defects in glomerular basement membranes. Extensive linkage analyses refined the localization of the gene to

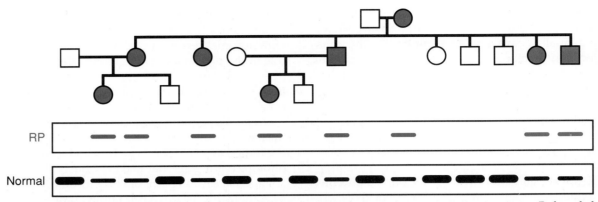

Figure 8–27. Demonstration of a rhodopsin mutation in a family with autosomal dominant retinitis pigmentosa. Red symbols indicate affected individuals. Below the pedigree are the results of diagnostic assays, in which allele-specific oligonucleotides (ASOs) for the mutant or normal rhodopsin sequence were used. For a discussion of ASO technology, see Chapter 5. (Adapted from Dryja TP, McGee TL, Reichel E, et al [1990] A point mutation of the rhodopsin gene in one form of retinitis pigmentosa. Nature 343:364–366.)

the middle of the X chromosome long arm, in Xq22. Positional cloning strategies had narrowed down the region of interest to perhaps 3 to 5 million base pairs. At about the same time, independent studies on genes encoding collagen chains demonstrated that whereas most collagen genes are autosomal, a gene for a type IV collagen α-chain mapped to the X chromosome, in band Xq22, thus leading to the suggestion that defects in this collagen chain gene might be responsible for X-linked Alport syndrome. Indeed, mutations in the collagen gene have now been demonstrated in several families of affected patients, thus verifying the genetic hypothesis and providing immediate diagnostic tools for the presymptomatic detection of this progressive disorder (Barker et al., 1990).

STATUS OF THE HUMAN GENE MAP

Both physical and genetic mapping strategies have contributed to the development of a human gene map that now includes nearly 2000 identified genes and more than 6000 cloned DNA segments. The number of mapped loci in the human genome has increased exponentially since the early 1980s. In addition, the depth of information at individual loci has increased as approaches for fine mapping and methods for large-scale cloning have been improved. Figure 8–28 shows the current gene map for two human chromosomes, the X chromosome and chromosome 7. (Similar maps for all of

the human chromosomes can be found in Appendix IV.) Both maps show only those loci at which an inherited condition has been described. For most or all of these, human gene mapping methods can be immediately translated into diagnostic assays for presymptomatic or prenatal detection. In addition, as the relevant disease genes are cloned and characterized, many by positional cloning strategies, an enormous increase in the understanding of the molecular basis of human genetic disease is expected to result. Neither map in Figure 8–28 shows the large number of genes assigned to these chromosomes for which no disease connection has yet been established. However, as illustrated by the candidate gene approach, the involvement of many of these genes in an inherited condition is expected to become apparent over time.

Much of the progress to date has been made in single-gene disorders, which is not surprising given the emphasis of current approaches on pedigree analysis and linkage detection (Table 8–4). However, in the future, it is likely that more progress will be made in unraveling the genetic components involved in conditions such as hypertension, behavioral disorders, and cancer (see Chapters 15 and 16). Gene mapping strategies, together with sophisticated methods for pedigree analysis, are just beginning to be applied to these more complex disorders.

With the focus on human gene mapping as part of the Human Genome Project, it is hoped

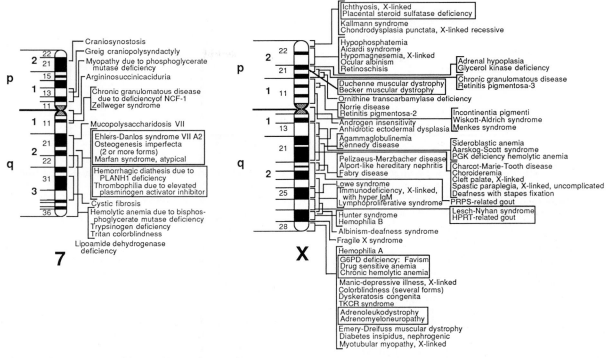

Figure 8–28. The current gene maps of chromosome 7 and the X chromosome, showing the regional location of genes involved in genetic disorders. Many of these disorders have been localized on the basis of genetic linkage analyses in family studies. Others have been placed on the map on the basis of knowledge of the biochemical or molecular defect. The "morbid anatomy" of all the human chromosomes is given in Appendix IV. (Courtesy of V. A. McKusick, Johns Hopkins University, updated from McKusick, 1990.)

that a complete map of all 50,000 to 100,000 human genes will be assembled by the year 2005. The combined approach of linkage analysis to assign a particular gene for an inherited disorder to a specific chromosomal region, followed by positional cloning strategies to identify the responsible gene and establish the molecular defect or defects, should continue to reap a bountiful harvest.

General References

Donis-Keller H (1991) Human gene mapping techniques: A laboratory manual. Stockton Press, New York.

Human Gene Mapping 10 (1989) Tenth International Workshop on Human Gene Mapping. Cytogenet Cell Genet 51:1–1148.

Human Gene Mapping 11 (1991) Eleventh International Workshop on Human Gene Mapping. Cytogenet Cell Genet 58:1–2200.

McKusick VA (1989) Mapping and sequencing the human genome. N Engl J Med 320:910–915.

McKusick VA (1990) Mendelian inheritance in man: Catalogs of autosomal dominant, autosomal recessive, and X-linked phenotypes, 9th ed. Johns Hopkins University Press, Baltimore.

Ott J (1985) Analysis of human genetic linkage. Johns Hopkins University Press, Baltimore.

White R, Lalouel JM (1988) Chromosome mapping with DNA markers. Sci Am 258:40–48.

Problems

1. The Huntington disease (HD) locus was found to be tightly linked to a DNA polymorphism on chromosome 4 by Gusella et al. (1983). However, in the same study, they ruled out linkage between HD and the MNSs polymorphism, which also map to chromosome 4. What is the explanation?

2. Linkage disequilibrium was an important observation in the positional cloning of the autosomal recessive cystic fibrosis gene. Referring to Chapter 4 as necessary, would you expect to find linkage disequilibrium for an autosomal dominant disease such as HD? Type 1 neurofibromatosis? Why or why not?

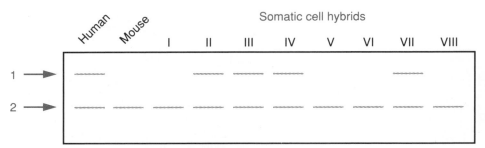

Southern blot data for question 3

3. The data shown were obtained with a human cDNA probe for gene Q in the same panel of rodent/human somatic cell hybrids analyzed in Figure 8–3 and Table 8–2. What do you conclude about fragment 1 in the Southern blot? Fragment 2? In reference to Table 8–2, where does the Q gene map?

4. Reeders et al. (1985) reported close linkage between a polymorphism in the α-globin locus on the short arm of chromosome 16 and autosomal dominant polycystic kidney disease, a common and progressive multiorgan condition, in a series of British and Dutch families, with the following data:

$$\theta = 0.00 \quad 0.01 \quad 0.10 \quad 0.20 \quad 0.30 \quad 0.40$$

Lod scores (Z) $-\infty$ 23.40 24.59 19.48 12.81 5.48

$$Z_{max} \quad \theta_{max}$$
$$25.85 \quad 0.05$$

How would you interpret these data?

In a subsequent study, a large family from Sicily with polycystic kidney disease was also investigated for linkage, with the following data (Kimberling et al., 1988):

$$\theta = 0.00 \quad 0.10 \quad 0.20 \quad 0.30 \quad 0.40$$

Lod scores (Z) $-\infty$ -8.34 -3.34 -1.05 -0.02

How would you interpret the data in this second study? What implications do these data have for use of linkage information in presymptomatic diagnosis and genetic counseling?

5. The following data were obtained in a study designed to test the hypothesis that a defect in a gene for γ crystallin, one of the major proteins of the eye lens, may be responsible for the inherited eye defect in Coppock's cataract, an autosomal dominant disorder (data from Lubsen et al., 1987). The filled-in symbols in the pedigree indicate family members with cataracts. The letters indicate DNA haplotypes at the polymorphic γ crystallin locus on chromosome 2, detected with a cDNA clone. What would you conclude from this study? What additional studies might be performed to confirm or reject the hypothesis?

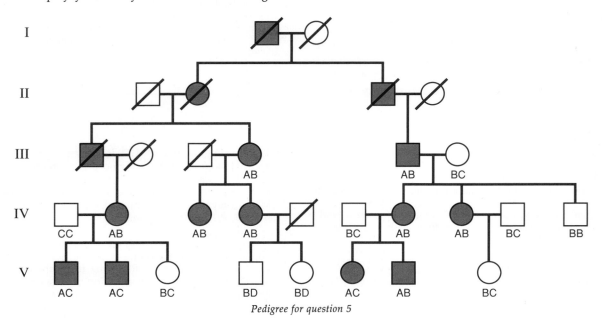

Pedigree for question 5

6. The following pedigree shows an example of molecular diagnosis in Wiskott-Aldrich syndrome, an X-linked immunodeficiency, by using a linked DNA polymorphism with a map distance of approximately 5 cM between the polymorphic locus and the Wiskott-Aldrich syndrome gene. What is the likely phase in the carrier mother? How did you determine this? What diagnosis would you make regarding the current prenatal diagnosis?

7. In the family described in Question 6, the maternal grandfather becomes available for DNA testing and shows allele *B* at the linked locus. How does this finding affect your determination of phase in the mother? What can you conclude about the affected son? What further studies might be performed to verify this? What diagnosis would you make now in regard to the current prenatal diagnosis?

8. Prenatal diagnosis is attempted for an autosomal recessive condition in a family with one previously affected child. A DNA polymorphism with alleles at 7, 9, or 12 kb is very closely linked to the disorder. DNA hybridization (Southern blot) data are obtained from available family members (shown below).
   a) What is the presumed genotype of the father at the linked marker locus?
   b) What is the phase in the mother? In the father?
   c) Which of the children are carriers of this disorder, and which are homozygous normal?
   d) What is the diagnosis in the current pregnancy? On what assumptions is this diagnosis based?

9. What are some of the implications of knowing the map position of a particular gene for medical genetics? In other words, why map genes?

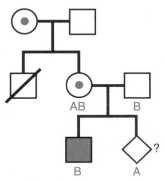

Pedigree for questions 6 and 7

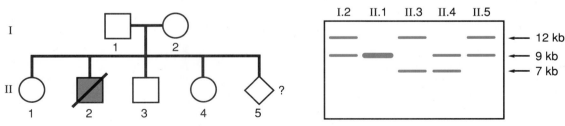

Pedigree and Southern blot data for question 8

CHAPTER 9

CLINICAL CYTOGENETICS: GENERAL PRINCIPLES AND AUTOSOMAL ABNORMALITIES

A new era in medical genetics opened in 1959 with two virtually simultaneous discoveries: the finding by Lejeune and his colleagues that "enfants mongoliens" (children with mongolism, now known as Down syndrome or trisomy 21) have 47 chromosomes instead of the usual 46 in their somatic cells, and the first observations, by Ford and colleagues and by Jacobs and Strong, of sex chromosome anomalies in patients with disorders of sexual development. It is now known that chromosome disorders form a major category of genetic disease, accounting for a large proportion of all reproductive wastage, congenital malformations, and mental retardation, as well as playing an important role in the pathogenesis of malignancy.

Specific chromosome abnormalities are responsible for 60 or more identifiable syndromes, which collectively are more common than all the Mendelian single-gene disorders together (Borgaonkar, 1989). They are present in an estimated 0.7 percent of live births, in about 2 percent of all pregnancies in women over 35 years old, and in fully 50 percent of all spontaneous first-trimester abortions.

In this chapter we discuss the numerical and structural abnormalities observed in human karyotypes and describe some of the best-known abnormalities of the autosomes. The sex chromosomes and their abnormalities are presented in the next chapter.

GENERAL PRINCIPLES OF CLINICAL CYTOGENETICS

Abnormalities of chromosomes may be either numerical or structural and may involve one or more autosomes, sex chromosomes, or both simultaneously. By far the most common type of clinically significant chromosome abnormality is **aneuploidy,** an abnormal chromosome number due to

201

an extra or missing chromosome, which is always associated with physical or mental maldevelopment, or both. **Reciprocal translocations** (exchange of segments between nonhomologous chromosomes) are also relatively common but usually have no phenotypic effect, although as explained later there may be an associated increased risk of abnormal offspring. The relative frequencies of numerical and structural abnormalities observed in spontaneous abortions, in fetuses of mothers over 35 years of age that are analyzed in amniocentesis, and in live births are presented in the box.

probably results from failure of one of the maturation divisions, in either ovum or, usually, sperm. The phenotypic expression of a triploid karyotype depends on the source of the extra chromosome set; triploids with an extra set of paternal chromosomes typically have an abnormal placenta and are classified as partial hydatidiform moles, but those with an additional set of maternal chromosomes are not so classified and are spontaneously aborted earlier in pregnancy. Tetraploids are always 92,XXXX or 92,XXYY, suggesting that tetraploidy results from failure of completion of an early cleavage division of the zygote.

Abnormal karyotype	First-trimester abortuses	Fetuses of mothers > 35 years	Live births
Total incidence	1/2	1/50	1/160
Percentage of abnormalities			
Numerical abnormalities (aneuploidy, polyploidy)	96%	85%	60%
Structural abnormalities			
balanced	—	10%	30%
unbalanced	4%	5%	10%

Some abbreviations commonly used in descriptions of chromosomes and their abnormalities and examples of abnormal karyotypes are listed in Table 9–1.

ABNORMALITIES OF CHROMOSOME NUMBER

A chromosome complement with any chromosome number other than normal is said to be **heteroploid.** An exact multiple of the haploid chromosome number (n) is called **euploid,** and any other chromosome number is **aneuploid.**

Triploidy and Tetraploidy

In addition to the diploid (2n) number characteristic of normal somatic cells, two other euploid chromosome complements, **triploid** (3n) and **tetraploid** (4n), are occasionally reported. Both triploidy and tetraploidy have been seen in fetuses, and a few triploid infants have been liveborn, though their survival has been brief. Triploidy

Aneuploidy

Aneuploidy is the most common and clinically significant type of human chromosome disorder, occurring in at least 3 to 4 percent of all clinically recognized pregnancies. Although by definition a person is aneuploid if he or she has fewer or more chromosomes than an exact multiple of the haploid set, most aneuploid patients have either **trisomy** (three instead of the normal pair of a particular chromosome) or, less often, **monosomy** (only one representative of a particular chromosome). Either trisomy or monosomy can have severe phenotypic consequences.

Trisomy can exist for any chromosome of the set, but trisomy for a whole chromosome is rarely compatible with life. By far the most common type of trisomy in liveborn infants is **trisomy 21** (karyotype 47,XX or XY,+21), the chromosome constitution seen in 95 percent of patients with Down syndrome (Fig. 9–1). Monosomy for an entire chromosome is almost always lethal; an important exception is monosomy for the X chromosome, described in Chapter 10.

The causes of aneuploidy are not well under-

Table 9–1. Some Abbreviations Used for Description of Chromosomes and Their Abnormalities and Representative Examples

Abbreviation	Meaning	Example	Condition
		46,XX	Normal female karyotype
		46,XY	Normal male karyotype
cen	centromere		
del	deletion	46,XX,del(5p)	Female with cri du chat syndrome due to deletion of part of short arm of one chromosome 5
der	derivative chromosome	der(1)	Translocation chromosome derived from chromosome 1 and containing the centromere of chromosome 1
dic	dicentric chromosome	dic(X;Y)	Translocation chromosome containing centromeres from both the X and the Y chromosomes
dup	duplication		
fra	fragile site	46,Y,fra(X)(q27.3)	Male with fragile X chromosome
i	isochromosome	46,X,i(Xq)	Female with isochromosome for the long arm of the X chromosome
ins	insertion		
inv	inversion	inv(3)(p25q21)	Pericentric inversion of chromosome 3
mar	marker chromosome	47,XX,+mar	Female with an extra, unidentified chromosome
mat	maternal origin	47,XY,+der(1)mat	Male with additional der(1) translocation chromosome inherited from his mother
p	short arm of chromosome		
pat	paternal origin		
q	long arm of chromosome		
r	ring chromosome	46,X,r(X)	Female with ring X chromosome
rcp	reciprocal translocation		
rob	Robertsonian translocation		
t	translocation	46,XX,t(2;8)(q21;p13)	Female with balanced translocation between chromosome 2 and chromosome 8, with breaks in 2q21 and 8p13
ter	terminus	46,X,Xq⁻(pter→q21:)	Female with partial deletion of the long arm from Xq21 to Xqter (nomenclature shows the portion of the chromosome that is present)
+	gain of	47,XX,+21	Female with trisomy 21
−	loss of	45,XX,−14,−21,+t(14q21q)	Normal female carrier of a Robertsonian translocation between the long arms of chromosomes 14 and 21; karyotype is missing a normal 14 and a normal 21
		4p⁻	Chromosome 4 with a portion of the short arm deleted
:	break	5qter→5p15:	Deleted chromosome 5 in a patient with cri du chat syndrome, with a deletion breakpoint in band p15
::	break and join	2pter→2q21::8p13→8pter	Description of der(2) portion of t(2;8)
/	mosaicism	46,XX/47,XX,+8	Female with two populations of cells, one with a normal karyotype and one with trisomy 8

Abbreviations from ISCN (1985) Report of the Standing Committee of Human Cytogenetic Nomenclature (1985). Karger, Basel.

stood, but it is known that whatever the underlying molecular mechanism, the most common chromosomal mechanism is meiotic **nondisjunction,** the failure of a pair of chromosomes to disjoin in the normal way during one of the two meiotic divisions, usually during meiosis I. The consequences of nondisjunction during meiosis I and meiosis II are different (Fig. 9–2). If the error occurs during meiosis I, the gamete with 24 chromosomes contains both the paternal and the maternal members of the pair. If it occurs during meiosis II, the gamete with the extra chromosome contains both copies of either the paternal or the maternal chromosome. (However, recombination almost certainly has taken place in the preceding meiosis I, resulting in some genetic differences between the chromatids and thus the corresponding daughter chromosomes; see Chapter 2.)

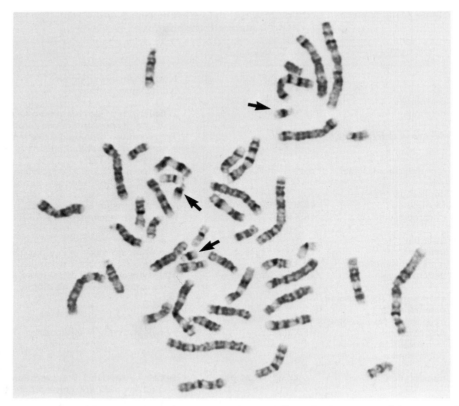

Figure 9–1. Chromosome spread from a patient with trisomy 21. Arrows indicate the three copies of chromosome 21. (Photomicrograph courtesy of Gloria Nie, Cytogenetics Laboratory, The Hospital for Sick Children, Toronto.)

To determine the parental origin of the error and the meiotic stage at which it occurred, as well as to learn whether an association exists between nondisjunction and recombination, both polymorphic DNA probes spanning the long arm of chromosome 21 and cytogenetic heteromorphisms of the short arm have been used. As shown in Figure 9–3, in many cases analysis of markers on the chromosomes of the parents and the aneuploid patient reveals the stage and parental origin of the error.

More complicated forms of multiple aneuploidy have been reported. A gamete occasionally has an extra representative of more than one chromosome. Nondisjunction can take place at two successive meiotic divisions or by chance in both male and female gametes simultaneously, resulting in zygotes with bizarre chromosome numbers, which are extremely rare except for the sex chromosomes. Nondisjunction can also occur in a mitotic division after formation of the zygote. If this happens at an early cleavage division, clinically significant **mosaicism** may result. In some malignant cell lines and some cell cultures, mitotic nondisjunction can lead to highly abnormal karyotypes.

ABNORMALITIES OF CHROMOSOME STRUCTURE

Structural rearrangements result from chromosome breakage, followed by reconstitution in an abnormal combination. Rearrangement can take place in many ways, all of which are more rare than aneuploidy; the most common type, a balanced translocation (either reciprocal or Robert-

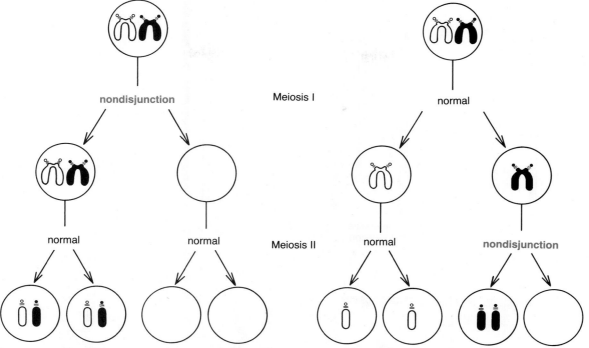

Figure 9–2. The different consequences of nondisjunction at meiosis I (left) and meiosis II (right). If the error occurs at meiosis I, the gametes either contain a representative of both members of the chromosome 21 pair or lack a chromosome 21 altogether. If nondisjunction occurs at meiosis II, the abnormal gametes contain two copies of one parental chromosome 21 (and no copy of the other) or lack a chromosome 21.

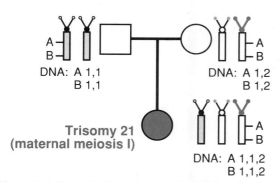

Figure 9–3. Determination of origin of nondisjunction in trisomy 21. In this family, the mother's two chromosome 21s can be distinguished by a chromosomal heteromorphism (see Fig. 6–2). Her daughter who has Down syndrome had inherited both of these heteromorphisms, demonstrating that the origin of her extra chromosome 21 is maternal. The mother and her daughter are heterozygous for the heteromorphism, as well as for two chromosome 21 DNA polymorphisms (loci A and B), demonstrating that the nondisjunction occurred in maternal meiosis I.

sonian, to be discussed), is present in about 1 in 500 newborns. Chromosome exchange occurs spontaneously at a low frequency and may also be induced by breaking agents (clastogens) such as ionizing radiation, some viral infections, and many chemicals. Like numerical abnormalities, structural rearrangements may be present in all cells of a person or in mosaic form.

Structural rearrangements are defined as **balanced,** if the chromosome set has the normal complement of genetic information, or **unbalanced,** if there is additional or missing information. Some rearrangements are stable, capable of passing through cell division unaltered, whereas others are unstable. To be stable, a rearranged chromosome must have normal structural elements, including a single functional centromere and two telomeres. Some of the types of structural rearrangements observed in human chromosomes are illustrated in Figure 9–4.

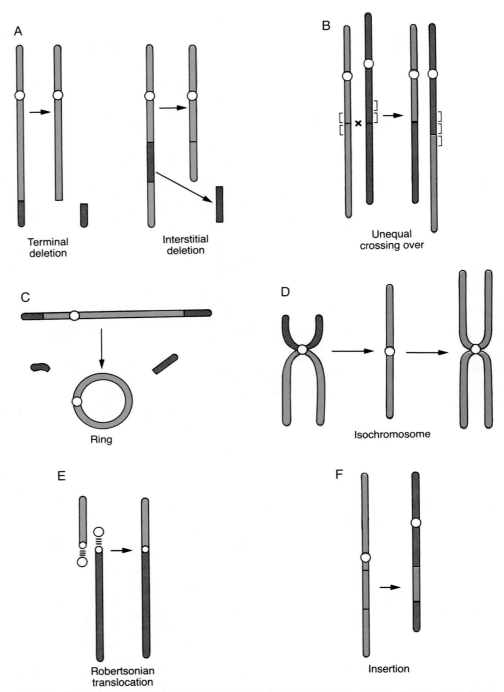

Figure 9–4. Structural rearrangements of chromosomes, described in the text. A. Terminal and interstitial deletions, each generating an acentric fragment. B. Unequal crossing over between segments of homologous chromosomes or between sister chromatids (duplicated or deleted segment indicated by the brackets). C. Ring chromosome with two acentric fragments. D. Generation of an isochromosome for the long arm of a chromosome. E. Robertsonian translocation between two acrocentric chromosomes. F. Insertion of a segment of one chromosome into a nonhomologous chromosome.

Unbalanced Rearrangements

In unbalanced rearrangements, the phenotype is likely to be abnormal because of deletion, duplication, or (in some cases) both. Duplication of part of a chromosome is comparable with partial trisomy; deletion leads to a partial monosomy. Any change that disturbs the normal balance of functional genes can result in abnormal development.

Deletion

Deletion is loss of a chromosome segment, resulting in chromosome imbalance (Fig. 9–4A). A carrier of a chromosomal deletion (with one normal homolog and one deleted homolog) is hemizygous for the genetic information on the corresponding segment of the normal homolog. The clinical consequences depend on the size of the deleted seg-

ment and the number and function of the genes that it contains.

A deletion may be terminal or interstitial. Deletions may originate simply by chromosome breakage and loss of the acentric segment. Alternatively, unequal crossing over between misaligned homologous chromosomes or sister chromatids may account for deletion in some cases (Fig. 9–4B). Deletions can also be generated by abnormal segregation from a balanced translocation or inversion, as described later.

High-resolution banding techniques can reveal deletions that are too small to be seen in ordinary metaphase spreads (Fig. 9–5). To be identifiable cytogenetically by high-resolution banding, a deletion must span at least 2000 to 3000 kb, but karyotypically undetectable deletions with phenotypic consequences have been detected by molecular techniques (Ledbetter and Cavenee, 1989). Small deletions within genes, or extending over

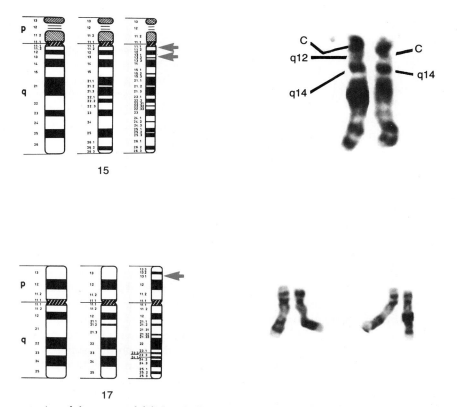

Figure 9–5. Demonstration of chromosomal deletions in "contiguous gene syndromes" by high-resolution banding. In each case, the homolog on the right is deleted. Top: Deletion of 15q11.2–q13.2 on one copy of chromosome 15 in Prader-Willi syndrome. (C = centromere.) Bottom: Deletion of the terminal short arm of one copy of chromosome 17 in Miller-Dieker syndrome. Chromosomes from 2 cells are shown. In both syndromes, loss of material from one homolog leads to segmental aneusomy, a partial imbalance of genetic material. (Photographs courtesy of David Ledbetter, Baylor College of Medicine.)

Table 9–2. Selected Examples of Segmental Aneusomy

Disorder	Deletion	Description
Langer-Giedion syndrome	8q24.11–q24.13	Mental retardation, microcephaly, dysmorphism, bone abnormalities
DiGeorge sequence	22q11	Absence of thymus and parathyroids
WAGR syndrome	11p13	Wilms tumor with aniridia, gonadoblastoma, and retardation; see Chapter 16
Retinoblastoma	13q14	Embryonic neoplasm of retinal cells, childhood cancer; see Chapter 16
Prader-Willi syndrome	15q11–q13	Dysmorphic syndrome; see Chapter 4
Angelman syndrome	15q11–q13	Dysmorphic syndrome; see Chapter 4
Miller-Dieker syndrome	17p13.3	Severe dysmorphic syndrome with lissencephaly and other malformations

Data excerpted from Harper PS, Frezal J, Ferguson-Smith MA, et al. (1989) Report of the committee on clinical disorders and chromosomal deletion syndromes. Human Gene Mapping 10: Tenth International Workshop on Human Gene Mapping. Cytogenet Cell Genet 51:563–611.

several contiguous genes, are recognized mechanisms of mutation (Chapter 6).

Numerous deletions have been identified in the investigation of dysmorphic patients and in prenatal diagnosis, but knowledge of the functional genes lost in the deleted segments and their relation to the phenotypic consequences is extremely limited at present. Several dysmorphic syndromes are associated with cytogenetically visible deletions (Table 9–2). The example of Prader-Willi and Angelman syndromes (described in Chapter 4) suggests that genomic imprinting, a process that marks maternal and paternal chromosomes differently, may lead to differences in phenotypic expression in patients with deletions that appear to be identical in extent but different in parental origin.

Duplications

Duplications, like deletions, can originate by unequal crossing over (Fig. 9–4B) or by abnormal segregation from meiosis in a carrier of a translocation or inversion. In general, duplication appears to be much less harmful than deletion. However, because duplication in a gamete results in chromosomal imbalance, and because the chromosome breaks that generate it may disrupt genes, duplication often leads to some phenotypic abnormality.

Although many duplications have been reported, very few of any one kind have been studied so far, and generalizations about the associated phenotypes would be premature. Nonetheless, certain phenotypes appear to be associated with duplications of particular chromosomal regions.

Ring Chromosomes

Ring chromosomes are formed when a chromosome undergoes two breaks and the broken ends of the chromosome reunite in a ring structure (Fig. 9–4C). If the centromere is within the ring, the two distal fragments, lacking a centromere, are lost. Ring chromosomes are quite rare but have been detected for every human chromosome.

Rings may undergo difficulties at mitosis, when the two sister chromatids of the ring chromosome attempt to disjoin at anaphase. There may be breakage of the ring followed by fusion, and larger and smaller rings may thus be generated. Because of this mitotic instability, it is not uncommon for ring chromosomes to be found in only a proportion of cells.

Isochromosomes

An isochromosome (Fig. 9–4D) is a chromosome in which one arm is missing and the other reduplicated. A person with 46 chromosomes carrying an isochromosome therefore has a single copy of the genetic material of one arm and three copies of the genetic material of the other arm or, in other words, is partially monosomic and partially trisomic. A person with two normal homologs in addition to the isochromosome is tetrasomic for the chromosome arm involved in the isochromosome (Fig. 9–6). Although the basis for isochromosome formation is not precisely known, at least two mechanisms have been documented: (1) misdivision through the centromere in meiosis II and (2) translocation of one arm of one chromosome to its

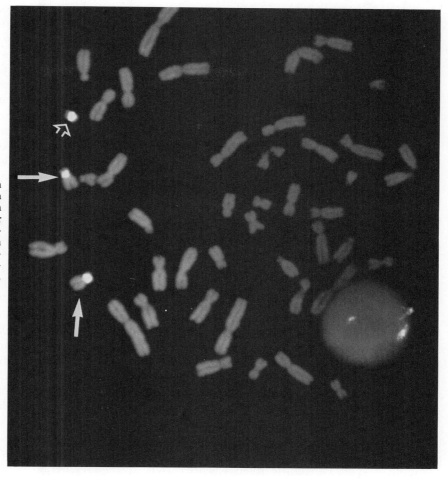

Figure 9–6. Identification of a marker chromosome as i(18p), an isochromosome for the short arm of chromosome 18, by molecular cytogenetic techniques with fluorescence in situ hybridization and a specific DNA probe for the centromere of chromosome 18. (Photograph courtesy of V. E. Powers, Stanford University.)

homolog (or sister chromatid) at the proximal edge of the other arm, adjacent to the centromere.

The most common isochromosome is an isochromosome of the long arm of the X chromosome, i(Xq), in some individuals with Turner syndrome (see Chapter 10). However, isochromosomes for a number of autosomes have also been described, including isochromosomes for the short arm of chromosome 18, i(18p) (Fig. 9–6), and for the short arm of chromosome 12, i(12p). Isochromosomes are also frequently seen in karyotypes of both solid tumors and hematological malignancies (Chapter 16).

Dicentric Chromosomes

A dicentric is a rare type of abnormal chromosome in which two chromosome segments (from differ-

ent chromosomes or from the two chromatids of a single one), each with a centromere, fuse end to end, with loss of their acentric fragments. Dicentrics, because of their two centromeres, tend to break at anaphase; if the two centromeres are close together, however, or if one becomes inactivated (Therman et al., 1974), a dicentric may be stable. Such chromosomes are sometimes called "pseudodicentrics." The most common pseudodicentrics involve one or both of the sex chromosomes (Chapter 10).

Balanced Rearrangements

Chromosomal rearrangements do not usually have a phenotypic effect if they are balanced, because all the genetic information is present even though it is packaged differently. However, structural rearrangements pose a threat to the subsequent generation, because carriers are likely to produce a high frequency of unbalanced gametes and therefore have an increased risk of having abnormal offspring with unbalanced karyotypes. There is also a possibility that one of the chromosome breaks will disrupt a gene, leading to mutation. This is a well-documented cause of X-linked diseases in female carriers of balanced X;autosome translocations (Chapter 10), and, as discussed in Chapter 8, can be a useful clue to the location of the gene responsible for a genetic disease. Balanced translocations are more common in institutionalized mentally retarded individuals, in couples who have had two or more spontaneous abortions, and in infertile males than in the general population.

Inversions

An inversion occurs when a single chromosome undergoes two breaks and is reconstituted with the segment between the breaks inverted. Inversions are of two types: **paracentric** (beside the centromere), in which both breaks occur in one arm, and **pericentric** (around the centromere), in which there is a break in each arm. Because paracentric inversions do not change the arm ratio of the chromosome, they can be identified only by banding, if at all. Pericentric inversions are easier

to identify cytogenetically because they may change the proportion of the chromosome arms as well as the banding pattern.

An inversion does not usually cause an abnormal phenotype in carriers, as it is a balanced rearrangement. Its medical significance is for the progeny; a carrier of either type of inversion is at risk of producing abnormal gametes that may lead to unbalanced offspring. The consequences of the two types of inversion are different (Fig. 9–7). When an inversion is present, a loop is formed when the chromosomes pair in meiosis I. Recombination, which is a normal feature of meiosis I, is somewhat suppressed within inversion loops, but it is not completely suppressed and is likely to occur with larger inversions. As shown in Figure 9–7, both gametes with balanced chromosome complements (either normal or possessing the inversion) and gametes with unbalanced complements are formed, depending on the location of recombination events. When the inversion is paracentric, the unbalanced recombinant chromosomes are typically acentric or dicentric and may not lead to viable offspring, although there have been rare exceptions. Thus the risk that a carrier will have a liveborn child with an abnormal karyotype is very low indeed.

A pericentric inversion, on the other hand, can lead to the production of unbalanced gametes with both duplication and deficiency of chromosome segments (Fig. 9–7). The duplicated and de-

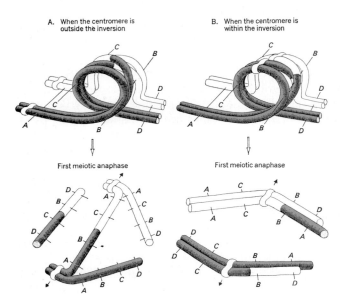

Figure 9–7. Crossing over within inversion loops formed at meiosis I in carriers of a chromosome with segment B-C inverted (order A-C-B-D, instead of A-B-C-D). A. Paracentric inversion. Gametes formed after the second meiosis contain either a normal (A-B-C-D) or a balanced (A-C-B-D) copy of the chromosome, because the acentric and dicentric products of the crossover are inviable (see bottom). B. Pericentric inversion. Gametes formed after the second meiosis may be normal, balanced, or unbalanced (see bottom). Unbalanced gametes contain a copy of the chromosome with a duplication or a deficiency of the material flanking the inverted segment (A-B-C-A or D-B-C-D). (From GENERAL GENETICS, 2/E by Adrian M. Srb and Ray D. Owen. Copyright ©1952, 1965 by W. H. Freeman and Company. Reprinted by permission.)

ficient segments are the segments that are distal to the inversion. Overall, the apparent risk of a carrier of a pericentric inversion producing a child with an unbalanced karyotype is 1 to 10 percent (Gardner and Sutherland, 1989). Each pericentric inversion, however, is associated with a particular risk, and large pericentric inversions are more likely than smaller ones to lead to viable recombinant offspring because the unbalanced segments in the recombinant progeny are smaller in the case of large inversions.

A pericentric inversion of chromosome 3, originally seen in a multigeneration kindred from Newfoundland (Allderdice et al., 1975), is one of the few for which sufficient data have been obtained to allow an estimate of the segregation of the inversion chromosome in the offspring of carriers. The inv(3)(p25q21) has since been reported from a number of North American centers, in families whose ancestors have been traced to Newfoundland. Carriers of the inv(3) chromosome are normal, but some of their offspring have a characteristic abnormal phenotype (Fig. 9–8) associated with a recombinant chromosome 3, in which there is duplication of the segment distal to 3q21 and deficiency of the segment distal to 3p25. Nine individuals who were carriers of the inversion have had 53 recorded pregnancies that resulted in 7 spontaneous abortions, 31 phenotypically normal children, and 15 children with multiple congenital anomalies (of whom 12 died in the first year of life; Allderdice et al., 1975). Although these data may not be typical because they are biased by the deliberate inclusion of carriers with poor reproductive histories, the high empiric risk of an abnormal pregnancy outcome in this group (22/53, or > 40 percent) indicates the importance of family chromosome studies to identify carriers and to offer genetic counseling and prenatal diagnosis.

The most common inversion seen in human chromosomes is a small pericentric inversion of chromosome 9, which is present in up to 1 percent of all individuals tested by cytogenetics laboratories. The inv(9)(p11q12) has no known deleterious effect on carriers and does not appear to be associated with a significant risk of miscarriage or unbalanced offspring; it is, therefore, generally considered a normal variant.

Translocations

Translocation involves the exchange of chromosome segments between nonhomologous chromosomes. There are two main types: reciprocal and Robertsonian.

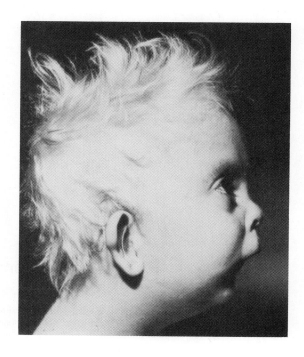

Figure 9–8. A child with an abnormal karyotype, offspring of a carrier of a pericentric inversion. See text for discussion. (From Allderdice PW, Brown N, Murphy DP [1975] Chromosome 3 duplication q21 → qter, deletion p25 → pter syndrome in children of carriers of a pericentric inversion inv(3)(p25q21). Am J Hum Genet 27:699–718.)

Reciprocal Translocations. This type of rearrangement results from breakage of nonhomologous chromosomes, with reciprocal exchange of the broken-off segments. Usually only two chromosomes are involved, and because the exchange is reciprocal, the total chromosome number is unchanged (Fig. 9–9). There are also rare complex translocations involving three or more chromosomes. Reciprocal translocations are usually harmless although, like other balanced structural

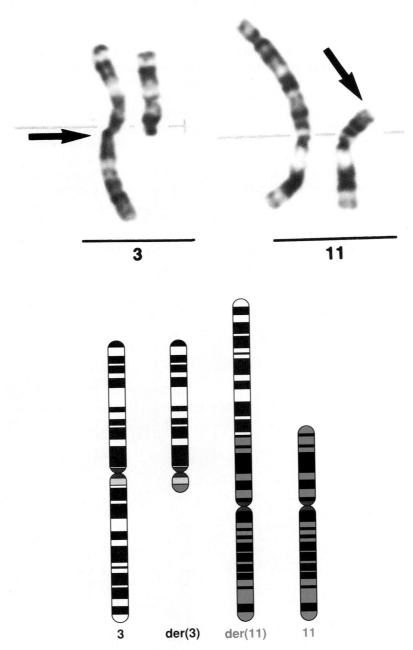

Figure 9–9. Partial karyotype of a patient with a balanced translocation between chromosome 3 and chromosome 11. The complete karyotype is 46,XX,t(3;11)(q12;p15.5). Arrows indicate the positions of the translocation breakpoints on the normal chromosomes 3 and 11. (Original karyotype courtesy of Tim Donlon, Cytogenetics Laboratory, Stanford University Medical Center.)

rearrangements, they are associated with a high risk of unbalanced gametes and abnormal progeny. Reciprocal translocations are relatively common and are found in approximately 1 in 500 newborns. They come to attention either during prenatal diagnosis or when the parents of an abnormal child with an unbalanced translocation are karyotyped.

When the chromosomes of a carrier of a bal-anced reciprocal translocation pair at meiosis, a quadriradial (cross-shaped) figure is formed, as shown in Figure 9–10. Usually at anaphase the chromosomes segregate from this configuration in one of three ways, described as **alternate, adjacent-1,** and **adjacent-2 segregation.** Alternate segregation, the usual type of 2:2 segregation, produces balanced gametes that have either a normal chromosome complement or the two translo-

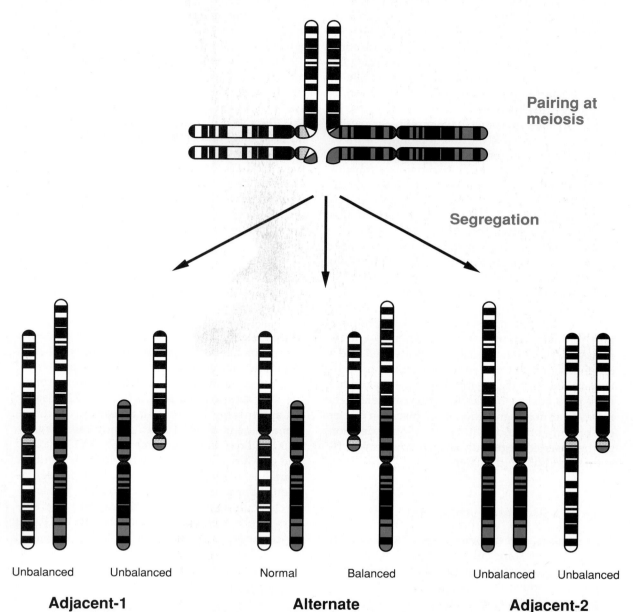

Pairing at meiosis

Segregation

| Unbalanced | Unbalanced | | Normal | Balanced | | Unbalanced | Unbalanced |

Adjacent-1   **Alternate**   **Adjacent-2**

Figure 9–10. Meiotic segregation in a reciprocal translocation between chromosome 3 and chromosome 11. See Figure 9–9 for partial karyotype and text for discussion.

cation chromosomes. In adjacent-1 segregation, homologous centromeres segregate, whereas in adjacent-2 segregation (which is rare), homologous centromeres pass to the same daughter cell. Both adjacent-1 and adjacent-2 segregation yield unbalanced gametes (Fig. 9–10). There are other possible meiotic complications, in particular the risk of nondisjunction, resulting in 3 : 1 or even 4 : 0 segregation.

Robertsonian Translocations. This type of rearrangement involves two acrocentric chromosomes that fuse near the centromere region with loss of the short arms (Fig. 9–4E). The resulting balanced karyotype has only 45 chromosomes, including the translocation chromosome, which in effect is made up of the long arms of two chromosomes. Because the short arms of all five pairs of acrocentric chromosomes have multiple copies of genes for ribosomal RNA, loss of the short arms of two acrocentric chromosomes is not deleterious.

Although a carrier of a Robertsonian translocation is phenotypically normal, there is a risk of unbalanced gametes and therefore of unbalanced offspring. The chief clinical importance of this type of translocation is that carriers of a Robertsonian translocation involving chromosome 21 are at risk of producing a child with translocation Down syndrome, the most common human structural abnormality (see discussion later in this chapter).

Insertions. An insertion is a nonreciprocal type of translocation that occurs when a segment removed from one chromosome is inserted into a different chromosome, either in its usual orientation or inverted (Fig. 9–4F). Because they require three chromosome breaks, insertions are relatively rare. Abnormal segregation in an insertion carrier can produce offspring with duplication or deletion of the inserted segment, as well as normal offspring and balanced carriers.

Marker Chromosomes

Very small marker chromosomes are occasionally seen in chromosome cultures, frequently in a mosaic state. They are usually in addition to the normal chromosome complement and are thus called **supernumerary chromosomes.** Although superficially it seems to be a numerical abnormality, a marker chromosome is also a structural rearrangement. Cytogeneticists find markers very hard to characterize specifically, even by high-resolution techniques, because they are usually so small that the banding pattern is ambiguous or nonapparent. Newer techniques of molecular cytogenetics involving fluorescence in situ hybridization with specific DNA probes (Chapter 8 and Fig. 9–6) may allow identification, however. Tiny marker chromosomes often consist of little more than centric heterochromatin. However, larger ones certainly contain some material from one or both chromosome arms, creating an imbalance for whatever genes are present. Because of the problem of identification, the clinical significance of a marker is difficult to assess, and the finding of a marker in a fetal karyotype can present a serious problem in assessment and genetic counseling.

One particular supernumerary chromosome, duplication of part of the long arm of chromosome 22, is associated with a rare dysmorphic syndrome known as the **cat-eye syndrome.** Patients with this extremely variable syndrome, in which the most common findings are coloboma of the iris and anal atresia, have a quadruple complement of the chromosome segment involved.

CLASSIFICATION AND INCIDENCE OF CHROMOSOME ANOMALIES

The incidence of different types of chromosomal aberration has been measured in a number of large population surveys (Tables 9–3, 9–4, and 9–5). The major numerical disorders of chromosomes are three autosomal trisomies (trisomy 21, trisomy 18, and trisomy 13) and four types of sex chromosomal aneuploidy: Turner syndrome (usually 45,X); Klinefelter syndrome (47,XXY); 47,XYY; and 47,XXX. Triploidy and tetraploidy account for a small percentage of cases, particularly in spontaneous abortions. The classification and incidence of chromosomal defects measured in these surveys can be used to summarize the fate of 10,000 conceptuses, as presented in Table 9–6.

Live Births

The overall incidence of chromosome abnormalities in newborns has been found to be about 1 in

Table 9–3. Incidence of Chromosomal Abnormalities in Newborn Surveys

Type of Abnormality	Number	Approximate Incidence
Sex Chromosome Abnormalities in 37,779 Males		
Total	98	1/385 male births
47,XXY	35	1/1080
47,XYY	35	1/1080
Other	28	1/1350
Sex Chromosome Abnormalities in 19,173 Females		
Total	29	1/660 female births
45,X	2	1/9600
47,XXX	20	1/960
Other	7	1/2740
Autosomal Numerical Abnormalities in 56,952 Infants		
Total	82	1/695 live births
Trisomy 21	71	1/800
Trisomy 18	7	1/8140
Trisomy 13	3	1/19,000
Triploidy	1	1/57,000
Structural Abnormalities in 56,952 Infants *(Autosomes and Sex Chromosomes)*		
Total	144	1/395 live births
Balanced rearrangements		
Robertsonian	51	1/1120
Other	59	1/965
Unbalanced rearrangements	34	1/1675
All Chromosome Abnormalities *(Autosomes and Sex Chromosomes)*	353	1/160 live births

Data from Hook EB, Hamerton JL (1977). The frequency of chromosome abnormalities detected in consecutive newborn studies, differences between studies, results by sex and by severity of phenotypic involvement. *In* Hook EB, Porter IH (eds) Population cytogenetics: Studies in humans. Academic Press, New York, pp. 63–79.

Table 9–4. Incidence of Down Syndrome in Liveborns and Fetuses in Relation to Maternal Age

Maternal Age (Years)	Incidence		
	At Birth	*At Amniocentesis (16 Weeks)*	*At Chorionic Villus Sampling (9–11 Weeks)*
15–19	1/1250	—	—
20–24	1/1400	—	—
25–29	1/1100	—	—
30	1/900	—	—
31	1/900	—	—
32	1/750	—	—
33	1/625	1/420	—
34	1/500	1/325	—
35	1/350	1/250	1/240
36	1/275	1/200	1/175
37	1/225	1/150	1/130
38	1/175	1/120	1/100
39	1/140	1/100	1/75
40	1/100	1/75	1/60
41	1/85	1/60	1/40
42	1/65	1/45	1/30
43	1/50	1/35	1/25
44	1/40	1/30	1/20
45 and over	1/25	1/20	1/10

Data from Hook et al. (1983) and Hook et al. (1988). Figures have been rounded and are approximate.

Table 9–5. Frequencies of Chromosome Abnormalities in Spontaneous Abortions

Type	Frequency (Approximate) (Percent)
Aneuploidy	
45,X	20
Autosomal monosomy	<1
Autosomal trisomy	
Total	52
Trisomy 16	16
Trisomy 18	3
Trisomy 21	5
Trisomy 22	5
Other trisomies	23
Triploidy	16
Tetraploidy	6
Structural Rearrangements	4

Data chiefly from Boué A, Boué J, Gropp A (1985) Cytogenetics of pregnancy wastage. Ann Rev Genet 14:1–57.

160 births (0.7 percent). The findings are summarized in Table 9–3, classified separately for specific numerical abnormalities of sex chromosomes and autosomes and for balanced and unbalanced structural rearrangements. Most of the autosomal abnormalities can be diagnosed at birth, but most sex chromosome abnormalities, with the exception of Turner syndrome, are not diagnosed until puberty. Balanced rearrangements are rarely identified clinically unless a carrier of a rearrangement gives birth to a child with an unbalanced chromosome complement and family studies are initiated; unbalanced rearrangements are likely to come to clinical attention for the usual reasons, dysmorphism and delayed physical and mental development.

Fetuses at Prenatal Diagnosis

Because prenatal diagnosis is usually performed for mothers over 35 years old, incidence data for fetal cytogenetic abnormalities are influenced by late maternal age, which increases the risk of trisomy. Two procedures are commonly used to provide fetal tissue for analysis: (1) amniocentesis at about the 16th week of gestation and (2) chorionic villus sampling (CVS) at about the 9th to 11th week (see Chapter 19). Because trisomy 21 accounts for about half of all abnormalities identified prenatally, the incidence of Down syndrome seen in live births, in amniocentesis, and in CVS at different maternal ages can provide a basis for comparison and an idea of the amount of fetal loss between the 11th and 16th weeks and between the 16th week and birth (Table 9–4). At all the maternal ages shown, there is some loss between the 11th and 16th weeks, as would be expected from the high rate of chromosome abnormality seen in spontaneous abortions (see next section), and an additional loss later in pregnancy. In fact, probably only 20 to 25 percent of trisomy 21 conceptuses survive to birth.

Table 9–6. Outcome of 10,000 Conceptions

Outcome	Conceptions	Spontaneous Abortions		Live Births
		No.	Percent	
Total	10,000	1500	15	8500
Normal Chromosomes	9200	750	8	8450
Abnormal Chromosomes				
Total	800	750	94	50
Triploid/tetraploid	170	170	100	—
45,X	140	139	99	1
Trisomy 16	112	112	100	—
Trisomy 18	20	19	95	1
Trisomy 21	45	35	78	10
Trisomy, other	209	208	99.5	1
47,XXY, 47,XXX, 47,XYY	19	4	21	15
Unbalanced rearrangements	27	23	85	4
Balanced rearrangements	19	3	16	16
Other	39	37	95	2

Spontaneous Abortions

The overall frequency of chromosome abnormalities in spontaneous abortions is at least 50 percent, and the kinds of abnormalities differ in a number of ways from those seen in liveborns (Table 9–5). The single most common abnormality in abortuses is 45,X (Turner syndrome), which is present in 18 percent of chromosomally abnormal spontaneous abortuses but in only 0.6 percent of chromosomally abnormal live births. The other sex chromosome abnormalities, which are quite common in live births, are rare in abortuses. Another difference is the distribution of kinds of trisomy; for example, trisomy 16 is the most common trisomy in abortuses but is not seen at all in live births.

Because the overall miscarriage (spontaneous abortion) rate (about 15 percent), the overall incidence of specific chromosome defects in abortuses, and their incidence in live births are known, one can estimate the proportion of all conceptuses of a given karyotype that are lost by spontaneous abortion (Table 9–6).

Recurrence Risk After Spontaneous Abortion of a Chromosomally Abnormal Fetus

Does a mother who has a spontaneous abortion in which the karyotype is abnormal have an increased risk of another such event? The answer may be no, at least for older women (Warburton et al., 1987). After an abortion of a fetus with a normal karyotype, a subsequent aborted fetus is also likely to have a normal karyotype (Table 9–7). Unexpectedly, however, after an abortion of a fetus with trisomy or other abnormal karyotype, the risk of trisomy in a second abortion appears not to be significantly increased when correction is made for maternal age. This is different from findings for younger women who have previously given birth to a trisomic infant or who have had a trisomic fetus detected prenatally. These younger women do appear to have a higher recurrence risk.

MOSAICISM

When a person has a chromosome abnormality, the abnormality is usually present in all his or her cultured cells. Sometimes, however, two or more different chromosome complements are detected. This situation is called **mosaicism.** Mosaicism may be either numerical (the most common type) or structural.

A common cause of mosaicism is nondisjunction in an early postzygotic mitotic division. For example, a zygote with an additional chromosome 21 might lose the extra chromosome in a mitotic division and continue to develop as a 46/47,+21 mosaic. The significance of a finding of mosaicism is often difficult to assess, especially if it is identified prenatally. The effects of mosaicism on development vary with the timing of the nondisjunctional event, the nature of the chromosome abnormality, the proportions of the different chromosome complements present, and the tissues affected. An additional problem is that the proportions of the different chromosome complements seen in the tissue being analyzed (for example, cultured amniocytes or lymphocytes) may not necessarily reflect the proportions present in other tissues or in the embryo during its early devel-

Table 9–7. Chromosome Analysis of Repeat Spontaneous Abortions

First Abortion Outcome	Second Abortion Outcome			
	Total	*Normal*	*Trisomy*	*Other Abnormality*
Total	273	173 (63%)	61 (22%)	39 (14%)
Normal	157 (58%)	122 (78%)	18 (11%)	17 (11%)
Trisomy	72 (26%)	33 (46%)	30 (42%)	9 (13%)
Other abnormality	44 (16%)	18 (41%)	13 (30%)	13 (30%)

Data from Warburton D, Kline J, Stein Z, et al. (1987) Does the karyotype of a spontaneous abortion predict the karyotype of a subsequent abortion?—Evidence from 273 women with two karyotyped spontaneous abortions. Am J Hum Genet 41:465–483.

opmental stages. In laboratory studies, cytogeneticists attempt to differentiate between true mosaicism, present in individuals, and **pseudomosaicism,** in which the mosaicism probably arose in cell culture. The distinction is not always easy or certain.

Clinical studies of the phenotypic effects of mosaicism have two main weaknesses. First, because people are hardly ever karyotyped without some clinical indications, clinically normal mosaic persons are rarely ascertained; second, there have been few follow-up studies of prenatally diagnosed mosaic fetuses. Nonetheless, it is generally the case that individuals who are mosaic for a given trisomy, such as mosaic Down syndrome, are less severely affected than nonmosaic trisomic individuals.

Mosaicism is relatively common in cytogenetic studies of chorionic villus cultures and can lead to major interpretive problems in prenatal diagnosis (Chapter 19).

STUDIES OF CHROMOSOMES IN HUMAN MEIOSIS

Although human ova are still resistant to cytogenetic analysis, a technique has been devised to allow the analysis of metaphase chromosomes in

---

Clinical Indications for Chromosome Analysis

Because of the complexity and cost of chromosome analysis, its use is ordinarily limited to cases with specific indications. Apart from the specific phenotypes mentioned in this chapter and in Chapter 10, in which chromosome analysis is a standard part of clinical evaluation, there are also some nonspecific general clinical indications that suggest a need for cytogenetic analysis:

1. **A number of problems of early growth and development.** Failure to thrive, developmental delay, dysmorphic facies, multiple malformations, short stature, ambiguous genitalia, and mental retardation are frequent findings in children with chromosome abnormalities, although not restricted to that group. Unless there is a definite nonchromosomal diagnosis, chromosome analysis should be performed for patients presenting with a combination of such problems.

2. **Stillbirth and neonatal death.** As noted earlier, the incidence of chromosome abnormalities is much higher among stillbirths than among live births. It is also elevated among infants who die in the neonatal period. Chromosome analysis should be performed for all stillbirths and neonatal deaths that might have a cytogenetic basis in order to identify a possible specific cause or, alternatively, to rule out chromosome abnormality as the reason for the loss. In such cases, karyotyping is essential for accurate genetic counseling and may provide important information for prenatal diagnosis in future pregnancies.

3. **Fertility problems.** Chromosome studies are indicated for women presenting with amenorrhea and for couples with a history of infertility or habitual abortion. A chromosome abnormality (usually a structural rearrangement or sex chromosome mosaicism) is seen in one or the other parent in a significant proportion (3 to 6 percent) of cases in which there have been two successive miscarriages or infertility.

4. **Family history.** A known or suspected chromosome abnormality in a first-degree relative is an indication for chromosome analysis under some circumstances. Chromosome analysis in phenotypically normal family members is obviously unnecessary when the proband is known to have Down syndrome with trisomy 21. On the other hand, if a patient has translocation Down syndrome, the parents' chromosomes should be analyzed; if one parent is found to be a translocation carrier, the study should then be extended to other family members.

human sperm by inducing fusion of sperm with hamster oocytes (Rudak et al., 1978). The technique is laborious, and so far only a few studies have been reported, but some information is available about the segregation of chromosomes in sperm from males with normal karyotypes as well as from carriers of some types of human structural aberrations. An alternative method is to use molecular cytogenetic techniques to measure aneuploidy directly in human sperm by detecting copies of a particular chromosome in interphase preparations (Pieters et al., 1990).

Among males with normal karyotypes, the reported incidence of aneuploidy in sperm is 1 to 5 percent. Male carriers of reciprocal translocations produce sperm with normal and balanced chromosome complements in approximately equal proportions, as expected, but about half the sperm have unbalanced karyotypes. This is in contrast to the observations in liveborn offspring of male translocation carriers, very few of whom have unbalanced chromosome sets. Further analysis and comparison of the findings in sperm, fetuses, and newborns await future research.

DISORDERS OF AUTOSOMES

AUTOSOMAL TRISOMIES

In the preceding section, the types of chromosome abnormalities were described and the reasons for their occurrence were briefly discussed. In this section, the major autosomal disorders of clinical significance are described. Although there are numerous rare chromosome disorders in which gain or loss of an entire chromosome or a chromosome segment has been reported, many of these either have been seen only in fetuses that were aborted spontaneously or involve relatively short chromosome segments. There are only three well-defined chromosome disorders compatible with postnatal survival in which there is trisomy for an entire autosome: **trisomy 21** (Down syndrome), **trisomy 18**, and **trisomy 13**.

Each of these autosomal trisomies is associated with growth retardation, mental retardation, and multiple congenital anomalies. Nevertheless, each has a highly distinctive phenotype. The developmental abnormalities characteristic of any one trisomic state must be determined by the extra dosage of the genes on the additional chromosome. Knowledge of the relation between the extra chromosome and the consequent developmental abnormality has been limited, but molecular analysis, especially in Down syndrome, is beginning to show that specific genes on the extra chromosome may be responsible for the abnormal phenotype. In general, any chromosomal imbalance, whether it involves addition or loss of genes, is expected to have a specific phenotypic effect determined by the dosage of the specific genes on the extra or missing chromosome segment (Epstein, 1986). We return to this subject in the next section.

Down Syndrome

Down syndrome, or trisomy 21, is by far the most common and best known of the chromosome disorders and is the single most common genetic cause of moderate mental retardation. About one child in 800 is born with Down syndrome, and among liveborn children or fetuses of mothers 35 years of age or older the incidence is far higher (Table 9–4). The syndrome was first described clinically by Langdon Down in 1866, but its cause remained a deep mystery for almost a century. Two noteworthy features of its population distribution drew attention: late maternal age, and the peculiar distribution within families— concordance in all monozygotic twins but almost complete discordance in dizygotic twins and other family members. Waardenburg suggested in 1932 that a chromosome abnormality could explain these observations, but at that time no one was prepared to believe that humans were really likely to have chromosome abnormalities. However, when techniques for detailed analysis of human chromosomes became available, Down syndrome was one of the first conditions to be examined chromosomally. In 1959 Lejeune and colleagues, as well as several other groups, were able to confirm that most children with Down syndrome have 47 chromosomes, the extra member being a small acrocentric chromosome that has since been designated chromosome 21 (Fig. 9–1).

The older term "mongolism," once used to refer to this condition, reflected the somewhat Oriental cast of countenance produced by the characteristic epicanthal folds and upslanting palpebral fissures. The term is now considered inappropriate and should not be used.

Phenotype

Down syndrome can usually be diagnosed at birth or shortly thereafter by its dysmorphic features, which vary among patients but nevertheless produce a distinctive phenotype (Fig. 9–11). Hypotonia may be the first abnormality noticed in the newborn. In addition to the dysmorphic features already mentioned, the patients are short in stature and have brachycephaly, with a flat occiput. The neck is short, with loose skin on the nape. The nasal bridge is flat, the ears are low-set and have a characteristic folded appearance, the eyes have Brushfield spots around the margin of the iris, and the mouth is open, often showing the furrowed, protruding tongue. The hands are short and broad, often with a single transverse palmar crease ("simian crease") and incurved fifth digits, or clinodactyly (Fig. 9–12). The feet show a wide gap between the first and second toes, with a furrow extending proximally on the plantar surface. The dermatoglyphics (patterns of the ridged skin) are highly characteristic.

The major cause for concern in Down syndrome is mental retardation. Even though in early infancy the child may not seem delayed in devel-

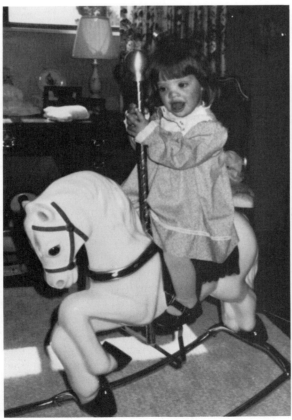

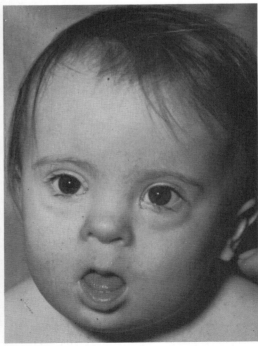

A   B

Figure 9–11. Two children with Down syndrome. (Left, courtesy of David Patterson, Eleanor Roosevelt Institute, Denver. Right, from Jones KL [1988] Smith's Recognizable patterns of human malformation, 4th ed. WB Saunders, Philadelphia.)

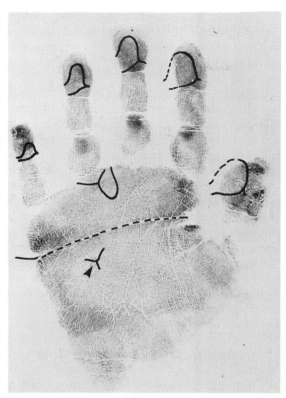

Figure 9-12. Characteristic dermal patterns of the palm of a child with Down syndrome: a single flexion crease (simian crease), axial triradius (arrow) in distal position, a pattern area on the palm between the third and fourth digits, and ulnar loops on all ten digits.

opment, the delay is usually obvious by the end of the first year. The intelligence quotient is usually 25 to 50 when the child is old enough to be tested. Nevertheless, many children with Down syndrome develop into happy and even self-reliant persons in spite of these limitations (Fig. 9-11).

Congenital heart disease is present in about one third of all liveborn Down syndrome infants and in a somewhat higher proportion of abortuses with the syndrome. Certain malformations are more common in Down syndrome than in other disorders, such as duodenal atresia and tracheoesophageal fistula. There is a fifteenfold increase in the risk of leukemia.

Prenatal and Postnatal Survival

About three quarters of all Down syndrome conceptuses are lost by spontaneous abortion either in the first trimester or, less frequently, later in pregnancy, and many liveborn children with the syndrome die in early postnatal life. The patients least likely to survive both prenatally and postnatally are those with congenital heart disease; about one fourth of the liveborn infants with heart defects die before their first birthday (Baird and Sadovnick, 1988). About half the patients survive to more than 50 years of age, and one in seven is still alive at age 68 (Baird and Sadovnick, 1989). Premature senility, associated with the neuropathological findings characteristic of Alzheimer disease (cortical atrophy, ventricular dilatation, and neurofibrillar tangles), affects Down syndrome patients at an age several decades earlier than the typical age of onset of Alzheimer disease in the general population.

The Chromosomes in Down Syndrome

The clinical diagnosis of Down syndrome usually presents no particular difficulty. Nevertheless, karyotyping is indicated for confirmation and to provide the basis for genetic counseling. Although the particular karyotype responsible for Down syndrome has little if any effect on the phenotype of the patient, it is essential for determination of the recurrence risk.

Trisomy 21. In about 95 percent of all patients, Down syndrome involves trisomy for chromosome 21 (Fig. 9-1), resulting from meiotic nondisjunction of the chromosome 21 pair (Figs. 9-2, 9-3). As noted earlier, the risk of having a child with trisomy 21 increases with maternal age, especially after the age of 30 years (Table 9-4). The meiotic error responsible for the trisomy usually occurs during maternal meiosis (about 95 percent of cases), predominantly in meiosis I, but can also occur in paternal meiosis (about 5 percent of cases), again usually in meiosis I (Stewart et al., 1988; Antonarakis et al., 1991).

Robertsonian Translocation. About 4 percent of Down syndrome patients have 46 chromosomes, one of which is a Robertsonian translocation between chromosome 21q and the long arm of one of the other acrocentric chromosomes (usually chromosome 14 or 22). The translocation chromosome replaces one of the normal acrocentrics, and the karyotype of a Down syndrome patient with a Robertsonian translocation between chromosomes 14 and 21 is therefore 46,XX or XY,− 14,+ t(14q21q). In effect, the patient is trisomic for 21q.

Unlike standard trisomy 21, translocation Down syndrome shows no relation to maternal age but has a relatively high recurrence risk in families when a parent, especially the mother, is a carrier of the translocation. For this reason, karyotyping of the parents and possibly other relatives is necessary before genetic counseling can be provided.

A carrier of a Robertsonian translocation involving chromosomes 14 and 21 has only 45 chromosomes; one chromosome 14 and one chromosome 21 are missing and are replaced by the translocation chromosome, t(14q21q). The gametes that can be formed by a carrier are shown in Figure 9–13. Theoretically, there are six possible types of gamete, but three of these appear unable to lead to viable offspring. Of the three viable types, one is normal, one is balanced, and one is unbalanced, having both the translocation chromosome and the normal chromosome 21. In combination with a normal gamete, this could produce a child with translocation Down syndrome (Fig. 9–14). Theoretically, the three types of gametes are produced in equal numbers, and thus the theoretical risk of a Down syndrome child should be 1 in 3. However, extensive population studies have

shown that unbalanced chromosome complements appear in only 15 percent of the progeny of carrier mothers and very few of the progeny of carrier fathers who have translocations involving chromosome 21.

21q21q Translocation. A 21q21q translocation chromosome is a chromosome made up of two chromosome 21 long arms, seen occasionally in Down syndrome carriers or patients. It is thought to originate as an isochromosome rather than by Robertsonian translocation. Although this is a rare abnormality, it is particularly important because all gametes of a carrier of such a chromosome must either contain the 21q21q chromosome, with its double dose of chromosome 21 genetic material, or lack it and have no chromosome 21 representative at all. The potential progeny inevitably have either Down syndrome or monosomy 21, which is rarely viable. In other words, an individual unfortunate enough to have this defect is unable to have normal children and will probably have only children with Down syndrome.

Mosaic Down Syndrome. About 1 percent of Down syndrome patients have mosaicism, usually for cell populations with either a normal or a trisomy 21 karyotype. It is likely that most mosaic Down patients derive from trisomy 21 zygotes, as mentioned previously. The phenotype may be milder than that of typical trisomy 21, but there is

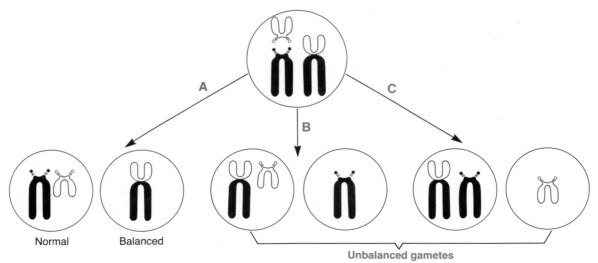

Normal   Balanced

Unbalanced gametes

Figure 9–13. Chromosomes of gametes that theoretically can be produced by a carrier of a Robertsonian translocation, t(14q21q). A. Normal and balanced complements. B. Unbalanced, one product with both the translocation chromosome and the normal chromosome 21, the reciprocal product with chromosome 14 only. C. Unbalanced, one product with both the translocation chromosome and chromosome 14, the reciprocal product with chromosome 21 only. See text for a description of the eventual fate of these gametes.

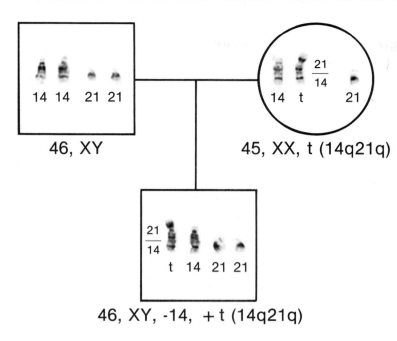

46, XY

45, XX, t (14q21q)

46, XY, -14, + t (14q21q)

Figure 9-14. Translocation 14q21q transmitted by a carrier mother to her child, who has Down syndrome. The father's chromosomes are normal. Only chromosomes 14, 21, and t(14q21q) are shown. (Courtesy of R. G. Worton, The Hospital for Sick Children, Toronto.)

wide variability in phenotypes among mosaic patients, possibly reflecting the variable proportion of trisomy 21 cells in the embryo during early development. The ascertained patients with mosaic Down syndrome probably represent the more abnormal cases, since very mildly affected persons are less likely to be karyotyped. Low-grade mosaicism in germinal tissue of a parent is one of the postulated causes of Down syndrome, especially among the patients born to mothers in the younger age groups or in the rare families with more than one trisomic child.

Partial Trisomy 21. Very rarely, Down syndrome is diagnosed in a patient in whom only a part of the long arm of chromosome 21 is present in triplicate, and a Down syndrome patient with no cytogenetically visible chromosome abnormality is even more rarely identified. These patients are of particular interest because they can show what region of chromosome 21 is likely to be responsible for the Down syndrome phenotype (the "critical region") and what regions can be triplicated without causing the phenotype. Detailed cytogenetic and molecular characterization of such patients has narrowed the critical segment to chromosome band 21q22 (Fig. 9 – 15). This region is expected to contain at least 50 to 100 genes.

What genes on chromosome 21, when ex-

pressed in triple dosage, might account for the pathogenesis of Down syndrome? Figure 9 – 15 shows the map positions of several genes on chromosome 21. The genes that may be within the critical region include those for superoxide dismutase (SOD1); cystathionine β-synthase, the enzyme that is deficient in homocystinuria (CBS); α A crystallin, a lens protein (CRYA1); and an oncogene, ETS2.

Attempts to correlate triple dosage of specific genes with specific aspects of the Down syndrome phenotype have been unsuccessful so far. One problem is that although rare patients have triplication of only a very small segment of chromosome 21, most patients have trisomy for the entire chromosome, not only the critical region. Earlier, when the familial Alzheimer disease gene was mapped to chromosome 21, a causal connection was assumed because the pathological changes characteristic of Alzheimer disease are also seen in Down syndrome patients. Although it is possible that these changes are due to the presence of the Alzheimer disease gene in triple dose, it is now known that this gene lies outside the Down syndrome critical region. Sorting out the genes crucial to the expression of Down syndrome from those that merely happen to be syntenic with them on chromosome 21 is a task for the future.

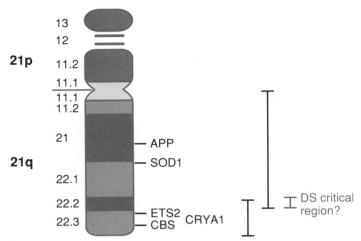

Figure 9–15. Schematic representation of chromosome 21, showing the localization of selected genes and the possible position of the "Down syndrome critical region" in 21q22.2–22.3, which, when present in three copies, seems to be responsible for at least some of the major phenotypic features in Down syndrome, such as the characteristic facies, lowered IQ, short stature, and heart defects. The two brackets illustrate the region of chromosome 21 triplicated in Down syndrome patients with only a partial trisomy of 21. Genes shown are APP, amyloid precursor protein; SOD1, superoxide dismutase-1; ETS2, the ets-2 oncogene; CBS, cystathionine-β-synthase; and CRYA1, α crystallin lens protein. (Adapted from Rahmani et al., 1989, and Korenberg et al., 1990.)

Etiology of Trisomy 21

Although the chromosomal basis of Down syndrome is clear, the reason for the chromosome abnormality is still poorly understood. The high percentage of all cases of trisomy 21 in which the abnormal gamete originated during maternal meiosis I suggests that something about maternal meiosis I, related to late maternal age, is the underlying cause. One obvious possibility is the "older egg" model: it has been suggested that the older the oocyte, the greater the chance that the chromosomes will fail to disjoin correctly. However, the cytogenetic and molecular analysis described earlier has shown that about 5 percent of all the nondisjunctional events that involve chromosome 21 happen in paternal rather than maternal meiosis, and these cases show advanced maternal age as well. A full explanation of chromosome 21 nondisjunction is thus not yet possible (Antonarakis et al., 1991; Epstein, 1989).

Risk of Down Syndrome

A frequent problem in genetic counseling, especially in prenatal genetics, is how to assess the risk of the birth of a Down syndrome child. Down syndrome can be detected prenatally by cytogenetic analysis of chorionic villus or amniotic fluid cells, and in fact about 80 percent of all prenatal diagnoses are performed because late maternal age gives rise to concern about the risk of Down syndrome in the fetus. A commonly accepted guideline is that a woman is eligible for prenatal diagnosis if the risk that her fetus has Down syndrome outweighs the risk that the procedure of amniocentesis or chorionic villus sampling used to obtain fetal tissue for chromosome analysis will lead to fetal loss (see Chapter 19). The risk depends chiefly on the mother's age but also on both parents' karyotypes.

The population incidence of Down syndrome in live births is currently estimated to be about 1 in 800, depending on the maternal age distribution for all births and the proportion of older mothers who make use of prenatal diagnosis and selective termination. At about age 30 the risk begins to rise sharply, reaching 1 in 25 births in the oldest maternal age group (Table 9–4). Even though younger mothers have a much lower risk, their birth rate is so much higher that more than half of the mothers of all Down syndrome babies are under 35 years old. The risk of Down syndrome due to translocation or partial trisomy is unrelated to maternal age, but there is some evidence that mothers of mosaic patients tend to be older than average; this evidence strengthens the view that many mosaics begin as trisomy 21 zygotes. The paternal age appears to have no influence on the risk.

Trisomy 18

In the United States and Canada, 50 percent or more of pregnant women aged 35 and over undergo prenatal diagnosis for fetal chromosome analysis, but only about 1 percent of the fetuses tested are found to have trisomy 21. Current approaches to more precise or efficient identification of fetuses at risk, by means of alpha-fetoprotein assay and ultrasonography, are discussed in Chapter 19. Methods to examine rare fetal cells found in the maternal circulation are being developed.

Recurrence Risk

The recurrence risk of trisomy 21 or some other autosomal trisomy, after one such child has been born in a family, is about 1 percent overall. For mothers under 30 years old, the risk is about 1.4 percent, and for older mothers, it is the same as the age-related risk; that is, there is an increase in risk for the younger mothers, but only the age-related for the older mothers. The reason for the increased risk for the younger mothers is not known. One possibility is that unrecognized germline mosaicism in one parent, with a trisomic cell line as well as a normal cell line, may be a factor. A history of trisomy 21 elsewhere in the family, although often a cause of maternal anxiety, does not appear to significantly increase the risk of having a Down syndrome child. The recurrence risk of translocation Down syndrome has already been discussed.

The phenotype of an infant with trisomy 18 is shown in Figure 9–16. The incidence of this condition in liveborn infants is about 1 in 8000 births. The incidence at conception is much higher, but about 95 percent of trisomy 18 conceptuses are aborted spontaneously. Postnatal survival is also poor; survival for more than a few months is rare, though affected children aged 15 years or more have been reported. About 80 percent of the patients are female, perhaps because of preferential survival. As in most other trisomies, late maternal age is a factor.

The features of trisomy 18 always include mental retardation and failure to thrive, and often include severe malformation of the heart. Hypertonia is a typical finding. The head has a prominent occiput, and the jaw recedes. The ears are low-set and malformed. The sternum is short. The fists clench in a characteristic way, the second and fifth digits overlapping the third and fourth (Fig. 9–16). The feet are rocker-bottom, with prominent calcanei. The dermal patterns are distinctive, with single creases on the palms and arch patterns on most or all digits. The nails are usually hypoplastic.

The trisomy 18 phenotype, like that of trisomy 21, can result from a variety of rare karyotypes other than complete trisomy. There may be a translocation involving all or most of chromosome 18, which may be either de novo or inherited from a balanced carrier parent. The trisomy may also be

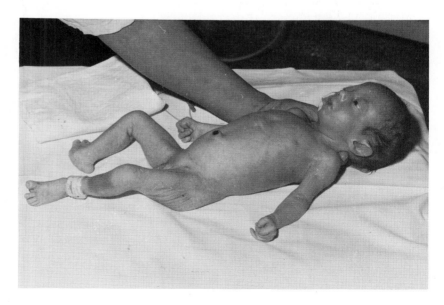

Figure 9–16. An infant with trisomy 18. Note the clenched fist with the second and fifth digits overlapping the third and fourth, rocker-bottom feet with prominent calcanei, dorsiflexion of the big toe, and large, low-set ears with simple helix. (Courtesy of D. H. Carr, McMaster University, Hamilton, Ontario.)

present in mosaic form, with variable but usually somewhat milder expression. The "critical region" for trisomy 18 has not yet been identified, but trisomy of the entire long arm alone produces the characteristic trisomy 18 phenotype.

Trisomy 13

The striking phenotype of trisomy 13 is shown in Figure 9–17. The incidence is about 1 in 25,000 births. Trisomy 13 is clinically severe, lethal in almost all cases by the age of six months. About half of trisomy 13 individuals die within the first month. Like most other trisomies, it is associated with late maternal age. The extra chromosome usually arises from nondisjunction in maternal meiosis I (Hassold et al., 1987). About 20 percent of the cases are caused by an unbalanced translocation. The recurrence risk is low; even when one parent of a translocation patient is a carrier of the translocation, the empiric risk that a subsequent liveborn child will have the syndrome is less than 2 percent.

The phenotype of trisomy 13 includes severe central nervous system malformations such as arhinencephaly and holoprosencephaly. Growth retardation and severe mental retardation are present. The forehead is sloping, there is ocular hypertelorism, and there may be microphthalmia, iris coloboma, or even absence of the eyes. The ears are malformed. Cleft lip and cleft palate are often present. The hands and feet may show postaxial polydactyly, and the hands clench with the second and fifth digits overlapping the third and fourth, as in trisomy 18. The feet are rocker-bottom. The palms often have simian creases. Internally there are usually congenital heart defects of specific types and urogenital defects, including cryptorchidism in males, bicornuate uterus and hypoplastic ovaries in females, and polycystic kidneys. Of this constellation of defects, the most distinctive at first glance are the general facial appearance with cleft lip and palate and ocular abnormalities, the polydactyly, the clenched fists, and the rocker-bottom feet.

AUTOSOMAL DELETION SYNDROMES

There are many reports of cytogenetically detectable deletions in dysmorphic patients, but most of these deletions have been seen in only a few patients and are not associated with recognized syndromes. As mentioned earlier, a number of microdeletion syndromes have been described (Table 9–2). In addition, there are two well-delineated autosomal deletion syndromes, a severe mental retardation syndrome associated with deletion of part of chromosome 4p (the 4p− syndrome), and the cri du chat (or 5p−) syndrome.

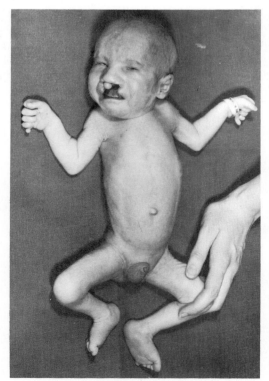

Figure 9–17. An infant with trisomy 13. Note particularly the bilateral cleft lip and polydactyly. (Courtesy of P. E. Conen, The Hospital for Sick Children, Toronto.)

Cri du Chat (5p−) Syndrome

The cri du chat syndrome, in which there is a deletion of the short arm of chromosome 5, was given its common name because a crying affected infant sounds just like a mewing cat. It accounts for about 1 percent of all institutionalized mentally retarded patients. The facial appearance, shown in Figure 9–18, is distinctive, with microcephaly, hypertel-

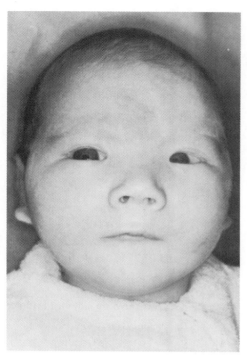

Figure 9–18. An infant with cri du chat syndrome, which results from deletion of part of chromosome 5p. Note characteristic facies with hypertelorism, epicanthus, and retrognathia.

orism, antimongoloid slant of the palpebral fissures, epicanthal folds, low-set ears sometimes with preauricular tags, and micrognathia.

Most cases of cri du chat syndrome are sporadic, but 10 to 15 percent of the patients are the

offspring of translocation carriers. An illustrative pedigree is shown in Figure 9–19.

The breakpoints and extent of the deleted segment of chromosome 5p vary in different patients, but the critical region, missing in all patients with the phenotype, has been identified as chromosome band 5p15. A number of DNA probes and genes have been demonstrated to be deleted from 5p— chromosomes. However, the basis for the relationship between monosomy for such genes and the clinical phenotype remains to be explained.

MENDELIAN DISORDERS WITH CYTOGENETIC EFFECTS

There are several rare single-gene syndromes, in addition to the relatively common fragile X syndrome (see Chapter 4), in which there is a characteristic cytogenetic abnormality (Table 9–8). In each disorder, a detailed chromosome study is an important element of diagnosis. This is especially true for the fragile X syndrome and for Bloom syndrome, in which a striking increase in **sister chromatid exchange** is found (Fig. 9–20). The nature of the chromosome defect and presumably the underlying molecular defect in chromosome replication or repair is different in each of these disorders.

Several of the chromosome breakage syndromes listed in Table 9–8 are associated with an

Figure 9–19. Pedigree of child with cri du chat syndrome whose mother was a carrier of a balanced translocation between chromosomes 5p and 9p. The mother had (1) the affected child, who received her deleted chromosome 5 and normal chromosome 9, (2) a retarded daughter, who received her normal chromosome 5 and the translocated chromosome 9 (and was therefore trisomic for the translocated segment of chromosome 5p), (3) a daughter carrying the balanced translocation, and, after amniocentesis and chromosome analysis, two sons: (4) a carrier of the balanced translocation and (5) a son with a normal karyotype.

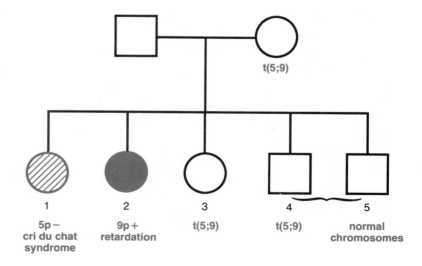

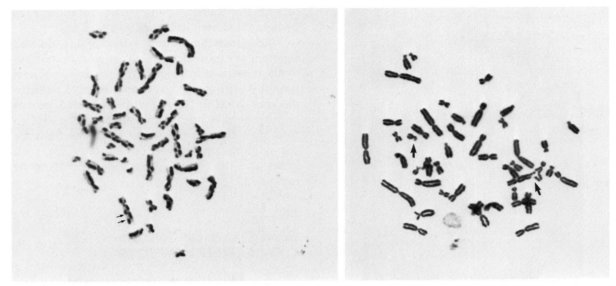

Figure 9–20. Characteristic chromosome abnormalities seen in two chromosomal instability syndromes. Left: high frequency of sister chromatid exchanges in chromosomes from a patient with Bloom syndrome. Two exchanges are indicated by the arrows. Right: chromosome breaks (arrows) and gaps in chromosomes from a patient with Fanconi anemia. See text for discussion. (Photomicrographs courtesy of Chin Ho, Cytogenetics Laboratory, The Hospital for Sick Children, Toronto.)

increased risk of malignancy. Further analysis of the correlation between decreased ability to replicate or repair DNA and increased risk of malignancies might be expected to provide insight into the relationship between mutagenesis and carcinogenesis.

CANCER CYTOGENETICS

An important field of cancer research is the delineation of cytogenetic changes in specific forms of cancer, and the relation of the breakpoints of the various structural rearrangements to oncogenes.

Table 9–8. Mendelian Disorders with Cytogenetic Effects

Disorder	Inheritance	Clinical Features	Cytogenetic Effects
Ataxia telangiectasia (multiple forms)	AR	Cerebellar ataxia, telangiectasia, growth retardation, Ig deficiencies, oculomotor apraxia, predisposition to malignancy	Chromatid-type damage; DNA repair defects
Bloom syndrome	AR	Low birth weight, dwarfism, malar hypoplasia, butterfly rash of face exacerbated by sunlight, predisposition to malignancy	High frequency of sister chromatid exchange (SCE) and chromosome breakage in culture (Fig. 9–20)
Fanconi anemia (multiple forms)	AR	Short stature, radial hypoplasia, anemia, pancytopenia, bronzing of skin, predisposition to leukemias or carcinomas	High frequency of chromosome breakage and nonhomologous interchange (Fig. 9–20)
Fragile X syndrome	X-linked	Mental retardation, macroorchidism, increased head circumference, large ears and chin (see Fig. 4–20)	Fragile site at Xq27.3 (see Fig. 4–21)
Roberts syndrome	AR	Limb reduction, severe growth deficiency, midfacial defect, mental retardation	Premature separation of centromeric heterochromatin in metaphase
Xeroderma pigmentosum (multiple forms)	AR	Sensitivity to sunlight, skin changes, mental deterioration, predisposition to malignancy	Defective excision repair of UV radiation–induced breakage, expressed as increased SCE rate after exposure to UV light or chemical carcinogens

AR = autosomal recessive.

The cytogenetic changes seen in cancer cells are numerous and diverse. Many are repeatedly seen in the same type of tumor. About 150 nonrandom chromosome changes involving all chromosomes except the Y chromosome have been identified in 43 types of neoplasia (Trent et al., 1989). In the future, the association of cytogenetic analysis with tumor type and with the effectiveness of therapy will be an important part of the management of patients with cancer. The types of chromosome changes seen in cancer and the role of chromosome abnormalities in the etiology or progression, or both, of different malignancies are discussed further in Chapter 16.

General References

Borgaonkar DS (1989) Chromosomal variation in man: a catalog of chromosomal variants and anomalies, 5th ed. Alan R. Liss, New York.

Epstein CJ (1986) The consequences of chromosome imbalance: Principles, mechanisms, and models. Cambridge University Press, New York.

Epstein CJ (1989) Down syndrome. *In* Scriver CR, Beaudet AL, Sly WS, Valle D (eds) The metabolic basis of inherited disease, 6th ed. McGraw-Hill, New York, pp. 291–326.

Gardner RJM, Sutherland GR (1989) Chromosome abnormalities and genetic counseling. Oxford University Press, New York.

Hook EB, Porter IH (eds) (1977) Population cytogenetics: Studies in humans. Academic Press, New York.

Ledbetter DH, Cavenee WK (1989) Molecular cytogenetics: Interface of cytogenetics and monogenic disorders. *In* Scriver CR, Beaudet AL, Sly WS, Valle D (eds) The metabolic basis of inherited disease, 6th ed. McGraw-Hill, New York, pp. 343–371.

Stewart GD, Hassold TJ, Kurnit DM (1988) Trisomy 21: Molecular and cytogenetic studies of nondisjunction. Adv Hum Genet 17:99–140.

Therman E (1988) Human chromosomes: Structure, behavior, effects, 2nd ed. Springer-Verlag, New York.

Problems

1. You send a blood sample from a dysmorphic infant to the chromosome laboratory for analysis. The laboratory's report states that the child's karyotype is 46,XY,18q−.
   a) What does this karyotype mean?
   b) The laboratory asks for blood samples from the clinically normal parents for analysis. Why?
   c) The laboratory reports the mother's karyotype as 46,XX and the father's karyotype as 46,XY,−7,−18,+t(7;18)(q35;q12). What does the latter karyotype mean? Referring to the normal chromosome idiograms in Appendix I, sketch the translocation chromosome or chromosomes in the father and in his son. Sketch these chromosomes in meiosis in the father. What kinds of gametes can he produce?
   d) In light of this new information, what does the child's karyotype mean now? What regions are monosomic? Trisomic? Given information from Chapter 3, estimate the number of genes present in the trisomic or monosomic regions.

2. A spontaneously aborted fetus is found to have trisomy 18.
   a) What proportion of fetuses with trisomy 18 are lost by spontaneous abortion?
   b) What is the risk that the parents will have a liveborn child with trisomy 18 in a future pregnancy?

3. A newborn child with Down syndrome, when karyotyped, is found to have two cell lines: 70 percent of her cells have the typical 47,XX,+21 karyotype, and 30 percent are normal 46,XX. When did the nondisjunctional event probably occur? What is the prognosis for this child?

4. Which of the following persons is or are expected to be phenotypically normal?
   a) A female with 45 chromosomes, including a Robertsonian translocation between chromosomes 14 and 21.
   b) A female with 46 chromosomes, including a Robertsonian translocation between chromosomes 14 and 21.
   c) A female with the karyotype 47,XX,+18.
   d) A male with deletion of a band on chromosome 4.
   e) A person with a balanced reciprocal translocation.
   What kinds of gametes can each of these individuals produce? What kinds of offspring might result, assuming that the other parent is chromosomally normal?

5. Discuss possible reasons why the recurrence risk of Down syndrome is higher for mothers under 30 years of age than for mothers over 35 years of age.

6. For each of the following, state whether chromosome analysis is indicated or not. For which family members, if any? For what kind of chromosome abnormality might the family in each case be at risk?
   a) A pregnant 29-year-old woman and her 41-year-old husband, with no history of genetic defects.
   b) A pregnant 41-year-old woman and her 29-year-old husband, with no history of genetic defects.
   c) A couple whose only child has Down syndrome.
   d) A couple whose only child has Duchenne muscular dystrophy.
   e) A couple who have two severely retarded boys with neurofibromatosis, an autosomal dominant disorder normally *not* associated with retardation.

CHAPTER
10

THE SEX CHROMOSOMES AND THEIR ABNORMALITIES

The X and Y chromosomes have long attracted attention and interest because they differ between the sexes, because they have their own specific patterns of inheritance, and because they are involved in primary sex determination. They are structurally quite distinct and are subject to different forms of genetic regulation, yet they pair in male meiosis. For all these reasons, they require special attention. In the previous chapter, we considered the general principles of clinical cytogenetics, as well as specific features of the major autosomal aneuploidy conditions. In this chapter, we review the common sex chromosome abnormalities and their clinical consequences, the current state of knowledge concerning the control of sex determination, and other Mendelian abnormalities of sexual differentiation.

THE CHROMOSOMAL BASIS FOR SEX DETERMINATION

It has been known for decades that human male and female cells have different sex chromosomes (Painter, 1921) and that the difference is visible in interphase as well as in mitosis (Barr and Bertram, 1949). Although Painter's discovery of the human sex chromosomes could not be exploited clinically

at the time because cytogenetic techniques were inadequate, the discovery of sex chromatin masses (**Barr bodies**) in interphase cells of females but not of males was soon followed by the development of a simple technique that allowed Barr bodies to be studied in buccal smears (Fig. 10–1). As a result, it was quickly recognized that although most females were "chromatin positive" and most males were "chromatin negative," there were exceptions. It was especially noteworthy that many short, infertile females with a condition known as Turner syndrome had no Barr bodies, whereas tall, infertile males with a condition known as Klinefelter syndrome did have Barr bodies.

Soon after cytogenetic analysis became feasible, the chromosomal basis for these discrepancies became apparent. Because the anomalous sex chromatin findings had suggested that the Turner and Klinefelter syndromes were characterized by unusual sex chromosome constitutions, they were two of the first conditions for which chromosome studies were performed. Patients with Klinefelter syndrome were found to have 47 chromosomes with two X chromosomes as well as a Y chromosome (karyotype 47,XXY; Jacobs and Strong, 1959), whereas most Turner syndrome patients were found to have only 45 chromosomes with a single X chromosome (karyotype 45,X; Ford et al.,

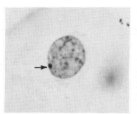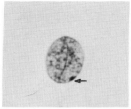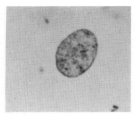

Figure 10–1. Sex chromatin (Barr bodies) in epithelial cells of human buccal mucosa. Arrows indicate the sex chromatin close to the nuclear membrane in female cells. A male cell (right) has no sex chromatin. (From Moore KL, Barr ML [1955] Smears from the oral mucosa in the determination of chromosomal sex. Lancet 2:57–58.)

1959). These findings promptly established the crucial role of the Y chromosome in normal male development.

The next step in the understanding of the human sex chromosomes was an explanation of sex chromatin in terms of **X inactivation**. As additional sex chromosome abnormalities were identified, the number of Barr bodies seen in interphase cells was observed to be always one less than the total number of X chromosomes per cell:

Sexual phenotype	Karyotype	Barr bodies
Male	46,XY; 47,XYY	0
	47,XXY; 48,XXYY	1
	48,XXXY; 49;XXXYY	2
	49,XXXXY	3
Female	45,X	0
	46,XX	1
	47,XXX	2
	48,XXXX	3
	49,XXXXX	4

The theory of X inactivation (the **Lyon hypothesis**) is that in somatic cells in normal females (but not in normal males), one X chromosome is inactivated, thus equalizing the expression of X-linked genes in the two sexes. The Barr body represents the late-replicating, inactive X chromosome (see Chapter 4). The replication asynchrony between active (early-replicating) and inactive (late-replicating) X chromosomes can be recognized cytogenetically by specialized banding procedures called "replication banding" (Fig. 10–2). In patients with extra X chromosomes, any X chromosome in excess of one is inactivated and forms a Barr body (see table above). Thus all diploid somatic cells in both males and females have a single active X chromosome, regardless of the total number of Xs or Ys present. X inactivation and its con-

sequences have been discussed in relation to X-linked disorders in Chapter 4.

Even though many abnormalities of the sex chromosomes have been defined and their clinical consequences reported in detail, there still remain mysteries about the precise role of the sex chromosomes in sexual differentiation. There are exceptions, not yet fully understood, to the rule that females are always XX and males always XY. These exceptions, which include XX males, XY females, and XX true hermaphrodites, suggest that the entire Y chromosome is not the sole determinant of phenotypic sex. Molecular analysis is currently being used to find an explanation for these unusual karyotype/phenotype combinations and to identify the gene or genes on the Y chromosome that are responsible for determining sex. Discrepancies between chromosomal sex and gonadal or phenotypic sex can also be caused by single-gene mutations, some X-linked and others autosomal.

EMBRYOLOGY OF THE REPRODUCTIVE SYSTEM

The embryology of the male and female reproductive systems is summarized in Figure 10–3. By the sixth week of development in both sexes, the primordial germ cells have migrated from their earlier extraembryonic location to the gonadal ridges, where they are surrounded by the sex cords to form a pair of primitive gonads. Up to this time, the developing gonad, whether chromosomally XX or XY, is bipotential.

The current concept is that development into an ovary or a testis is determined by the coordinated action of a sequence of genes that leads to ovarian development when no Y chromosome is present or to testicular development if a Y is

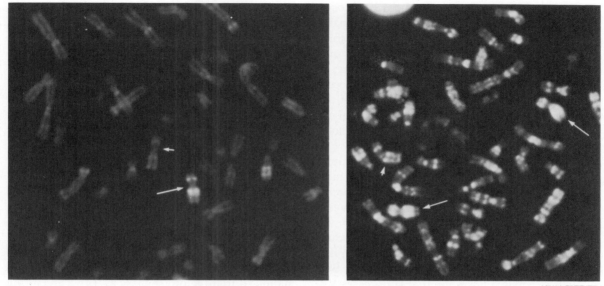

Figure 10–2. Replication banding and late replication of the inactive X chromosome in peripheral lymphocytes from a normal 46,XX female (left) and a 47, XXX female (right). Brightly staining chromosomal regions are those that replicate late in the S phase. Active X chromosomes (small arrow) replicate synchronously with the rest of the karyotype. Inactive X chromosomes (long arrows) replicate late. (Figure on right from Latt SA et al. [1976] BrdU-33258 Hoechst analysis of DNA replication in human lymphocytes with supernumerary or structurally abnormal X chromosomes. Chromosoma 57:135–153.)

present. The ovarian pathway is followed unless a gene on the short arm of the Y, designated TDF (testis-determining factor), acts as a switch, diverting development into the male pathway. The search for the major testis-determining gene is one of the leading current problems in medical genetics, and we return to it later.

In the presence of a Y chromosome, the medullary tissue forms typical testes with seminiferous tubules and Leydig cells, which, under the stimulation of human chorionic gonadotropin from the placenta, become capable of androgen secretion. The spermatogonia, derived from the primordial germ cells by 200 or more successive mitoses, form the walls of the seminiferous tubules together with supporting Sertoli cells.

If no Y chromosome is present, the gonad, by default, forms an ovary; the cortex develops, the medulla regresses, and oogonia begin to develop within follicles. The oogonia are derived from the

Figure 10–3. Schematic of the gonads and genital ducts, described in the text.

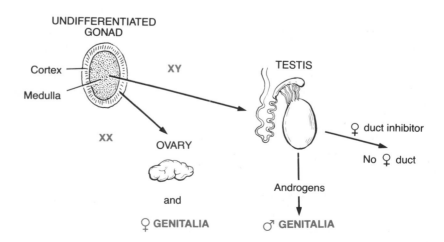

primitive germ cells by a series of about 30 mitoses, far fewer than the number required for spermatogenesis. Beginning at about the end of the third month, the oogonia enter meiosis I, but this process is arrested at a stage called **dictyotene,** in which the cell remains until ovulation occurs many years later (see Chapter 2). Many of the oogonia degenerate before birth, and only about 400 mature into ova during the 30 years or so of sexual maturity of the female.

While the primordial germ cells are migrating to the genital ridges, thickenings in the ridges indicate the developing genital ducts, the **mesonephric** (formerly called Wolffian) and **paramesonephric** (formerly called Müllerian) ducts. In the male, the Leydig cells of the fetal testes produce androgen, which stimulates the mesonephric ducts to form the male genital ducts, and the Sertoli cells produce a hormone that suppresses formation of the paramesonephric ducts. In the female (or in an embryo with no gonads), the

mesonephric ducts regress, and the paramesonephric ducts develop into the female duct system.

In the early embryo, the external genitalia consist of a genital tubercle, paired labioscrotal swellings, and paired urethral folds. From this undifferentiated state, male external genitalia develop under the influence of androgens, or, in the absence of a testis, female external genitalia are formed regardless of whether an ovary is present.

THE Y CHROMOSOME

The structure of the Y chromosome and its role in sexual development have been analyzed at the molecular level (Fig. 10–4). In male meiosis, the X and Y chromosomes normally pair by segments at the ends of their short arms and undergo recombination in that region (see Fig. 2–14). The pairing segment includes the **pseudoautosomal region** of the X and Y chromosomes, so called because the X-

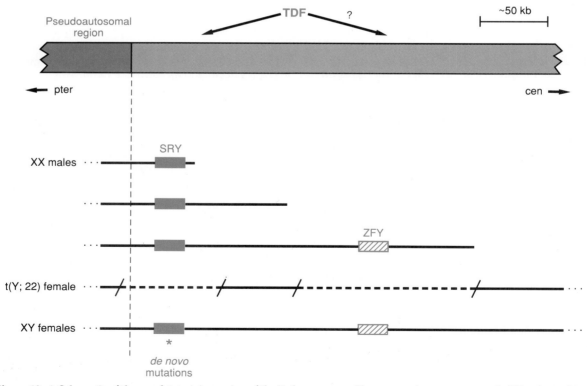

Figure 10–4. Schematic of the sex-determining region of the Y chromosome. Chromosomal rearrangements in XX males and in a female with a t(Y;22) have been key to the assignment of the sex-determining region to a location near the pseudoautosomal boundary. Point mutations (*) in the SRY gene in 46,XY females provide direct evidence that this gene may be the same as TDF. (Based on data of Page et al., 1987; Sinclair et al., 1990; Berta et al., 1990; Jager et al., 1990.)

and Y-linked copies of this region are homologous to one another, like pairs of autosomes.

The Major Testis-Determining Gene

As a result of recombination in meiosis I, sequences in the pseudoautosomal region of the X and Y chromosomes normally exchange (Fig. 10–5). In rare instances, however, genetic recombination occurs between the X and Y short arms outside of the pseudoautosomal region, and this

aberrant exchange mechanism can produce two rare abnormalities: **XX males** and **XY females.** XX males are phenotypic males with a 46,XX karyotype who usually possess some Y chromosomal sequences translocated to the short arm of the X. These sequences are not visible cytogenetically but have been revealed by molecular analysis (Fig. 10–5; Ferguson-Smith, 1966; Petit et al., 1987). Similarly, phenotypic females with a 46,XY karyotype have lost the testis-determining region of the Y chromosome. Each of these sex-reversal disorders occurs with a frequency of approximately 1 in 20,000 births.

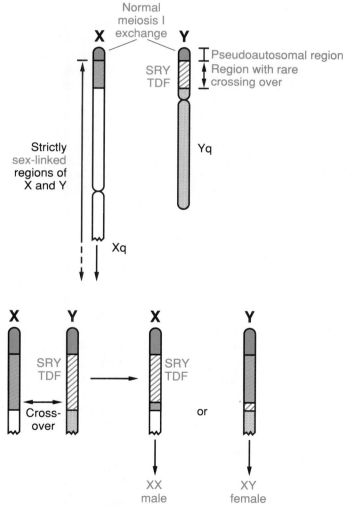

Figure 10–5. Etiology of XX male phenotype by aberrant exchange between X- and Y-linked sequences. X and Y chromosomes normally recombine within the pseudoautosomal segment in male meiosis. If recombination occurs below the pseudoautosomal boundary, between the X-specific and Y-specific portions of the chromosomes, sequences responsible for male sexual differentiation may be translocated from the Y to the X. Fertilization by a sperm containing such an X chromosome leads to an XX male.

Different deletions of the pseudoautosomal region and of the sex-specific region of the Y chromosome have been used in an effort to map the precise location of the primary testis-determining region on the short arm of the Y chromosome. Examining an XX male with the smallest identified segment of Y chromosomal material and a female who carried a Y;22 translocation but lacked a small region of Yp, Page and colleagues (1987) identified a region approximately 140 kb long (equivalent to only 0.2 percent of the entire Y chromosome) that was believed likely to encode at least part of the TDF gene (Fig. 10–4). DNA sequences contained in this region are highly conserved in other mammals, and a homologous segment was identified on the X chromosome. The Y-linked sequence was called ZFY because it potentially encodes a so-called "zinc-finger" protein that, by analogy to other zinc-finger proteins, is thought to bind to nucleic acids in a sequence-specific manner and thus potentially to regulate gene expression.

Initially, the ZFY sequence was accepted as a strong candidate for the long-sought major testis-determining gene, TDF, but more recent studies have cast serious doubt on this interpretation. The presence of an X-linked homologous gene (known as ZFX), the absence of ZFY-like sequences on the sex chromosomes of marsupials, reports of XX males with Y chromosome sequences closer to the pseudoautosomal boundary but without ZFY sequences (Palmer et al., 1989), and failure of expression of the mouse homolog of ZFY in the embryonic testes of mice (Koopman et al., 1989) all argue that ZFY and TDF are distinct and that ZFY cannot by itself induce male sexual differentiation (Burgoyne, 1989). Another strong candidate locus, termed the "sex-determining region on the Y" (SRY), was identified by Goodfellow and colleagues (Sinclair et al., 1990). This gene lies between the pseudoautosomal boundary and ZFY on the short arm of the Y chromosome and is present in several XX males or XX hermaphrodites (described later in this chapter) who do not have ZFY sequences (Fig. 10–4). Deletion of the SRY gene (as well as the ZFY gene) in the female patient with the Y;22 translocation mentioned earlier leaves open the question of which (or both) of these two genes may be responsible for inducing maleness (Page et al., 1990). Most recently, however, three female 46,XY patients have been found who have no cytological alterations of the Y chro-

mosome but who have mutations in the SRY coding sequence (Fig. 10–4), thus strongly implicating SRY in male sex determination (Berta et al., 1990; Jager et al., 1990). Nonetheless, a secondary role for ZFY cannot be ruled out. Thus the identity and the precise localization of the true testis-determining gene or genes remain to be proved. In the meantime, the story serves as an excellent illustration of the importance of examining a few or even one unusual patient for establishing genetic principles of extraordinary theoretical and practical significance.

THE X CHROMOSOME

A number of genes and regions of the X chromosome have special roles in sex determination or X inactivation (Fig. 10–6). Although in female somatic cells one X is inactivated, several regions of the short arm and at least one on the long arm contain genes that escape inactivation and continue to be expressed from both X chromosomes in females. A gene in the pseudoautosomal segment remains active, and at least two genes outside but near the pseudoautosomal region also remain partly active; for example, the gene for steroid sulfatase, or STS (deficiency of which causes the X-linked disorder ichthyosis), lies not within the pseudoautosomal region but just proximal to it and remains almost fully active, even on the "inactive" X (Shapiro et al., 1979). Genes in at least two other regions of the short arm and on the long arm near the X inactivation center (described later) are also expressed from both active and inactive X chromosomes (Schneider-Gadicke et al., 1989; Brown and Willard, 1990; Fisher et al., 1990). One of these, the X-linked gene homologous to the Y-linked ZFY gene discussed earlier, has been proposed to play a role in sex determination (Burgoyne, 1989). The clinical significance of genes that escape inactivation is uncertain because, of the identified noninactivated genes, only STS is associated with a known X-linked clinical disorder. These genes, however, are candidates to explain clinical symptoms in cases of X chromosome aneuploidy, because their gene products in such cases may be either under- or overexpressed in relation to normal females.

As described in an earlier section and in Chapter 4, the chromosome-wide basis for X inac-

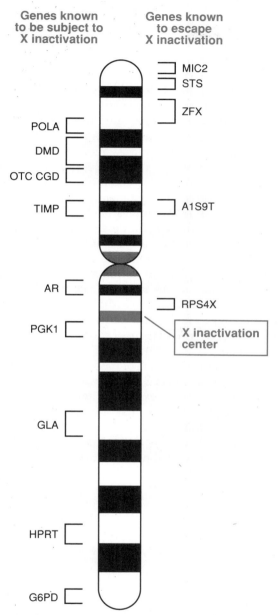

**Genes known
to be subject to
X inactivation**

**Genes known
to escape
X inactivation**

POLA

DMD

OTC CGD

TIMP

AR

PGK1

GLA

HPRT

G6PD

MIC2

STS

ZFX

A1S9T

RPS4X

X inactivation
center

Figure 10–6. Schematic of X chromosome. Only a few important gene loci are indicated. In total, more than 200 X-linked disorders are known, many of which have been assigned to particular locations on the chromosome. Selected genes that are known to be subject to X inactivation are shown at the left. Genes that escape inactivation and are expressed from both active and inactive Xs are shown on the right. The position of the X inactivation center in Xq13 is shown in red. (Based on Brown and Willard, 1990; Brown et al., 1991; Fisher et al., 1990.)

tivation is well established. Supporting evidence has come from the study of individual genes; in contrast to the few noninactivated genes just mentioned, at least 40 X-linked genes have been shown to be subject to inactivation. From the study of structurally abnormal, inactivated X chromosomes, it has been proposed that a DNA region in proximal Xq, in band Xq13 (Fig. 10–6), contains an **X inactivation center,** a locus that must be present on an X chromosome for inactivation to occur. The molecular basis for inactivation and the role of the X inactivation center are unknown and remain subjects of intense investigation (Brown et al., 1991).

Although X inactivation is normally random in female somatic cells, there are exceptions. In almost all patients with structural abnormalities of an X chromosome, the structurally abnormal chromosome is inactivated, presumably reflecting selection against unbalanced cells that could cause abnormalities. Because of this preferential inactivation of the abnormal X, X chromosome anomalies are tolerated better than similar abnormalities of autosomes and consequently are more frequently observed. Nonrandom inactivation is also observed in the case of X;autosome translocations. If such a translocation is balanced, the normal X chromosome is preferentially inactivated, and the two parts of the translocated chromosome remain active, again probably reflecting selection against cells in which autosomal genes have been inactivated. In the unbalanced offspring of a balanced carrier, however, only the translocation product carrying the X inactivation center is present and this chromosome is invariably inactivated; the normal X is always active. These nonrandom patterns of inactivation have the general effect of minimizing, but by no means eliminating, the clinical consequences of the particular chromosomal defect. Normal X chromosomes can also show nonrandom inactivation. In the extraembryonic membranes, the paternal X is the one that is preferentially inactivated; the basis or significance of this parental bias is unknown.

One consequence sometimes observed in balanced carriers of X;autosome translocations is that the break itself may cause a mutation by disrupting a gene on the X chromosome at the site of the translocation. The only normal copy of the particular gene (on the normal X) is inactivated in most or all cells because of nonrandom X inactivation of the normal X, thus allowing expression in a female of an X-linked trait normally observed only in hemizygous males. Several X-linked genes (including the gene that, when abnormal, results in Duchenne or Becker muscular dystrophy) have been mapped to specific regions of the X chromosome when a typical X-linked phenotype has been found in a female who then proved to have an X;autosome translocation (see Chapter 8). The general clinical message of these findings is that if a female patient manifests an X-linked phenotype normally seen only in males, high-resolution chromosome analysis is indicated. The finding of a balanced translocation can both explain the phenotypic expression and show the gene's probable map position on the X chromosome.

CLINICAL DISORDERS OF THE SEX CHROMOSOMES

Sex chromosome abnormalities, like abnormalities of the autosomes, can be either numerical or structural and can be present in all cells or in mosaic form. Their incidence in live-born children, in fetuses examined prenatally, and in spontaneous abortions was compared in Chapter 9 with the incidence of similar abnormalities of the autosomes and is summarized in Table 10–1. X and Y chromosome aneuploidy is relatively common, and sex chromosome abnormalities are among the

most common of all human genetic disorders, with an overall frequency of about 1 in 500 births. The phenotypes associated with these chromosomal defects are, in general, less severe than those associated with comparable autosomal disorders because X inactivation, and the apparent low gene content of the Y, minimize the clinical consequences of sex chromosome imbalance. By far the most common sex chromosome defects in live-born infants and in fetuses are the trisomic types (XXY, XXX, and XYY), but all three are rare in spontaneous abortions. In contrast, monosomy for the X (Turner syndrome) is relatively rare in live-born infants but is the most common chromosome anomaly reported in spontaneous abortions.

Structural abnormalities of the sex chromosomes are less common; the defect most frequently observed is an isochromosome of the long arm of the X ("isoXq") seen in complete or mosaic form in about 10 to 15 percent of females with Turner syndrome. Mosaicism is more common for sex chromosome abnormalities than for autosomal abnormalities, and in some patients it is associated with relatively mild expression of the associated phenotype.

As a group, disorders of the sex chromosomes tend to occur as isolated events without apparent predisposing factors, except for an effect of late maternal age in the cases that originate in errors of maternal meiosis I. Because almost all patients with sex chromosome abnormalities have only mild developmental abnormalities, a parental de-

Table 10–1. Incidence of Sex Chromosome Abnormalities

Sex	Disorder	Karyotype	Approximate Incidence
Male	Klinefelter syndrome	47,XXY	1/1000 males
		48,XXXY	1/25,000 males
		Others (48,XXYY, 49,XXXYY, mosaics)	1/10,000 males
	XYY syndrome	47,XYY	1/1000 males
	Other X or Y chromosome abnormalities		1/1500 males
	XX males	46,XX	1/20,000 males
			Overall incidence: 1/400 males
Female	Turner syndrome	45,X	1/10,000 females
		46,X,i(Xq)	1/50,000 females
		Others (deletions, mosaics)	1/15,000 females
	Trisomy X	47,XXX	1/1000 females
	Other X chromosome abnormalities		1/3000 females
	XY females	46,XY	1/20,000 females
	Androgen insensitivity	46,XY	1/20,000 females
			Overall incidence: 1/650 females

Data adapted from Hirschhorn (1987), Hook and Warburton (1983), Hook (1985), and Hook and Cross (1987), and from Table 9–3.

Table 10–2. Follow-Up Observations on Patients with Sex Chromosome Aneuploidy

Disorder	Karyotype	Phenotype	Sexual Development	Intelligence	Behavior Problems
Klinefelter syndrome	47,XXY	Tall male (see text)	Infertile; atrophic testes	Educational problems (65%)	May have poor psychosocial adjustment
XYY syndrome	47,XYY	Tall male	Normal	Normal	Frequent
Trisomy X	47,XXX	Female, usually tall	Usually normal	Educational problems (70%)	Occasional
Turner syndrome	45,X	Short female, distinctive features (see text)	Infertile; streak gonads	Normal	Rare

Data from Ratcliffe SG, Paul N (eds) (1986) Prospective studies on children with sex chromosome aneuploidy. March of Dimes Birth Defects Foundation, Birth Defects Original Article Series 22(3). Alan R. Liss, New York.

cision regarding potential termination of a pregnancy in which the fetus is found to have this type of defect can be a difficult one.

Sex Chromosome Aneuploidy

The four well-defined syndromes associated with sex chromosome aneuploidy have already been briefly mentioned, but their importance in clinical medicine as causes of infertility or abnormal development, or both, justifies a more detailed description.

The effects of these chromosome abnormalities on development have been studied in a long-term multicenter study that was initiated in the 1960s and still continues. To avoid the bias inherent in studying development in cases unusual enough to be referred to a medical center for assessment, only cases determined by screening of newborns or by prenatal diagnosis have been used. The major conclusions of the study are summarized in Table 10–2.

Klinefelter Syndrome (47,XXY)

The phenotype of Klinefelter syndrome, the first human sex chromosome abnormality to be reported, is shown in Figure 10–7. The patients are tall and thin, with relatively long legs. They appear physically normal until puberty, when signs of hypogonadism become obvious. The testes remain small, and the secondary sexual characteristics remain underdeveloped. Klinefelter patients are almost always infertile.

The incidence is about 1 in 1000 male live births (1 in 2000 total births) and 1 in 300 spontaneous abortions. Even though the phenotype seems benign in comparison with that in autoso-

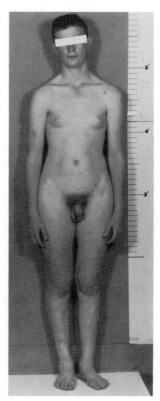

Figure 10–7. Phenotype of a male with 47,XXY Klinefelter syndrome. Note long limbs and relatively small genitalia. Gynecomastia, present in this patient, is not a constant feature. (Photograph courtesy of Murray Barr, University of Western Ontario, London, Ontario.)

mal trisomies, half of all 47,XXY conceptions are lost prenatally.

About 15 percent of Klinefelter patients have mosaic karyotypes. As a group, such mosaic patients have variable phenotypes; some may have normal testicular development. The most common mosaic karyotype is 46,XY/47,XXY, probably as a consequence of loss of one X chromosome in an XXY conceptus during an early postzygotic division. As predicted by the finding that 47,XXY Klinefelter patients have a Barr body, one of the two X chromosomes is inactivated.

In a combined cytogenetic and molecular investigation of the parental origin and meiotic stage of the nondisjunctional error responsible for the syndrome, it was found that about half the cases result from errors in paternal meiosis I, one third from errors in maternal meiosis I, and the remainder from errors in meiosis II or from a postzygotic mitotic error leading to mosaicism. Maternal age is increased in the cases associated with maternal meiosis I errors, but not in the other cases (Jacobs et al., 1988).

Although there is wide phenotypic variation among patients with this and other sex chromosome aneuploidies, just as there is in the general population, some consistent phenotypic differences have been identified between patients with Klinefelter syndrome and chromosomally normal males. Their score on certain intelligence performance tests (IQ tests) is slightly but significantly reduced. Two thirds of the patients have educational problems, especially dyslexia, whereas fewer than one quarter of normal persons have learning difficulties. Puberty occurs at the normal age, but testicular size remains well below average. Gynecomastia, though emphasized as a typical finding in the early literature, is usually absent. Many of the affected boys have relatively poor psychosocial adjustment.

There are several variants of Klinefelter syndrome, with a karyotype other than 47,XXY, including 48,XXYY, 48,XXXY, and 49,XXXXY. As a rule, the additional X chromosomes cause a correspondingly more abnormal phenotype (even though the extra X chromosomes are inactive), with a greater degree of dysmorphism, more defective sexual development, and more severe mental impairment. An unexpected observation in 49,XXXXY patients (and in their female counterparts, with 49,XXXXX karyotypes) is that the phenotype is similar in many respects to that of Down syndrome. This observation argues against the widely held view that the phenotype of Down syndrome strictly depends on the triple dosage of genes on chromosome 21 and suggests instead a more general delay in development related to chromosome imbalance.

47,XYY Syndrome

Although the 47,XYY chromosome constitution is not associated with an obviously abnormal phenotype, it became of great medical and scientific interest after the observation that the proportion of XYY males was much higher in the population of a maximum security prison, especially among the tallest inmates, than in the general population (Jacobs et al., 1968). About 3 percent of males in prisons and mental hospitals have a 47,XYY karyotype; among the group over 6 feet tall, the incidence is much higher (more than 20 percent). Among all live male births, the frequency of the 47,XYY karyotype is about 1 in 1000.

The origin of the error that leads to the XYY karyotype must be paternal nondisjunction at meiosis II, producing YY sperm. The less common XXYY and XXXYY variants, which share the features of the XYY and Klinefelter syndromes, probably also originate in the father, in a sequence of nondisjunctional events at both meiosis I and meiosis II.

XYY males identified in newborn screening programs without ascertainment bias are tall and have an increased risk of behavioral problems, in comparison with chromosomally normal males. They have normal intelligence and are not dysmorphic. Fertility is normal, and there appears to be virtually no increased risk that a 47,XYY male will have a chromosomally abnormal child.

Parents whose child is found, prenatally or postnatally, to be XYY are often extremely concerned about the behavioral implications. Indeed, some physicians believe that the information should be withheld when the identification is made postnatally. Inability to predict the outcome in individual cases makes identification of an XYY fetus one of the most severe genetic counseling problems faced in prenatal diagnosis programs.

Trisomy X (47,XXX)

Trisomy X and the rarer tetrasomy X (48,XXXX) and pentasomy X (49,XXXXX) syndromes are the counterparts in the female of Klinefelter syndrome in the male. Trisomy X females, though usually above average in stature, are not phenotypically abnormal. Some are first identified in infertility clinics and others in institutions for the mentally retarded, but probably many remain undiagnosed. The follow-up studies have shown that XXX females develop pubertal changes at an appropriate age, although there are reports of precocious puberty in some patients. Some have borne children, virtually all of whom are chromosomally normal. There is a significant deficit in performance on IQ tests, and about 70 percent of the patients have serious learning problems.

In 47,XXX cells, two of the X chromosomes are inactivated and late-replicating (Fig. 10–2), as suggested originally by the finding of two Barr bodies. Almost all cases result from errors in maternal meiosis, and of these the majority are in meiosis I. There is an effect of late maternal age, restricted to those patients in whom the error was in maternal meiosis I (May et al., 1990).

The tetrasomy X syndrome is associated with more serious retardation in both physical and mental development, and the pentasomy X syndrome, like XXXXY, usually includes severe developmental retardation with multiple physical defects reminiscent of Down syndrome.

Turner Syndrome (45,X and Variants)

Unlike patients with other sex chromosome aneuploidies, females with Turner syndrome can often be identified at birth or before puberty by their distinctive phenotypic features (Fig. 10–8). Turner syndrome is much less common than other sex chromosome aneuploidies. The incidence of the Turner syndrome phenotype is approximately 1 in 5000 live female births.

The most frequent chromosome constitution in Turner syndrome is 45,X (sometimes written in the literature as 45,XO) with no second sex chromosome, either X or Y. However, about 50 percent of cases have other karyotypes. About one quarter of Turner syndrome cases involve mosaic karyo-

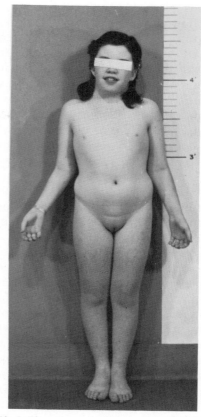

Figure 10–8. Phenotype of a female with 45,X Turner syndrome. For details, see text. (From Barr ML [1960] Sexual dimorphism in interphase nuclei. Am J Hum Genet 12:118–127.)

types, in which only a proportion of cells are 45,X. The most common karyotypes and their relative frequencies are as follows (Hook and Warburton, 1983):

45,X	53%
45,X/46,XX mosaics	15%
46,X,i(Xq)	10%
45,X/46,X,i(Xq) mosaics	8%
46,XXq⁻ or 46,XXp⁻ deletions	6%
Other 45,X/? mosaics	8%

The chromosome constitution is clinically significant; for example, patients with an isoXq are like classic 45,X patients, whereas patients with a deletion of Xp have short stature and congenital malformations, and those with a deletion of Xq often have only gonadal dysfunction.

The typical abnormalities in Turner syndrome include short stature, gonadal dysgenesis (usually streak gonads), characteristic unusual facies, neck webbing, low posterior hairline, broad chest with widely spaced nipples, and an elevated frequency of renal and cardiovascular anomalies. At birth, infants with this syndrome often have edema of the dorsum of the foot, a useful diagnostic sign. Many patients have coarctation of the aorta. Lymphedema may be present in fetal life, causing cystic hygroma (visible by ultrasound), which is the cause of the neck webbing seen postnatally. Intelligence is usually average or above average. However, patients often display a deficiency in spatial perception, perceptual motor organization, or fine motor execution. As a consequence, the nonverbal IQ is significantly lower than the verbal IQ.

The very high frequency of 45,X in spontaneous abortions has already been mentioned. This single abnormality accounts for 18 percent of all chromosomally abnormal spontaneous abortions and is present in an estimated 1.5 percent of all conceptuses (see Chapter 9). Usually the single X is maternal in origin; in other words, the meiotic error is usually paternal. The basis for the unusually high frequency of X or Y chromosome nondisjunction in paternal meiosis is unknown. Furthermore, it is not clear why the 45,X karyotype is usually lethal in utero but is apparently fully compatible with postnatal survival.

As adults, many Turner syndrome patients are distressed by their infertility and short stature. Although estrogen therapy can lead to the development of the internal and external genitalia, secondary sexual characteristics, and menses, it does not correct infertility, which is an almost constant feature that results from early germ cell atresia. The possible value of low doses of estrogen, androgen, and growth hormone in the treatment of short stature in Turner syndrome is currently under investigation. Thus far, few if any studies involving large numbers of patients have provided data on the impact of these agents on final adult height, although it is clear that each drug may affect short-term growth rate.

Although the vast majority of 45,X patients are phenotypic females, very rarely a 45,X chromosome set is found in a phenotypic male who has testes but is sterile. The 45,X males may have begun life as 45,X/46,XY mosaics in whom the XY line was lost, at least in the tissue studied, or may have an unrecognized Y;autosome translocation

involving the TDF locus. There are also a few rare cases of 46,XY females with Turner syndrome stigmata. In all such cases, a portion of the Y chromosome is deleted (Levilliers et al., 1989; Fisher et al., 1990).

Disorders of Sexual Development with Normal Chromosomes

For some newborn infants, determination of sex is difficult or impossible because the genitalia are ambiguous, with anomalies that tend to make them resemble those of the opposite chromosomal sex. Such anomalies may vary from mild hypospadias in males (a developmental anomaly in which the urethra opens on the underside of the penis or on the perineum) to enlarged clitoris in females. Such problems do not necessarily indicate a cytogenetic abnormality of the sex chromosomes but may be due to single-gene defects or to nongenetic causes. Nonetheless, determination of the child's karyotype is an essential part of the investigation of such patients.

True Hermaphroditism

A true hermaphrodite has both testicular and ovarian tissue and usually has ambiguous genitalia. The typical karyotype is 46,XX, but about 10 percent of patients are 46,XY.

A small percentage of true hermaphrodites are chimeras whose tissues are composed of a mixture of XX and XY cells. Unlike a mosaic, in whom the cell lines are derived from a single zygote, a chimera is composed of cells derived from different zygotes. Chimerism can occur when dizygotic twins exchange hematopoietic stem cells in utero or, very rarely, when two separate zygotes are fused into one individual. If the original zygotes were of different sexes, true hermaphroditism may result. The first twin chimera to be described was a true hermaphrodite with different-colored eyes.

XX true hermaphroditism has been studied in Blacks in southern Africa, where its incidence is relatively high (Ramsay et al., 1988). The condition does not have single-gene inheritance (except as noted later), and in contrast to findings in most

XX males, the patients have no detectable Y chromosome material. Failure to demonstrate Y-specific DNA sequences in the patients indicates that this type of true hermaphroditism is distinct from the most common form of 46,XX maleness. However, there is one report of XX males and XX true hermaphrodites coexisting in the same pedigree, indicating a common etiology (de la Chapelle, 1988). Thus it appears that 46,XX true hermaphroditism has more than one cause.

Pseudohermaphroditism

Pseudohermaphrodites are "pseudo" because, unlike true hermaphrodites, they have gonadal tissue of only one sex. Male pseudohermaphrodites are karyotypically 46,XY, or mosaics with an XY cell line, and female pseudohermaphrodites are 46,XX. In either case, the external genitalia are ambiguous or characteristic of the opposite chromosomal sex.

The causes of pseudohermaphroditism in males include dysgenesis of the gonads during embryological development, abnormalities of gonadotropins, inborn errors of testosterone biosynthesis, and abnormalities of androgen target cells. These disorders are heterogeneous both genetically and clinically, and, in some cases, they may correspond to milder manifestations of the same cause underlying true hermaphroditism. One specific cause, an X-linked syndrome known as **androgen insensitivity syndrome,** is discussed in the next section.

Female pseudohermaphroditism is usually due to **congenital adrenal hyperplasia,** an autosomal recessive disorder of cortisol biosynthesis. The external genitalia in female fetuses can also become masculinized if the fetal circulation contains excessive amounts of either male or female sex hormones, which may originate either in the fetus, as in congenital adrenal hyperplasia, or in the mother.

In a number of malformation syndromes with normal chromosomes, ambiguous genitalia or hypospadias are frequent or occasional features. One example is the Smith-Lemli-Opitz syndrome, an autosomal recessive condition characterized by mental retardation, abnormal facies, skeletal anomalies, and cryptorchidism and hypospadias in males (Fig. 10–9).

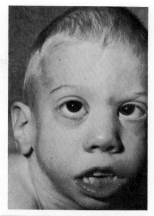

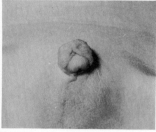

Figure 10–9. Smith-Lemli-Opitz syndrome. Facies and genitalia of a 5-year-old patient. Dysmorphic facies, hypospadias and cryptorchidism in males, failure to thrive, and mental retardation are characteristic of this autosomal recessive syndrome. (From Jones KL [1988] Smith's Recognizable patterns of human malformation, 4th ed. WB Saunders, Philadelphia, p. 105.

ANDROGEN INSENSITIVITY SYNDROME

There are several forms of androgen insensitivity resulting in male pseudohermaphroditism, one of which is an X-linked defect of receptor function known as the complete androgen insensitivity syndrome (formerly known as **testicular feminization**). In this disorder, affected persons are chromosomal males (karyotype 46,XY) with apparently normal female external genitalia, who have a blind vagina and no uterus or uterine tubes (Fig. 10–10). The incidence of androgen insensitivity is about 1 in 20,000 live births. Axillary and pubic hair is sparse. As the alternative name "testicular feminization" indicates, testes are present either within the abdomen or in the inguinal canal, where they are sometimes mistaken for hernias in infants who otherwise appear to be normal females. Although the testes secrete androgen normally, there is end-organ unresponsiveness to androgens resulting from absence of androgen receptors in the cytosol of the appropriate target

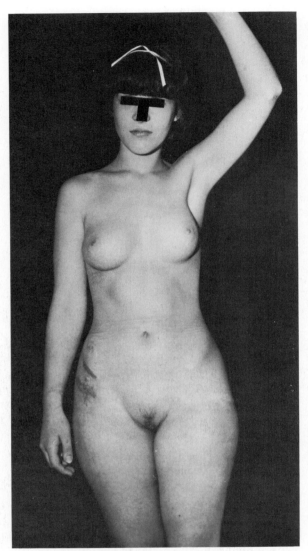

Figure 10–10. Complete androgen insensitivity syndrome (testicular feminization) in a 46,XY individual. Note female body contours, absence of axillary hair, sparse pubic hair, and breast development. (Photograph courtesy of L. Pinsky, McGill University.)

some with milder expression, may be allelic to the classical form (Pinsky and Kaufman, 1987). The molecular defect has been determined in several cases and ranges from a complete deletion of the AR gene on the X chromosome (see Fig. 5–7) to point mutations in the steroid-binding domain of the androgen receptor protein.

CONGENITAL ADRENAL HYPERPLASIA

Congenital adrenal hyperplasia (CAH) is a group of autosomal recessive disorders arising from specific defects in enzymes of the adrenal cortex required for cortisol biosynthesis, and resulting in virilization of female infants. Although any one of several enzymatic steps may be defective in CAH, by far the most common defect is deficiency of 21-hydroxylase, which has an incidence of about 1 in 12,500 births. Deficiency of 21-hydroxylase blocks the normal biosynthetic pathway, causing overproduction of the precursors, which are then shunted into the pathway of androgen biosynthesis, causing abnormally high androgen levels. Female infants homozygous for 21-hydroxylase deficiency are born with ambiguous genitalia, often requiring surgical correction. Affected male infants have normal external genitalia and may go unrecognized in early infancy. Later in childhood, in both sexes, androgen excess leads to rapid growth and accelerated skeletal maturation. Of patients with classic 21-hydroxylase deficiency, 25 percent have the simple virilizing type and 75 percent have a salt-losing type that is clinically more severe and may lead to neonatal death. A screening test developed to identify the condition in newborns, in which heel-prick blood specimens are blotted onto filter paper, is now in use in many countries. It is valuable in prevention of the serious consequences of the salt-losing defect in early infancy and in prompt diagnosis of affected males as well as affected females.

An allelic, nonclassical form of 21-hydroxylase deficiency, which does not cause pseudohermaphroditism, has a frequency of up to 3 percent in some ethnic groups; its onset is typically in adult life, with physical signs of androgen excess (New et al., 1989).

The 21-hydroxylase locus is on the short arm of chromosome 6, within the HLA major histocompatibility complex (see Chapter 14). Not only is the gene genetically linked to HLA, but different forms of CAH show associations with different

cells. The receptor protein, specified by the normal allele at the X-linked androgen receptor (AR) locus, has the role of forming a complex with testosterone and dihydrotestosterone. If the complex fails to form, the hormone cannot enter the nucleus, become attached to chromatin, and stimulate the transcription of messenger RNAs required for differentiation in the male direction.

Several variants of androgen insensitivity,

HLA haplotypes, suggesting that the different mutations originated on specific haplotype backgrounds (see Chapter 8). This information can be of use in prenatal diagnosis of CAH, with DNA methods and genetic linkage analysis.

HYDATIDIFORM MOLES

Occasionally in an abnormal pregnancy the placenta is converted into a mass of tissue resembling a bunch of grapes or a hydatid cyst. This is due to abnormal growth of the chorionic villi, in which the epithelium proliferates and the stroma undergoes cystic cavitation. Such an abnormality is called a mole. (The word "mole" simply means mass.) Although not strictly a defect of the sex chromosomes or of sex determination, moles reflect abnormal chromosomal mechanisms that affect early embryonic development and are thus included in this chapter.

A mole may be complete, with no fetus or normal placenta present, or partial, with remnants of placenta and perhaps a small atrophic fetus. The origins of the two types differ. In most **complete moles,** the chromosomes are all paternal in origin, the karyotype is 46,XX, and with rare exceptions all genetic markers are homozygous. The interpretation is that the mole originates when a single 23,X sperm fertilizes an ovum that lacks a nucleus, and its chromosomes then double. The absence of any maternal contribution is thought to be responsible for the very abnormal development, with hyperplasia of the trophoblast and grossly disorganized or absent fetal tissue.

About half of all cases of choriocarcinoma (a malignancy of fetal, not maternal, tissue) develop from hydatidiform moles. Given the present knowledge of the association of homozygosity with malignant change (see Chapter 16), it may be that homozygosity for markers in complete moles is related to their risk of malignant transformation.

Partial moles are triploid; the extra chromosome set is usually paternal but may be maternal. In both cases fetal development is severely abnormal, but the defects are different. An extra paternal set results in abundant trophoblast but poor embryonic development, whereas an extra maternal set results in severe retardation of embryonic growth with a small, fibrotic placenta. The speci-

ficity of the effect is a further example of genetic imprinting (Reik, 1989).

General References

Chandley AC (1986) The genetics of human reproduction. Experientia 42:1109–1117.
de la Chapelle A (1988) The complicated issue of sex determination. Am J Hum Genet 43:1–3.
Griffin JE, Wilson JD (1989) The androgen resistance syndromes: 5α-reductase deficiency, testicular feminization, and related disorders. *In* Scriver CR, Beaudet AL, Sly WS, Valle D (eds) The metabolic basis of inherited disease, 6th ed. McGraw-Hill, New York, pp. 1919–1944.
Lyon MF (1988) X chromosome inactivation and the location and expression of X-linked genes. Am J Hum Genet 42:8–16.
New MI, White PC, Pang S, et al (1989) The adrenal hyperplasias. *In* Scriver CR, Beaudet AL, Sly WS, Valle D (eds) The metabolic basis of inherited disease, 6th ed. McGraw-Hill, New York, pp. 1881–1917.
Pinsky L, Kaufman M (1987) Genetics of steroid receptors and their disorders. Adv Hum Genet 16:299–472.
Ratcliffe SG, Paul N (eds) (1986) Prospective studies on children with sex chromosome aneuploidy. March of Dimes Birth Defects Foundation, Birth Defects Original Article Series 22(3). Alan R. Liss, New York.
Simpson JL (1990) Disorders of gonads and internal reproductive ducts. *In* Emery AEH, Rimoin DL (eds) Principles and practice of medical genetics, 2nd ed. Churchill Livingstone, Edinburgh, pp. 1593–1617.

Problems

1. In a woman with a 47,XXX karyotype, what types of gametes would theoretically be formed and in what proportions? What are the theoretical karyotypes and phenotypes of her progeny? (Actually, a triple-X woman almost always has children with normal karyotypes only.)

2. One of your patients is a girl with severe hemophilia A, an X-linked recessive disorder.
    a) You are advised to arrange for chromosome analysis of this child. Why? What mechanisms can allow the occurrence of an X-linked recessive phenotype in a female?
    b) The laboratory reports that the child has an X;autosome translocation, with a breakpoint in the X chromosome at Xq28. How could this explain her phenotype?

3. The birth incidences of 47,XXY and 47,XYY males are approximately equal. Is this what you would expect on the basis of the possible origins of the two abnormal karyotypes? Explain.

4. How can a person with an XX karyotype differentiate as a male?

5. A baby girl presents with bilateral inguinal masses that are thought to be hernias but are found to be testes in the inguinal canals. What karyotype would you expect to find in the child? What is her disorder? What genetic counseling would you offer to the parents?

6. A baby girl with ambiguous genitalia is found to have 21-hydroxylase deficiency of the salt-wasting type. What karyotype would you expect to find? What is the disorder? What genetic counseling would you offer to the parents?

7. What are the expected clinical consequences of the following deletions? If the same amount of DNA is deleted in each case, why might the severity of each be different?
   a) 46,XX,13p$^-$
   b) 46,XYq$^-$
   c) 46,XX,5p$^-$
   d) 46,XXq$^-$

8. Discuss the clinical consequences of X chromosome inactivation. Provide possible explanations for the fact that persons with X chromosome aneuploidy are clinically not completely normal.

CHAPTER 11

THE HEMOGLOBINOPATHIES: MODELS OF MOLECULAR DISEASE

MUTATION → ALTERED PROTEIN → ABNORMAL FUNCTION → DISEASE

In the next two chapters, we describe how mutations cause disease. The trail of molecular and biochemical events that leads from a mutant gene to a clinical illness is often instructive about normal function; moreover, knowledge of these events is the foundation of rational therapy for genetic diseases. The study of phenotype at the level of proteins and metabolism constitutes the discipline of biochemical or metabolic genetics. Indeed, single-gene diseases that are classified as "biochemical" or "metabolic" are simply those disorders in which biochemical abnormalities have already been identified. Human biochemical genetics was established by Sir Archibald Garrod, who introduced the term **inborn errors of metabolism** in 1902 to describe lifelong diseases that arise because the genetic deficiency of a specific enzyme causes a block in a normal metabolic pathway. In albinism, one of the prototypic defects studied by Garrod, deficiency of the enzyme tyrosinase in the hair, skin, and eye prevents the synthesis of the pigment melanin, and the consequences are readily seen. Another enzyme defect examined by Garrod, pentosuria, illustrates a different princi-

ple: mutations that produce biochemical defects do not necessarily cause disease; they may result only in clinically benign biochemical traits that are detected coincidentally, often by screening tests.

As already noted in Chapters 6 and 8, variation in DNA sequences within the population is universal; such variants may not alter the phenotype. Thus when a nucleotide change in the coding region does not affect the quantity or function of a polypeptide, or when mutations affect proteins that are apparently nonessential, the phenotype is normal. In contrast, a genetic disease occurs when changes in the DNA of essential genes reduces the amount or function (or both) of the gene products (messenger RNA [mRNA] and protein) to below required levels. So far, those single-gene diseases in which the molecular defect has been identified result from alterations in DNA sequences that control gene expression or encode the structure of a protein. Although other types of DNA are also potential targets for mutation (e.g., the genes for ribosomal RNA and transfer RNA that encode RNA rather than protein products, or sequences that are structurally important to the chromosome,

247

such as centromeric or telomeric DNA), no diseases are known to result from variation in these sequences. The repetitive nature of these genes and sequences may preclude a pathological effect of mutation in any one of them. In addition, these molecules play such a central role that defects in them may be lethal.

The pathogenesis of a genetic disease cannot be understood completely unless the primary biochemical abnormality caused by the mutation is known. A specific protein deficiency has been demonstrated in about 500 of the approximately 4500 single-gene diseases (both autosomal and X-linked) presently recognized (Costa et al., 1985; McKusick, 1990). Although it is impressive that the basic defect has been elucidated in so many disorders, it is sobering to reflect that there is probably not a single genetic disease in which the pathophysiology is entirely understood. Sickle cell disease is among the best characterized, but the knowledge of even this disorder is incomplete, despite the fact that it was the first "molecular disease" to be recognized (Pauling et al., 1949). Nevertheless, the study of genetic disease at its various phenotypic levels (the protein, the cell, the tissue, and the whole body) has not only provided a wealth of important information about specific disorders but has also greatly increased our understanding of the normal biological processes that are disrupted by the mutations.

This chapter describes the hemoglobins, perhaps the best understood of all human proteins, discussing both their normal biology and their genetic defects. Chapter 12 reviews representative diseases that are caused by mutations in other types of proteins, and presents a general approach for understanding how proteins are altered by genetic disease.

HEMOGLOBINS AND THEIR DISEASES

The disorders of human hemoglobins, or the **hemoglobinopathies,** occupy a unique position in medical genetics for several reasons. They are easily the most common genetic diseases in the world, and they cause substantial morbidity. The World Health Organization (1982) estimated that approximately 5 percent of the world population are carriers of genes for clinically important disorders of hemoglobin and that about one third of a million severely affected homozygotes or compound heterozygotes are born each year (Weatherall et al., 1989). Moreover, because hemoglobin was one of the first protein structures to be deduced and because the human globin genes were the first disease-related genes to be cloned, their molecular pathology is better understood than perhaps any other group of genetic diseases. These insights are of immediate relevance to medical practice. One of the first clinical applications of molecular biology was the use by Kan and Dozy (1978) of a restriction fragment length polymorphism (RFLP) for the prenatal diagnosis of sickle cell disease, and a disorder of hemoglobin synthesis, thalassemia, is likely to be one of the first conditions to be treated by gene transfer therapy (Chapter 13). The globins also cast light on the process of evolution at both the molecular and the population levels and provide a model of gene action during development. For all these reasons, the genetic background of the human hemoglobins merits examination in some detail.

Structure and Function of Hemoglobin

Hemoglobin is the oxygen carrier in vertebrate red blood cells and is also found in some invertebrates and in the root nodules of legumes. The molecule is tetrameric. Each subunit is composed of a polypeptide chain, globin, and a prosthetic group, heme, which is an iron-containing pigment that combines with oxygen and gives the molecule its oxygen-transporting ability.

Human Hemoglobins and Their Genes. The hemoglobin molecule consists of two each of two different types of polypeptide chain. In normal adult hemoglobin (hemoglobin A, or Hb A), these globin chains are designated α and β (the structure of the β-globin gene is described in Chapter 3). The four chains are folded and fitted together to form a globular tetramer with a molecular weight of approximately 64,500 (Fig. 11–1), a structure that, for Hb A, is abbreviated as $\alpha_2\beta_2$. The two kinds of chains are almost equal in length, the α chain having 141 amino acids and the β chain 146. Because the α and β chains are encoded by genes at separate loci (the α locus on chromosome 16 and the β locus on chromosome 11; see Chapter 3), a mutation affects one chain or the other but not both.

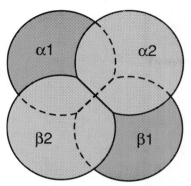

Figure 11–1. Representation of a tetrameric $\alpha_2\beta_2$ molecule of normal adult hemoglobin (Hb A). There are two α and two β chains, each associated with a heme moiety. As hemoglobin shifts from the oxygenated to the deoxygenated state, critical movement of the chains occurs at the $\alpha_1 : \beta_2$ contacts. Substitutions at the subunit interfaces can alter oxygen affinity (e.g., Hb Kempsey and Hb Kansas; see text) or the stability of the molecule.

The chains resemble one another markedly both in amino acid sequence (primary structure) and in three-dimensional configuration (tertiary structure).

In addition to Hb A, there are five other normal human hemoglobins, each of which has a tetrameric structure comparable to that of Hb A in consisting of two α or α-like chains and two non-α chains. The subunit composition of these hemoglobins, the developmental period in which they are expressed, and the chromosomal locations of the eight genes that encode the chains of which they are composed are shown in Figure 11–2. The genes for the α and α-like chains are clustered in tandem arrangement on chromosome 16, and those for the β and β-like chains are on chromosome 11. There are two identical α-globin genes, designated α_1 and α_2, instead of a single one on each copy of chromosome 16; these two loci are expressed equally. Within the β gene complex, a close homology exists between the β and δ globins, which differ in only 10 of their 146 amino acids. The two γ globins differ from one another in just one amino acid, and from the β chain in 38. The

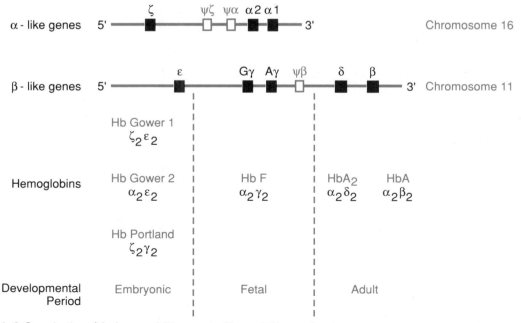

Figure 11–2. Organization of the human globin genes and hemoglobins produced in each stage of human development. (Redrawn from Stamatoyannopoulos G, Nienhuis AW [1987] Hemoglobin switching. *In* Stamatoyannopoulos G, Nienhuis AW, Leder P, Majerus PW [eds] The molecular basis of blood diseases. WB Saunders, Philadelphia, pp. 66–105.)

expression of the ζ (zeta), ϵ (epsilon), γ (gamma), and δ (delta) genes is described below.

Features of Globin Structure Relevant to the Hemoglobinopathies. Several aspects of globin structure have been highly conserved during evolution and are central to an understanding of the hemoglobinopathies. Above all, evolution has preserved the tertiary structure of the globin polypeptide, so that virtually all globins examined have the seven or eight helical regions (depending on the chain) designated A to H in Figure 11–3. This conformation is conserved despite extensive divergence of the sequence. In fact, only two amino acid residues have been conserved in all globins throughout nature: the histidine to which the iron of heme is covalently linked (residue F8 in Fig. 11–3), and a phenylalanine (residue CD1 in Fig. 11–3) that wedges the porphyrin of heme into its "pocket" in the folded protein. About 35 other internal sites along the chain are almost invariably occupied by nonpolar residues, forming a hydrophobic shell that excludes water from the interior of the molecule. In contrast, polar (hydrophilic) residues tend to be arrayed on the surface of the molecule, in contact with water. Amino acid substitutions that change the polarity of a residue are likely to be deleterious and therefore will not be conserved through evolution.

The study of the structure and evolution of hemoglobin indicates that certain types of mutations are likely to be pathogenic. Thus a mutation that alters globin conformation, substitutes for highly conserved amino acids, or disrupts the hydrophobic shell by replacing one of the nonpolar residues is likely to cause a hemoglobinopathy. The preservation of globin conformation reflects the axiom that form is one of the major determinants of protein function, and many mutations alter hemoglobin function through their effect on conformation. The fact that many sites are alike in all four major chains (α, β, δ, and γ) of human globin exemplifies how selection places rigid constraints on some types of changes in specific proteins. Like all proteins, globin has "sensitive areas," in which mutations cannot occur without affecting function, and "insensitive areas," in which variation is tolerated more freely.

Developmental Expression of Globin Genes

The ontogeny of the globin genes is depicted in Figure 11–4. The change in the expression of the various genes during development, referred to as globin switching, is a classic example of the ordered regulation of gene expression in development (Stamatoyannopoulos and Nienhuis 1987). The genes in each of the two globin gene clusters (Fig. 11–2) are expressed sequentially, and there is equimolar production of the α-like and β-like globin chains.

Interestingly, the temporal switches of globin synthesis are accompanied by changes in the major site of erythropoiesis. Embryonic globin synthesis occurs in the yolk sac from the third to eighth weeks of gestation, with the production of the transitory embryonic hemoglobins containing the α-like ζ globins and β-like ϵ globins (Fig. 11–2). In combination with each other and the α or γ chains, these two embryonic globins form the three embryonic hemoglobins: Hb Gower 1 ($\zeta_2\epsilon_2$), Hb Gower 2 ($\alpha_2\epsilon_2$), and Hb Portland ($\zeta_2\gamma_2$). At about the fifth week of gestation, the major site of hematopoiesis begins to move from the yolk sac to

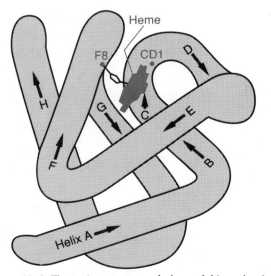

Figure 11–3. The tertiary structure of a hemoglobin molecule. The molecule has eight helical regions, designated A to H. Two highly conserved and critical residues are shown: at position F8, the histidine to which the iron of heme is covalently linked, and at CD1, the phenylalanine that wedges the porphyrin ring of heme into the heme "pocket" of the folded protein. See discussion of Hb Hammersmith and Hb Hyde Park, which have substitutions for the CD1 Phe and F8 His, respectively.

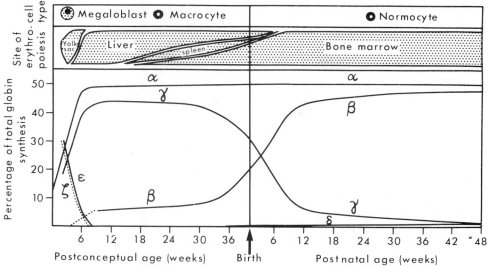

Figure 11–4. Development of erythropoiesis in the human fetus and infant. Types of cells responsible for hemoglobin synthesis, organs involved, and types of globin chain synthesized at successive stages are shown. (Redrawn from Wood WG [1976] Haemoglobin synthesis during human fetal development. Br Med Bull 32: 282–287.)

the fetal liver. Concomitantly, the synthesis from the α-globin cluster switches from ζ to α globin, whereas that of the β-globin cluster changes from ε to γ synthesis, to form the major fetal hemoglobin, $\alpha_2\gamma_2$ (Hb F).

Hb F is the predominant hemoglobin throughout fetal life and constitutes approximately 70 percent of total hemoglobin at birth, but in adult life Hb F represents less than 1 percent of the total hemoglobin. Although β chains can be detected in early gestation, their synthesis becomes significant only near the time of birth; by 3 months of age, almost all the hemoglobin present is of the adult type, Hb A. Synthesis of the δ chain begins in late fetal life and continues after birth, but Hb A$_2$ ($\alpha_2\delta_2$) never accounts for more than about 2 percent of adult hemoglobin. The mechanism of regulation of chain production is of potential therapeutic importance in the thalassemias (see Chapter 13).

The Locus Control Region. The expression of the β-globin gene is only partly controlled by the promoter and two enhancers in the immediate flanking DNA (see Chapter 3). Several studies have shown that normal expression of genes in the β-globin cluster requires additional sequences from a domain called the locus control region (LCR), located 6 to 20 kb upstream of the ε-globin gene. The LCR is responsible for high-level ex-

pression of the β-globin gene in the appropriate tissues, and also for the correct timing of expression during development (van Assendelft et al., 1989; Enver et al., 1990). The clinical significance of the LCR is twofold. First, and not surprisingly, patients who have deletions of the LCR fail to express the genes of the β-globin cluster (Kioussis et al., 1983). Second, and of wider significance, the LCR is likely to be an essential ingredient for gene therapy of disorders of the β-globin cluster (see Chapter 13).

Gene Dosage, Ontogeny, and Clinical Disease. The differences in gene dosage (four α- and two β-globin genes per diploid genome) and ontogeny of the α and β globins are important to an understanding of the pathogenesis of many hemoglobinopathies. Mutations in the β-globin gene are more likely to cause disease because a single mutation will affect 50 percent of the β chains, whereas a single α-chain mutation affects only 25 percent of the α-chains. On the other hand, β-globin mutations have no prenatal consequences, because γ globin is the major β-like globin before birth, and Hb F constitutes three quarters of the total hemoglobin at term. Because α chains are the only α-like components of all hemoglobins 6 weeks after conception (Fig. 11–4), α-globin mutations cause severe disease in both fetal and postnatal life.

GENETIC DISORDERS OF HEMOGLOBIN

The hereditary disorders of hemoglobin can be divided into three broad groups:

1. **Structural variants** that alter the globin polypeptide without affecting its rate of synthesis.
2. **Thalassemias,** in which there is decreased synthesis of one or more of the globin chains, re-sulting in an imbalance in the relative amounts of the α and β chains. (The oversimplification of this classification is demonstrated by the fact that a few rare variants are effectively synthesized but are highly unstable, and thus they cause thalassemias because they distort the $\alpha:\beta$ chain ratio).

3. **Hereditary persistence of fetal hemoglobin (HPFH),** a group of clinically benign conditions that are of interest because they impair the perinatal switch from γ- to β-globin synthesis.

Table 11–1. The Major Classes of Hemoglobin Structural Variants

Name	Molecular Basis of Mutation	Change in Polypeptide	Pathophysiological Effect of Mutation	Inheritance
Variants Causing Hemolytic Anemia				
Hemoglobins with novel physical properties				
Hb S	Single nucleotide substitution	β 6 Glu→Val	Deoxygenated Hb S polymerizes→sickle cells→vascular occlusion and hemolysis	AR
Hb C	Single nucleotide substitution	β 6 Glu→Lys	Oxygenated Hb C tends to crystallize→less deformable cells→mild hemolysis; the disease in Hb S:Hb C compounds is like mild sickle cell disease	AR
Unstable hemoglobins				
Hb Hammersmith	Single nucleotide substitution	β 42 Phe→Ser	An unstable Hb→Hb precipitation→hemolysis; also low O_2 affinity	AD
Hemoglobins with Altered O_2 Transport				
Hb Hyde Park (a Hb M)	Single nucleotide substitution	β 92 His→Tyr	Substitution makes oxidized heme iron resistant to methemoglobin reductase→Hb M, which cannot carry O_2→cyanosis (asymptomatic) in carriers	AD
Hb Kempsey	Single nucleotide substitution	β 99 Asp→Asn	Substitution keeps the Hb in its high O_2-affinity structure→less O_2 to tissues→polycythemia	AD
Hb Kansas	Single nucleotide substitution	β 102 Asn→Thr	Substitution keeps the Hb in its low O_2-affinity structure→asymptomatic cyanosis in carriers	AD
Variants with Thalassemia Phenotypes				
Hb E	Single nucleotide substitution	β 26 Glu→Lys	Mutation→an abnormal Hb and decreased synthesis (abnormal RNA splicing)→mild thalassemia	AR
Hb Lepore	Homologous, unequal crossing over between the δ- and β-chains	A $\delta\beta$ fusion protein, the normal length of a non-α globin	Decreased synthesis→severe thalassemia in homozygotes, or in genetic compounds with β-thalassemia alleles	AR

Hemoglobin Structural Variants

Most of the variant hemoglobins result from point mutations in one of the globin structural genes, but a few are formed by other, more complex, molecular mechanisms. More than 400 abnormal hemoglobins have been described, and approximately half of these are clinically significant. The hemoglobin structural variants can be divided into three classes (Table 11–1), depending on the clinical phenotype:

1. Variants that cause **hemolytic anemia.** The great majority of hemoglobin mutants that cause hemolytic anemia are unstable, but two of the best-known variants that cause hemolysis, sickle cell globin and Hb C, do so because they assume unusual, rigid structures.

2. Mutants with **altered oxygen transport,** due either to increased or decreased oxygen affinity, or to the formation of methemoglobin, which is incapable of reversible oxygenation.

3. Structurally abnormal globins that cause **thalassemia** because, as just mentioned, the mutation in the coding region also impairs the rate of synthesis or the stability of the globin polypeptide.

The structural mutants described in this chapter (Table 11–1) have been chosen for discussion because they are representative of these groups and because they illustrate principles of general significance.

Hemolytic Anemias

HEMOGLOBINS WITH NOVEL PHYSICAL PROPERTIES: SICKLE CELL DISEASE

Sickle cell hemoglobin (Hb S) was the first abnormal hemoglobin to be detected and is of great clinical importance. It is due to a change in only 1 of the 146 amino acids in β globin: a substitution of valine for glutamic acid at the sixth position of the polypeptide. This point mutation, which can be abbreviated as β 6 Glu→Val (a shorthand for summarizing mutations used throughout the book), results from a single nucleotide change (A→T) in the codon (Fig. 11–5). Homozygosity for this mutation is the cause of **sickle cell disease,** a serious disorder that in some parts of the world is relatively common. The disease has a characteristic geographic distribution, occurring most frequently in equatorial Africa and less commonly in the

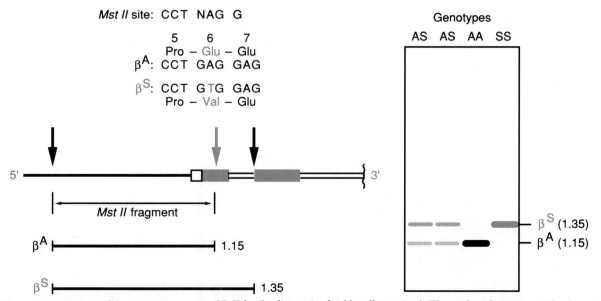

Figure 11–5. The use of the restriction enzyme *Mst*II for the diagnosis of sickle cell anemia. **A.** The nucleotide sequence of codons 6 to 8 of β-globin, and the corresponding amino acids, are shown. The recognition sequence of *Mst*II is also shown for comparison. Only the β^A gene will be cut at this position. **B.** The *Mst*II cleavage sites (arrows) in the 5' region of the β-globin gene, showing the different fragments obtained from a β^A and a β^S gene. **C.** Representation of a Southern blot showing the DNA fragments observed after *Mst*II cleaved DNA from normal persons (genotype *A/A*), persons with the sickle trait (genotype *A/S*), and persons with sickle cell disease (genotype *S/S*) is probed with a β-globin cDNA. (Redrawn from Chang JC, Kan YW [1982] A sensitive new prenatal test for sickle cell anemia. N Engl J Med 307:30–32.)

Mediterranean area and India and in countries to which people from these regions have migrated (Chapter 7). About 1 in 600 American Blacks is born with this disease, which is often fatal in early childhood although longer survival is becoming more common.

Clinical Features. Sickle cell disease is a severe hemolytic condition characterized by a tendency of the red cells to become grossly abnormal in shape (i.e., sickled) under conditions of low oxygen tension (Fig. 11–6). Patients with sickle cell disease generally present in the first 2 years of life with anemia (hemoglobin levels ranging from 6 to 10 g/dL), failure to thrive, splenomegaly, repeated infections, and, episodically, the so-called "hand–foot" syndrome: painful swelling of the hands or feet that results from the occlusion of the capillaries in the small bones of the extremities, a type of sickle cell "crisis." Crises also occur in older patients and are due to vascular obstruction and painful infarcts in various tissues including not only bones but also spleen and lungs. Recurrent infarction in the spleen leads to its resorption during childhood, with a concomitant loss of immune function. Splenic hypofunction is one cause of an increased susceptibility to certain bacterial infections, including pneumococcal sepsis. The effect of the disease on life span is variable, and mortality may not be increased if good medical care is available; infection is the major cause of death at all ages (Weatherall et al., 1989).

Heterozygotes, who are said to have **sickle cell trait,** are clinically normal, although their red cells will sickle when subjected to very low oxygen pressure in vitro. Occasions when this might happen in vivo are very unusual, although heterozygotes appear to be at risk for splenic infarction, especially when flying at high altitudes in airplanes with reduced cabin pressure. The heterozygous state is present in approximately 8 percent of American Blacks, but in areas where the gene frequency is high (e.g., West Central Africa), up to 25 percent of the newborn population are heterozygotes.

The Molecular Pathology of Hb S. The abnormality of sickle cell hemoglobin was identified in 1949 by Pauling and associates. They designated sickle cell disease as the prototype of the "molecular diseases" after they demonstrated that Hb A and Hb S were readily distinguishable from one another by electrophoresis and concluded that their globin molecules were different. They also observed that the hemoglobin of persons with sickle cell trait behaved like a mixture of normal and sickle cell hemoglobin. The structure of sickle cell hemoglobin was, in their words, "a clear case of a change produced in a protein by an allelic change in a single gene" (Pauling et al., 1949). Ingram (1956) then discovered that the abnormality in sickle cell hemoglobin was a replacement of 1 of the 146 amino acids in the β chain of the hemoglobin molecule. All the clinical manifestations of sickle cell hemoglobin are consequences of this single change in the β-globin gene. This was the first demonstration *in any organism* that a mutation in a structural gene could cause an amino acid substitution in the corresponding protein.

Because the abnormality of Hb S is localized in the β chain, the formula for sickle cell hemoglobin may be written as $\alpha_2\beta_2^S$, or more precisely, as

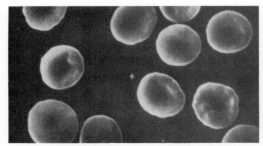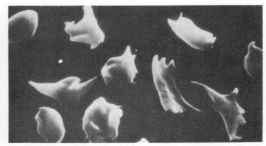

Figure 11–6. Both pictures show a scanning electron micrograph of red cells from a patient with sickle cell disease. The classic sickle shape is produced only when the cells are in the deoxygenated state (right). Oxygenated cells are on the left. (From Kaul DK, Fabry ME, Windisch P, et al. [1983] Erythrocytes in sickle cell anemia are heterogeneous in their rheological and hemodynamic characteristics. J Clin Invest 72:22–31.)

$\alpha_2{}^A\beta_2{}^S$. A heterozygote has a mixture of the two types of hemoglobin, A and S. The relationship of clinical status, hemoglobin types, and genes can be summarized as follows:

and cellular pathology is summarized in Figure 11–7.

Management. Ironically, despite the fact that the molecular basis of this disease has been known

Clinical Status	Hemoglobin	Hemoglobin Composition	Genotype
Normal	Hb A	$\alpha_2{}^A\beta_2{}^A$	$\alpha\alpha/\alpha\alpha$ β/β
Sickle cell trait	Hb A, Hb S	$\alpha_2{}^A\beta_2{}^A$, $\alpha_2{}^A\beta_2{}^S$	$\alpha\alpha/\alpha\alpha$ β/β^S
Sickle cell disease	Hb S	$\alpha_2{}^A\beta_2{}^S$	$\alpha\alpha/\alpha\alpha$ β^S/β^S

Sickling and Its Consequences. Hemoglobin molecules containing the mutant β subunits are normal in their ability to perform their principal function of binding oxygen (provided they have not polymerized, as described next), but in deoxygenated blood, they are only one fifth as soluble as normal hemoglobin. The relative insolubility of deoxyhemoglobin S is the physical basis of the sickling phenomenon. Under conditions of low oxygen tension, the sickle hemoglobin molecules aggregate in the form of rod-shaped polymers or fibers, which distort the shape of the erythrocyte (Fig. 11–7) to a sickle shape. These misshapen erythrocytes are less deformable than normal and, unlike normal red cells, cannot squeeze in single file through capillaries, thereby blocking blood flow and causing local hypoxia. The molecular

longer than that of any other single gene defect, current treatment is only supportive. Although there is a general appreciation of the events that lead to sickling, the molecular details have yet to be worked out, and no specific therapy that prevents or reverses the process in vivo has been identified. The potential use of gene therapy for this disease is discussed in Chapter 13.

Prenatal diagnosis for couples known to be carriers of the gene can be performed with chorionic villus biopsy samples at the ninth to twelfth weeks of pregnancy (reviewed in Chapter 19). The restriction enzyme *Mst*II recognizes the specific site of the sickle mutation, thereby providing a direct diagnostic test that distinguishes affected homozygotes, carriers, and normal persons (Fig. 11–5).

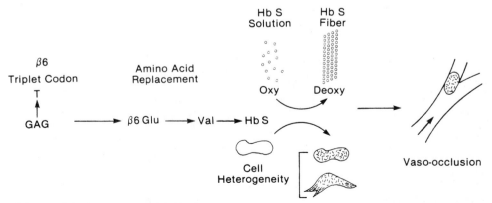

Figure 11–7. Scheme of the pathogenesis of sickle disease. (Redrawn from Ingram V [1986] Sickle cell disease—molecular and cellular pathogenesis. *In* Bunn HF, Forget BG [eds] Hemoglobin: Molecular, genetic and clinical aspects. WB Saunders, Philadelphia, pp. 453–501.)

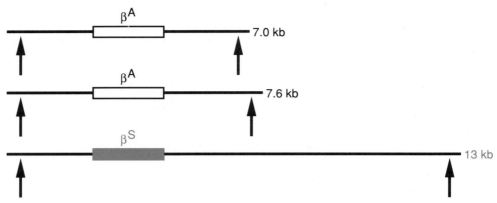

Figure 11-8. The *Hpa*I restriction fragment length polymorphism adjacent to the β^S gene. (From Kan YW, Dozy AM [1978] Polymorphism of DNA sequence adjacent to human beta-globin structural gene: Relationship to sickle mutation. Proc Natl Acad Sci USA 75:5631-5635.)

Multiple Origins of the Hb S Mutation. In a landmark paper, Kan and Dozy (1978) described a polymorphism in the DNA sequence adjacent to the β-globin gene, about 5 kb beyond the 3' end (Fig. 11-8). In some African populations, the 13 kb *Hpa*I fragment is so frequently associated with the sickle hemoglobin gene, rather than with the normal allele, that it was initially the major marker

of sickle cell disease in many at-risk families. About 60 percent of Black Americans who have the sickle mutation have the variant *Hpa*I site. This was the first example of the potential of RFLP analysis for clinical application.

Not all ethnic groups in which the sickle mutation is present have the gene in a 13 kb *Hpa*I fragment as do West Africans. In India, Saudi Ara-

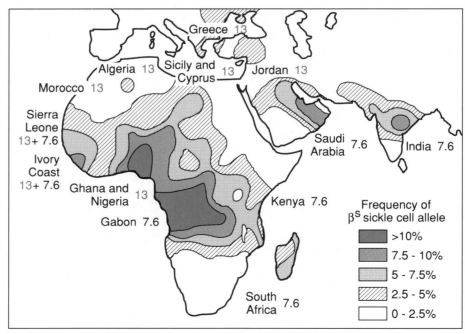

Figure 11-9. The distribution of the sickle-cell gene in relation to *Hpa*I fragments 7.6 kb and 13 kb in length. The mutation associated with the 13 kb fragment originated in West Africa and spread from there. The mutation associated with the 7.6 kb fragment arose separately and probably had multiple origins. (Redrawn from Kan YW [1978] The Harvey Lectures, Series 76. Academic Press, New York, pp. 75-93.)

bia, South Africa, Gabon, and Kenya, the mutation is typically associated with a 7.6 kb fragment (Fig. 11–9). These findings imply that the sickle mutation occurred in West Africa on a chromosome that already had a mutant *HpaI* site and that it arose independently at least once elsewhere. The protection that the sickle cell gene confers against malaria in heterozygotes, discussed in Chapter 7, accounts for the high frequency that the gene has reached in malarial areas of the world.

HEMOGLOBINS WITH NOVEL PHYSICAL PROPERTIES: HEMOGLOBIN C

Hemoglobin C was the second hemoglobin variant to be identified, and coincidentally, like Hb S, it is also due to a substitution at the sixth position of the β chain, the glutamic acid being replaced by lysine (β 6 Glu→Lys). Hb C appears to be less soluble than Hb A, and it tends to crystallize in red cells, reducing their deformability in capillaries and causing a mild hemolytic disorder.

The β^C gene is frequent in West Africa and in descendants of people of this region (about 1 percent of American Blacks are carriers). Thus it is not uncommon to find Hb C individuals who have a β^S allele or a thalassemia allele at the other β-globin locus. Persons who are genetic compounds for the β^C and β^S mutations (Hb SC disease) have a hemolytic disorder that is milder than sickle cell anemia and may have no clinical problems until, unexpectedly, a serious complication develops as a result of vascular occlusion, particularly a retinopathy.

AN UNSTABLE HEMOGLOBIN: Hb HAMMERSMITH

The unstable hemoglobins, represented here by Hb Hammersmith, are almost invariably due to point mutations that cause denaturation of the globin polypeptide (Perutz, 1987). The denatured globin chains are insoluble and precipitate to form inclusions (Heinz bodies) that contribute to damage of the red cell membrane and cause hemolysis. The amino acid substitution in Hb Hammersmith (β 42 Phe→Ser) is particularly noteworthy because the substituted phenylalanine residue (residue CD1 in Fig. 11–3) is one of the two amino acids that are conserved in all globins. Thus it is not surprising that substitutions at this position produce serious disease. The role of the bulky phenylalanine is to wedge the heme into its pocket in β globin. Its replacement with serine, a smaller residue that leaves a gap, allows the heme to drop out of its pocket. In addition to its instability, Hb Hammersmith has a low oxygen affinity, which causes cyanosis.

Variants with Altered Oxygen Transport

Mutations that alter the ability of hemoglobin to transport oxygen, although rare, are of general interest because they illustrate how a mutation can impair one set of functions of a protein (in this case, hemoglobin binding and release) that is the responsibility of one domain and yet leave relatively intact the other properties of the molecule; for example, the mutations to be described generally have little or no effect on hemoglobin stability.

METHEMOGLOBINS (Hb M)

Oxyhemoglobin is the form of hemoglobin that is capable of reversible oxygenation; its heme iron is in the reduced (or ferrous) state. The heme iron tends to oxidize spontaneously to the ferric form, and the resulting molecule, referred to as methemoglobin, is incapable of reversible oxygenation. If significant amounts of methemoglobin accumulate in the blood, cyanosis results. Maintenance of the heme iron in the reduced state is the role of the enzyme methemoglobin reductase. In several mutant globins (either α or β), substitutions in the region of the heme pocket affect the heme–globin bond in a way that makes the iron resistant to the reductase. Although heterozygotes for these mutant hemoglobins are cyanosed, they are asymptomatic. Homozygosity for this condition is unknown, presumably because the homozygous state is lethal. One example of a β-chain methemoglobin is Hb Hyde Park (β 92 His→Tyr), in which the conserved histidine (residue F8 in Fig. 11–3) to which heme is covalently bound has been replaced by tyrosine. Methemoglobinemia can also originate by a genetically distinct mechanism, through a deficiency of the reductase enzyme; in this case, however, the inheritance is autosomal recessive rather than autosomal dominant.

HEMOGLOBINS WITH ALTERED OXYGEN AFFINITY

Mutations that alter oxygen affinity are of significance because they demonstrate the importance of subunit interaction for the normal function of a multimeric protein like hemoglobin. In the Hb A tetramer, the chains are in an

$$\alpha_1 \alpha_2$$
$$\beta_2 \beta_1$$

arrangement. The $\alpha_1 : \beta_2$ interface has been very highly conserved throughout evolution because it is subject to significant movement between the chains when the hemoglobin shifts from the oxygenated (relaxed) to the deoxygenated (tense) form of the molecule. Predictably, substitutions in residues at the $\alpha_1 : \beta_2$ interface have serious pathological effects because they prevent the oxygen-related movement between the chains. The β-globin mutants Hb Kempsey and Hb Kansas are instructive because although both mutations disturb the $\alpha_1 : \beta_2$ interface, the molecular and clinical effects are the inverse of one another. In Hb Kempsey (β 99 Asp $\rightarrow$ Asn), the mutation "locks" the hemoglobin into the relaxed structure, which has high oxygen affinity, and causes polycythemia. Carriers of Hb Kansas (β 102 Asn$\rightarrow$Thr), on the other hand, have cyanosis, because the mutation inhibits the formation of the relaxed (oxygenated) structure, so that the hemoglobin has a lowered oxygen affinity. However, one carrier of Hb Kansas is healthy enough to be an excellent tennis player, suggesting that he can extract a larger-than-normal fraction of oxygen from blood (Perutz, 1987).

Variant Hemoglobins with Thalassemia Phenotypes

HEMOGLOBIN E: AN ABNORMAL BETA-GLOBIN POLYPEPTIDE WITH REDUCED mRNA SYNTHESIS

With the exception of Hb E, structurally abnormal hemoglobins that also cause thalassemia because they are synthesized at a reduced rate are relatively uncommon. This β-globin mutant (β 26 Glu$\rightarrow$Lys) is remarkable for its frequency, its allelic interaction with other β-globin mutants, and its effect on RNA splicing (Table 11–1; see Fig. 11–17). It is probably the most common structurally abnormal hemoglobin in the world, occurring at high frequency in Southeast Asia, where there are at least 1 million homozygotes and 30 million heterozygotes (Weatherall et al., 1989).

Although Hb E homozygotes are asymptomatic and only mildly anemic, genetic compounds with the Hb E mutation and different β-thalassemia alleles have abnormal phenotypes that are largely determined by the severity of the other allele. Hb E is also notable because its mutation, although located in the coding region, reduces normal splicing of the β^E-globin RNA, producing a mild thalassemia phenotype. Discussion of the effect of this mutation on splicing is deferred to a later discussion on RNA splicing mutants that cause β-thalassemia.

LEPORE HEMOGLOBINS: FUSION GENES

Some patients with moderate to severe β-thalassemia have been found to have an unusual non-α chain that consists of the N-terminal half (50 to 80 residues) of a normal δ chain fused to the C-terminal half (60 to 90 residues) of a normal β chain, which together form a new $\delta\beta$ fusion chain, termed Hb Lepore. These variants have arisen by a process of homologous unequal crossing over (see Chapter 6), which is possible because the two genes are highly homologous (differing in only 10 of their 146 amino acids) and contiguous on chromosome 11 (Fig. 11–10). Misalignment based on the sequence homology between the δ gene of one chromatid and the β gene of the corresponding chromatid, occurring during meiosis, could happen as a relatively rare accident. Crossing over between the two similar genes would then be possible, resulting in the formation of two products: (1) a fusion gene beginning as a δ and ending as a β, and (2) a reciprocal product with a normal δ and a normal β gene, as well as a fusion gene coding for a β segment followed by a δ segment (Fig. 11–10). The first is a Lepore gene; the second is an "anti-Lepore" gene (Table 11–2). Homologous unequal crossing over as a general mechanism in evolution is presented in Chapter 6.

The Molecular Basis of Human Hemoglobin Variants

As Table 11–2 shows, although most hemoglobin variants are caused by single nucleotide substitutions that produce a missense mutation in one codon, other molecular mechanisms have been recognized. These other mutant hemoglobins demonstrate the diverse ways in which the primary sequence of a protein can be altered.

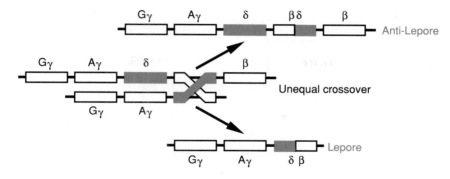

Figure 11–10. Model for the origin of a Lepore gene by unequal crossing over. The adjacent δ and β genes differ at only 10 of their 146 residues. If mispairing occurs, followed by intergenic crossing over, two hybrid genes result: one with a deletion of part of each locus (a Lepore gene) and one with a corresponding duplication (an anti-Lepore gene). (Redrawn from Weatherall DJ, Clegg JB [1981] The thalassemia syndromes, 3rd ed. Blackwell Scientific Publications, Oxford.)

The various molecular mechanisms underlying single nucleotide substitutions are discussed in Chapter 6. Of particular note is the increased frequency with which the dinucleotide CpG is mutated to TpG, which has been observed in studies of both polymorphisms and disease-causing mutations such as Hb Brigham (Table 11–2). A few mutant globins with two amino acid substitutions are known; this situation undoubtedly reflects the high frequency of carriers of the sickle gene, because in most cases one of the two mutations is that for sickle cell globin. Thus in Hb C$_{Harlem}$, a second mutation probably occurred within a β^S allele.

As discussed earlier, homologous but unequal crossing over between similar genes on different chromatids is believed to explain the origin of Hb Lepore, and the discovery of anti-Lepore hemoglobins (see Fig. 11–10) such as Hb Miyada supports this hypothesis. Whereas the misalign-

Table 11–2. The Molecular Basis of Hemoglobin Variants*

Abnormality in Globin Chain	Example	Affected Residues	Inferred or Demonstrated Mechanism
Single amino acid substitution	Hb Brigham	β chain: 100 Pro→Leu CCG→CTG	C→T substitution reflects increased frequency with which CpG mutates to TpG
Two amino acid substitutions in one polypeptide chain	Hb C$_{Harlem}$	β chain: 6 Glu→Val and 73 Asp→Asn	A second mutation has occurred in a mutant gene
Fusion hemoglobins	Hb Lepore Hb Miyada (an anti-Lepore Hb)	a $\delta\beta$ fusion chain a $\beta\delta$ fusion chain	Homologous recombination and unequal crossing over between *different* genes
Small deletions	Hb Gun Hill	β chain: a 5 amino acid deletion	Homologous recombination and unequal crossing over within *same* gene
Elongated polypeptide	Hb Constant Spring	α chain: an additional 31 amino acids	Substitution in stop codon: UAA or UAG to CAA or CAG→readthrough to next stop codon in reading frame
	Hb Tak	β chain: an additional 11 residues	Frameshift near end of chain allows readthrough to a downstream stop in new frame

* Derived in part from Bunn FH (1987) Human hemoglobins: Normal and abnormal. *In* Nathan DG, Oski FA (eds) Hematology of infancy and childhood, 3rd ed. WB Saunders, Philadelphia, pp. 613–640.

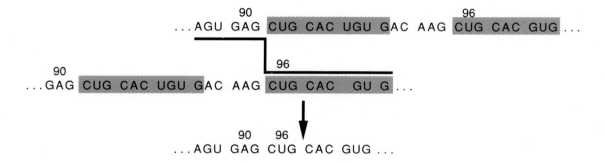

Hb Gun Hill - β $^{91-95}$ deleted

Figure 11–11. The proposed mechanism for the origin of Hb Gun Hill, a hemoglobin β-chain structural variant with a deletion of residues 91 to 95. Unequal crossing over between chromosome pairs may have occurred, as a result of mispairing between two nearly identical nucleotide sequences (in red) that are in the region of codons 90 to 98 of the β-globin gene. The crossover shown here would delete codons 91 to 95.

ment that generated the Lepore and anti-Lepore globins occurred between *different* genes (β and δ), Hb Gun Hill is probably the result of a misalignment between two similar sequences in the *same* gene. A deletion of 15 base pairs (which, 15 being a multiple of 3, maintains the normal β-globin reading frame) has occurred in a region where two nearly identical nine-nucleotide sequences occur near each other in the β-globin gene (Fig. 11–11). The similarity of these repeat sequences presumably allows them to misalign during meiosis, and subsequent unequal crossing over deletes one of the repeats and the intervening five base pairs.

In contrast to deleted hemoglobins such as Lepore and Gun Hill, other variants have extended globin chains. An α-chain mutant, Hb Constant Spring (α 142 Stop→Gln), has a 31-residue extension that results from a mutation in the normal stop codon, allowing translation to continue downstream to the next stop codon (at position 173).

Hb Constant Spring:

α	Arg	Stop!					
	CGU	UAA	GCU	GGA	...	GAA	UAA
	141		143				173
	CGU	CAA	GCU	GGA	...	GAA	UAA
α^{cs}	Arg	Gln	Ala	Gly	...	Glu	Stop!

Other elongated chains have small deletions or additions that change the reading frame, so that the protein continues until the next stop codon in the new frame is reached. In Hb Tak, for example, there is a two base pair insertion (either the AC

insertion shown or a CA insertion between residues 146 and 147) that extends the β-globin chain by 11 residues.

Hb Tak:

β	His	Stop!					
	CAC	UAA	GCU	CGC	...		
	146		148				157
		AC					
	CAC	U	AAG	CUC	...	UAU	UAA
β^{Tak}	His	Thr	Lys	Leu	...	Tyr	Stop!

As other genetic disorders are described at a molecular level, one often has a sense of déjà vu on recognizing alterations similar to those seen in hemoglobin variants. The same can be said about the molecular disturbances that are described below in other hemoglobin defects such as the thalassemias.

Thalassemia: An Imbalance of Globin-Chain Synthesis

The thalassemias, collectively the most common human single-gene disorders, are a heterogeneous group of diseases of hemoglobin synthesis in which the mutation reduces the level of synthesis of either the α or β chain (Weatherall et al., 1989). The reduction leads to a distortion of the α:β chain ratio, which in turn causes the pathophysiology. The chain that is produced at the normal rate is in relative excess; in the absence of a complementary chain with which to form a tetramer, the excess normal chains eventually precipitate in the cell, damaging the membrane and leading to premature destruction of the red cell. In addition, the defect in hemoglobin synthesis produces a hypochromic, microcytic anemia.

In recent years much progress has been made in clarifying the molecular and genetic basis of the thalassemias (Orkin, 1987; Weatherall et al., 1989; Kazazian, 1990). Two main groups are defined: the **α-thalassemias,** in which α-chain synthesis is reduced or absent, and the **β-thalassemias,** in which β-chain synthesis is impaired. A genetic and clinical complication is that it is not unusual for alleles for both types of thalassemia, as well as for structural hemoglobin abnormalities, to coexist in an individual and to interact. Because there are many mutant globin alleles, they interact to produce a wide variety of complex hematological problems. In this discussion we risk oversimplification by mentioning only some of the most common and best known types.

Both α- and β-thalassemia have a high frequency in diverse populations, presumably because of the protective advantage against malaria conferred on carriers, analogous to the heterozygote advantage of sickle hemoglobin carriers. (The phenomenon of heterozygote advantage, and other explanations for the high frequency of a gene in a population, are discussed in Chapter 7.) Alpha-thalassemia, however, is more prevalent and widely distributed. There is a characteristic distribution of the thalassemias in a band around the Old World: in the Mediterranean, the Middle East, and parts of Africa, India, and Asia. The name is derived from the Greek word for sea, *thalassa,* and signifies that the disease was first discovered in persons of Mediterranean origin. In most countries, thalassemia carriers are sufficiently numerous to pose the important problem of differential diagnosis from iron deficiency anemia, and to be a relatively common source of referral for homozygote detection in prenatal diagnosis.

The Alpha-Thalassemias

Genetic disorders of α-globin production affect the formation of *both* fetal and adult hemoglobins (Figs. 11–2, 11–4) and therefore cause intrauterine as well as postnatal disease. In the absence of α-globin chains with which to associate, the chains from the β-globin cluster are free to form a homotetrameric hemoglobin. Hemoglobin with a γ_4 composition is known as Hb Bart's, and the β_4 tetramer is called Hb H. Because neither of these hemoglobins is capable of releasing oxygen to tissues in normal conditions, they are completely ineffective oxygen carriers. Consequently, infants with severe α-thalassemia and high levels of Hb Bart's suffer severe intrauterine hypoxia and are born with massive generalized fluid accumulation, a condition called hydrops fetalis. In milder α-thalassemias, an anemia develops because of the gradual precipitation of the Hb H in the erythrocyte. This leads to the formation of inclusions in the mature red cell, and the removal of these inclusions by the spleen damages the cells, leading to their premature destruction.

Deletions of the Alpha-Globin Genes. The most common forms of α-thalassemia are the result of deletions. The reason for the frequency of this type of abnormality in mutants of the α and not the β chain is revealed by comparison of these genes and their local chromosomal contexts (Fig. 11–2). Not only are there two identical α genes on each chromosome 16, but the intron sequences around the two α genes are also highly homologous. These regions of extended homology undoubtedly reflect the size of the duplication unit that generated the pair of α genes.

The arrangement of tandem regions of homology in and around the α genes facilitates misalignment, homologous pairing, and recombination between the α1 gene domain on one chromosome and the corresponding α2 gene region on the other, as shown in Figure 11–12. Evidence that this explanation for the deletions is correct is provided by reports of rare normal individuals with a triplicated α gene complex (Fig. 11–12). Deletions or other alterations of one, two, three, or all four of these genes cause a correspondingly severe hematological abnormality, as tabulated in Table 11–3.

Although the α-thalassemias are distributed throughout the world, the homozygous deletion type of α-thalassemia leading to hydrops fetalis is largely restricted to Southeast Asians. This heterogeneity of incidence has a clear molecular basis. The heterozygous state, called α-thalassemia trait (two normal and two mutant α genes), can result from either of two genotypes ($-\alpha/-\alpha$ or $--/\alpha\alpha$). The latter is relatively common in

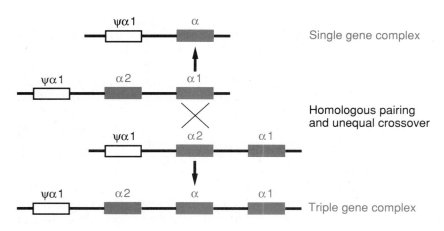

Single gene complex

Homologous pairing
and unequal crossover

Triple gene complex

Figure 11–12. The probable mechanism of the most common form of α-thalassemia, which is due to deletions of one of the two α-globin genes on a chromosome. Misalignment, homologous pairing, and recombination between the α1 gene on one chromosome and the α2 gene on the homologous chromosome results in the deletion of one α gene. (Redrawn from Orkin SH [1987] Disorders of hemoglobin synthesis: The thalassemias. *In* Stamatoyannopoulos G, Nienhuis AW, Leder P, Majerus PW (eds) The molecular basis of blood diseases. WB Saunders, Philadelphia, pp. 106–126.)

Southeast Asians, and offspring may consequently receive two (−−/−−) chromosomes. In other groups, however, heterozygosity is usually the result of the (−α/−α) genotype, from which there is virtually no possibility of transmitting the hydrops fetalis genotype. In some populations, such as Melanesians and certain East Indians, the frequency of the (−α) haplotype is actually greater than that of normal (αα) α-globin chromosomes.

Nondeletion Forms of Alpha-Thalassemia. These occur less commonly than the deletion genotypes just described. Only one type of nondeletion α-thalassemia illustrates a novel mechanism of mutation that has not also been described in β-thalassemia (reviewed in the next section). Four α-chain termination mutations, including the structural variant Hb Constant Spring (Table 12–2), cause α-thalassemia, apparently because of a pronounced instability of the mutant mRNA.

The Beta-Thalassemias

The β-thalassemias share many features with α-thalassemia. Decreased β-globin production causes a hypochromic, microcytic anemia, and the imbalance in globin synthesis leads to precipitation of the excess α chains, which in turn leads to damage of the red cell membrane. In contrast to α globin, however, the β chain is important only in the postnatal period (Fig. 11–4). Consequently, the onset of β-thalassemia is not apparent until a few months after birth, when β globin would normally replace γ globin as the major non-α chain, and only the synthesis of the major adult hemoglobin, Hb A, is reduced. The excess α chains are insoluble, so that they precipitate in red cell precursors and are destroyed in the bone marrow; this process causes ineffective erythropoiesis (Fig. 11–13). Because the δ gene is intact, Hb A$_2$ production continues, and in fact elevation of the Hb A$_2$ level is unique to β-thalassemia heterozygotes. The Hb F level is also increased, not because of a reactivation of the γ globin gene expression that was switched off at birth, but because of selective survival and perhaps also increased production of the minor population of adult red cells that contain Hb F.

In contrast to α-thalassemia, the β-thalasse-

Table 11–3. Clinical States of Alpha-Thalassemia Genotypes

Clinical Condition	Number of Functional α Genes	Genotype	α-Chain Production
Normal	4	αα/αα	100%
Silent carrier	3	αα/α−	75%
α-thalassemia trait (mild anemia, microcytosis)	2	α−/α− or αα/−−	50%
Hb H (β$_4$) disease (moderately severe hemolytic anemia)	1	α−/−−	25%
Hydrops fetalis or homozygous α-thalassemia (Hb Bart's: γ$_4$)	0	−−/−−	0%

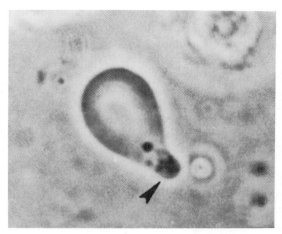

Figure 11–13. Visualization of one pathological effect of the deficiency of β-chains in β-thalassemia: the precipitation of the excess normal α chains to form a Heinz body in the red cell. Phase microscopy of a wet preparation of scrapings from the spleen of a patient with homozygous β-thalassemia, showing an α-chain inclusion body (arrow) within a teardrop-shaped red cell. Such inclusions are removed from the erythrocyte by reticuloendothelial cells, damaging the cell membrane and causing premature destruction of the cell. (From Nathan DG [1972] Thalassemia. N Engl J Med 286:586–594.)

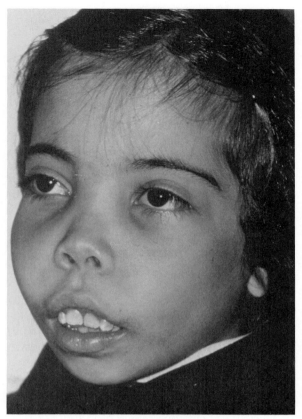

Figure 11–14. The typical facial appearance of a child with untreated β-thalassemia. Note prominent cheek bones and the protrusion of the upper jaw that results from the expansion of the marrow cavity in the bones of the skull and face. (Photograph courtesy of N. Olivieri, The Hospital for Sick Children, Toronto.)

mias are usually due to single base-pair substitutions rather than deletions. There is such great variety in β-thalassemia alleles that persons carrying two such genes, though commonly called homozygotes, are more likely to be compounds with two different β-globin mutations. As a general rule, individuals with two β-thalassemia alleles ("homozygotes") have **thalassemia major**, a condition characterized by severe anemia and requiring lifelong medical management. When the β-thalassemia alleles allow so little production of β globin that no Hb A is present, the condition is designated **$β^0$-thalassemia.** If some Hb A is detectable, the patient is said to have **$β^+$-thalassemia.** Although homozygotes have clinical pictures of severity that vary according to the combined effect of the two alleles present, survival into adult life was, until recently, unusual.

The Clinical Phenotype. Infants affected with homozygous β-thalassemia present with anemia once the postnatal production of Hb F decreases, generally before 2 years of age. The severe hemolytic anemia (Hb usually <5 gm/L) leads to failure to thrive, jaundice, hepatosplenomegaly, and an expansion of the bone marrow that causes distinctive skeletal changes that are evident, in addition to other features, as thalassemic facies (Fig. 11–14). The red cells in peripheral blood are all markedly hypochromic and variable in size and shape. Treatment of the thalassemias is presently based on correction of the anemia and the increased marrow expansion by blood transfusion, and on control of the consequent iron accumulation by the administration of chelating agents. However, bone marrow transplantation for patients early in the course of their disease has been recently shown to have great promise (Lucarelli et al., 1990).

Carriers of one β-thalassemia allele are clinically well and are said to have **thalassemia minor.** Such individuals have hypochromic, microcytic red cells and may have a slight anemia that can initially be misdiagnosed as iron deficiency. The diagnosis of thalassemia minor can be supported by hemoglobin electrophoresis, which generally reveals an increase in the level of Hb A_2 ($α_2δ_2$).

MOLECULAR BASIS OF BETA-THALASSEMIA: A PANORAMA OF POINT MUTATIONS

Almost every type of abnormality that can reduce the synthesis of an mRNA or protein has been identified as a cause of β-thalassemia. More than 80 β-globin substitutions that cause β-thalassemia have been defined (Kazazian, 1990); the locations in the gene of representative mutations are shown in Figure 11–15. Many of the mutants decrease the abundance of the normal β-globin mRNA, and they are of three types: (1) promoter mutants; (2) RNA splicing mutants, the most common and certainly the most interesting; and (3) mRNA capping or tailing mutants. Other forms of β-thalassemia have defects in the coding region—nonsense or frameshift mutations—that lead to the synthesis of a short, unstable polypeptide. Unexpectedly, a few hemoglobin structural variants (i.e., with mutations in the coding region) also impair transcription of the β-globin gene, as exemplified by Hb E, which was described earlier. Comprehensive overviews of the molecular basis of β-thalassemia have been published (Orkin 1987; Weatherall et al., 1989). Table 11–4 summarizes the major types of gene defects that result in β-thalassemia.

Deletions That Cause Beta-Thalassemia. In contrast to α-thalassemia, deletions are an infrequent cause of simple β-thalassemia. The only common deletion in any racial group is a 619 base pair partial deletion of the 3′ end of the gene in patients of Asian Indian origin (Table 11–4). Hb Lepore, discussed earlier as a Hb variant, is due to unequal crossing over that produces an approximately 7 kb deletion in and between the δ and β genes.

Complex Thalassemias and the Hereditary Persistence of Fetal Hemoglobin. Although deletions of the β-globin gene alone, which cause simple β-thalassemia, are relatively uncommon, numerous larger deletions that remove the β locus or other genes of the β-globin cluster, or both, have been described. The thalassemias that result from these deletions are called complex, and they are named according to the genes deleted—that is, δβ⁰-thalassemia and $^{A}\gamma\delta\beta^{0}$-thalassemia, and so on. This discussion focuses entirely on deletions that are 3′ to the γ genes (Fig. 11–16); these deletions are of particular interest because they impair the perinatal switch from γ- to β-globin synthesis.

Patients with deletions that leave at least one of the γ genes intact have one of two clinical presentations, depending on the deletion: δβ⁰ thalas-

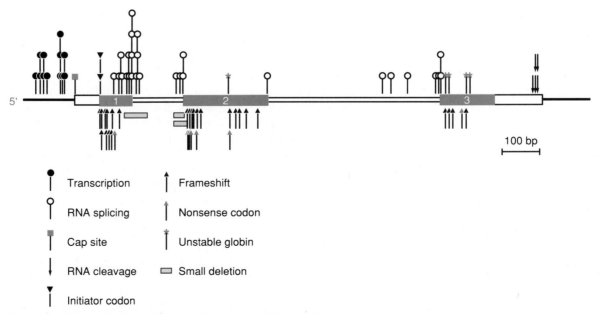

Figure 11–15. Point mutations that cause β-thalassemia. Note the distribution of mutations throughout the gene, and the fact that the mutations affect virtually every process required for the production of normal β-globin. (Redrawn from Kazazian HH [1990] The thalassemia syndromes: Molecular basis and prenatal diagnosis in 1990. *In* Miescher LA, Jaffé ER (eds) Seminars in Hematology 27(3). WB Saunders, Philadelphia, pp. 209–228.)

Table 11–4. The Molecular Basis of Beta-Thalassemia

Type	Example	Phenotype	Affected Population
Deletions			
Fusion proteins	Hb Lepore, a 7 kb deletion → a $\delta\beta$ fusion protein	β^0, β^{Lepore}	Italian
β-globin gene deletions	619 base pair deletion	β^0	Indian
Defective mRNA Synthesis			
RNA splicing defects (see Fig. 11–17)	Abnormal acceptor site of intron 1: $\underline{A}G \rightarrow \underline{G}G$	β^0	Black
Promoter mutants	*Mutation in the ATA box* $-31\ -30\ -29\ -28$ $-31\ -30\ -29\ -28$ $\underline{A}$ T A A $\rightarrow$ $\underline{G}$ T A A	β^+	Japanese
Abnormal RNA cap site	A → C transversion at the mRNA cap site	β^+	Asian
Polyadenylation signal defects	AA$\underline{T}$AAA→AA$\underline{C}$AAA	β^+	Black
Nonfunctional mRNAs			
Nonsense mutations	*codon 39* gln → stop! $\underline{C}$AG → $\underline{U}$AG	β^0	Mediterranean (especially Sardinian)

Frameshift mutations	*codon 16: 1 bp deletion*
	   15 16 17 18 19
	normal trp gly lys val asn
	   UGG GGC AAG GUG AAC
	   UGG _GCA AGG UGA
	mutant trp ala arg stop!
		β^0	Indian

Coding Region Mutations That Also Alter Splicing			
Neutral mutations	*codon 24* gly → gly GG$\underline{U}$ → GG$\underline{A}$	β^+	Black
Missense mutations	*Hb E: codon 26* glu → lys $\underline{G}$AG → $\underline{A}$AG	β^+, β^E (Hb A 60%, Hb E 40%)	Southeast Asian

Derived in part from Weatherall et al. (1989) and Orkin (1987).

semia, or a clinically benign state called **hereditary persistence of fetal hemoglobin (HPFH).** Homozygotes with either of these conditions are viable because the remaining γ gene or genes remain active after birth, instead of switching off as would normally occur. As a result, Hb F ($\alpha_2\gamma_2$) synthesis continues postnatally at a high level, compensating for the absence of Hb A. Because γ chains are the only products from the β-globin cluster in these patients, both groups have 100 percent Hb F. The clinically benign nature of HPFH is due to a greater production of γ chains, reflected in a higher level of Hb F in heterozygotes (17 to 35 percent Hb F) than is generally seen in

heterozygotes for $\delta\beta^0$-thalassemia (5 to 18 percent Hb F; Weatherall et al., 1989). Figure 11–16 shows that the deletions that cause $\delta\beta^0$-thalassemia overlap with those that cause HPFH, and it is not clear why HPFH patients have higher levels of γ-gene expression. The more fundamental question, which also remains unanswered, is why either group of patients have postnatal γ-gene expression at all. The elucidation of the molecular basis of the postnatal γ-gene expression, and of the differential γ-gene expression in HPFH and $\delta\beta$-thalassemia, is likely to provide some insight into the mechanisms that regulate gene expression in the β-globin cluster during development.

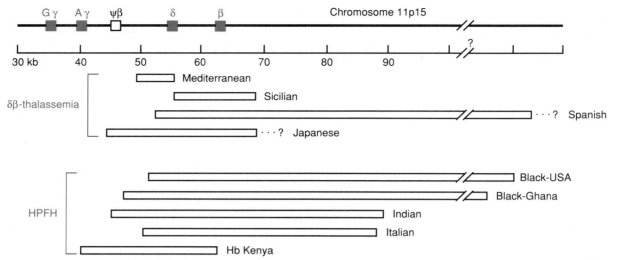

Figure 11–16. Location and size of deletions of various δβ-thalassemia and HPFH mutations. Note the overlap between the deletions responsible for these two types of conditions. (Redrawn from Stamatoyannopoulos G, Nienhuis AW [1987] Hemoglobin switching. *In* Stamatoyannopoulos G, Nienhuis AW, Leder P, Majerus PW (eds) The molecular basis of blood diseases. WB Saunders, Philadelphia, pp. 66–105.)

A few patients with HPFH have, not deletions, but rather single base-pair substitutions (nondeletion HPFH) in the upstream regulatory region of either the $^A\gamma$ or $^G\gamma$ genes. In Greek $^A\gamma$ HPFH, for example, there is a G→A change a few bases 5′ to a CCAAT box (a promoter element; see Chapter 3) of the $^A\gamma$ gene. These mutations are presumed to alter the affinity of regulatory (DNA-binding) proteins required for the postnatal repression of γ-gene expression. Individuals with nondeletion HPFH are clinically normal; their genetic condition is recognized incidentally during hematological studies undertaken for other reasons.

Defective mRNA Synthesis. The great majority of β-thalassemia patients with defective mRNA synthesis have abnormalities in RNA splicing. More than two dozen defects of this type have been described (Kazazian, 1990); the effect of these mutations on splicing is often unexpectedly complex. Apart from their importance with regard to their combined clinical burden, they have also contributed extensively to the recognition of the sequences that determine where splicing occurs during RNA processing (introduced in Chapter 3).

The splice defects fall into three groups, depending on the region of the unprocessed RNA in which the mutation is located:

Group 1. Splice junction mutations: in the 5′ intron donor or 3′ intron acceptor sites, or their surrounding consensus sequences

Group 2. Intron mutations: that activate cryptic splice sites that compete with the correct site

Group 3. Exon mutations: that affect splicing by activating cryptic splice sites that compete with the correct site

Splice Junction Mutations. This group includes mutations at the 5′ donor or 3′ acceptor splice junctions of the introns or in the consensus sequences surrounding the junctions. The critical nature of the conserved GT dinucleotide at the 5′ intron donor site, and of the AG at the 3′ intron receptor site (conserved in the introns of virtually all genes), is apparent from the complete loss of normal splicing seen in all patients carrying mutations with changes in these dinucleotides. An example of an acceptor site mutation, found in patients of Mediterranean origin, is shown in Figure 11–17, in which the AG at the 3′ end of intron 2 has been changed to GG, producing a β^0-thalassemia allele. The inactivation of the normal acceptor site elicits the use of other acceptor-like sequences elsewhere in the RNA precursor (Orkin, 1987).

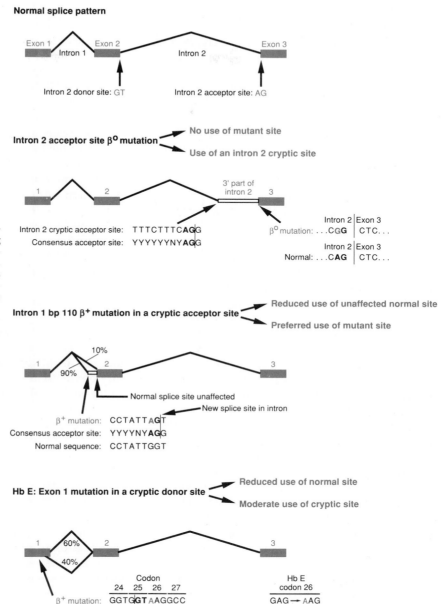

Figure 11-17. Examples of mutations that disrupt normal splicing of the β-globin gene to cause β-thalassemia. In the intron 2 defect, the normal splice acceptor site is altered, aborting all normal splicing; the result is the use of a cryptic site in the intron. In the intron 1 defect, the mutation creates an acceptor splice site that is preferred to the normal acceptor site by the splicing apparatus. In the Hb E defect, the mutation in codon 26 in exon 1 activates a cryptic donor splice site that competes quite effectively with the normal donor site.

These alternative sites are termed **cryptic splice sites** because they are normally not used by the splicing apparatus when the correct site is available. Cryptic donor or acceptor slice sites, as described shortly, can be found in either exons or introns and may be used alone or in competition with other cryptic sites or the normal splice site.

The A→G acceptor site mutation shown in Figure 11–17 results in the use of a cryptic acceptor site upstream from the normal site, in intron 2. The cryptic site conforms perfectly to the consensus acceptor splice sequence (where Y = either pyrimidine, T or C). RNA made from this mutant gene cannot encode β globin because the third exon has been enlarged at the 5' end, as a result of the inclusion of the intron 2 sequences in the alternatively spliced mRNA. Perhaps not surprisingly, several other mutations also result in the use of the same intron 2 cryptic splice site.

The importance of the consensus sequences surrounding the donor or acceptor dinucleotides is illustrated by the impact of mutations in bases adjacent to the dinucleotides. For example, mutations in the fifth or sixth nucleotide of the donor sequence of intron 1 impair the production of β-globin mRNA. In contrast to mutations in the dinucleotides, however, some splicing still occurs at the correct site in these consensus sequence mutations, so that the phenotypes are those of β^+-thalassemia.

Intron Mutations. A mutation within an intron cryptic splice site can sometimes enhance its use and concomitantly reduce splicing at the correct site, which remains perfectly intact. An example of the preferential use of a cryptic site, as a consequence of a mutation in it, is shown in Figure 11–17. A substitution of G→A in base pair 110 of intron 1 activates a cryptic acceptor site by creating an AG dinucleotide and increasing the resemblance of the site to the consensus sequence. The globin mRNA thus formed is elongated (19 extra nucleotides) at the 5' side of exon 2; a premature stop codon is introduced into the transcript. A β^+-thalassemia phenotype results because the correct acceptor site is still used, although at a reduced level, 10 percent (Spritz et al., 1981). As a generalization, cryptic site mutations are often "leaky," and β-globin mutations of this type frequently allow enough use of the normal splice site to produce a β^+-thalassemia phenotype.

Exon Mutations That Affect Splicing. Although it is conceptually useful to distinguish between mutations in the coding region that directly alter the protein and those outside the coding region that cause disease by affecting the quantity of the specific mRNA, the structural variant Hb E illustrates that both problems sometimes result from a single mutation. This dual effect is possible because mutations in exons can also activate cryptic splice sites, thereby interfering with normal RNA processing. As shown in Tables 11–1 and 11–4, the missense mutation that produces Hb E also activates a cryptic donor site in exon 1, making it more similar to the consensus sequence. Moderate use is made of this alternative splicing pathway, but the majority of RNA is still processed from the correct site, and a mild β^+-thalassemia is the result. A similar defect causing mild β^+-thalassemia has been found in codon 24, but notably, this mutation does not change the encoded amino acid (both GGT and GGA code for glycine); this is an example of a translationally silent mutation that is not neutral in its effect (Table 11–4).

Nonfunctional mRNAs. A nonfunctional mRNA is one that cannot direct the synthesis of a complete polypeptide because the mutation generates a stop codon, which prematurely terminates translation (see Chapter 6). In some patients with β-thalassemia, the failure in translation is due to a single nucleotide substitution that creates a nonsense mutation. In other cases, frameshift mutations result from small insertions or deletions that are not multiples of three nucleotides (i.e., one codon). Both types of nonfunctional mRNA mutations cause β^0-thalassemia because no β globin can be made.

One of the nonsense mutations, a C→T transition that creates a stop in codon 3 (Table 11–4), is common in Mediterranean populations, particularly on the island of Sardinia. Unexpectedly, this mutation has also been found to be associated with reduced levels of the β-globin mRNA, indicating that there is a previously unsuspected relationship between translation and transcription. This example illustrates that one of the benefits of characterizing the molecular pathology of human disease is the recognition of previously unknown biological phenomena.

Frameshifts that cause β-thalassemia occur early enough in the coding sequence that a stop codon is encountered downstream in the new reading frame, well before the normal termination signal. In contrast, frameshifts near the carboxyl terminus of the protein allow most of the mRNA to be translated normally, or to produce elongated globin chains such as Hb Tak, referred to earlier (Table 11–2). An example of a β^0-thalassemia frameshift mutation is shown in Table 11–4, in which a 1 base pair deletion in codon 16 switches the reading frame so that a stop is encountered only three codons later in the new frame.

Defects in Capping and Tailing of Beta-Globin mRNA. All messenger RNAs undergo posttranscriptional modifications outside the coding region that are necessary for their normal stability or function (Chapter 3). The critical nature of two of these changes, the capping of the RNA at its extreme 5' end (at the cap site) and the polyadenylation of the 3' end of the message, is indicated by two unique but informative patients with β^+-thalassemia (Table 11–4). One Asian patient was discovered to have an A→C transversion in the first nucleotide of the message (the cap site is a purine in 90 percent of eukaryotic messages; Wong et al., 1987). This mutation may impair the addition of the cap, a 7-methylguanosine, thus exposing the RNA to degradation. The polyadenylation of mRNA occurs after its enzymatic cleavage, and the signal for the cleavage site, AAUAAA, is found near the 3' end of most eukaryotic mRNAs. A patient with a substitution that changed the signal sequence to AACAAA produced only a minor fraction of β-globin mRNA that was polyadenylated at the normal position.

CONCLUSION

In retrospect, it is fortunate that the hemoglobinopathies were the first group of genetic diseases to be examined at a molecular level, because they exhibit such a diversity of molecular pathology. Most other genetic conditions have been found to result from mechanisms of altered gene function that have already been recognized, in some form, in a hemoglobin disorder. Thus although the he-

---

The Hemoglobinopathies: Models of Interallelic and Intergenic Interaction

GENETIC COMPOUNDS AT THE BETA-GLOBIN LOCUS

Clinical heterogeneity is frequently due to genetic heterogeneity. One mechanism by which different mutations can produce phenotypic variation is demonstrated by **genetic compounds** at the β-globin locus. Two or more of the most common β-globin mutations, such as the mutations leading to Hb C, Hb S, or Hb E, and some of the thalassemia alleles are sometimes present at relatively high frequencies in the same population. Consequently, it is not uncommon to find people in certain parts of the world (e.g., Africa) who are genetic compounds (an alternative term is "compound heterozygotes") for different mutations at the β-globin locus, and who have clinical phenotypes that result from the interaction of the two different mutant alleles. For example, patients with both sickle cell (β^S) and β-thalassemia alleles have phenotypes that vary in severity depending on the particular β-thalassemia mutation that they have inherited; those with a severe thalassemia allele have a disorder that resembles sickle cell disease. A similar situation prevails with Hb E:β thalassemia genetic compounds.

MODIFICATION OF CLINICAL EXPRESSION BY INTERACTION BETWEEN ALPHA- AND BETA-GLOBIN MUTANTS

The geographic distributions of many of the common α- and β-globin mutant alleles frequently overlap (e.g., in the Mediterranean). As a result, occasional patients who have coinherited mutations at both the α- and β-globin loci are recognized. The study of such patients has indicated that significant modification of the biochemical and clinical phenotype of mutations at one locus can occur when the other locus also has a mutant allele. For example, β-thalassemia homozygotes who also inherit an α-thalassemia allele sometimes have less severe disease. The imbalance of globin chain synthesis that occurs in β-thalassemia, reflecting the relative excess of α chains, is ameliorated by the decrease in α-chain production that results from the α-thalassemia mutation. This example of gene interaction illustrates, at a molecular level, why the same mutant gene may have variable phenotypic effects in different individuals, even different affected members of a single family. Variable expressivity and penetrance in other disorders may sometimes be due to comparable interactions between gene products.

moglobinopathies are paradigms for the genetic and mutational basis of "molecular disease," the biochemical pathology of each disease reflects different and often unique aspects of the structure and function of the protein altered by the mutation. The next chapter extends the concepts learned from the hemoglobinopathies, and by describing some of the most important genetic diseases that are understood at a biochemical and molecular level, provides an overview of the pathophysiology that results from mutations in various classes of proteins.

General References

Bunn HF, Forget BG (1986) Hemoglobin; molecular, genetic, and clinical aspects. WB Saunders, Philadelphia.

Kazazian HH Jr (1990) The thalassemia syndromes: Molecular basis and prenatal diagnosis in 1990. *In* Miescher LA, Jaffé ER (eds) Seminars in Hematology 27(3). WB Saunders, Philadelphia, pp. 209–228.

McKusick VA (1990) Mendelian inheritance in man, 9th ed. Johns Hopkins University Press, Baltimore.

Orkin SH (1987) Disorders of hemoglobin synthesis: the thalassemias. *In* Stamatoyannopoulos G, Nienhuis AW, Leder P, Majerus PW (eds) The molecular basis of blood diseases. WB Saunders, Philadelphia, pp. 106–126.

Perutz MF (1987) Molecular anatomy, physiology, and pathology of hemoglobin. *In* Stamatoyannopoulos G, Nienhuis AW, Leder P, Majerus PW (eds) The molecular basis of blood diseases. WB Saunders, Philadelphia, pp. 127–178.

Schechter AN, Noguchi CT, Rodgers GP (1987) Sickle cell disease. *In* Stamatoyannopoulos G, Nienhuis AW, Leder P, Majerus PW (eds) The molecular basis of blood diseases. WB Saunders, Philadelphia, pp. 179–218.

Stamatoyannopoulos G, Nienhuis AW (1987) Hemoglobin switching. *In* Stamatoyannopoulos G, Nienhuis AW, Leder P, Majerus PW (eds) The molecular basis of blood diseases. WB Saunders, Philadelphia, pp. 66–105.

Weatherall DJ, Clegg JB, Higgs DR, Wood WG (1989) The hemoglobinopathies. *In* Scriver CR, Beaudet AL, Sly WS, Valle D (eds) The metabolic basis of inherited disease, 6th ed. McGraw-Hill, New York, pp. 629–663.

Problems

1. A child dies of hydrops fetalis. Draw a pedigree with genotypes that illustrates to the carrier parents the genetic basis of the infant's thalassemia. Explain why a Melanesian couple whom they met in the hematology clinic, who also have the α-thalassemia trait, are unlikely to have a similarly affected infant.

2. Why are most β-thalassemia patients likely to be genetic compounds? In what situations might you anticipate that a β-thalassemia patient would be likely to have two identical β-globin alleles?

3. Tony, a young Italian boy, is found to have moderate β-thalassemia, with a Hb of 7 gm/dL (normal amounts are 10 to 13 gm/dL). When you perform a Northern blot of his reticulocyte RNA, you unexpectedly find three β-globin mRNA bands, one of normal size, one larger than normal, and one smaller than normal.

   What mutational mechanisms could account for the presence of three bands like this in a β-thalassemia patient? In *this* patient, the fact that the anemia is mild suggests that a significant fraction of normal β-globin mRNA is being made. What types of mutation would allow this to occur?

4. A man is heterozygous for Hb M Saskatoon, a hemoglobinopathy in which the normal amino acid His is replaced by Tyr at position 63 of the β-chain. His mate is heterozygous for Hb M Boston, in which His is replaced by Tyr at position 58 of the α-chain. Heterozygosity for either of these mutant alleles produces methemoglobinemia. Outline the possible genotypes and phenotypes of their offspring.

5. A child has a paternal uncle and a maternal aunt with sickle cell disease. What is the probability that the child has sickle cell disease?

6. A woman has sickle cell trait and her mate is heterozygous for Hb C. What is the probability that their child has no abnormal hemoglobin?

7. Match the following:

——— complex β-thalassemia	1. Detectable Hb A
——— β^+-thalassemia	2. Three
——— number of α-globin genes missing in Hb H disease	3. β-thalassemia
——— two different mutant alleles at a locus	4. α-thalassemia
——— prenatal diagnosis of sickle cell disease	5. High-level β-chain expression
——— insoluble β-chains	6. α-thalassemia trait
——— number of α-globin genes missing in hydrops fetalis with Hb Bart's	7. Genetic compound
——— locus control region	8. $\delta\beta$ genes deleted
——— $\alpha-/\alpha-$ genotype	9. Four
——— increased Hb A_2	10. Restriction enzyme *Mst*II

CHAPTER
12

THE MOLECULAR AND BIOCHEMICAL BASIS OF GENETIC DISEASE

MUTATION→ALTERED PROTEIN→ABNORMAL FUNCTION→DISEASE

The examination of the molecular and biochemical basis of genetic disease that began with the hemoglobinopathies (Chapter 11) is extended in this chapter to other proteins and their corresponding diseases. The chapter is divided in two sections. In the first section, "Diseases Due to Mutations in Different Classes of Proteins," we describe several major genetic diseases that illustrate how mutations in different classes of proteins disrupt cell and organ function. Although the hemoglobins have taught geneticists much about inherited disease, different lessons have often come from the study of other disorders, including enzymopathies such as phenylketonuria, receptor defects including the one responsible for familial hypercholesterolemia, conditions that affect molecular transport (for example, cystic fibrosis), and mutations in structural proteins, including disorders of dystrophin in Duchenne muscular dystrophy and the defects of collagen that cause osteogenesis imperfecta.

In the second section, "How Proteins Are Altered in Genetic Disease," we present a general approach for understanding how proteins are altered by genetic disease, and we provide a framework for classifying these diverse effects. The increase in medical knowledge, exemplified by molecular genetics, necessitates that medical science be taught, as much as possible, in terms of concepts and principles. There are more than 500 single-gene traits in which the biochemical defect is partly or largely understood, and it would be impossible to remember the molecular pathology and pathophysiology of each one, or even of every biochemical category of disease. Furthermore, because there are at least 3000 known diseases in which the biochemical defect remains to be identified and between 50,000 and 100,000 genes, many of which will be shown in the coming decades to be implicated in genetically determined conditions, there is a great need for general frameworks into which new knowledge can be placed. We outline the mechanisms by which mutations impair the synthesis, processing, or molecular associations of proteins, and the consequent effects on protein function. The relationships between a molecular defect and the location and nature of its clinical pathology are also examined.

271

DISEASES DUE TO MUTATIONS IN DIFFERENT CLASSES OF PROTEINS

Proteins carry out an astounding number of different functions, some of which are presented in Table 12–1. As the list indicates, mutations in virtually every class of protein can lead to genetic disease. The recognition that a disease results from abnormality in a protein of a particular class is often useful in understanding its pathogenesis and inheritance, and in devising therapy. In this section, we describe important genetic diseases that affect representative proteins from each of the groups. For the most part, we have chosen to use common or important diseases for illustration, but

Table 12–1. Some Functional Classes of Proteins, With Corresponding Diseases

Function		Examples of Proteins Affected by Mutations (Disease)	Inheritance
Enzymes	Literally hundreds, in all areas of metabolism, including		
	Amino acids	• phenylalanine hydroxylase (PKU)	AR
	Carbohydrates	• galactose-1-phosphate uridyl transferase (galactosemia)	AR
	Organic acids	• methylmalonyl-CoA mutase (methylmalonic aciduria)	AR
	Lipids	• medium chain acyl CoA dehydrogenase (MCAD deficiency)	AR
	Complex lipids	• hexosaminidase A (Tay-Sachs disease)	AR
	Purines	• adenosine deaminase (severe combined immunodeficiency)	AR
	Porphyrins	• porphobilinogen deaminase (acute intermittent porphyria)	AD
Transport	Interorgan	• hemoglobin (the thalassemias, hemoglobin variants)	AR
	Organelle membrane	• a lysosomal cystine transport protein (cystinosis)	AR
	Intracellular transport	• a copper transport protein (Menkes syndrome)	XR
	Epithelial membrane	• a protein involved in chloride transport in lung, sweat gland and pancreas (cystic fibrosis)	AR
Structure of cells and organs	Extracellular	• types I and II collagen (osteogenesis imperfecta)	AR, AD
		• type III collagen (Ehlers-Danlos syndrome type IV)	AD
	Cell membrane and cytoskeleton	• the red cell membrane skeleton protein, spectrin (hereditary spherocytosis)	AD
		• dystrophin (Duchenne/Becker muscular dystrophy)	XR
	Organelle	• a protein required for peroxisome biogenesis (Zellweger syndrome)	AR
Extracellular homeostasis	Immune protection	• proteins of the complement system (e.g., complement C3 deficiency → recurrent bacterial infections)	AD, AR
	Hemostasis	• Factor VIII (hemophilia A)	XR
	Protease inhibition	• alpha₁-antitrypsin (deficiency → lung and liver disease)	AR
Control of growth and differentiation	Tumor suppressors	• Rb protein (retinoblastoma and osteosarcoma)	AD
	Oncogenes	• c-*abl* proto-oncogene (translocation to chromosome 22 → a hybrid oncogene → chronic myelogenous leukemia)	Somatic mutation
Intercellular metabolism and communication	Light receptors	• rhodopsin (one form of AD retinitis pigmentosa)	AD
		• green and red light opsins (X-linked color blindness)	XR
	Hormones	• growth hormone (dwarfism)	AR
		• insulin (rare forms of adult-onset diabetes mellitus)	AD
	Hormone receptors	• vitamin D receptor, a DNA binding protein (hypocalcemic vitamin D dependency rickets [type II])	AR
		• androgen receptor (testicular feminization)	XR
		• insulin receptor (leprechaunism)	AR
	Signal transducers	• the stimulatory guanine nucleotide-binding protein of adenylate cyclase (pseudohypoparathyroidism)	AD
		• defective cyclic AMP response to vasopressin (diabetes insipidus)	XR
	Metabolite receptors	• low-density lipoprotein receptor (familial hypercholesterolemia)	AD

The protein classification has been adapted and modified from Stryer L (1981) Biochemistry, 2nd ed. WH Freeman, San Francisco. AD = autosomal dominant; AR = autosomal recessive; XR = X-linked recessive.

rarer conditions are described when they best demonstrate a principle. Not every disease listed in Table 12–1 is reviewed here. The interested reader can find a wealth of information on genetic diseases that are understood at the biochemical level in the comprehensive reference *The Metabolic Basis of Inherited Disease* (Scriver et al., 1989). The treatment of genetic disease, including that of many of the conditions described in this chapter, is presented in Chapter 13.

ENZYME DEFECTS

Enzymes are the catalysts that mediate, with great rapidity, the chemical reactions that occur in biological systems. Apart from the recently discovered catalytic ribonucleic acids (RNAs) involved in RNA processing, enzymes are proteins. The diversity of substrates on which enzymes act is only superficially indicated in Table 12–1; the list includes only a few important enzymopathies, which presently number in the hundreds. One of the best-known groups of inborn errors of metabolism, the hyperphenylalaninemias that arise from deficient activity of phenylalanine hydroxyl-

ase, is discussed first; several additional enzyme defects of significance are then briefly examined. In a summary section, general features of the pathophysiology of enzymopathies are presented.

Aminoacidopathies

The Hyperphenylalaninemias

The abnormalities that lead to an increase in the blood level of phenylalanine, most notably **phenylketonuria**, or PKU (see box, Chapter 4), illustrate almost every principle of biochemical genetics of relevance to enzyme defects. Indeed, PKU has been justifiably termed the epitome of inborn errors of metabolism (Scriver et al., 1989).

Phenylketonuria (PKU). Classic PKU, an autosomal recessive disorder of phenylalanine catabolism, results from mutation in phenylalanine hydroxylase, the enzyme that converts phenylalanine to tyrosine (Fig. 12–1). The discovery of PKU by Fölling in 1934 marked the first demonstration of a genetic defect as a cause of mental retardation. Because phenylalanine cannot be degraded by patients with PKU, it accumulates in body fluids,

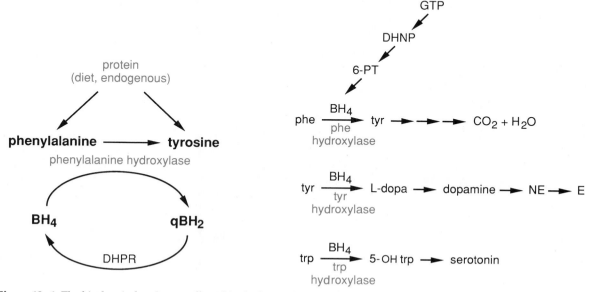

Figure 12–1. The biochemical pathways affected in the hyperphenylalaninemias. BH_4 = tetrahydrobiopterin; qBH_2 = quininoid dihydrobiopterin, the oxidized product of the hydroxylation reactions, which is reduced to BH_4 by dihydropteridine reductase (DHPR); phe = phenylalanine; tyr = tyrosine; trp = tryptophan; L-dopa = L-dihydroxyphenylalanine; NE = norepinephrine; E = epinephrine; 5-OH trp = 5-hydroxytryptophan; GTP = guanosine triphosphate; DHNP = dihydroneopterin triphosphate; 6-PT = 6-pyruvoyltetrahydropterin.

damaging the developing central nervous system in early childhood, and interfering with the function of the mature brain. A small fraction is metabolized by alternative pathways, producing increased amounts of phenylpyruvic acid (a keto acid and the compound responsible for the name of the disease) and other minor metabolites, which are excreted in the urine. Ironically, despite the fact that the enzymatic defect has been known for decades, the exact biochemical mechanism by which the increase in phenylalanine damages the brain is still unknown. The neurological damage due to the metabolic block in classic PKU may be largely avoided by dietary modifications that prevent phenylalanine accumulation. The management of PKU is a paradigm of the treatment of many metabolic diseases whose outcome can be improved by preventing accumulation of an enzyme substrate and its derivatives, and it is described further in Chapter 13.

Newborn Screening. Population screening of newborns for PKU is done widely. PKU is the prototype of genetic diseases for which mass newborn screening is appropriate (see Chapter 18): the disorder is relatively common (approximately 1/10,000 live births); treatment, if begun early in life, is effective; and without treatment, severe retardation is inevitable. The screening test is performed a few days after birth, usually before the infant leaves the hospital. A droplet of blood is obtained from a heel prick, dried on filter paper, and sent to central laboratories for assay of blood phenylalanine levels. Positive test results must be confirmed quickly because delays in the initiation of treatment have profound effects on the intellectual outcome of PKU patients.

Benign Hyperphenylalaninemia. Whereas PKU results from a virtually complete loss of phenylalanine hydroxylase activity (less than 1 percent), less severe phenotypes result when there is some residual phenylalanine hydroxylase activity. If the residual activity is about 5 percent of control levels, the plasma phenylalanine concentration is only about tenfold above normal (about 1 mM) when the patient is on a normal diet, much lower than the concentrations found in classic PKU (2 to 3 mM). This moderate increase in phenylalanine does not damage the brain, and affected individuals, who are said to have benign hyperphenylalaninemia, come to clinical attention only because they are identified by newborn screening. Their normal phenotype has been the best indication of the "safe" level of plasma phenylalanine (less than 1 mM) that must not be exceeded in the treatment of patients with classic PKU.

GENETIC HETEROGENEITY IN THE HYPERPHENYLALANINEMIAS

The Molecular Defects in Phenylalanine Hydroxylase (PAH). Only four alleles account for the great majority of defects at the PAH locus in individuals of northern European descent (Table 12–2). The most common mutation, a defect in the exon 12 donor splice site, causes skipping of the 12th exon during RNA splicing. The aberrant

Table 12–2. Phenylalanine Hydroxylase (PAH) Gene: RFLP Haplotypes, Mutations, and Clinical Phenotypes

PAH RFLP Haplotype	Northern Europe: Frequency on Chromosomes with Normal PAH Alleles*	Northern Europe: Frequency on Chromosomes with a Mutant PAH Allele*	Northern Europe: Mutation Associated with Haplotype	Clinical Phenotype of Homozygotes
1	35%	18%	261Arg → Gln	Benign hyperphenylalaninemia
2	5%	20%	408Arg → Trp	Classic PKU
3	3%	38%	Exon 12 donor splice site GT → AT	Classic PKU
4	32%	14%	158Arg → Gln	Mild PKU

* These are not all the haplotypes found in northern Europe, but they account for almost 90% of the mutant PAH alleles in the population. Based on data from Scriver et al. (1989), Okano et al. (1990a), and Okano et al. (1990b).

mRNA thus formed contains a premature translational stop and generates a truncated and unstable protein.

In northern Europe, the four principal alleles are largely restricted to specific haplotypes (Table 12–2), although more than 40 restriction fragment length polymorphism (RFLP) haplotypes around the PAH gene have now been identified (Scriver et al., 1989). As discussed in Chapter 8, the fact that a mutation is often associated with a particular haplotype *in a specific population* facilitates the identification of the mutation in an affected individual, making possible prenatal diagnosis, carrier testing, and analysis of the allele frequency in the population. The association of a specific mutation with a particular haplotype in different population subgroups suggests that the mutation originally occurred on a chromosome with that haplotype (see Chapter 8); in the case of PKU, the data suggest single origins for several alleles in northern Europe. Examination of other populations indicates that the four common northern European mutations do not necessarily occur on chromosomes with the same haplotypes as in northern Europe (Rey et al., 1988). Consequently, one cannot assume that a particular haplotype is associated with a particular mutation, except in well-defined populations.

In groups other than northern Europeans, there is substantial genetic heterogeneity in the PAH mutant population (Rey et al., 1988; Scriver et al., 1989; Okano et al., 1990a, 1990b). For example, in mixed populations of southern and northern European ancestry in France, only two thirds of the mutant alleles are found on the four haplotypes that predominate in Denmark (Rey et al., 1988), the remainder being accounted for by 12 other haplotypes. Consequently, on the basis of haplotype analysis, in most populations the majority of patients with PAH mutations are **genetic compounds** (i.e., have two different abnormal alleles), a finding entirely in agreement with enzymatic and clinical observations of phenotypic heterogeneity in PAH defects.

Defects in Tetrahydrobiopterin (BH₄) Metabolism. It was initially thought that all children with hereditary hyperphenylalaninemia had a primary deficiency of PAH. It is now clear, however, that in about 1 to 3 percent of these patients the PAH gene is normal, and their hyperphenylalaninemia is the result of a genetic defect in the formation of the cofactor of PAH, tetrahydrobiopterin (BH_4) (Fig. 12–1). BH_4-deficient patients were first recognized because, despite the successful administration of a low-phenylalanine diet, they developed profound neurological problems in the first year of life. This poor outcome is due to the requirement of two other enzymes, tyrosine hydroxylase and tryptophan hydroxylase, for the BH_4 cofactor. Both of these hydroxylases are critical for the synthesis of monoamine neurotransmitters such as dopa, norepinephrine, epinephrine, and serotonin (Fig. 12–1).

BH_4-deficient patients have defects either in one of the steps in the biosynthesis of BH_4 from guanosine triphosphate (GTP) or in the regeneration of BH_4 by dihydropteridine reductase (DHPR) (Fig. 12–1). It is critical to recognize these conditions because their treatment differs markedly from that for classic PKU. For this reason, all hyperphenylalaninemic infants should be screened for BH_4 deficiency. Apart from controlling the blood phenylalanine levels, the object of therapy for these patients is to try to normalize the neurotransmitters in the brain by administering the products of tyrosine hydroxylase and tryptophan hydroxylase, L-dopa and 5-hydroxytryptophan, respectively. Like classic PKU, these disorders are inherited as autosomal recessive traits.

Maternal PKU. The generally successful treatment of PKU allows affected homozygotes to lead an independent life and have near-normal prospects for marriage and parenthood. Because phenylketonurics who have been effectively managed from birth function well in so many ways, it was disconcerting to discover that almost all the offspring of female phenylketonurics not on a low-phenylalanine diet are abnormal, with mental retardation (92 percent), microcephaly, growth impairment, and malformations, particularly of the heart (Lenke and Levy, 1980). Most of these children are heterozygotes. Their retardation is due not to their own genetic constitution but to the highly teratogenic effect of elevated levels of phenylalanine in the maternal circulation. Accordingly, it is imperative that PKU women planning pregnancies commence a low-phenylalanine diet before conceiving.

Prenatal Diagnosis of Defects That Cause Hyperphenylalaninemia. The cloning of the human phenylalanine hydroxylase gene allowed prenatal diagnosis of classic PKU, which was not previously possible because PAH is not expressed in amniocytes (see Chapter 19). Fetal diagnosis is now feasible in most families with at least one affected child by taking advantage of the linkage disequilibrium that exists between specific alleles and certain PAH RFLP haplotypes in some populations, as outlined earlier. Characterization of the mutations in a family permits more specific molecular diagnosis. Prenatal diagnosis is also available for all the defects that lead to BH_4 deficiency.

Defects in Purine Metabolism

Lesch-Nyhan Syndrome

Between the extremes of phenotype produced by the complete functional deficiency of a protein and mutations that produce no clinical abnormalities, a variety of clinical phenotypes of intermediate severity may be found. A dramatic illustration of such phenotypic variation is provided by individuals with deficiency of the X-linked enzyme hypoxanthine guanine phosphoribosyltransferase (HPRT) (Fig. 12–2). Patients with no residual HPRT activity have a remarkable phenotype called the Lesch-Nyhan syndrome, characterized by choreoathetosis (a movement disorder), spasticity, variable mental retardation, uric acid overproduction that causes gout, and, most striking, self-mutilation. The neurological abnormalities may result from changes in brain purine levels produced by the disease, consistent with the theory that some purines are putative neurotransmitters. In contrast to Lesch-Nyhan patients, persons with levels of HPRT activity ranging from approximately 1 to 30 percent of normal present only with gout, as a result of uric acid overproduction, and with none of the more dramatic neurological findings. Partial HPRT deficiency of this type, however, accounts for less than 2 percent of all adult male patients with gout. Patients with HPRT deficiency also illustrate how loss of normal feedback inhibition on the regulation of a metabolic pathway can have pathophysiological consequences, an important principle of biochemical genetic disease (Fig. 12–2).

Lysosomal Storage Diseases

Lysosomes are membrane-bound organelles containing an array of hydrolytic enzymes involved in

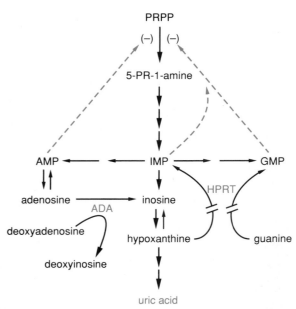

Figure 12–2. An outline of the purine synthetic pathway. In the absence of HPRT, the ability to reutilize hypoxanthine and guanine to make IMP and GMP is lost. As a consequence, the normal feedback inhibition by IMP and GMP (broken arrows) on an early step in purine synthesis is greatly reduced, and the de novo synthesis of purines, and ultimately uric acid, is increased (heavy central arrows). PRPP = phosphoribosylpyrophosphate; AMP = adenosine monophosphate; IMP = inosine monophosphate; GMP = guanosine monophosphate; ADA = adenosine deaminase; HPRT = hypoxanthine guanine phosphoribosyltransferase.

the degradation of a variety of biological macromolecules. Genetic defects of these hydrolases lead to the accumulation of their substrates inside the lysosome, resulting in cellular dysfunction and, eventually, cell death. The gradual accumulation of the substrate is responsible for the one uniform clinical feature of these diseases: their unrelenting progression. In most of these conditions, substrate storage is manifested clinically as an increase in the mass of the affected tissues and organs. When the brain is affected, as is often the case, the picture is one of neurodegeneration. The clinical phenotypes often make the diagnosis of a storage disease straightforward and usually suggest the disease category, if not the specific disorder.

Another prominent feature of lysosomal storage diseases is their clinical and genetic heterogeneity. Different defects in one gene (**allelic heterogeneity**) may cause both severe phenotypes with onset in infancy and disorders with onset in adult life, as well as a range of intermediate presentations. The **clinical heterogeneity** is usually due to very small variations in the amount of residual enzyme activity. Alternatively, a single phenotype may result from defects in separately encoded enzymes (**locus heterogeneity**) that act at different steps in a catabolic pathway. More than two dozen lysosomal hydrolase deficiencies, all of which are recessive in inheritance, have been described.

Tay-Sachs Disease

Tay-Sachs disease is one of a group of heterogeneous lysosomal storage diseases, the G_{M2} gangliosidoses, that result from the inability to degrade a

sphingolipid, G_{M2} ganglioside (Fig. 12–3; Sandhoff et al., 1989). The biochemical lesion is a marked deficiency of hexosaminidase A (hex A). Although the enzyme is ubiquitous, the disease has its clinical impact almost solely on the brain, the predominant site of G_{M2} ganglioside synthesis. Catalytically active hex A is the product of a three-gene system encoding the α and β subunits of the enzyme (the HEXA and HEXB genes, respectively), and an activator protein that must associate with the substrate and the enzyme before the latter can cleave the terminal N-acetyl-β-galactosamine residue from the ganglioside (Fig. 12–3).

The clinical presentations of defects in the three genes are indistinguishable, but they can be differentiated by enzymatic analysis. Mutations in the HEXA gene affect the α subunit and disrupt hex A activity to cause Tay-Sachs disease (or less severe variants of hex A deficiency). Most Tay-

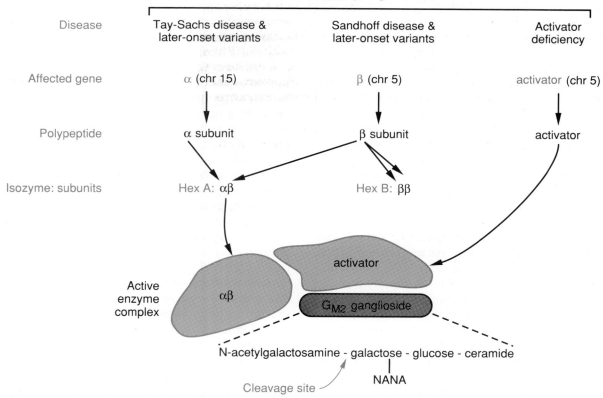

Figure 12–3. The three-gene system required for hexosaminidase A activity, and the diseases that result from defects in each of the genes. The function of the activator protein is to bind the ganglioside substrate and present it to the enzyme. (Modified from Sandhoff K, Conzelmann E, Neufeld EF, et al. [1989] The G_{M2} gangliosidoses. *In* Scriver CR, Beaudet AL, Sly WS, Valle D [eds] The metabolic basis of inherited disease, 6th ed. McGraw-Hill, New York, pp. 1807–1839.)

Table 12–3. Mutant Hexosaminidase A Alleles in Ashkenazi Jewish and Other Populations

Mutation	Effect on Gene Product	Frequency in Ashkenazi Jews	Estimated Frequency in Non-Ashkenazi	Homozygous Phenotype
4 bp insertion (exon 11)	Premature stop codon	79%	15%–20%	Tay-Sachs disease
Exon 12 splice junction: G → C	Defective mRNA splicing	18%	<1%	Tay-Sachs disease
269 Gly → Ser	<3% residual activity	3%	1%	Adult-onset G_{M2} gangliosidosis
Other alleles	Variable	<1%	>80%	Variable

Derived from Triggs-Raine BL, Feigenbaum ASJ, Natowicz M, et al. (1990) Screening for carriers of Tay-Sachs diseases among Ashkenazi Jews. N Engl J Med 323:6–12; and Sandhoff K, Conzelmann E, Neufeld EF, et al. (1989) The G_{M2} gangliosidoses. *In* Scriver CR, Beaudet AL, Sly WS, Valle D (eds) The metabolic basis of inherited disease, 6th ed. McGraw-Hill, New York, pp. 1807–1839.

Sachs alleles lead to a profound deficiency of the α subunit mRNA and of hex A activity (Table 12–3; see Figs. 6–15 and 6–17). Defects in the HEXB gene, or in the gene encoding the activator protein, impair the activity of both hex A and hex B (Fig. 12–3) to produce Sandhoff disease and activator protein deficiency (which is very rare), respectively.

The clinical course of Tay-Sachs disease is particularly tragic. Affected infants appear normal until about 3 to 6 months of age but then gradually undergo progressive neurological deterioration until death at 2 to 4 years. The effects of neuronal cell death can be seen directly in the form of the so-called cherry-red spot in the retina, which is the prominent red macular fovea centralis surrounded by a pale macula.

Multiple alleles have been identified at the HEXA locus and are responsible for remarkable clinical heterogeneity in hex A deficiency. In later-onset variants of the disease, there are small but definite amounts of functioning residual enzyme, and the age of onset of symptoms is roughly proportional to the residual activity. In the adult-onset form, the presentation commonly includes lower motor neuron dysfunction and ataxia due to spinocerebellar degeneration, but in contrast to the infantile disease, vision and intelligence usually remain normal.

Population Genetics. About 1 in 27 Ashkenazi Jews is a carrier of a Tay-Sachs allele, and the incidence of affected infants is 100 times higher than in other populations (Sandhoff et al., 1989). Either founder effect or heterozygote advantage have been considered to be the most likely expla-nations. Molecular analysis has shown, unexpect-edly, that three alleles account for 99 percent of the mutations in all Ashkenazi Jewish patients and carriers (Table 12–3) (Triggs-Raine et al., 1990). It therefore appears that a full interpretation of the high frequency of the disease in the Ashkenazi Jewish population is not yet possible. The presence of three alleles does not necessarily confirm the heterozygote advantage hypothesis, since they may each owe their frequency to founder effect. A practical benefit of the molecular characterization of the disease is the greater precision that it will lend to carrier screening in the Ashkenazi Jewish population.

The Mucopolysaccharidoses

Mucopolysaccharides, or glycosaminoglycans (GAGs), are polysaccharide chains synthesized by connective tissue cells as normal constituents of many tissues. They are made up of long disaccha-ride repeating units; the nature of the two sugar molecules is the distinguishing feature of a specific GAG. The degradation of these macromolecules requires the stepwise removal of the monosaccha-ride unit at the end of the chain by an enzyme specific to the monosaccharide and the bond in-volved. A series of enzymes is thus required for the degradation of any one GAG, and a single enzyme often participates in the catabolism of more than one GAG.

The mucopolysaccharidoses are a heteroge-neous group of storage diseases in which muco-polysaccharides accumulate in lysosomes as a re-sult of a deficiency of one of the enzymes required for their degradation (Table 12–4). In a specific mucopolysaccharidosis, one or more GAGs may accumulate if the defective enzyme is required for their catabolism. The nondegraded GAGs appear in the urine, in which they can be detected by screening tests. These disorders, like many other genetic diseases, include examples of both locus and allelic heterogeneity.

The first two mucopolysaccharidoses to be recognized were X-linked recessive **Hunter syndrome** in 1917 and the more severe autosomal recessive **Hurler syndrome** in 1919. Each of these conditions was originally called "gargoylism" because of the coarseness of the facial features of affected individuals (Fig. 12–4). Affected children are mentally retarded, have skeletal abnormalities and short stature, and have other abnormalities listed in Table 12–4.

Hurler syndrome is due to a severe deficiency of α-L-iduronidase. A clinically distinct disorder, **Scheie syndrome,** was originally thought to involve a different locus, principally because of its much milder phenotype. However, the Scheie and Hurler syndromes are allelic, but the α-L-iduronidase mutations that cause Scheie syndrome may be associated with higher residual activity. An intermediate phenotype, Hurler/Scheie syndrome, may, in at least some cases, be a genetic compound of Hurler and Scheie alleles. It could also result from two alleles with activity intermediate between Hurler and Scheie alleles.

The difference in the pattern of inheritance of the autosomal Hurler and X-linked Hunter syndromes indicated that they were due to defects in different proteins. This difference was demonstrated in another way by Neufeld and her col-

Table 12–4. Examples of Mucopolysaccharidoses

Syndrome	Clinical Features	Enzyme Defect; Stored/Excreted Mucopolysaccharide	Genetics	Comment
Hurler	Diagnosed at 6–18 months, corneal clouding, skeletal changes on X-ray called dysostosis multiplex, hepatosplenomegaly, coarse facies, stiff joints, nasal discharge, hydrocephalus, death <10 years	α-L-iduronidase; dermatan sulfate, heparan sulfate	AR	Probably due to any allele that abolishes the activity of the enzyme; most patients are likely to be genetic compounds
Scheie	Onset after age 5 years, normal intelligence and life span, corneal clouding, stiff joints, valvular heart disease, visual impairment	α-L-iduronidase; dermatan sulfate, heparan sulfate	AR	Complementation tests show that this milder phenotype involves the same gene locus as Hurler syndrome
Hurler/Scheie	Intermediate phenotype between Hurler and Scheie syndrome	α-L-iduronidase; dermatan sulfate, heparan sulfate	AR	Some cases are probably genetic compounds of Hurler and Scheie alleles
Hunter	Similar to Hurler syndrome but with slower progression, no corneal clouding, and a unique pebbly skin lesion	Iduronate sulfatase; dermatan sulfate, heparan sulfate	XR	A milder phenotype without central nervous system disease also occurs, with a much less aggressive somatic course
Sanfilippo A	Hyperactivity and retardation, progressive neurodegeneration; mild somatic features → underdiagnosis	Heparan N-sulfatase; heparan sulfate	AR	On the whole, the most severe of the four very similar types of Sanfilippo syndrome
Sanfilippo B	Similar to Sanfilippo A syndrome	α-N-acetylglucosaminidase; heparan sulfate	AR	Probably the most heterogeneous of the four types of the syndrome, even within a family

AR = autosomal recessive; XR = X-linked recessive.
Modified from Neufeld EF, Muenzer J (1989) The mucopolysaccharidoses. *In* Scriver CR, Beaudet AL, Sly WS, Valle D (eds) The metabolic basis of inherited disease, 6th ed. McGraw-Hill, New York, pp. 1565–1587.

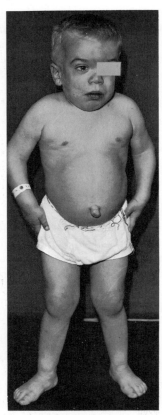

Figure 12–4. A child with Hurler syndrome, showing the typical coarse facial features. At 5 years of age, he is only as tall as a typical 3-year-old. (From Smith DW [1982] Recognizable patterns of human malformation, 3rd ed. WB Saunders, Philadelphia.)

leagues, who showed in cell culture that although fibroblasts from patients of either type accumulated mucopolysaccharides in the culture medium, the accumulation could be corrected by cocultivation of both cell types in the same culture dish. The interpretation, which proved correct, was that the lysosomal enzyme deficient in one mutant cell type was taken up from the medium, into which it had been released by the other cell type. This simple experiment was a powerful demonstration that the two diseases affected different proteins. In contrast, cocultivation of Scheie and Hurler cells failed to induce any biochemical correction, indicating, as enzyme assays later showed, that they were due to defects in the same protein.

The observation that a cell can take up the lysosomal enzyme that it lacks from the extracellular fluid offers hope that the transplantation of normal cells into patients with storage diseases

may allow correction of the biochemical defect in the rest of the body. Encouraging initial results have been obtained in some mucopolysaccharidosis patients treated by bone marrow transplantation (see Chapter 13).

Another mucopolysaccharidosis, **Sanfilippo syndrome,** illustrates the locus heterogeneity that can underlie a relatively homogeneous clinical phenotype. An important clinical feature of Sanfilippo patients is that intellectual and behavioral abnormalities are evident well before physical changes, which tend to be mild. Initially regarded as a single entity, this syndrome can result from one of four enzyme deficiencies, two of which are outlined in Table 12–4. The clinical phenotypes of individual patients provide little basis for suggesting which enzyme (and, therefore, which gene) is defective.

Complementation Analysis of Human Genetic Disease

In the cocultivation experiments just described, the geneticists examined an issue that commonly arises in the study of patients with genetic disease: do two individuals with what appears to be the same disorder have defects in the same gene? If mutual correction occurs, the genetic defects are said to complement one another, and the affected genes must be different. Experiments of this type are called **complementation tests.** Their utility lies in the fact that they require no knowledge of the affected genes or proteins, but only the ability to examine the cells for the correction of a mutant phenotype: in the case of the mucopolysaccharide storage diseases, the reduction of mucopolysaccharide accumulation. Complementation analysis has been used to dissect the genetic basis of many human genetic diseases.

If there is doubt that the corrective factor can be transferred through the culture medium, the different cells can be fused to form a heterokaryon, in which both nuclei are inside a single cell (Chapter 8). Experiments of this type have demonstrated that **xeroderma pigmentosum** (XP), a rare disease associated with a 2000-fold increased frequency of sunlight-induced skin cancer, is caused by mutation in one of at least nine genes (which probably all encode enzymes) important for DNA excision repair. People with mild defects may have only a heightened sensitivity to sunlight, whereas severely affected patients are subject to severe sunburn in infancy, abnormal freckling and skin atrophy, and ultimately, in the worst cases, various tumors (carcinomas, melanomas, and internal neoplasms) as well.

On occasion, complementation tests in heterokaryons yield positive results even if the muta-

tions in the two groups of mutant cells affect the same gene. In this instance, the complementation is said to be *intragenic* (vs. *intergenic*) and demonstrates that the patients have allelic mutations. Intragenic complementation occurs only when the affected proteins are homomultimers, indicating that the mutant subunit from one allele interacts

Enzyme Deficiencies and Disease: General Concepts

The following concepts are fundamental to understanding and treating enzymopathies:

1. **Enzymopathies are almost always recessive.** Most enzymes are produced in quantities significantly in excess of minimal biochemical requirements, so that heterozygotes with about 50 percent of residual activity are clinically normal. In fact, many enzymes may maintain normal substrate and product levels with activities of less than 10 percent. The enzymes of porphyrin synthesis are exceptions, an observation which is understandable when it is recognized that they can each limit the rate of porphyrin synthesis (discussed later in this chapter).

2. **Substrate accumulation or product deficiency.** Because the function of an enzyme is to convert a substrate to a product, all of the pathophysiological consequences of enzymopathies can be attributed either to the accumulation of the substrate, to the deficiency of the product, or to some combination of the two (Fig. 12–5).

3. **Diffusible versus macromolecular substrates.** A important distinction can be made between enzyme defects in which the substrate is a "small" molecule, such as phenylalanine, that can be readily distributed throughout body fluids by diffusion or transport, and defects in which the substrate is a macromolecule, such as a mucopolysaccharide, that remains trapped within its organelle or cell. The pathology of the macromolecular diseases is confined to the tissues in which the substrate accumulates, whereas the site of the disease in the small molecule disorders is often unpredict-

able because the unmetabolized substrate, or its derivatives, can move freely throughout the body, damaging cells that may normally have no relationship to the affected enzyme.

4. **Loss of multiple enzyme activities.** A single patient may have defects in more than one enyzme. There are several possible mechanisms: (a) several enzymes may utilize the same cofactor (e.g., BH_4 deficiency); (b) two or more enzymes may share a common subunit or an activating, processing, or stabilizing protein (e.g., the G_{M2} gangliosidoses); (c) multiple enzymes may be processed by a common modifying enzyme, and in its absence they may not become active, or their uptake into an organelle may be impaired (e.g., I-cell disease, described below in the section "How Proteins Are Altered in Genetic Disease"); and (d) a group of enzymes may be absent or ineffective if the organelle in which they are normally found is defective (e.g., the disorders of peroxisome biogenesis discussed below).

5. **Phenotypic homology.** The pathological and clinical features resulting from an enzyme defect are often shared by (a) diseases due to deficiencies of other enzymes that function in the same area of metabolism (e.g., the mucopolysaccharidoses) and (b) the different diseases that may result from partial and complete defects of the enzyme. Partial defects often present with clinical abnormalities that are a subset of those found with the complete deficiency, although the etiological relationship between the two diseases may not be immediately obvious (e.g., partial HPRT deficiency and Lesch-Nyhan syndrome).

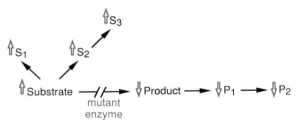

Figure 12-5. A model metabolic pathway showing that the potential effects of an enzyme deficiency include accumulation of the substrate (S) or derivatives of it (S1, S2, S3), or deficiency of the product (P) or compounds (P1, P2) made from it. In some cases, the substrate derivatives are normally only minor metabolites that are formed at increased rates when the substrate accumulates (e.g., phenylpyruvate in PKU).

with the mutant subunit from the other allele in a way that improves the function of the multimeric protein.

DEFECTS IN RECEPTOR PROTEINS

The recognition of a class of diseases due to defects in receptor molecules began with the identification, by Goldstein and Brown in 1974, of the low-density lipoprotein (LDL) receptor as the polypeptide affected in familial hypercholesterolemia (see box in Chapter 4). Their discovery has cast much light on normal cholesterol metabolism and on the biology of cell surface receptors in general. LDL receptor deficiency is representative of a number of disorders now recognized to result from receptor defects, some of which are listed in Table 12-1.

Familial Hypercholesterolemia: A Genetic Hyperlipoproteinemia

The genetic hyperlipoproteinemias are of clinical significance because of their role in myocardial infarction, a major cause of death and disability. Hyperlipoproteinemias are characterized by elevated levels of plasma lipids (cholesterol, triglycerides, or both) and specific plasma lipoproteins. A number of distinct single-gene forms with different biochemical and clinical phenotypes have been defined, although in some cases the phenotypes have not yet been completely characterized. At each locus there may well be more than one mutant allele.

Familial hypercholesterolemia is one of several disorders grouped as familial type 2 hyperlipoproteinemia. It is characterized by elevation of

plasma cholesterol carried by LDL, the principal cholesterol transport protein in plasma (Goldstein and Brown, 1989). The disease is due to mutations in the structural gene encoding the LDL receptor, a cell surface protein responsible for binding LDL and delivering it to the cell interior (Hobbs et al., 1990). Both heterozygotes and homozygotes develop premature heart disease as a result of atheromas (deposits of LDL-derived cholesterol in the coronary arteries), xanthomas (cholesterol deposits in skin and tendons; see Fig. 4-8), and arcus corneae (deposits of cholesterol around the periphery of the cornea). Few diseases have been as thoroughly characterized: the sequence of pathological events from the affected locus to its effect on individuals and populations has been well documented.

Genetics. Familial hypercholesterolemia is

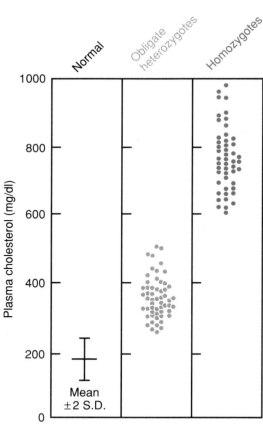

Figure 12-6. Gene dosage in LDL deficiency: the distribution of total plasma cholesterol levels in 49 patients homozygous for deficiency of the LDL receptor, in their parents (obligate heterozygotes), and in normal controls. (Redrawn from Goldstein JL, Brown MS [1989] Familial hypercholesterolemia. *In* Scriver CR, Beaudet AL, Sly WS, Valle D [eds] The metabolic basis of inherited disease, 6th ed. McGraw-Hill, New York, pp. 1215–1250.)

inherited as an autosomal dominant trait. Both homozygous and heterozygous phenotypes are known, and a clear gene dosage effect is evident: the disease presents earlier and much more severely in homozygotes than in heterozygotes (see Fig. 4–8), reflecting the greater reduction in the number of LDL receptors and the greater elevation in plasma LDL-cholesterol (Fig. 12–6). Homozygotes may have clinically significant coronary heart disease in childhood, and few live beyond the third decade. Although the homozygous form is rare (1 person in one million), the heterozygous form, with a population frequency of at least 1 in 500, is one of the most common human single-gene disorders. Because of the genetic nature of

familial hypercholesterolemia, it is important to make the diagnosis in the approximately 5 percent of survivors of myocardial infarction who are heterozygotes. However, only about 1 in 20 individuals in the general population with increased plasma cholesterol and a type 2 hyperlipoprotein pattern has familial hypercholesterolemia, whereas most have an uncharacterized hypercholesterolemia of multifactorial origin.

Cholesterol Uptake by the LDL Receptor. Normal cells obtain cholesterol, an essential lipid component of membranes and a precursor of steroid hormones and bile salts, either by de novo synthesis or by the uptake from plasma of exogenous cholesterol bound to LDL. The uptake proc-

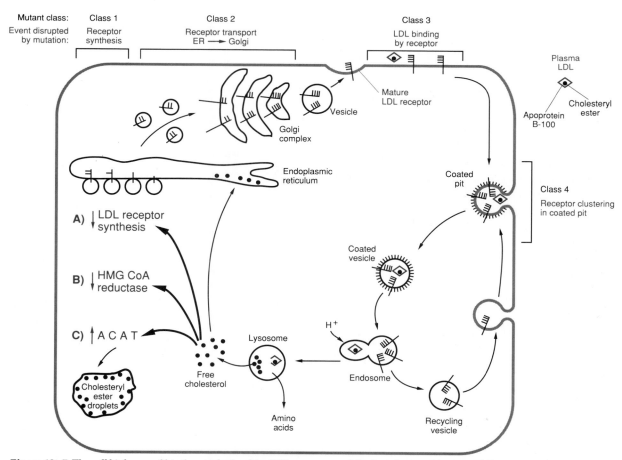

Figure 12–7. The cell biology and biochemical role of the LDL receptor, and the four classes of mutations that alter its function. After synthesis in the endoplasmic reticulum, the receptor is transported to the Golgi apparatus and subsequently to the cell surface. Normal receptors are localized to clathrin-coated pits, which invaginate, creating coated vesicles and then endosomes, the precursors of lysosomes. Normally, intracellular accumulation of free cholesterol is prevented because the increase in free cholesterol (A) decreases the formation of LDL receptors, (B) reduces de novo cholesterol synthesis, and (C) increases the storage of cholesteryl esters. The biochemical phenotype of each class of mutant is discussed in text. (Modified from Brown MS, Goldstein JL [1985] The LDL receptor and HMG-CoA reductase—two membrane molecules that regulate cholesterol homeostasis. Curr Top Cell Regul 26:3–15.)

ess is mediated by the LDL receptor, which recognizes apoprotein B-100, the protein moiety of LDL. The LDL receptors on the cell surface are localized to depressed regions (coated pits) lined by the protein clathrin (Fig. 12–7). Receptor-bound LDL is brought into the cell by invagination of the coated pits, which ultimately evolve into lysosomes in which LDL is hydrolyzed to release free cholesterol. The increase in free intracellular cholesterol reduces endogenous cholesterol formation by suppressing the rate-limiting enzyme of the synthetic pathway (3-hydroxy-3-methylglutaryl coenzyme A reductase, or HMG CoA reductase). Cholesterol not required for cellular metabo-

lism or membrane synthesis may be re-esterified for storage as cholesteryl esters, a process stimulated by the activation of acyl CoA:cholesterol acyltransferase (ACAT). The increase in cholesterol also reduces synthesis of the receptor (Fig. 12–7).

Structure of the LDL Receptor. The mature LDL receptor has five distinct structural domains that, for the most part, have distinguishable functions. Some of these regions are encoded by single exons or by groups of exons that encode regions that are homologous to domains in other polypeptides (Fig. 12–8). Analysis of the effect on the receptor of mutations in the various domains has

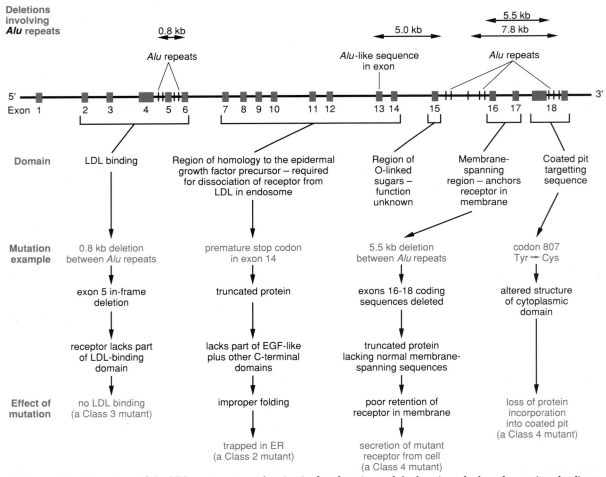

Figure 12–8. The structure of the LDL receptor gene showing its five domains and the location of selected mutations leading to familial hypercholesterolemia. The sizes of various deletions are indicated by the horizontal bars above the gene (with exons indicated in red). Mutations in the exons of the various domains have effects on the receptor consistent with the role of the domain in the biology of the receptor. Exons, introns, and *Alu* repeats are only approximately to scale. (Modified from Goldstein JL, Brown MS [1989] Familial hypercholesterolemia. *In* Scriver CR, Beaudet AL, Sly WS, Valle D [eds] The metabolic basis of inherited disease, 6th ed. McGraw-Hill, New York, pp. 1215–1250.)

played an important part in establishing the function of many of the domains. These studies exemplify the important contribution that genetic analysis can make in determining the structure-function relationships of a protein.

Effect of Mutations on the LDL Receptor. Fibroblasts cultured from affected patients have been used to characterize the mutant receptors and the resulting disturbances in cellular cholesterol metabolism. At least 18 different mutations have been identified, but they can be grouped into four classes, depending on which step of the normal cellular itinerary of the receptor is disrupted by the mutation (Fig. 12–7; Goldstein and Brown, 1989; Hobbs et al., 1990). Class 1 mutations are null alleles that prevent the synthesis of any detectable receptor; they are the most common type of disease-causing mutations at this locus. Some class 1 alleles are due to deletions, whereas others produce normal amounts of LDL-receptor mRNA and presumably have defects that impair the formation or stability of the polypeptide. In the remaining three classes, the receptor is synthesized normally, but its function is impaired.

Mutations in classes 2 and 4 (Fig. 12–7) define features of the polypeptide critical to its subcellular localization. The relatively common class 2 mutations are designated *transport-deficient* because the LDL receptors accumulate at the site of their synthesis, the endoplasmic reticulum, instead of being transported to the Golgi complex. These alleles are predicted to prevent proper folding of the protein, an apparent requisite for exit from the endoplasmic reticulum.

Class 3 mutant receptors reach the cell surface but are incapable of binding LDL (Fig. 12–7). Consequently, these alleles have enabled researchers to identify the LDL-binding domain (Fig. 12–8). In one mutant of this type, an unequal crossover that is due to misalignment and recombination between *Alu* repeat sequences has deleted part of the LDL-binding domain. Homologous recombination between *Alu* repeats has been found to be a general cause of deletions, both in this gene and in others (see Chapter 6).

Class 4 mutations impair localization of the receptor to the coated pit, and consequently the bound LDL is not internalized (Fig. 12–7). These mutations alter or remove the cytoplasmic domain at the carboxyl terminus of the receptor, demonstrating that this region normally targets the receptor to the coated pit. One such allele, a cysteine for tyrosine substitution in exon 17 (Fig. 12–8), is thought to alter the conformation of the cytoplasmic domain of the receptor, thereby interfering with its binding to a protein that directs incorporation into the coated pit.

Pathogenesis of Atherosclerotic Plaques in Familial Hypercholesterolemia. Despite the impressive knowledge of the normal biology of the LDL receptor and its molecular defects in familial hypercholesterolemia, the mechanisms by which the elevation in LDL leads to formation of atherosclerotic plaques in arteries is unclear. In homozygotes, the increased LDL is cleared from the extracellular fluid by *receptor-independent* pathways, including uptake by scavenger cells such as macrophages. Studies of macrophages in vitro show that excess cholesterol is stored as cholesterol ester droplets, producing the foam cell appearance typically seen in xanthomas and atherosclerotic plaques, but the in vivo relevance of this work is presently uncertain.

DEFECTS IN MEMBRANE TRANSPORT

Cystic Fibrosis

Since the 1960s, cystic fibrosis (CF) has been one of the most publicly visible of all human genetic diseases (see box, Chapter 4). It is the most common fatal autosomal recessive genetic disorder of children in Caucasian populations, with an incidence of approximately 1 in 2000 Caucasian births and a carrier frequency of about 1 in 22. The basic physiological defect is not yet fully determined; however, with the isolation of the affected gene by Tsui, Riordan, Collins, and their associates (Rommens et al., 1989; Riordan et al., 1989; Kerem et al., 1989), it is likely to be identified in the near future. The cloning of the CF gene by linkage analysis and positional cloning (or "reverse genetic") strategies (see Chapter 8) was the first delivery on the promise that molecular biology would put the genes involved in hereditary diseases into the hands of medical scientists, even if nothing was initially known about the location of the affected locus, or the function of its normal product.

Phenotype. The lungs and exocrine pancreas are the major organs affected by the disease.

Chronic obstructive lung disease develops as a result of thick secretions and recurrent infections, and deficiencies of pancreatic enzymes (lipase, trypsin, chymotrypsin) prevent normal digestion. Intense management of the lung disease appears to prolong life, and digestion and nutrition can be largely restored by pancreatic enzyme supplements. Death results from pulmonary failure and infection. At present, only about half the patients survive to 26 years of age, but the clinical course is variable. About 15 percent of CF patients have enough residual pancreatic exocrine function for normal digestion and are designated **pancreatic sufficient** (PS). Moreover, CF-PS patients have better growth and pulmonary function and a superior overall prognosis than do the majority, who are **pancreatic insufficient** (PI). The clinical heterogeneity of the pancreatic disease is at least partly due to allelic heterogeneity, a point to be discussed shortly. The genital tract is also affected in CF; only 2 to 3 percent of males and somewhat more than 10 percent of females are fertile (Boat et al., 1989).

In most patients the diagnosis can be based on the pulmonary or pancreatic findings and on an elevated level of sweat chloride (more than 60 mEq/L), an abnormality reflected in the salty taste of the skin. Less than 2 percent of patients have normal sweat chloride but an otherwise typical clinical picture; in these cases, molecular analysis can be used to ascertain whether they have mutations at the CF locus.

The CF Gene and the CFTR Protein. The CF gene on chromosome 7q31 spans about 250 kb of DNA, and the coding region, with at least 27 exons, is predicted to encode a large integral membrane protein of about 170 kilodaltons. On the basis of the physiological abnormalities in transmembrane ion transport, the polypeptide encoded by the CF gene has been named the CFTR (CF transmembrane conductance regulator) protein. The polypeptide is composed of two repeated motifs, each of which has six putative membrane-spanning regions adjacent to a putative nucleotide (ATP)-binding fold (NBF). The two motifs are separated by a cytoplasmic region that may have a regulatory function and is thus named the R-domain (Fig. 12–9). The putative ATP-binding domains were recognized by their homology to the active sites of a superfamily of proteins that couple ATP hydrolysis to the transport of molecules into

or out of cells (Riordan et al., 1989; Hyde et al., 1990).

The Biochemical Defect. The basic biochemical defect is unknown. Although mutations in CFTR must be directly responsible for CF, it is not yet clear how the observed defects in chloride permeability are produced because the normal function of the CFTR is not fully understood. In the sweat gland, respiratory tract, and lymphocytes of CF patients, the conductive flow of chloride is defective. On the basis of its sequence, it was thought that the CFTR protein itself may be not a chloride channel (Hyde et al., 1990) but the transporter of a molecule that regulates the channel (Ringe and Petsko, 1990). However, recent studies (Anderson et al., 1991; Kartner et al., 1991) suggest that CFTR is a cyclic AMP–activated chloride channel. It is also uncertain whether the abnormalities in Na^+ transport, exemplified by the high sweat Na^+ concentration, are secondary to the defect in Cl^- permeability or are also a direct consequence of the CFTR defect.

THE GENETICS OF CF

Mutations in the CFTR Polypeptide. The first CF mutation identified, a deletion of a phenylalanine residue at position 508 (ΔF508) in the first ATP-binding fold (NBF1; Fig. 12–9) is the most common defect, accounting for about 70 percent of all CF alleles (Kerem et al., 1989; Lemna et al., 1990). Mutations of all types except major deletions or rearrangements have been found throughout the coding region, including other small deletions, insertions that cause frameshifts, nonsense and missense mutations, and point mutations that affect RNA processing. A complete absence of CFTR function is known to be compatible with life because patients who are homozygous for nonsense and splicing mutations have been recognized (Cutting et al., 1990b). Thus the fact that patients with gross alterations in the gene have not been identified is unexpected and unexplained.

Many of the missense mutations in NBF1 and NBF2 involve amino acid residues that are highly conserved in homologous ATP-binding proteins, indicating that they play some critical role (Fig. 12–9; Cutting et al., 1990a; Dean et al., 1990; Kerem et al., 1990a; Zielenski et al., 1991). Although the apparent concentration of mutations in the two ATP-binding domains may reflect the attention that these regions have received in initial studies, there is some suggestion of an uneven distribution of mutations throughout the gene. For example, in one set of 11 non-ΔF508 alleles, the frequency of mutations in NBF1 was approximately sixfold greater than in NBF2 (Kerem et al., 1990a); in addition, missense mutations in the R-domain have yet to be described (Davies, 1990). The large number of mutations in NBF1 may reflect the presence of mutational hot spots in some

of its DNA sequences. For example, four independent missense mutations have been identified in codon 549: Ser→Asn, Ser→Ile, and two different substitutions leading to Ser→Arg. Some of the most significant alleles are shown in Figure 12–9.

Correlations Between Genotype and Phenotype. Linkage and molecular analyses have firmly established that all CF is due to mutation in the chromosome 7 CFTR locus and not in any other gene. Consequently, the clinical heterogene-

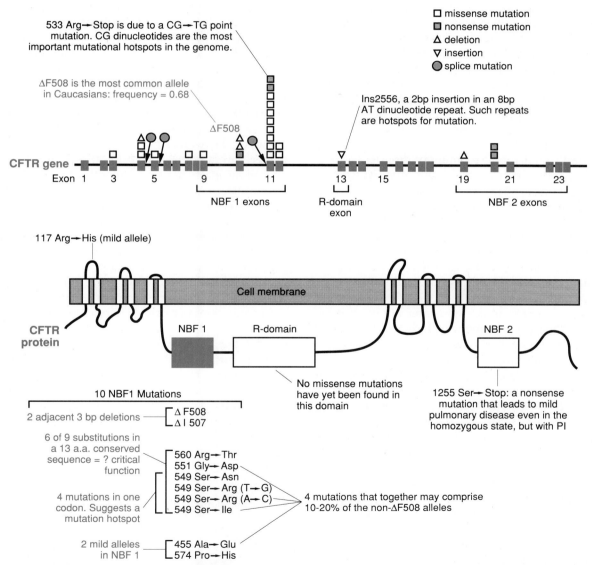

Figure 12–9. Selected mutations in the CFTR gene and their effects on the protein. Unless otherwise noted, all the mutations cause pancreatic insufficiency (PI). Alleles associated with PI do not necessarily cause severe lung disease (e.g., 1255 Ser→Stop). The exons, introns, and domains of the protein are not drawn to scale. (Based on data from Cutting et al., 1990a; Dean et al., 1990; Kerem et al., 1990a; Sangiuolo et al., 1991; White et al., 1990; and Zielenski et al., 1991.)

ity in CF must arise from allelic heterogeneity, the effects of other modifying loci, or nongenetic factors. Many alleles can now be confidently assigned a clinical phenotype (Fig. 12–9). Patients homozygous for the common ΔF508 mutation are almost exclusively of the PI phenotype (Table 12–5), as are those with the similar mutation, a deletion of an isoleucine residue at position 507 (ΔI507; Kerem et al., 1990a). On the other hand, the 20 percent of patients with a PS phenotype are expected to carry a mild mutation on at least one chromosome (Table 12–5).

Both the ΔF508 and ΔI507 mutations are in NBF1, and mutations in this domain, much of which is highly conserved, generally but not invariably result in the PI phenotype. Thus two NBF1 mutations, 455 Ala→Glu and 574 Pro→His, each produce the PS phenotype when they form a genetic compound with the severe allele ΔF508. Remarkably, two patients with nonsense mutations in each copy of the CFTR gene have been found to have mild pulmonary disease, yet both have severe pancreatic insufficiency (Cutting et al., 1990b). One possible explanation of this phenotype is that in the lung, the absence of the CFTR polypeptide may be less detrimental than a defective protein that may affect ion transport.

The CF Gene in Populations. At present it is not possible to account for the high CF gene frequency of 1 in 45 that is observed in Caucasian populations (see Chapter 7). The disease is much less frequent in non-Caucasians, although it has been reported in American Indians, Blacks, and Asians (e.g., approximately 1 in 90,000 Hawaiians of Asian descent).

The ΔF508 allele is the only one found to date that is common in virtually all Caucasian populations (CF Genetic Analysis Consortium, 1990). Haplotype analysis of Caucasian populations indicates that most alleles, and in particular the ΔF508 allele, have a strict haplotype correlation and therefore have a single origin (Kerem et al., 1989). Direct DNA analysis by the sequencing of amplified genomic DNA (see Chapter 5) has been used to determine the frequency of the ΔF508 allele in various parts of Europe (CF Genetic Analysis Consortium, 1990). The frequency of this allele appears to vary significantly in different populations, from 0.88 in Denmark to 0.45 in southern and central Italy.

In populations in which the ΔF508 allele frequency is approximately 0.70 among all mutant alleles, about 50 percent of patients are homozygous for the ΔF508 allele, and an additional 40 percent have genetic compound genotypes for ΔF508 and another allele (Table 12–5). In addition, approximately 70 percent of CF carriers have the ΔF508 mutation (Lemna et al., 1990). Except for ΔF508, most of the more than 50 CF mutations that have been found at the CFTR locus are rare (Davies, 1990), although four mutations that together may account for 10 to 20 percent of the remaining alleles have been identified (Fig. 12–9; Kerem et al., 1990a). In addition, some non-ΔF508 alleles may have relatively high frequencies in certain populations.

Population Screening. The complex issues that are raised by considering population screening for CF are discussed in Chapter 18. At present, it is generally agreed that universal screening should not be considered until at least 95 percent of the mutations in carriers can be detected (Workshop on Population Screening for the Cystic Fibrosis Gene, 1990). However, population screening may not be feasible if dozens or hundreds of rare mutations make up the remaining 30 percent of alleles that are not due to ΔF508.

Genetic Analysis of Families of Patients, and Prenatal Diagnosis. The high frequency of the ΔF508 allele is useful when CF patients with-

Table 12–5. **The Genotype of 293 Cystic Fibrosis Patients with respect to ΔF508**

	ΔF508/ΔF508	**ΔF508/Other Allele**	**Other Allele/Other Allele**
Number of patients	151	117	25
% of all patients	52%	40%	8%
% with PI	99%	72%	36%
% with PS	1%	28%	64%
Age at diagnosis (±SD)	1.8 ± 3.3 years	4.4 ± 5.9 years	8.4 ± 8.3 years

Adapted from Kerem E, Corey M, Kerem B-S, et al. (1990) The relationship between genotype and phenotype in cystic fibrosis: Analysis of the most common mutation (ΔF508). N Engl J Med 323:1517–1522.

PI = pancreatic insufficiency; PS = pancreatic sufficiency.

out a family history present for DNA diagnosis. The identification of the ΔF508 allele, in combination with haplotype analysis, can be used to predict the status of family members for (1) confirmation of disease status (e.g., in a newborn or a sibling with an ambiguous presentation), (2) carrier detection, and (3) prenatal diagnosis. Because of the fortuitous association of the major CF mutation with a specific haplotype, linkage analysis can be performed for almost all families at risk, and, together with the increasing knowledge of specific mutations other than ΔF508, accurate diagnosis is possible in virtually all families (Lemna et al., 1990).

For fetuses with a 1-in-4 risk, prenatal diagnosis by DNA analysis at 8 to 10 weeks, with tissue obtained by chorionic villus biopsy, is the method of choice (see Chapter 19). Biochemical methods of prenatal diagnosis based on the measurement of intestinal enzymes (e.g., intestinal alkaline phosphatase) in amniotic fluid are also reasonably accurate, with a false-positive rate of 2 to 5 percent and a false-negative rate of 2 to 10 percent (Boat et al., 1989). This method would now be used only when the index case is not available or when time to perform mutational or genetic linkage studies in the family is insufficient.

Molecular Genetics and The Treatment of CF. At present, the treatment of CF is directed toward controlling pulmonary infection and improving nutrition. The identification of the affected gene offers the realistic hope that the basic physiological abnormalities in the disease will soon be understood at a molecular level. It may then be possible to design pharmacological interventions that would directly correct the abnormal biochemical phenotype. Alternatively, gene transfer therapy may be possible in CF, but significant obstacles remain to be overcome (discussed in Chapter 13).

DISORDERS AFFECTING STRUCTURAL PROTEINS

Duchenne and Becker Muscular Dystrophies: Defects in Dystrophin

Like cystic fibrosis, Duchenne muscular dystrophy (DMD) has long received attention from the general and medical communities because it is a severe, untreatable, relatively common disorder as-

sociated with relentless clinical deterioration (see box, Chapter 4). The isolation of the gene affected in this X-linked disorder, and the characterization of its protein (named "dystrophin" because of its association with DMD), has given insight into every aspect of the disease, greatly improved the genetic counseling of affected families, and suggested strategies for treatment (Harper, 1989; Worton and Gillard, 1991).

The Clinical Phenotype of DMD. Affected boys are normal for the first year or two of life but develop muscle weakness at age 3 to 5 years, when they begin to have difficulty climbing stairs and in rising from a sitting position (Fig. 12–10). The child is confined to a wheelchair by the age of 12 and is unlikely to survive beyond the age of 20. Patients die of respiratory failure or, because the

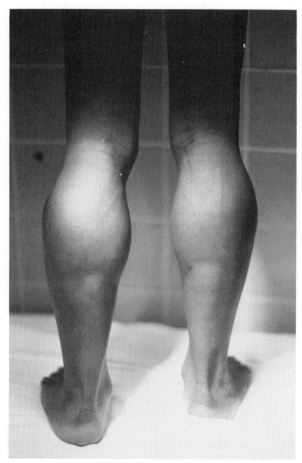

Figure 12–10. Pseudohypertrophy of the calves in a 8-year-old boy with DMD, due to the replacement of normal muscle tissue with connective tissue and fat. (Courtesy of R. H. A. Haslam, The Hospital for Sick Children, Toronto.)

myocardial muscle is also affected, of cardiac failure. In the preclinical and early stages of the disease, the serum creatine kinase level is grossly elevated (50 to 100 times the upper limit of normal) because of its release from diseased muscle. The brain is the only other clinically affected organ; on average, there is a modest decrease in IQ of about 20 points.

Becker Muscular Dystrophy (BMD). BMD is also due to mutations in the dystrophin gene, but the Becker alleles produce a phenotype that is much milder. Patients are said to have BMD if they are still walking after the age of 16 years. There is significant variability in the progression of the disease, and some patients remain ambulatory for many years.

THE GENETICS OF DMD AND BMD

Inheritance. DMD has an incidence of about 1 in 3300 live male births, with a calculated mutation rate of 10^{-4}, an order of magnitude higher than those of most other genetic diseases. In fact, given a production of about 8×10^7 sperm per day, a normal male produces a sperm with a new mutation in the DMD gene every 10 to 11 seconds! In Chapter 4, DMD is presented as a typical X-linked recessive that is lethal in males, so that one third of cases are predicted to be new mutants and two thirds of patients have carrier mothers (see also Chapter 18). The great majority of carrier females have no clinical manifestations, although about 70 percent have an elevated level of serum creatine kinase. However, in accordance with random inactivation of the X chromosome, the normal X chromosome appears to be inactivated in a critical proportion of cells in some female heterozygotes, and about 8 percent of adult female carriers have significant muscle weakness, which in some leads to serious proximal muscle disability. In rare instances, females have been reported with DMD; some have X;autosome translocations, others have only one X chromosome (Turner syndrome) with a DMD mutation on that chromosome, and a rare group consists of heterozygous monozygotic twins (see Chapter 17).

BMD accounts for about 15 percent of the mutations at the locus. An important genetic distinction between these allelic phenotypes is that whereas DMD is a genetic lethal, the reproductive fitness of males with BMD is quite high (up to about 70 percent of normal), so that they can transmit the gene to their daughters. Consequently, a high proportion of BMD cases are inherited, and few (about 10 percent) represent new mutations.

The DMD Gene and Its Product. The most remarkable feature of the DMD gene is its size, estimated to be 2300 kb, or 1.5 percent of the X chromosome. This huge gene and that for neurofibromatosis, type 1 (NF1), are the largest known in any species, by an order of magnitude. The high mutation rate can therefore be at least partly explained from the fact that the locus is a large target for mutation. The gene, with at least 70 exons, produces a large mRNA transcript (14 kb) that encodes dystrophin, a 400-kilodalton protein. In accordance with the specific tissues clinically affected by the disease, dystrophin is most abundant in skeletal and cardiac muscle and is found in lesser amounts in the brain. The protein has several distinct domains (Fig. 12–11), some of which show homology to other structural proteins. It is thought that dystrophin is critical to the maintenance of the structural integrity of muscle membrane.

Molecular Analysis of DMD and BMD. Most molecular defects in DMD patients are deletions, which account for more than 60 percent of the mutations (Figs. 12–11, 12–12). The types of defects that have been demonstrated to date are listed in Table 12–6. The distribution of the deletions in the gene is not random; they are clustered in one of two regions, either in the 5' half of the gene or in a central region that appears to encompass a deletion hot spot (Fig. 12–11). The reasons for this focal distribution are unknown. The major explanation for the fact that a patient with a deletion may nevertheless have the milder BMD phenotype is that the deletion has removed one or more exons with an integral number of codons, so that there is no change in the translational reading frame (Monaco et al., 1988; Gillard et al., 1989). Such patients therefore make a dystrophin molecule lacking some of the amino acids encoded by the central deletion, but with the normal amino and carboxyl termini.

Characterization of the dystrophin protein by Western blotting (see Fig. 5–11) and immunofluorescence (Fig. 12–13) demonstrates that DMD patients have little or no dystrophin, whereas in almost all BMD patients the protein is present, although generally at reduced levels.

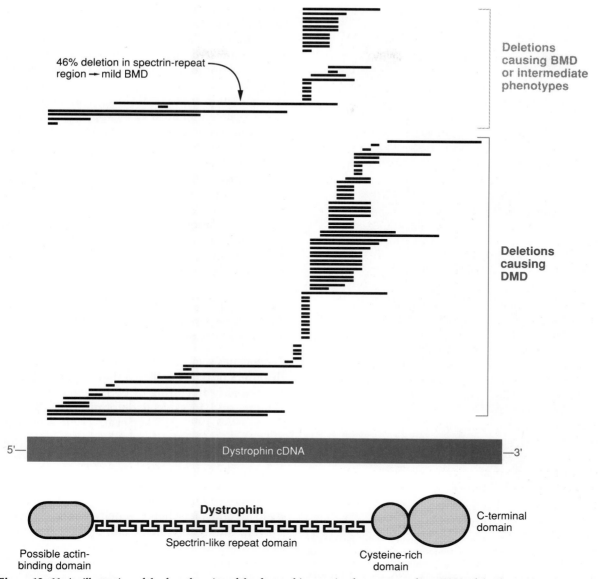

Figure 12-11. An illustration of the four domains of the dystrophin protein, the corresponding cDNA of the dystrophin gene, and the distribution of deletions in patients with BMD and DMD. The domains of the protein are not drawn to scale.

THE CLINICAL APPLICATION OF MOLECULAR GENETICS TO MUSCULAR DYSTROPHY

Prenatal Diagnosis and Carrier Detection. With molecular techniques, prenatal diagnosis is possible for at least 90 percent of known female carriers, with at least 95 percent accuracy (see Chapter 19). In the 60 to 70 percent of families in whom the mutation results from a deletion or du-plication, the presence or absence of the defect can be assessed directly from examination of the fetal DNA by Southern blotting or polymerase chain reaction (PCR) analysis. In most other families in which the defect has not yet been defined, linked markers allow prenatal diagnosis. Identification of carrier or noncarrier status is possible in approximately 75 percent of female relatives of an affected boy, by using DNA methods and serum creatine kinase measurement (see Chapter 18). In

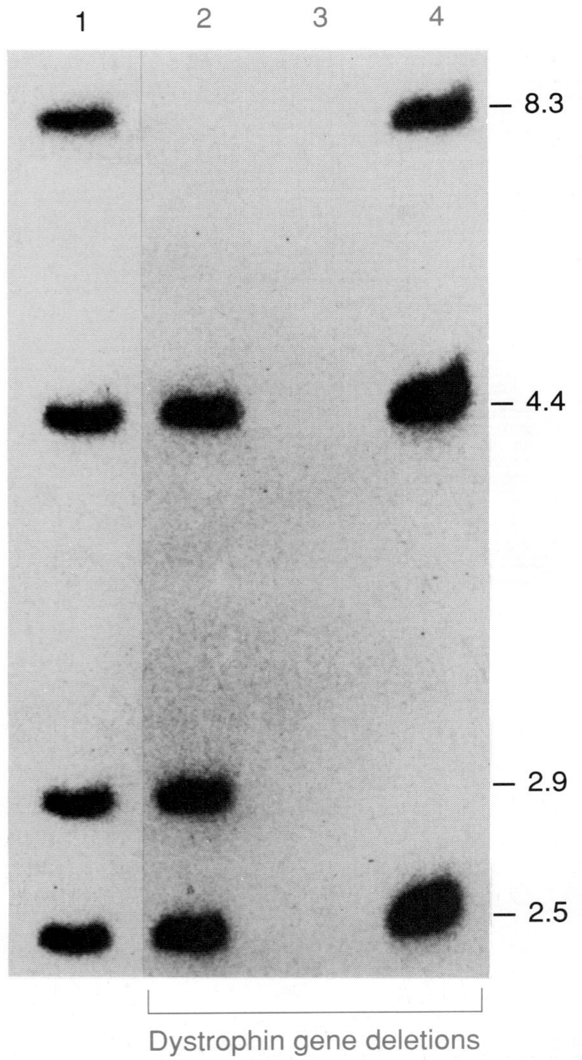

Dystrophin gene deletions

Figure 12–12. Deletions of various segments of the dystrophin gene in patients with DMD, demonstrated by Southern blot analysis with a probe from the middle (the spectrin repeat region) of the cDNA. Lane 1 = normal DNA, showing the four bands that hybridize to the cDNA probe used; lanes 2–4 = DNA from three unrelated patients. Two patients have different deletions that remove a single band, whereas one patient (lane 3) has a deletion for the entire region of the gene homologous to the probe. (Courtesy of P. N. Ray and R. G. Worton, The Hospital for Sick Children, Toronto.)

somes in which recombination between the only available markers has occurred.

Maternal Mosaicism. If a boy with DMD is the first affected member of his family, and if his mother is not found to carry the mutation in her lymphocytes, the usual explanation is that he has a new mutation at the DMD locus. However, about 5 to 15 percent of such cases appear to be due to maternal germline mosaicism (Bakker et al., 1989), in which case the recurrence risk is significant (see Chapter 4).

Therapy. At present, only symptomatic treatment is available for DMD. The possibilities for rational therapy for DMD have greatly increased with the isolation of the dystrophin gene and the understanding of its normal role in the myocyte. Some of the therapeutic considerations are discussed in Chapter 13.

Osteogenesis Imperfecta: Heterogeneous Mutations in Collagen Genes

Osteogenesis imperfecta is a group of inherited disorders of type I collagen that predispose a patient to easy fracturing of bones, even with little trauma, and to skeletal deformity (Fig. 12–14; Byers, 1989, 1990; Prockop et al., 1990). A remarkable range of clinical variation has been recognized, from a lethal perinatal form to only a mild increase in fracture frequency. The four major phenotypes are outlined in Table 12–7. The clinical heterogeneity can be at least partly explained by locus and allelic heterogeneity: the phenotypes vary according to which chain of type I procollagen is affected, and according to the type and location of the mutation in the locus. The combined incidence of all forms of the disease is about 1 in 10,000.

Normal Collagen Structure in Relation to Osteogenesis Imperfecta. Certain features of normal type I collagen are essential to appreciating the pathogenesis of this disease. Type I collagen is the major structural protein of bone and other fibrous tissues. The type I procollagen molecule is formed from two $pro\alpha1(I)$ chains (encoded on chromosome 17) and one similar but distinct $pro\alpha2(I)$ chain (encoded on chromosome 7; Fig. 12–15). The triple helical (collagen) section is composed of 338 tandemly arranged Gly-X-Y repeats; proline is often in the X position, and hy-

the remaining 25 percent, carrier detection may not be accurate because of (1) cases in which phase (the assignment of normal and mutant alleles to each of the two X chromosomes) cannot be determined, (2) missing samples from critical family members, and (3) the transmission of X chromo-

Table 12-6. Causes of Duchenne/Becker Muscular Dystrophy

Mechanism	Frequency	Phenotype
Molecular Defects		
Gene deletion (1 exon to whole gene)	>60%	DMD or BMD
Partial duplication of the gene	6%	DMD or BMD
Contiguous gene deletion	Rare	DMD plus other phenotypes depending on other genes deleted
Expression in Females		
Nonrandom X inactivation	Rare	DMD or BMD
Turner syndrome (45,X)	Rare	DMD or BMD
X;autosome translocation	Rare	DMD or BMD

droxyproline or hydroxylysine is often in the Y position. Glycine, the smallest amino acid, is the only residue compact enough to occupy the axial position of the helix, and consequently mutations resulting in substitutions to other residues are highly disruptive to the helical structure.

Several features of procollagen maturation are of special significance to the pathophysiology of osteogenesis imperfecta. First, the assembly of the individual chains into the triple helix begins at the C-terminal and moves toward the N-terminal. Consequently, mutations in the C-terminal part of the molecule are more disruptive because they interfere earlier with the propagation of the triple

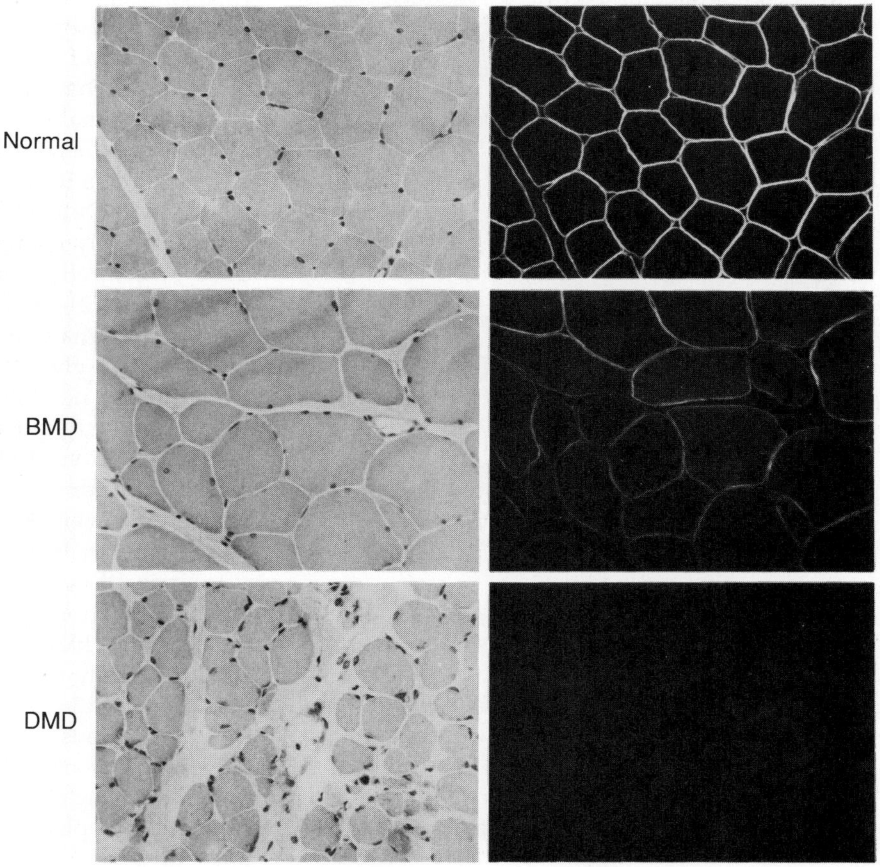

Figure 12-13. Microscopic visualization of the effect of mutations in the dystrophin gene in a patient with BMD and a patient with DMD. Left column = hematoxylin and eosin staining of muscle. Right column = immunofluorescence microscopy staining with an antibody specific to dystrophin. Note the localization of dystrophin to the myocyte membrane in normal muscle, the reduced quantity of dystrophin in BMD muscle, and the complete absence of dystrophin from the myocytes of the DMD muscle. The amount of connective tissue between the myocytes in the DMD muscle is increased. (Courtesy of K. Arahata, National Institute of Neuroscience, Tokyo.)

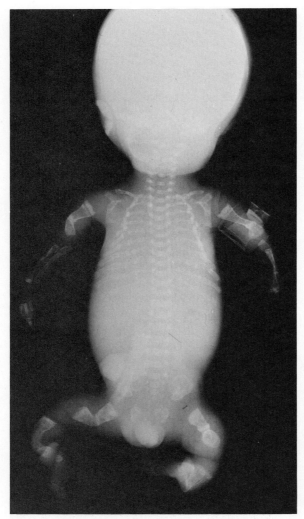

Figure 12–14. Radiograph of a premature (26 weeks' gestation) infant with the perinatal lethal form (Type II) of osteogenesis imperfecta. The skull is relatively large and unmineralized, and was soft to palpation. The thoracic cavity is small, the long bones of the arms and legs are short and deformed, and the vertebral bodies are flattened. All the bones are undermineralized. (Courtesy of T. Costa, The Hospital for Sick Children, Toronto.)

of collagen fibrils. As a result of all of these abnormalities, not only is the number of fibrils reduced, but many of those that are secreted are defective. In bone, the abnormal chains and the reduced number lead to decreased mineralization (Fig. 12–16).

MOLECULAR ABNORMALITIES OF COLLAGEN IN OSTEOGENESIS IMPERFECTA

More than 50 mutations affecting the synthesis or structure of type I collagen have already been found in patients with osteogenesis imperfecta, and the clinical heterogeneity has been shown to reflect even greater heterogeneity at the molecular level. To some extent, it is now possible to predict the phenotype that will result from a specific type of molecular defect (Fig. 12–17).

Type I Defects. The great majority of patients with Type I osteogenesis imperfecta have mutations that severely impair the *production* of type I collagen, represented as the pro$\alpha 1^0$ allele in Fig. 12–16. Typically, it is the pro$\alpha 1$(I) chain that is affected. Few of these defects have yet been characterized at the level of the gene, but they are presumably analogous to the mutations that cause thalassemia (i.e., promoter mutations, splice mutations, and so forth; see Chapter 11).

Type II Defects. The more severe Type II disease invariably results from mutations that produce *structurally abnormal* pro$\alpha 1$ and pro$\alpha 2$ chains (Figs. 12–16, 12–17). The great majority of these patients have substitutions in the triple helix that replace a glycine with a more bulky residue. Substitutions near the carboxyl terminus of the chain invariably cause the lethal form of the disease, irrespective of the nature of the substituting residue. Residues with large or charged side chains, however, are highly disruptive no matter where they are located.

Type III and IV Defects. The few Type III and IV mutations that have been characterized indicate that, like the Type II form, these phenotypes generally result from structurally defective pro$\alpha 1$ or pro$\alpha 2$ chains (Byers, 1990). Frequently, the substitutions are located toward the N-terminal end of the molecule (Fig. 12–17). However, if the substituting residue is relatively small, such as serine, even replacements near the carboxyl terminus can cause Types III and IV osteogenesis imperfecta.

helix (Fig. 12–16). Second, the posttranslational modification (e.g., proline hydroxylation, glycosylation) of procollagen continues on any part of a chain not assembled into the triple helix. Thus when triple helix assembly is slowed by a mutation, the unassembled sections of the chains that are amino terminal to the defect are overmodified, thus slowing their secretion into the extracellular space and contributing to their instability. Overmodification may also interfere with the formation

Table 12–7. Summary of the Genetic, Biochemical, and Molecular Features of the Types of Osteogenesis Imperfecta

Type	Phenotype	Inheritance	Biochemical Defect	Gene Defect
Type I	**Mild:** blue sclerae, brittle bones, but no bony deformity. Often, presenile deafness.	AD	Common: All the Type I collagen made is *normal* (from the normal allele), but the quantity is reduced by half	Common: Null alleles that impair the production of proα1(I) chains, such as defects that interfere with mRNA synthesis
Type II	**Perinatal lethal:** severe skeletal abnormalities (fractures, deformities), dark sclerae, death within 1 month	AD* (new mutation)	Common: Production of *abnormal* type I collagen molecules due to substitution of the Gly in Gly-X-Y of the triple helical domain, toward the COOH-terminal part of the protein (Fig. 12–17)	Common: Missense mutations in the glycine codons of the genes for the α1 and α2 chains of type I collagen
Type III	**Progressive deforming:** fractures, often at birth, progressive bony deformity, limited growth, blue sclerae, dentinogenesis imperfecta, hearing loss	AD*	Gly substitutions in the triple helix, in general, towards the NH₂-terminal part of the protein (Fig. 12–17)	Missense mutations in the glycine codons of the genes for the α1 or α2 chains of type I collagen
Type IV	**Normal sclerae, deforming:** mild to moderate bony deformity, short stature, fractures, hearing loss, dentinogenesis imperfecta	AD	Gly substitutions in the triple helix, in general, towards the NH₂-terminal part of the protein (Fig. 12–17)	Missense mutations in the glycine codons of the genes for the α1 or α2 chains. Exon-skipping mutations in 5′ end of the α2 chain gene

Modified from Byers PH (1989) Disorders of collagen biosynthesis and structure. *In* Scriver CR, Beaudet AL, Sly WS, Valle D (eds) The metabolic basis of inherited disease, 6th ed. McGraw-Hill, New York, pp. 2805–2842; and Byers PH (1990) Brittle bones – fragile molecules: Disorders of collagen structure and expression. Trends Genet 6:293–300.
* = rare cases are autosomal recessive.

The Genetics of Osteogenesis Imperfecta.

Most of the mutations that cause the disease are autosomal dominant, but a few are autosomal recessive. At least some of the mechanisms by which different patterns of inheritance arise from different mutations in a single molecule have been revealed by characterization of the biochemical defects. More generally, this disease illustrates the genetic complexities that result when mutations alter structural proteins, particularly those composed of multiple different subunits.

The relatively mild phenotype and dominant

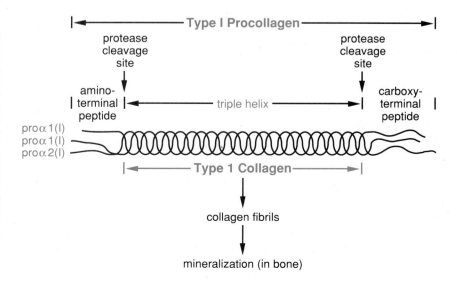

Figure 12–15. The structure of type I procollagen. Each collagen chain is made as a procollagen triple helix that is secreted into the extracellular space. The amino- and carboxyl-terminal domains are cleaved extracellularly to form collagen; mature collagen fibrils are then assembled and, in bone, mineralized. Note that type I procollagen is composed of two proα1(I) chains and one proα2(I) chain. (Redrawn from Byers PH [1989] Disorders of collagen biosynthesis and structure. *In* Scriver CR, Beaudet AL, Sly WS, Valle D [eds] The metabolic basis of inherited disease, 6th ed. McGraw-Hill, New York, pp. 2805–2842.)

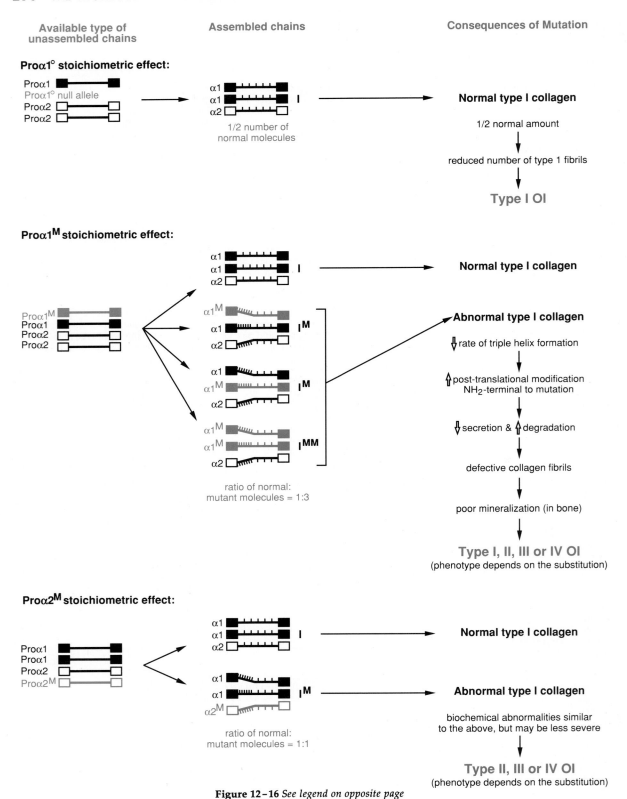

Figure 12–16 *See legend on opposite page*

Substitutions for Glycine in Proα1(I) Chain

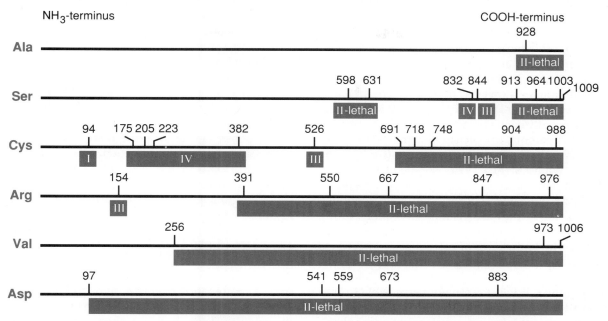

Figure 12–17. The phenotypic effect of substitutions in the proα1 chain of type I collagen. I, II, III, and IV = Types I–IV osteogenesis imperfecta. The numbers above the linear representation of the collagen molecules are the glycine residues that have been substituted by the amino acid noted to the left of each line. Note that, in general, the phenotypic effect of substitutions near the carboxyl terminus is more severe but that the effect also depends on the nature of the residue that replaces glycine. (Redrawn from Byers PH [1990] Brittle bones—fragile molecules: Disorders of collagen structure and expression. Trends Genet 6:293–300.)

inheritance of Type I osteogenesis imperfecta are consistent with the fact that although only half the normal number of molecules is made, they are of normal quality (Fig. 12–16). The more severe consequences of producing structurally defective proα1 chains (vs. none) partly reflect the stoichiometry of type I collagen, which is two proα1 chains to one proα2 chain (Fig. 12–16). Accordingly, if one proα1 chain is abnormal, three of four type I molecules have at least one abnormal chain; in contrast, if a proα2 chain is defective, only one of two molecules is affected. Mutations such as the proα1 missense allele (proα1^M) shown in Figure 12–16 are thus **dominant negative alleles** because they impair the contribution of both the normal proα1 allele and the normal pro α2 alleles.

In other words, the effect of the mutant allele is amplified because of the polymeric nature of the collagen molecule (Byers, 1989). The effect of dominant negative alleles is one general way by which mutations in a multimeric protein cause dominantly inherited diseases. In addition, the dominant negative effect also explains the observation that in some dominantly inherited diseases such as osteogenesis imperfecta, it is actually better to have a mutation leading to *no* gene product than one leading to an *abnormal* gene product.

Although mutations that produce structurally abnormal proα2 chains reduce the number of normal type I collagen molecules by one half (vs. three quarters in structurally abnormal proα1 chains; Fig. 12–16), this reduction is nevertheless suffi-

Figure 12–16. The pathogenesis of the major classes of type I procollagen mutants. Column 1: the types of procollagen chains available for assembly into a triple helix. Column 2: the effect of type I procollagen stoichiometry on the ratio of normal to defective collagen molecules formed in mutants with proα1 chain versus proα2 mutations. The small vertical bars on each procollagen chain indicate the posttranslational modification (see text). Column 3: the effect of the mutations on the biochemical processing of collagen. Proα1^M = a proα1 chain with a missense mutation; proα2^M = a pro α2 chain with a missense mutation; proα1^0 = a proα1 chain null allele.

cient, in the case of some mutations, to cause the severe perinatal lethal phenotype (Table 12–7; Byers, 1990).

Most infants with the Type II perinatal lethal form of osteogenesis imperfecta have a *new* dominant mutation, and consequently, the likelihood of recurrence in the family is very low. In occasional families, however, more than one sibling is affected with the Type II disease. Such recurrences have recently been recognized to be most often the result of parental mosaicism that affects the germline as well as some somatic tissues (Cohn et al., 1990; Wallis et al., 1990; see pedigree in Fig. 4–31). Thus although true autosomal recessive cases of the Type II form have been identified (Byers, 1989), they are the minority (Byers, 1990).

Clinical Management and Prenatal Diagnosis. The knowledge of osteogenesis imperfecta that is currently emerging has useful applications to prognosis. If a patient's molecular defect can be determined, it will eventually be possible to predict, at least to some extent, the natural history of the disease. In addition, the demonstration that a defect is inherited from an affected parent (autosomal dominant), from two unaffected but heterozygous parents (autosomal recessive), or as a new mutation will allow accurate recurrence risks to be calculated. Prenatal diagnosis in Type II osteogenesis imperfecta, the perinatal lethal form, may be performed by examination of skull and limb length by ultrasonography in the second trimester. In addition, the identification of specific mutations makes possible first-trimester diagnosis through the use of chorionic villus biopsy and DNA analysis.

PHARMACOGENETIC DISEASES

Pharmacogenetics is the special area of biochemical genetics that deals with variation in drug response and the contribution of genetics to such variation. In broad terms, pharmacogenetics can be said to encompass any genetically determined variation in response to drugs: for instance, the effect of barbiturates in precipitating attacks of porphyria in people with the gene for acute intermittent porphyria (see later in this chapter) or the effect of alcohol use by pregnant women on the incidence of fetal alcohol syndrome (see Fig.

17–5). In a narrower sense, pharmacogenetics can be restricted to those genetic variations that are revealed only by response to drugs or other chemicals. Some examples of pharmacogenetic variations are described briefly in this section.

The origin of polymorphisms for drug response and the mechanisms by which they are maintained pose a problem. They obviously have not developed in response to drugs, since they antedate the drugs concerned. The handling of and the response to drugs require many specific biochemical reactions, and the enzymes involved may participate in the metabolism of ordinary food substances.

Recognizing that there is normal variation in response to drugs, pharmacologists define the "potency" of a drug by the dose that produces a given effect in 50 percent of the population. For genetic traits, continuous variation is usually best explained on the basis of multifactorial inheritance or by a combination of genetic and environmental factors, as discussed in detail in Chapter 15. But response to drugs can also show discontinuous variation, with sharp distinctions between different degrees of response. The finding of a bimodal or trimodal population distribution of activity of a drug-metabolizing enzyme may indicate that the enzyme is coded by genes at a polymorphic locus.

Glucose-6-Phosphate Dehydrogenase (G6PD) Deficiency

Deficiency of G6PD, a ubiquitous X-linked enzyme, is the most common disease-producing enzyme defect of humans, estimated to affect 400 million people worldwide; one allele, the *A* variant, is found in 1 in 20 Black males in the United States. With over 300 variants described, G6PD deficiency also appears to be the most genetically heterogeneous disorder yet recognized (Luzzatto and Mehta, 1989). The high gene frequency of G6PD variants in some populations appears to reflect the fact that G6PD deficiency, like sickle cell hemoglobin and thalassemia, confers some protection against malaria (see Chapter 7). This enzymopathy originally came to attention when the antimalarial drug primaquine was found to induce hemolytic anemia in Black males, who were subsequently found to have G6PD deficiency.

The mechanism of the drug-induced hemolysis is reasonably clear. One of the products of G6PD, nicotinamide-adenine dinucleotide phosphate (NADPH), is the major source of reducing equivalents in the red blood cell. NADPH protects the cell against oxidative damage by regenerating reduced glutathione from the oxidized form. In G6PD deficiency, oxidant drugs such as primaquine deplete the cell of reduced glutathione, and the consequent oxidative damage leads to hemolysis. Additional offending compounds include sulfonamide antibiotics, sulfones such as dapsone (widely used in the treatment of leprosy and *Pneumocystis carinii* infection), naphthalene (moth balls), and a few others. The role of some drugs in producing hemolysis in G6PD deficiency is ambiguous because of the uncertain significance of other genetic factors (such as genetically determined ethnic and individual variation in pharmacokinetics) and nongenetic determinants (such as infection, which itself can induce hemolysis in severe variants of G6PD deficiency).

Favism, a severe hemolytic anemia that results from ingestion of the broad bean *Vicia faba* and that has been known since ancient times in parts of the Mediterranean, is due to extreme G6PD deficiency. The enzyme defect makes the cells vulnerable to oxidants in fava beans (Pythagoras, the Greek mathematician, warned his followers of the danger of eating these beans). In areas where severe deficiency variants like the Mediterranean allele are prevalent, they are a major cause of both neonatal jaundice and congenital nonspherocytic hemolytic anemia.

The normal and common abnormal variants of G6PD are listed in Table 12–8. The common deficiency alleles of American Blacks and of the Mediterranean region migrate electrophoretically at the same rate as A and B variants but have much lower activities, and so are called A$^-$ and B$^-$ variants, respectively. Although G6PD deficiency is far more common in males, an appreciable number (at least 1 in 400) of American Black females are genetically A$^-$/A$^-$, and are clinically susceptible to drug-induced hemolysis.

The A$^-$ Variant Has Decreased Stability. In addition to reduced catalytic activity, instability of the A$^-$ variant is a major factor in the pathological response to drug ingestion. Synthesis of the A$^-$ protein is unaffected by the mutation, but because the molecule is relatively unstable, its abundance decreases more quickly than normal as the red cell ages. (Remember that the mature red cell is anucleate, and thus new protein synthesis is limited.) After drug ingestion, patients with this allele have hemolysis only as long as it takes (usually about a week) to destroy the fraction of older red cells that have lost, through aging, a critical amount of G6PD activity. Even if the drug administration is continued, the hemolytic phase comes to an end because the young cells produced in response to hemolysis have sufficient newly synthesized G6PD A$^-$ to prevent oxidative damage.

The Acetylation Polymorphism

This important pharmacogenetic polymorphism was first discovered during the treatment of tuberculosis with the drug isoniazid. After a test dose, the rate of disappearance of isoniazid from plasma shows a bimodal distribution in the population, allowing the identification of individuals as rapid or slow acetylators (inactivators of the drug). Slow inactivators are homozygous for a recessive gene, and rapid inactivators are normal homozygotes or heterozygotes. It is now clear that the slow and rapid inactivation phenotypes are due to two major alleles of the enzyme hepatic arylamine *N*-acetyltransferase, the product of a gene that maps to chromosome 8. Slow acetylators have a substantial decrease in the quantity of the arylamine *N*-acetyltransferase in the liver (Grant et al., 1990). The frequencies of the two alleles have marked

Table 12–8. Common G6PD Phenotypes

G6PD Type	Allele Symbol	Electrophoretic Mobility	Enzyme Activity (~% Normal)	Approximate Population Distribution
B	Gd^B	Normal	100%	Normal
B$^-$	Gd^{B-}	Normal	4%	Common in Mediterranean region
A	Gd^A	Fast	90%	20% of American Black males
A$^-$	Gd^{A-}	Fast	15%	10% of American Black males

ethnic differences: for example, a minority (5 to 20 percent) of Asian populations have the slow acetylation phenotype, whereas 50 percent of American Blacks and up to 65 percent of Caucasians are slow acetylator homozygotes (Clark, 1985).

Significance. In addition to its effect on isoniazid inactivation, the acetylation phenotype affects the disposition of a wide variety of other drugs and xenobiotics (Grant and Spielberg, 1991). For example, rapid acetylators not only have a higher failure rate with weekly isoniazid therapy for tuberculosis but also require larger doses of hydralazine to control hypertension and of dapsone to treat leprosy and other infections. Conversely, slow acetylators are at increased risk of developing a drug-induced systemic lupus erythematosus–like syndrome while receiving hydralazine, hematological adverse drug reactions after isoniazid treatment, and sulfonamide-induced idiosyncratic adverse responses. In addition, slow acetylators exposed to carcinogenic arylamines (e.g, benzidine) have an increased incidence of bladder cancer (Evans, 1989) (see Chapter 16).

Screening. A simple test for acetylator phenotype has been developed on the basis of the urinary excretion of the caffeine metabolite 5-acetylamino-6-formylamino-3-methyluracil (AFMU). Accurate genotype identification can now be determined from a single urine sample after consumption of a caffeinated beverage, a feature that will allow screening of individuals who may be exposed to the relevant compounds (Grant and Spielberg, 1991).

Genetic Problems in Anesthesia

Malignant Hyperthermia

Malignant hyperthermia is an autosomal dominant condition in which there may be a dramatic adverse response to the administration of all commonly used inhalational anesthetics (e.g., halothane) and muscle relaxants such as succinylcholine chloride, with development of a very high temperature, sustained muscle contraction, and attendant hypercatabolism. The condition is an important if not a common cause of death in anesthesia, with an incidence that is higher in children (1 in 12,000) than in adults (1 in 40,000). Because

calcium ion is the chief regulator of muscle contraction and metabolism, the basic defect has long been suspected to lie in calcium ion metabolism or transport. The malignant hyperthermia gene maps to the long arm of chromosome 19 (McCarthy et al., 1990) and linkage analysis indicates that the mutant protein is likely to be the calcium ion release channel (also called the ryanodine receptor) in the sarcoplasmic reticulum (MacLennan et al., 1990). The cloning of the affected gene will allow linkage studies and mutant analysis to be used for establishing which members of affected families are at risk. The need for special precautions when at-risk persons require anesthesia is obvious. Dantrolene sodium is effective in preventing or reducing the severity of the response if an unsuspected attack occurs, and alternative anesthetics can be given to patients at risk.

Serum Cholinesterase and Succinylcholine Sensitivity

Serum cholinesterase is an enzyme of human plasma that has the property of hydrolyzing choline esters, such as acetylcholine. Its normal function is obscure, but its complete absence is fully compatible with normal health; hence it cannot play a major physiological role. A widely used muscle relaxant, succinylcholine (suxamethonium), is composed of two molecules of acetylcholine and is normally hydrolyzed by cholinesterase, a process that thereby reduces the amount of succinylcholine that reaches the motor end plates; this hydrolysis is allowed for in the dose given to the average patient. However, in European populations, about 1 in 3300 persons is homozygous for an atypical cholinesterase allele (Whittaker, 1986) and, being unable to degrade succinylcholine at the normal rate, responds abnormally to its administration with prolonged apnea lasting from 1 to several hours and requires artificial respiratory support.

Genetics. The major determinants of cholinesterase activity in the plasma are two codominant alleles, known as the "usual" (U) and "atypical" (A) alleles. Another allele, the K variant (La Du et al., 1990), is also common, but K/K homozygotes have no increase in succinylcholine sensitivity. Genetic compounds of the A and K alleles, on the other hand, are sometimes sensitive and sometimes not, but the factor or factors responsible for this variation are unclear. Cholinesterase deficiency is usually due to homozygosity for the atypical allele; the enzyme produced by homozygotes is qualitatively altered and has lower activity than the usual type. Serum cholinesterase phenotypes cannot be determined with certainty on the basis of cholinesterase levels in serum because the values thus obtained show considerable overlap. However, normal and abnormal phenotypes can be distinguished through the use of an inhibitor of cholinesterase, dibucaine (Nupercaine), a well-known local anesthetic. The "dibucaine number" of a serum sample is its percentage inhibition by dibucaine. The following relationships exist:

the clinical significance of the K variant, and improved pedigree analysis and genetic counseling (La Du et al., 1990).

In more general terms, succinylcholine sensitivity is an example of a significant pharmacogenetic problem in which rational therapy must take into account wide, genetically determined individual differences in response. The role of drug metabolism in mutagenesis, carcinogenesis, teratogenesis, cytotoxic damage, or autoimmune diseases has attracted attention (Grant and Spielberg, 1991). The management of patients with toxic reactions to drugs or chemicals should include, when possible, evaluation of the pharma-

Name of Allele	Homozygous Phenotype	Homozygote Dibucaine Number	Amino Acid Substitution	Allele Frequency
Usual	Normal	~80%	—	0.870
K variant	Normal	~80%	539 Ala→Thr	0.113
Atypical	Dibucaine resistant	~20%	70 Asp→Gly	0.017

Based on data from McGuire et al. (1989) and La Du et al. (1990).

The identification of the specific substitutions that are present in the cholinesterase alleles will allow accurate typing of patients, determination of

cogenetic status of the patient and members of the family, and appropriate genetic counseling about potential risks of certain drugs.

HOW PROTEINS ARE ALTERED IN GENETIC DISEASE

In this section we present a general approach for understanding and classifying the many effects that mutations have on proteins. We examine the pathogenesis of genetic disorders in terms of (1) the mechanisms by which mutations impair the formation of biologically active proteins (Table 12–9), (2) the effect of mutation on protein function (Fig. 12–18), (3) the relationship between the location of the mutant protein and the site of pathology, and (4) the relationship between the molecular abnormality of a protein and the resulting clinical phenotype. The approach to be described allows the student of genetics to recognize whether a new disease and its mutations establish novel principles of the genetic pathology of proteins or merely represent additional examples of well-recognized phenomena.

HOW MUTATIONS DISRUPT THE FORMATION OF BIOLOGICALLY NORMAL PROTEINS

To develop a biologically active protein, information must be transferred from the nucleotide sequence of the structural gene through to the polypeptide, which assumes forms of increasing maturity that are depicted in the central column of Table 12–9. Many of the maturational processes to which the polypeptide is subjected are entirely dependent on its primary amino acid sequence (Table 12–9, second column) and consequently may be disrupted by mutations in the structural gene of the protein. Diseases due to abnormalities in these processes, termed **primary abnormalities,** are presented in the first column of Table

Table 12–9. How Proteins Are Altered in Genetic Disease

Primary Abnormalities in steps directly dependent on the DNA sequence of the structural gene		Secondary Abnormalities in modifying events, or in the synthesis of associated molecules required for function	
Disease Example	**Affected Step**	**Modifying Event**	**Disease Example**
NUCLEOTIDE SEQUENCE			
Thalassemias in which decreased mRNA is due to deletions, or defects in regulatory or splice sites **HPFH:** increased transcription	Transcription, RNA splicing	Regulation of transcription	**Acute intermittent porphyria:** drugs that induce cytochrome P450 decrease free heme → induction of ALA synthetase → symptoms
MESSENGER RNA			
Thalassemias due to nonfunctional mRNAs with nonsense or frameshift mutations	Translation	Regulation of protein synthesis	**Acute intermittent porphyria:** heme affects both transcription and translation of ALA synthetase
UNFOLDED POLYPEPTIDE			
Hb Hammersmith: the heme pocket is deformed → conformational instability **Class 2 LDL receptor mutants:** abnormal folding	Polypeptide folding (secondary and tertiary structure)	Posttranslational modifications (e.g., glycosylation, hydroxylation)	**Ehlers-Danlos syndrome type VI:** lysyl hydroxylase deficiency → poorly cross-linked collagen
THREE-DIMENSIONAL CONFORMATION			
Methylmalonic aciduria: a defect in the leader sequence in one allele of methylmalonyl CoA mutase	Subcellular localization due to information in the amino acid sequence	Subcellular localization due to posttranslational modifications of the polypeptide	**I-cell disease:** failure to add a recognition marker to lysosomal enzymes
Many collagen defects → OI by impairing collagen helix assembly **Hb Kansas, Hb Kempsey:** impaired subunit interaction	For multimeric proteins: • subunit association • subunit interaction	Formation of multiprotein complexes and organelles	**Zellweger syndrome,** a defect in peroxisome biogenesis
LOCALIZATION AND ASSEMBLY*			
Cystathionine synthase deficiency: poor pyridoxal phosphate binding → homocystinuria in 50% of patients	Cofactor or prosthetic group binding (noncovalent or covalent)	Cofactor or prosthetic group synthesis or transport	**Mutations in vitamin B$_{12}$ metabolism** → methylmalonic aciduria, homocystinuria, or both
		Cofactor binding or removal (covalent)	**Holocarboxylase synthase deficiency; biotinidase deficiency**
B1 **allele of Tay-Sachs disease:** mutations may affect only the protein's function, as in active site mutations in enzymes	BIOLOGICAL FUNCTION		
G6PD, the A⁻ variant: many mutations alter conformation → instability → degradation → decreased CRM	Proteolytic degradation	Regulation of protein degradation	No examples yet known
DEGRADED PROTEIN			

* Which of these two steps occurs first varies with the type of protein.

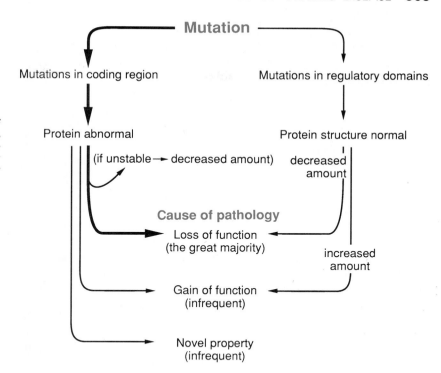

Figure 12–18. A general outline of the mechanisms by which mutations produce pathology. Mutations in the coding region result in structurally abnormal proteins that have a loss or gain of function, or a novel function that causes disease. Mutations in regulatory domains can cause only a loss or a gain of function. Mutations in either the coding region or regulatory domains can decrease the amount of the protein.

12–9. Virtually every step required for the formation of a biologically active protein is vulnerable to mutation.

In some instances, however, the biogenesis of a functional protein may depend not only on its primary structure but also on modifying events that are mediated by *other* proteins. These events may include alterations in the synthesis of the protein, posttranslational modifications of its structure, or the synthesis of polypeptides or other molecules that associate with the protein to make it biologically active (such as the cofactors required for the catalytic activity of many enzymes). When these modifying or associative events (Table 12–9, fourth column) fail to occur, the loss of function of the protein is due to a **secondary abnormality.** Of course, when a secondary abnormality is recognized to have altered a protein in a genetic disease, there must be a primary defect in the structural gene of some other protein, even though the clinical or biochemical phenotype of the patient initially suggests otherwise. Diseases that exemplify the molecular and clinical pathology that results from failure of modifying events are listed in the last column of Table 12–9.

In the remainder of this section, we elaborate on the biochemical events and diseases listed in Table 12–9. The steps and modifying events re-

quired for the formation of a functional protein are discussed briefly, and their importance is illustrated by examples of genetic diseases, many of which are described in Chapter 11 or in the first section of this chapter, that are known to disrupt them.

Abnormalities That Affect the Rates of mRNA and Protein Synthesis

Primary Abnormalities Affecting mRNA or Protein Synthesis

In Chapter 11, the mutations that cause β-thalassemia were outlined to illustrate the range of molecular abnormalities that can reduce the synthesis of an mRNA or its encoded protein. In rare instances, mutations can act to increase the quantity of an mRNA or to change the timing of its expression, as shown by the defects that cause hereditary persistence of fetal hemoglobin (HPFH).

Secondary Abnormalities Affecting mRNA or Protein Synthesis

Acute Intermittent Porphyria. When the rate of production of a protein is regulated rather

Disease Example	Affected Step	Modifying Event	Disease Example
	Nucleotide Sequence		
Thalassemias in which decreased mRNA is due to deletions, or defects in regulatory or splice sites. HPFH: increased transcription	Transcription	Regulation of transcription	Acute intermittent porphyria: drugs that induce cytochrome P450 decrease free heme→induction of ALA synthetase→symptoms
	Messenger RNA		
Thalassemias due to nonfunctional mRNAs with nonsense or frameshift mutations	Translation	Regulation of protein synthesis	Acute intermittent porphyria: heme affects both transcription and translation of ALA synthetase
	Unfolded Polypeptide		

than constitutive, abnormalities in the regulatory events may have pathological consequences. A remarkable disease that affects the synthesis of heme, and in which altered regulation of gene expression is central to the pathophysiology, is acute intermittent porphyria.

The primary defect in this disease is a deficiency of porphobilinogen (PBG) deaminase, an enzyme in the biosynthetic pathway of heme (Fig. 12–19). All patients with acute intermittent porphyria, whether their disease is clinically latent (about 90 percent of patients) or clinically expressed (about 10 percent), have an approximately 50 percent reduction in the enzymatic activity of PBG deaminase, which is consistent with the autosomal dominant nature of the disorder. Clinical expression of the disease occurs in response to

events that decrease the concentration of heme in the liver cell. Many drugs — for example, barbiturates, some steroid hormones, and numerous other chemicals — increase the synthesis of hepatic cytochromes P450, a class of heme-containing proteins. As a result, the cellular level of heme falls, reducing the feedback inhibition of heme on δ-aminolevulinic acid synthase, the rate-limiting step in the heme synthesis pathway (Fig. 12–19). The expression of the synthase is increased by both transcriptional and translational mechanisms. Thus the relative heme deficiency caused by the combination of the defect in PBG deaminase and the decrease in heme pools is responsible for a *secondary* increase in the synthase to levels above the normal range (Kappas et al., 1989). The fact that half of the normal activity of PBG deami-

Clinically latent AIP

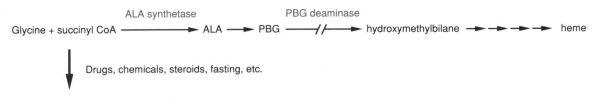

Drugs, chemicals, steroids, fasting, etc.

Clinically expressed AIP: post-pubertal neurologic symptoms

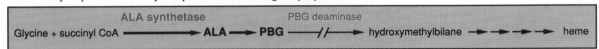

Figure 12–19. The pathogenesis of acute intermittent porphyria (AIP). Patients with AIP who are either clinically latent or clinically affected have about half the control levels of porphobilinogen (PBG) deaminase. When the activity of hepatic δ-aminolevulinic acid (ALA) synthase is increased in carriers by exposure to inducing agents (drugs, chemicals, etc.), the synthesis of ALA and PBG is increased. The residual PBG deaminase activity (approximately 50 percent of control) is overloaded, and the accumulation of ALA and PBG causes clinical disease. (Redrawn from Kappas A, Sassa S, Galbraith RA, Nordmann Y [1989] The porphyrias. *In* Scriver CR, Beaudet AL, Sly WS, Valle D [eds] The metabolic basis of inherited disease, 6th ed. McGraw-Hill, New York, pp. 1305–1365.)

nase is inadequate to cope with the metabolic load in some situations accounts for the dominant expression of the condition. The nervous system is the principal target. Because the peripheral, autonomic, and central nervous systems are all affected, the clinical manifestations are diverse, and this disease is one of the great mimics in clinical medicine, the presentation ranging from acute abdominal pain to psychosis.

bins, and in half of these a hydrophobic residue, leucine, has been replaced by a polar residue, arginine.

Another frequent cause of conformational alteration in hemoglobin is the introduction of proline into one of the eight major α helices of the molecule (see Fig. 11–3). The explanation is that proline introduces a kink that usually disrupts the tertiary structure of the α helix. There are, of

Disease Example	Affected Step	Modifying Event	Disease Example
	Unfolded Polypeptide		Ehlers-Danlos syndrome Type VI: lysyl hydroxylase deficiency→poorly cross-linked collagen
Hb Hammersmith: the heme pocket is deformed→conformational instability; Class 2 LDL receptor mutants: abnormal folding	Polypeptide folding (secondary and tertiary structure)	Posttranslational modifications (e.g., glycosylation, hydroxylation)	
	Three-Dimensional Conformation		

Abnormalities That Affect Protein Structure

Primary Abnormalities That Alter Protein Conformation

In general, two features are essential for the normal biological function of a protein: (1) a normal conformation and (2) the presence of certain amino acids that play specific functional roles. A mutation can alter one or both of these features. The conformation of a protein, or the three-dimensional arrangement of its atoms, is the principal determinant of its biological function. Apart from changes in protein structure resulting from posttranslational modifications, conformation is determined entirely by the primary amino acid sequence. It follows that changes in the amino acid sequence can alter conformation and thus function. An additional and common consequence of altered conformation is a decrease in protein stability.

One of the most common causes of conformational disruption in globular proteins, such as hemoglobin, is the insertion of a hydrophilic (or polar) amino acid into the hydrophobic (or nonpolar) interior of the protein, which leaves a gap in the nonpolar lining of the interior, making the protein unstable. This type of substitution has occurred in about one fifth of the unstable hemoglo-

course, many other types of conformational disruption, due to substitutions, that cause instability (Perutz, 1987).

Secondary Abnormalities That Affect Protein Structure: Defects in Posttranslational Modifications

During or after translation, many proteins are covalently modified in ways that are essential to their normal function. When the modification is reversible, it may regulate the biological activity of the modified protein. There are presently only a few examples of mutations in enzymes responsible for *regulatory* posttranslational modifications, but given the frequency and importance of such forms of regulation, it seems likely that additional examples will be recognized. Some forms of **glycogen storage disease, Type VI,** which affects liver and muscle, are of this class. Some Type VI patients have defects in liver glycogen phosphorylase, the enzyme that degrades glycogen by removing glucose residues from the glycogen polysaccharide; others have a deficiency of the phosphorylase kinase required to activate the phosphorylase. Both X-linked and autosomal forms of liver phosphorylase kinase deficiency have been recognized; they are presumably due to mutations in X-linked and autosomal subunits of the enzyme, respectively.

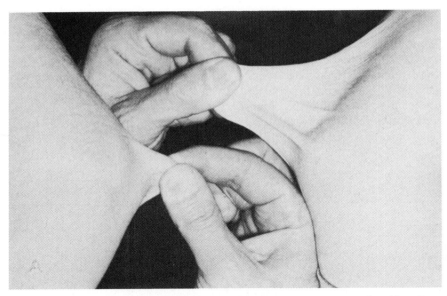

Figure 12–20. The hyperextensible skin of a patient with the Ehlers-Danlos syndrome. (Reproduced from Byers PH, Holbrook KA [1979] Heritable disorders of connective tissue. *In* Cohen AS [ed] The science and practice of clinical medicine, vol. 4: Rheumatology and immunology. Grune and Stratton, New York, p. 344.)

Ehlers-Danlos Syndrome. In many instances, the posttranslational modifications of a protein are permanent. A disease that results from the deficiency of a permanent posttranslational modification of collagen is Ehlers-Danlos syndrome, Type VI. Ehlers-Danlos syndrome is a heterogeneous group of connective tissue diseases characterized by skin fragility, joint hypermobility, and skin hyperextensibility (Fig. 12–20). In two types the basic defect has been found to be in the structural gene of the collagen I or III chains, these being the predominant collagens of the affected tissues. In the Type VI disorder, however, the disease results from defective posttranslational modification of collagens I and III, due to a deficiency of the enzyme lysyl hydroxylase. The hydroxylation of some of the lysine residues of collagen is essential for the formation of normal intermolecular cross links between collagen molecules, a process that stabilizes the collagen fibrillar network.

Abnormalities That Affect Subcellular Localization or Multiprotein Assembly

Once a polypeptide has folded into its correct conformation, it has to be directed to its appropriate cellular or extracellular location before it can assume a physiological role. In addition, a protein may require association with other proteins, or other types of molecules, before it can function normally. Whether localization or assembly with other molecules occurs first varies with the type of protein.

Primary Defects That Impair Cellular Trafficking

Methylmalonic Aciduria. Some proteins are directed to their appropriate cellular locale by virtue of information contained in the primary amino acid sequence. For example, most mitochondrial proteins are encoded by nuclear genes and must therefore be translocated from the cytoplasm to the mitochondria. For this purpose, they have a short amino-terminal leader sequence that allows them to be recognized by a receptor on the mitochondrial membrane and to be imported into the organelle. A mutation that illustrates the importance of correct subcellular localization has been identified in a patient with an autosomal recessive disorder of organic acid catabolism, methylmalonic aciduria. Methylmalonic acid is an organic acid intermediate in the catabolism of several amino acids and a few other compounds. It is converted by the enzyme methylmalonyl CoA mutase

Disease Example	Affected Step	Modifying Event	Disease Example
Three-Dimensional Conformation			
Methylmalonic aciduria: a defect in leader sequence in one allele of methylmalonyl CoA mutase	Subcellular localization due to information in amino acid sequence	Subcellular localization due to posttranslational modifications of the polypeptide	I-cell disease: failure to add a recognition marker to lysosomal enzymes
Many collagen defects→ osteogenesis imperfecta impair collagen helix assembly Hb Kansas, Hb Kempsey: impaired subunit interaction	For multimeric proteins: • subunit association • subunit interaction	Formation of multiprotein complexes and organelles	Zellweger syndrome: a defect in peroxisome biogenesis
Localization and Assembly			

(MM-CoA mutase) to succinyl-CoA, an intermediate of the citric acid cycle (Fig. 12–21). Mutations in the MM-CoA mutase structural gene, or in the formation of adenosylcobalamin, the vitamin B_{12} cofactor of the enzyme, lead to clinically heterogeneous presentations, usually associated with metabolic acidosis. The most severely affected patients present in the first weeks of life with lethargy, failure to thrive, and recurrent vomiting (Rosenberg and Fenton, 1989).

MM-CoA mutase entry into the mitochondria is mediated by a 32 amino acid leader sequence (or transit peptide; Fig. 12–21). In one patient, a mutation introduced a termination codon into the leader sequence (Ledley et al., 1990). However, translation initiates downstream from this stop

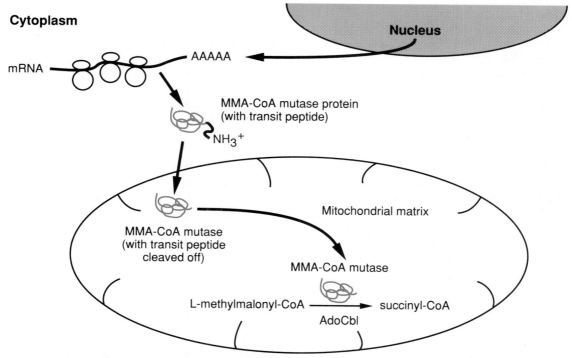

Figure 12–21. Most mitochondrial proteins, including methylmalonyl-CoA (MMA-CoA) mutase, are encoded by nuclear genes. The protein is directed through the mitochondrial membrane by an amino-terminal transit peptide. The peptide is removed in the mitochondria. AdoCbl = adenosylcobalamin.

codon to create an MM-CoA mutase precursor protein that lacks the leader peptide, and is thus not taken up by mitochondria. The occurrence of methylmalonic aciduria in this patient demonstrates that inappropriate subcellular localization can prevent the formation of a functional gene product. It should be noted, however, that most cases of mutase deficiency are due to point mutations that impair its catalytic activity but not its mitochondrial localization.

Secondary Defects That Impair Cellular Trafficking

I-Cell Disease. In contrast to mitochondrial and membrane proteins that are directed to their place of cellular residence by information contained in the primary amino acid sequence, other proteins are localized on the basis of posttranslational modifications. This is true of the acid hydrolases found in lysosomes, and in fact the existence and the mechanism of this form of cellular trafficking were unrecognized until I-cell disease, a severe autosomal recessive lysosomal storage disease, was investigated in the early 1970s (Wiesmann et al., 1971; Hickman and Neufeld, 1972). Cultured skin fibroblasts of patients with I-cell disease contain numerous abnormal lysosomes, or inclusions, throughout the cytoplasm (hence called inclusion-cells or I-cells).

In I-cell disease, many of the acid hydrolases normally present in lysosomes are grossly deficient within cells, but are found in excess in body fluids and in the medium of cells cultured from patients. The hydrolases in this condition are victims of a defect in a posttranslational modification that is required for their uptake by lysosomes. A typical hydrolase is a glycoprotein with mannose residues, some of which are phosphorylated. The mannose-6-phosphate residues are essential for recognition of the hydrolases by receptors on the cell and lysosomal membrane surface. In I-cell disease, there is a defect in the enzyme that transfers a phosphate group to the mannose residues. The fact that many enzymes are affected is consistent with the diversity of clinical abnormalities. The disorder has a range of pleiotropic effects, involving facial features, skeletal changes, severe growth retardation, and mental retardation. Affected children typically survive for only 5 to 7 years.

Mutations That Alter the Association of Proteins With Other Proteins

A newly synthesized protein may not become biologically active until it associates with other molecules. If the associated molecule is a protein, the result is a multimer or a more complex protein aggregate. Either identical or different polypeptides can combine to form a biologically active molecule. Not suprisingly, many mutations are known to interfere with these molecular interactions, thereby preventing the normal function of the protein.

Primary Mutations That Disrupt Subunit Assembly or Interaction in Multimeric Proteins

If a protein is composed of subunits, mutation may prevent their association by altering the subunit interfaces. This problem is seen in the defects of procollagen chain assembly in many of the mutations in type I collagen that cause the perinatal lethal (Type II) form of osteogenesis imperfecta (Table 12–7). If the mutation completely prevents assembly, or if the assembled protein is highly destabilized by poor subunit interaction as a consequence of the mutation, dissociation and degradation of the subunits (both mutant and normal) occur, as with the mutant proα1(I) chain (the proα1^M allele) shown in Figure 12–16.

Even when a mutation does not disturb subunit association, it may disturb critical interactions between the monomers, thereby impairing function. Two of the best-documented examples are the β-globin mutants Hb Kempsey and Hb Kansas, which, as described in Chapter 11, have mutations at the $\alpha_1 : \beta_2$ interface that prevent the normal movement of the α_1 and β_2 subunits that is required for normal binding and release of oxygen.

Secondary Functional Deficiencies Due to Failure to Form Multiprotein Complexes

The function of a protein may be reduced secondarily because other polypeptides, with which it normally forms a multiprotein complex, have primary genetic defects that prevent their synthesis. In the absence of the multiprotein structure, the component polypeptides may be subject to premature proteolysis. In other instances, the unassociated polypeptides may be present and functional but in the wrong cellular location, where their function is physiologically irrelevant. This principle is illustrated by defects of peroxisome biogenesis, the most severe of which is Zellweger syndrome.

Zellweger Syndrome: A Defect in Peroxisome Biogenesis. Severely affected infants with this autosomal recessive disease present in the neonatal period with dysmorphic features, including abnormal facies, profound neurological impairment, abnormalities in other major organs (e.g., the liver and kidney), and poor growth. Death usually occurs within the first few months. The pathology of this condition is characterized by an absence of normal peroxisomes, easily demonstrated in liver biopsy samples. This disease, and two other clinically similar but less abnormal phenotypes in which peroxisomes are also deficient, are the only examples in medicine of disorders resulting from the loss of the functions of an entire organelle.

The severe effects of Zellweger syndrome attest to the importance of peroxisomes, and the study of affected children provides an opportunity to understand their pathology as well as normal peroxisomal biosynthesis and function. At least five genes have been shown by complementation analysis to be affected in patients with the Zellweger syndrome (Roscher et al., 1989), but these genes and their products have not yet been identified. Their normal role may be to participate in the posttranslational import of proteins into the peroxisome after synthesis in the cytoplasm. Studies have shown that the peroxisomal membrane proteins in these diseases can be detected in unusual structures, larger-than-normal peroxisomes, that appear to be (nearly) empty membrane "ghosts."

In disorders of peroxisomal biogenesis, there is a *secondary* deficiency of many of the enzymes normally located inside the organelle. The deficient enzymes are synthesized normally but are prematurely degraded, probably because of their mislocation in the cytosol, where they may be vulnerable to proteolysis. Other unimported peroxisomal enzymes are stable, and their intracellular concentration can actually be increased. Catalase, for example, is entirely cytosolic in Zellweger syndrome and accumulates to twice its normal level. The cytosolic location of catalase is one of the most useful biochemical markers of these diseases. Another is the accumulation of very long-chain fatty acids, reflecting the fact that their oxidation normally begins in the peroxisome.

Mutations That Impair the Binding, Availability, or Removal of Cofactors or Prosthetic Groups

Certain proteins acquire biological activity only after they associate with nonprotein prosthetic groups or cofactors that play a critical role in the protein's function. Heme, the oxygen-binding moiety of hemoglobin, is a good example. Others include the cofactors that are required for the catalytic activity of some enzymes. Numerous mutations that interfere with ligand binding, synthesis, transport, or removal from a protein (when the binding is covalent) have been characterized. The nature of these defects makes them among the

Disease Example	Affected Step	Modifying Event	Disease Example
Localization and Assembly (which of these two steps occurs first varies with the type of protein)			
Cystathionine synthase deficiency: poor pyridoxal phosphate binding→homocystinuria in 50%	Cofactor or prosthetic group binding (noncovalent or covalent)	Cofactor or prosthetic group synthesis or transport	Mutations in vitamin B_{12} metabolism→methylmalonic aciduria and/or homocystinuria
		Cofactor binding or removal (covalent)	Holocarboxylase synthase deficiency; biotinidase deficiency
	Biological Function		

most responsive of all genetic diseases to specific biochemical therapy, particularly when the cofactor or its precursor is a water-soluble vitamin that can safely be given in large amounts.

Primary Mutations That Impair Cofactor Binding to the Protein

Homocystinuria Due to Cystathionine Synthase Deficiency. Homocystinuria due to cystathionine synthase deficiency (Fig. 12–22) was one of the first aminoacidopathies to be recognized (Carson et al., 1963). The clinical phenotype is often dramatic (and can be confused with the Marfan syndrome, a disorder of connective tissue), and in many cases treatment can be very effective. Perhaps most notably, it was one of the first genetic diseases shown to be vitamin responsive: pyridoxal phosphate is the cofactor of the enzyme, and the administration of large amounts of pyridoxine, the vitamin precursor of the cofactor, often ameliorates the biochemical abnormality (see Chapter 13).

The most common clinical features of this autosomal recessive condition (dislocation of the optic lens, mental retardation, osteoporosis, lengthening and thinning of the long bones, and thromboembolism of both veins and arteries) represent the pleiotropic effects of the enzyme deficiency, but how the biochemical abnormalities produce any component of the unusual phenotype is essentially unknown (Mudd et al., 1989). However, the accumulation of homocysteine is believed to be central to much, if not all, of the pathology. In many patients with homocystinuria, the affinity of the mutant enzyme for pyridoxal phosphate has been shown to be reduced, indicating an alteration in the conformation of the protein that affects this critical site.

Secondary Abnormalities in Protein Function Due to Inadequate Synthesis, Transport, Attachment, or Removal of Associated Molecules

In the example of homocystinuria, the binding of an associated molecule to a protein is impaired by mutations affecting the protein. In other diseases, on the other hand, loss of function of the protein may be secondary because of decreased availability of the associated molecule, which is due to primary genetic defects in its transport or synthesis or, when the bond is covalent, in its enzymatic attachment to or removal from the protein.

Defects in Associative Small Molecule Synthesis or Transport. Disorders of this class are well illustrated by types of homocystinuria that are the result, not of cystathionine synthase deficiency, but of various secondary defects in another enzyme, methionine synthase. As depicted in Figure 12–22, there are two pathways for the disposal of homocysteine: one through cystathionine synthase, the other involving the remethylation of homocysteine to methionine by methionine synthase. As shown, the cofactor of methionine

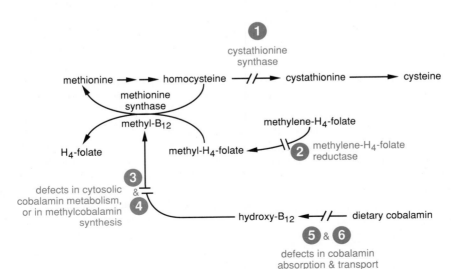

Figure 12–22. The six types of genetic defects that can cause homocystinuria. (1) Classical homocystinuria is due to defective cystathionine synthase. (2) In methylene-H_4-folate reductase defects, the decrease in methyl-H_4-folate impairs the function of methionine synthase. (3) Several different defects in the intracellular metabolism of cobalamins lead to a secondary decrease in the synthesis of methylcobalamin (methyl-B_{12}) and thus the function of methionine synthase. (4) Some disorders directly affect methyl-B_{12} formation. (5) Cobalamin intestinal absorption is abnormal in some patients. (6) Other patients have abnormalities in the major extracellular transport protein, transcobalamin II. Hydroxycobalamin = hydroxy-B_{12}.

Disease Example	Affected Step	Modifying Event	Disease Example
	Biological Function		
Mutations may affect only protein's function, as in active site mutations in enzymes (e.g., the *B1* allele of Tay-Sachs disease)			
Many mutations alter conformation→instability→degradation→decreased CRM (e.g., G6PD, the A⁻ variant)	Proteolytic degradation	Regulation of protein degradation	No examples yet known
	Degraded Protein		

synthase, methylcobalamin, is the product of a complex series of biochemical events. Although there are no reports of patients with a primary deficiency of methionine synthase, numerous disorders of vitamin B_{12} (cobalamin) transport or metabolism reduce the availability of methylcobalamin. Each of these conditions can therefore secondarily impair the function of methionine synthase. Many of these diseases also reduce the formation of adenosylcobalamin, the cofactor of methylmalonyl-CoA mutase (Fig. 12–21), and methylmalonic aciduria is consequently noted in such patients.

Several defects affect the intestinal absorption of cobalamin or its transport from the intestine to other cells; others disrupt specific steps in cobalamin biochemistry (Fig. 12–22). The clinical presentation of these disorders is variable, but includes megaloblastic anemia, developmental delay, and failure to thrive. These conditions are often partially or completely treatable with high doses of vitamin B_{12} (cobalamin). All are autosomal recessive.

Defects in Ligand Attachment or Removal. Two autosomal recessive diseases of biotin metabolism exemplify conditions belonging to this group. Of all the enzyme cofactors, biotin is unique in that it is permanently bound by covalent bonds to its apoenzymes (all four of which are carboxylases). Consequently, an enzyme, holocarboxylase synthetase, is required to attach the biotin to the carboxylase apoenzyme, and another, biotinidase, is needed to remove the biotin when the carboxylase is degraded, so that the biotin may be recycled. Absence of either the synthetase or biotinidase results in inadequate formation of the four carboxylases. Patients with these primary defects in biotin metabolism therefore develop sec-

ondary abnormalities of the four carboxylases, and it is the loss of the carboxylase activities that leads to clinical illness. The carboxylases are important for the catabolism of various organic acids, and the clinical presentation of these autosomal recessive conditions generally includes acidosis. Developmental delay is also a frequent occurrence. Patients with either type of biotin defect respond excellently to high doses of biotin.

Mutations That Principally Affect the Function of the Protein and Little Else

In this overview, we have described many properties of polypeptides that can be altered by mutation. In some instances, however, the protein may be quite normal apart from the loss of a single function. Mutant proteins in this category illustrate the importance of the second fundamental component required for the biological function of a protein (in addition to normal conformation): the presence of specific critical amino acids. Enzymes, for example, may have mutations in residues that constitute part of the active site; apart from impaired catalytic ability, such molecules may be relatively normal.

A mutation that alters the active site and apparently little else is one of the rarer alleles (the *B1* variant) that causes Tay-Sachs disease, referred to earlier. Whereas most Tay-Sachs alleles cause a profound deficiency of the α subunit protein (Table 12–3), the α subunit made in the *B1* variant (178 Arg→His) behaves like normal hex A in virtually every way, except for its nearly complete inability to cleave the natural substrate, G_{M2} ganglioside.

Structural Gene Mutations May Decrease the Stability of the Mutant Protein

As mentioned repeatedly, many mutations decrease the stability of the affected protein, often to the extent that little or none of the polypeptide can be detected. Occasionally, however, a mutation may have a more modest effect on stability and produce few other serious effects. In such instances, the instability contributes to the pathology by producing a time-dependent loss of the protein, as in the A⁻ variant of G6PD, described earlier.

THE EFFECT OF MUTATION ON PROTEIN FUNCTION

The effects of mutations on protein function are outlined in Figure 12–18. By definition, deleterious mutations cause pathology by changing the function of a protein, either by coding for an abnormality in structure or, less often, by altering a regulatory domain to change the number of normal protein molecules produced.

Loss-of-Function Mutations

The most common outcome of mutation, in either the coding or the regulatory region, is a loss of function of the protein (Fig. 12–18). Apart from any direct effect on function, a structurally abnormal protein may be unstable, so that its cellular concentration is decreased and its function secondarily reduced. Regardless of the specific reason for the loss of function, the clinical phenotype will be the same, as exemplified by the β-thalassemias. Most of the conditions already discussed belong to this category.

Gain-of-Function Mutations

Mutation can also alter the biochemical phenotype by enhancing the function of a protein, either by increasing its amount or by increasing the ability of each molecule to perform a normal function. However, more is not necessarily better, and disease may result. Although mutations that cause gain of function are uncommon, they may provide insight into the regulation of the expression of a gene or the molecular mechanism of a protein's function. Few variants of this class have come to clinical attention, presumably because a protein with increased function does not usually cause pathology. These mutations must be distinguished from those that lead to the acquisition of a *new* function by the mutant protein (to be discussed).

A subset of patients with the autosomal dominant form of **von Willebrand disease** exemplify gain-of-function mutations that cause disease. This condition is the most common inherited bleeding disorder, affecting 1 in 125 individuals, if all allelic variants and all degrees of severity are considered (Sadler, 1989). Most cases result from a simple quantitative deficiency of von Willebrand factor (vWF), a multifunctional protein that contributes to normal hemostasis in several ways, including binding platelets to the endothelium of vessel walls. The vWF of some hyperfunctional mutant alleles appears to have an increased affinity for platelets, presumably due to mutations in the domain of the vWF that normally binds to a glycoprotein on the platelet membrane (Ruggeri and Zimmerman, 1987). Bleeding may result from the fact that circulating platelets with vWF already bound to them cannot also bind to the vWF attached to the endothelium of vessel walls. This example illustrates the complexities of some mutations: an overall loss of the hemostatic function of the vWF in these variants is caused by the increased function of one domain of the protein.

Equally infrequent are regulatory mutants that increase the amount of mRNA made at a gene locus, or that alter the developmental expression of the locus, such as the mutations responsible for hereditary persistence of fetal hemoglobin (see Chapter 11).

Novel Property Mutations

In a few important diseases, some or all of the pathology results from the acquisition of a **novel property** due to the change in the amino acid sequence, rather than from loss of normal function. The classic disease illustrating a mutation of this type is sickle cell anemia. As discussed in Chapter 11, the ability of sickle hemoglobin to transport oxygen is normal. In contrast to normal hemoglobin, however, sickle hemoglobin chains aggregate when deoxygenated, ultimately forming the polymeric fibers that deform the red blood cell (see Fig. 11–6). This behavior has not been observed with any other mutant (or normal) hemoglobin molecule. The fact that mutations of this class are infrequent is not surprising. Many amino acid substitutions will be detrimental to the function or stability of a protein that has been finely tuned by evolution, but only rarely will a mutation introduce a new characteristic of pathological significance.

Alpha$_1$-Antitrypsin (α_1-AT) Deficiency

Another example of a mutation that confers new properties on a protein is provided by some variants of α_1-AT deficiency, an important autosomal recessive condition that leads to chronic obstructive lung disease and cirrhosis of the liver. The α_1-AT locus, on chromosome 14, is expressed principally in the liver, which secretes α_1-AT into plasma. Although α_1-AT inhibits a wide spectrum of proteases, its major physiological role is to bind and inhibit elastase, particularly elastase released from neutrophils in the lower respiratory tract (Cox, 1989).

Substantial genetic variability has been found in α_1-AT, over 75 genetic variants, called protease inhibitor (PI) types, having been identified (see Chapter 6). However, only about a dozen of these alleles lead to an increased risk of lung or liver disease, and only the Z allele is relatively common. In Caucasian populations, α_1-AT deficiency affects about 1 in 2500 persons, and 3 percent are carriers. The reason for the relatively high frequency of the Z allele in Caucasian populations is unknown, although analysis of DNA haplotypes suggests a single origin with subsequent spread in northern Europe. Given its increased risk of emphysema, α_1-AT deficiency is an important health problem, affecting 100,000 people in the United States alone.

The mutation in the Z allele (342 Glu→Lys) slows the rate of elastase inhibition by α_1-AT. However, the hepatic pathology of the Z protein appears to reflect a unique property: its tendency to aggregate in the rough endoplasmic reticulum of hepatocytes. Whereas normal α_1-AT is rapidly secreted from the liver, Z/Z patients have only about 15 percent of the normal plasma concentration of α_1-AT. The aggregation of the Z protein

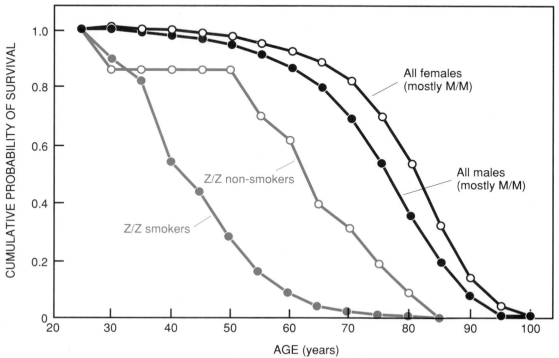

Figure 12–23. The effect of smoking on the survival of patients with alpha$_1$-antitrypsin deficiency. The curves show the cumulative probability of survival to specified ages of smokers, with or without alpha$_1$-antitrypsin deficiency. (Redrawn from Larrson C [1978] Natural history and life expectancy in severe alpha$_1$-antitrypsin deficiency, Pi Z. Acta Med Scand 204:345–351.)

appears to be responsible for its entrapment in the rough endoplasmic reticulum of hepatocytes. The molecular basis of this aggregation or insolubility is unclear, but Glu 342 appears to be critical to the normal folding or stability, or both, of the molecule. The presence of stored α_1-AT in the liver is thought to be responsible for the liver disease. About 17 percent of homozygotes present with neonatal jaundice, and approximately 25 percent of this group go on to develop cirrhosis.

α_1-AT Deficiency as an Ecogenetic Disease

The lung disease is due to the decreased plasma level of α_1-AT, which alters the normal balance between elastase and α_1-AT and allows progressive degradation of the elastin of alveolar walls. The progression of the emphysema is greatly augmented by smoking and is a powerful example of the effect that environmental factors may have on the phenotype of a genetic disease. Thus for persons with the Z/Z genotype, survival after age 60 is approximately 60 percent in nonsmokers, but only about 10 percent in smokers (Fig. 12–23). One molecular explanation for the effect of smoking is that the active site of α_1-AT, at methionine 358, is oxidized by both cigarette smoke and inflammatory cells, thus reducing its affinity for elastase by 2000-fold (Crystal et al., 1989).

The field of **ecogenetics,** illustrated by α_1-AT deficiency, is concerned with the interaction between environmental factors and different human genotypes. This area of medical genetics is likely to be one of increasing importance as genotypes are identified that entail an increased risk of disease upon exposure to certain environmental agents (for example, drugs, industrial chemicals, and viruses). In addition, genetic variation that may not by itself produce disease will be subject to increasing scrutiny in the search for the genetic contribution to non-Mendelian disorders, such as diabetes mellitus (Chapter 15).

THE LOCATION OF THE MUTANT PROTEIN AND THE SITE OF THE PATHOPHYSIOLOGY

Proteins can be divided into two general classes: **housekeeping proteins,** which are present in vir-

tually every cell and have fundamental roles in the maintenance of cell structure and function, and **specialty proteins,** which are produced in only one or a limited number of cell types and have unique functions that contribute to the individuality of the cells in which they are expressed. However, the distinction may not be absolute. A protein with a housekeeping role in most cells may be present at a higher level in a few tissues in which it has a more specialized function. Most tissues of higher eukaryotes, such as humans, express 10,000 to 15,000 genes. As many as 90 percent of the mRNA species found in a tissue are also present in many other tissues and encode the shared household proteins. The remaining 10 percent or so encode the specialty proteins of the tissue.

Mutations in Tissue-Specific Proteins

Mutation in a tissue-specific protein typically produces a disease restricted to that tissue (e.g., thalassemia affects primarily the red blood cell and its precursors), although there may be secondary effects on other tissues. However, mutations in tissue-specific proteins can also produce their primary clinical abnormalities in other cells and organs and, ironically, may even leave unaffected the tissue that lacks the mutant protein. For example, in PKU, mental retardation is the only significant pathological effect of deficiency of phenylalanine hydroxylase, which is found not in the brain but solely in the liver and kidneys. Thus one cannot necessarily infer that pathology in an organ results from a mutation in a gene expressed principally or only in that organ, or in that organ at all.

Mutations in Housekeeping Proteins

The clinical effects of mutations in a housekeeping protein are frequently limited to one or a few tissues, often tissues in which the protein is abundant and serves a specialty function. This situation is illustrated by two urea cycle enzymes: argininosuccinate synthetase and argininosuccinate lyase. The urea cycle is a liver-specific pathway that converts ammonia, which is neurotoxic, to urea. Argininosuccinate synthetase and lyase are expressed in all cells (where they participate in arginine biosynthesis), but their level of expression is substantially higher in the site of the urea cycle, the liver, than elsewhere. The major clinical effects of either enzymopathy (acute or chronic encephalopathy) are due to hyperammonemia from the loss of urea cycle function.

Combined Effects

In some disorders, loss of the housekeeping function causes one facet of the clinical presentation and loss of the tissue-specific function produces other features. For example, the purine metabolism enzyme HPRT (see Fig. 12–2) is normally present in all cells but is expressed at a higher level in the brain, where purines are putative neurotransmitters. In severe HPRT deficiency, which causes the Lesch-Nyhan syndrome (described earlier), overproduction of uric acid throughout the body causes gout and renal stones, whereas deficiency of the enzyme in the central nervous system leads to a movement disorder, spasticity, mental retardation, and self-mutilation. In contrast, moderate HPRT deficiency leads only to gout and nephrolithiasis and has no central nervous system effects.

THE RELATIONSHIP BETWEEN THE MOLECULAR PATHOLOGY OF PROTEINS AND THE CLINICAL PHENOTYPE

Two generalizations can be made about the relationship between the molecular pathology of mutant proteins and the clinical phenotype of the resulting diseases:

1. **Different mutations in a single gene may produce very different clinical phenotypes.** In other words, genetic heterogeneity at a locus (allelic heterogeneity) is often responsible for clinical heterogeneity. A dramatic illustration of this point is provided by the β-globin structural mutants described in Chapter 11 (see Table 11–1): the clinical presentations of the various mutations are often so different that from a clinical perspective alone, it is not at all obvious that they all affect a single pro-

tein. Some of the variation in clinical presentation predictably reflects the *specific* property of the protein that has been most perturbed (for example, the oxygen-binding function of hemoglobin in the polycythemias). In other cases, such as sickle cell disease, the molecular pathology is not due to a change in a normal function of the protein, and the effects of the mutation are largely unpredictable.

For some proteins, such as hex A (the enzyme deficient in Tay-Sachs disease), the phenotype caused by total loss of function is the same whether the loss is due to absence of the protein or to a defect that cripples catalysis without affecting quantity. For other proteins, it may be important whether the mutation results primarily in normal quantities of an abnormal protein or reduction in quantity of a normal protein. Thus thalassemia mutations lead to an underproduction of globin chains, whereas point mutations that do not substantially reduce the amount of a globin chain produce quite different phenotypes (for example, methemoglobinemia).

Most clinical phenotypes may result from one of many different mutations that have a similar effect on protein function. In contrast, the only β-globin mutation that has been found to cause sickle cell disease is the β 6 Glu→Val substitution. This occurrence of a specific disease with a unique point mutation is remarkable and at present represents one of the few illustrations of this phenomenon in medical genetics.

2. **The biochemical and clinical consequences of a mutation are often unpredictable.** No one would have foreseen that the sickle mutation would lead to polymerization of deoxygenated hemoglobin S or that the only significant consequence of phenylalanine hydroxylase deficiency would be mental retardation. Equally unexpected was the discovery that point mutations in the visual pigment rhodopsin are responsible for many cases of a slow degenerative disorder of the retina, autosomal dominant retinitis pigmentosa (Dryja et al., 1990). Patients with this condition have relatively normal vision for many years, at least partly because rhodopsin encoded by the unaffected allele participates normally in the conversion of a light photon into a nerve impulse in the retina; it is unclear whether the mutant rhodopsin molecules can function normally in the visual process. How the defects in the mutant allele lead to the slow but inexorable destruction of the photore-

ceptor cells, with loss of vision in adulthood, is also unknown.

CONCLUSION

As the biochemical pathology of an increasing number of genetic diseases is gradually untangled, and as the genetic components of the common multifactorial diseases are characterized, new and unforeseen pathophysiological mechanisms will be recognized. The understanding of genetic disease at a molecular level not only contributes to the knowledge of normal human biology but is also the foundation of effective treatment for these disorders. The principles applied in the treatment of genetic disease are presented in Chapter 13, with examples that include many of the conditions that have been described here and in Chapter 11.

General References

Harris H (1980) The principles of human biochemical genetics, 3rd ed. Elsevier North-Holland, Amsterdam.

McKusick VA (1972) Heritable disorders of connective tissue, 4th ed. CV Mosby, St. Louis.

Meyer UA (1990) Molecular genetics and the future of pharmacogenetics. Pharm Ther 46:349–355.

Meyer UA, Zanger UM, Grant D, Blum M (1990) Genetic polymorphisms of drug metabolism. Adv Drug Res 19:198–241.

Scriver CR, Childs B (1989) Garrod's inborn factors and disease. Oxford University Press, New York.

Scriver CR, Beaudet AL, Sly WS, Valle D (eds) (1989) The metabolic basis of inherited disease, 6th ed. McGraw-Hill, New York.

Valle D, Mitchell GA (1988) Inborn errors of metabolism in the molecular age. Prog Med Genet 7:100–129.

Problems

1. One mutant allele at the LDL receptor locus (leading to familial hypercholesterolemia) encodes an elongated protein that is about 50,000 daltons larger than the normal 120,000-dalton receptor. Indicate at least three mechanisms that could account for this abnormality. Approximately how many extra nucleotides would need to be translated to add 50,000 daltons to the protein?

2. In discussing the nucleotide changes found to date in the coding region of the cystic fibrosis gene, we stated that some of the changes (the missense changes) found so far are only "putative" mutations. What criteria would one need to fulfill before knowing that a nucleotide change is a mutation and not a polymorphism?

3. Johnny, 2 years of age, is failing to thrive. Investigations show that although he has clinical findings of CF, his sweat chloride is normal. The sweat chloride is normal in fewer than 2 percent of CF patients. His pediatrician and parents want to know if DNA analysis can determine whether or not he indeed has CF.
   a) Would DNA analysis be useful in this case? Briefly outline the steps involved in obtaining a DNA diagnosis for CF.
   b) If he has CF, what is the probability that he is homozygous for the ΔF508 mutation? (Assume that 85 percent of CF mutations could be detected at the time you are consulted and that his parents are from Northern Europe, where the ΔF508 allele has a frequency of 0.70).
   c) If he does not have the ΔF508 mutation, does this disprove the diagnosis? Explain.

4. James is the only person in his kindred affected by DMD. He has one unaffected brother, Joe. DNA analysis shows that James has a deletion in the DMD gene and that Joe has received the same maternal X chromosome but without a deletion. What genetic counseling would you give the parents regarding the recurrence risk of DMD in a future pregnancy?

5. DMD has a high mutation rate but shows no ethnic variation in frequency. Use your knowledge of the gene and the genetics of DMD to suggest why this disorder is equally common in all populations.

6. In patients with osteogenesis imperfecta, explain why the missense mutations at glycine positions in the triple helix of Type I collagen are confined to a limited number of other amino acid residues (Ala, Ser, Cys, Arg, Val, Asp).

7. Electrophoresis of red blood cell hemolysates shows that some females have two G6PD bands, but males have a single band. Explain this observation and the possible pathological and genetic significance of the finding of two bands in a Black American female.

8. A 2-year-old infant, the child of first cousin parents, has unexplained developmental delay. A survey of various biochemical parameters indicates that he has a deficiency of four lysosomal enzymes. Explain how a single autosomal recessive mutation might cause the loss of function of four enzyme activities. Why is it most likely that the child has an autosomal recessive condition, if he has a genetic condition at all?

CHAPTER 13

THE TREATMENT OF GENETIC DISEASE

In the coming decades, the impact of molecular biology and protein engineering on the treatment of genetic disease may be as great as that of DNA polymorphisms and positional cloning on general medical genetics in the preceding decade. In this chapter, therefore, we not only provide an overview of the standard therapies used in the management of genetic disease but also outline some of the new strategies that may be used in the future. In particular, we emphasize therapies that reflect the genetic approach to medicine. As with all therapy, the objective of treating genetic disease is to eliminate or ameliorate the effects of the disorder on not only the patient but also the family. In addition, the family must be informed about the risk that the disease may occur in other members. The latter responsibility, genetic counseling, is a major component of the management of hereditary disorders and is dealt with separately in Chapter 18. The preferred treatment of many single-gene diseases will eventually be gene transfer therapy, if the procedure can be made safe and effective. However, even when copies of a normal gene can be transferred into the patient to effect permanent cure, the family will need ongoing genetic counseling, carrier testing, and prenatal diagnosis, in many cases over several generations. For the present, we are left with replacing the de-fective protein, improving its function, or minimizing the consequences of its deficiency. A number of excellent overviews of the treatment of genetic disease have been published, including those by Valle (1987), Beaudet and colleagues (1989), Rosenberg (1990), and Desnick (1991).

THE PRESENT STATE OF TREATMENT OF GENETIC DISEASE

Multifactorial Diseases

For most multifactorial diseases (see Chapter 15), both the genetic and environmental components of the etiology are poorly understood. However, when an environmental contribution is recognized, an opportunity for effective intervention is available because exposure to the environmental factor can often be modified. Thus cigarette smoking is an environmental factor that all patients with emphysema should avoid. At least one mechanism by which cigarette smoke leads to emphysema has been disclosed by the study of the single-gene disorder alpha$_1$-antitrypsin (α_1-AT) deficiency. As described in the preceding chapter, cigarette smoke oxidizes the critical methionine residue at the active site of α_1-AT, which reduces

317

by 2000-fold its ability to inhibit elastase. Thus smoking produces a substantial acquired loss of α_1-AT function.

The general impression that genetic diseases are invariably difficult to treat is contradicted by data on disorders of multifactorial inheritance in newborns that may be cured by surgery, a form of phenotypic modification. These conditions include congenital heart defects, cleft lip and palate, and pyloric stenosis. Remarkably, these three structural abnormalities affect nearly 1.5 percent of all live-born infants, who make up approximately 30 percent of all newborns with genetic disease (Rosenberg, 1990). In about half of these patients, the diseases are curable by a single operation; a cure is therefore possible in at least 10 to 15 percent of infants with a genetically determined disorder. However, the treatment of inherited disease is rarely so beneficial, although it often improves the quality of life. For multifactorial disorders that typically present in adolescence or adult life, such as essential hypertension, diabetes, coronary artery disease, and schizophrenia and other major psychoses, the imperfections of treatment reflect ignorance of the etiology.

Single-Gene Diseases

The treatment of single-gene diseases is sadly deficient at present. A recent survey of 351 disorders showed that with current therapy, the life span can be restored to normal in only about 15 percent of single-gene conditions, reproductive capability in 11 percent, and social adaptation in 6 percent (Hayes et al., 1985). However, one bright note was identified by the analysis: the success of treatment is greatest for disorders in which the basic biochemical defect is known (Fig. 13–1). Even in this favored group, however, the treatment was completely corrective for phenotypic dysfunction in only 12 percent, partially corrective in 40 percent, and of no effect in the remainder. Thus research to elucidate the genetic and biochemical basis of hereditary disease does have an impact on the patient, although even in biochemically defined disorders, current therapy fails to restore normal health to the great majority of patients.

The present unsatisfactory state of treatment of genetic disease is due to numerous factors, in-

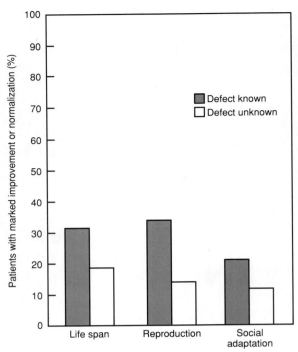

Figure 13–1. The effect of treatment of genetic diseases on three disease manifestations. Although the response to treatment is poor both for diseases of unknown cause and those in which the biochemical defect is known, the results are better in the latter group. (Adapted from Hayes A, Costa T, Scriver CR, Childs B [1985] The effect of Mendelian disease on human health. II: Response to treatment. Am J Med Genet 21:243–255.)

cluding the following three:

1. The mutant locus in more than 80 percent of genetic diseases (Hayes et al., 1985) is unknown, and knowledge of the pathophysiology in those diseases in which the affected gene or biochemical abnormality is known is inadequate. In phenylketonuria (PKU), for example, despite years of study, the mechanisms by which the elevation in phenylalanine impairs brain development and function are still poorly understood. For diseases such as cystic fibrosis and Duchenne muscular dystrophy, in which the affected protein has only recently been identified, much work is required before the normal function of the polypeptide is determined and the disease process fully elucidated.

2. Some mutations act early in development or cause irreversible pathology before they are diagnosed. These problems can be anticipated in

some cases if there is a family history of a genetic disease or if carrier screening identifies couples at risk. In the latter case, prenatal treatment is sometimes possible, for both medical (Pang et al., 1990) and surgical (Harrison et al., 1990) conditions.

3. The initial cases of a disease to be recognized are usually severely affected ones, which are often less amenable to treatment than more mildly affected ones. In the milder cases, the mutant protein may retain some residual function that can be increased by one of several strategies, as described later.

SPECIAL CONSIDERATIONS IN TREATING GENETIC DISEASE

The Need for Long-Term Assessment of Treatment

In genetic disease, perhaps more than in other areas of medicine, treatment initially judged as successful may eventually be shown to be imperfect. There are at least three facets to this problem. First, treatment may initially appear to be successful, only to be shown by longer observation to have subtle inadequacies. Thus although well-managed children with PKU have escaped severe retardation and have normal or near-normal IQs (see below), they often manifest subtle learning disorders and behavioral disturbances that impair their academic performance (Scriver et al., 1989). Similarly, in galactosemia patients (described in Chapter 6), learning disabilities like those observed in treated PKU patients have been recognized (Segal, 1989).

Second, successful treatment of the pathological changes in one organ may be followed by unexpected problems in tissues not previously observed to be clinically involved, because the patients did not survive long enough. For example, despite conscientious treatment, most females with galactosemia have ovarian failure that appears to result from continued galactose toxicity. The detection of the later manifestations may require many years of observation after the initial therapy. Another disease that illustrates this phenomenon is **cystinosis,** which is caused by cystine accumulation in the lysosome due to a defect in cystine efflux (see Table 12–1). The cystine stor-

age initially leads to renal failure. As patients who receive renal transplants grow older, however, morbidity results from hypothyroidism, from islet cell disease that causes diabetes, and from various neurological abnormalities (Gahl et al., 1989). A final example is provided by mutations in the retinoblastoma gene (see Chapter 16). Patients successfully treated for the eye tumor in the first years of life are at increased risk of developing an independent malignancy, osteosarcoma, after the first decade. Ironically, therefore, treatment that successfully prolongs life provides a new opportunity for the clinical expression of the basic defect, particularly in conditions in which the mutant gene is normally expressed in many tissues, thus providing more potential targets for the development of pathology.

Third, therapy that is problem free in the short term may produce serious side effects in the long term. For example, clotting factor infusion in hemophilia sometimes results in the formation of antibodies to the infused protein, and blood transfusion in thalassemia invariably produces iron overload, which can be managed but with difficulty.

Genetic Heterogeneity and Treatment

The optimal treatment of single-gene defects often requires an unusual degree of diagnostic precision, at the level of the affected molecule. As stated repeatedly in early chapters, genetic heterogeneity (allelic heterogeneity or locus heterogeneity) is a common characteristic of genetic diseases. For proper management, it is often critical not simply to treat a biochemical abnormality but to identify precisely the basic biochemical defect, as opposed to a secondary defect such as those outlined in Table 12–9. For example, abnormalities in phenylalanine hydroxylase and in the enzymes of biopterin metabolism both produce hyperphenylalaninemia, but the treatment of the two types of defects is quite different. Even allelic mutations may require different management: the clinically distinct β-globin disorders, thalassemia, and sickle cell disease, illustrate this concept.

The study of allelic variants of enzyme defects has shown that alleles that retain small amounts of residual enzyme activity often cause much less severe disease than null alleles. The contrast between patients with classic PKU (with virtually no residual enzyme activity) and those with benign hyperphenylalaninemia (with about 5 percent activity) illustrates this principle. The corollary of this observation is that effective treatment of classic PKU by gene or enzyme transfer would require the delivery of only small amounts of phenylalanine hydroxylase.

Allelic heterogeneity has additional implications for therapy. Some alleles produce a protein that is decreased in abundance but has residual function. Strategies designed to increase the expression or stability of the partially functional protein may be effective in correcting the biochemical defect. In contrast, nothing is to be gained by increasing the abundance of a mutant protein with no residual function. In fact, increased expression of a functionless mutant protein may be detrimental because it may exert a dominant negative effect (see Chapter 12) if it interacts with the product of the normal allele, or with other proteins, to impair their function. This consideration is also relevant to efforts to transfer a normal gene into a patient with a genetic disease. For example, in osteogenesis imperfecta, patients with null alleles may be easier to treat by gene transfer than those with qualitatively abnormal collagen chains that reduce the effective contribution of the transferred gene (see Fig. 12–16).

TREATMENT STRATEGIES

Genetic disease can be treated at many levels, at various steps away from the mutant gene (Fig. 13–2). In the remainder of this chapter, we describe the rationale used or proposed for treatment at each of these levels. In general, diseases described earlier in the book are used as examples, although new disorders are presented when necessary to illustrate a specific approach. None of the current treatments are necessarily mutually exclusive, although successful gene transfer therapy would render other therapies superfluous. Treatment "at the level of the clinical phenotype" (Fig. 13–2) is a category meant to include all the types of medical or surgical intervention that are not unique to the management of genetic disease. Often this is the only therapy available and, in

some cases, may be all that is necessary, as is the case, for example, with some surgically correctable malformations. Finally, the importance of educating the patient—not only to achieve understanding of the disease, its genetic implications, and the treatment but also to ensure compliance with therapy that may be inconvenient and lifelong—cannot be overemphasized.

Treatment of Metabolic Abnormalities

The most successful disease-specific approach to the treatment of genetic disease has been at the level of the metabolic abnormality. In fact, this concept is familiar to those who are aware of the need for dietary compensation for the inability of humans and other higher primates to synthesize ascorbic acid (vitamin C). The principal strategies used to manipulate metabolism in the treatment of inborn errors are listed in Table 13–1. The necessity for patients with pharmacogenetic diseases, such as glucose-6-phosphate dehydrogenase deficiency, to avoid certain drugs and chemicals is described in Chapter 12.

Dietary Restriction

Dietary restriction is one of the oldest and most effective methods of managing genetic disease. Its advantage is that it can be highly effective; its drawback is that it usually requires lifelong compliance with a restricted and often artificial diet. This dietary constraint is onerous for the family as well as the patient, especially in adolescence. Many of the diseases treatable in this manner involve amino acid catabolic pathways, and therefore severe restriction of normal dietary protein is usually necessary. Essential nutrients such as amino acids, however, cannot be withheld entirely; their intake must be sufficient for anabolic needs. Patients with mild enzymatic defects (i.e., "leaky" mutant alleles) can tolerate more of the offending compound; consequently, the diet is less restrictive, and compliance may be better. In other cases, the dietary precursor to the offending substrate is not an essential nutrient (e.g., galactose), and it can be eliminated from the diet altogether. Diseases involving more than two dozen loci are presently managed in this way.

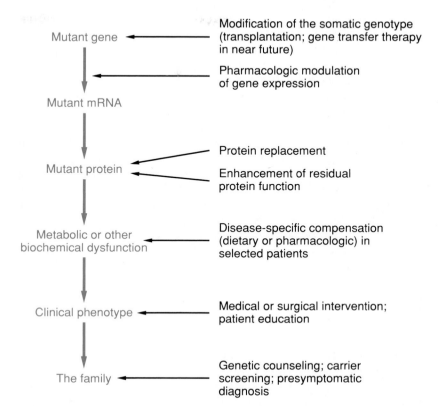

Level of intervention

Treatment strategy

Mutant gene ← Modification of the somatic genotype (transplantation; gene transfer therapy in near future)

← Pharmacologic modulation of gene expression

Mutant mRNA

Mutant protein ← Protein replacement

← Enhancement of residual protein function

Metabolic or other biochemical dysfunction ← Disease-specific compensation (dietary or pharmacologic) in selected patients

Clinical phenotype ← Medical or surgical intervention; patient education

The family ← Genetic counseling; carrier screening; presymptomatic diagnosis

Figure 13–2. The various levels of treatment that are relevant to genetic disease, with the corresponding strategies used at each level. (Adapted from Valle D [1987] Genetic disease: An overview of current therapy. Hosp Pract 22(7): 167–182.)

A diet restricted in phenylalanine largely circumvents the neurological damage in **classic PKU** (Scriver et al., 1989) (see Chapter 12). Phenylketonuric children are normal at birth because the maternal enzyme protects them during prenatal life. The results of treatment are best when the diagnosis is made soon after birth and treatment is begun promptly. If the child is fed a normal diet in the first months of life, irreversible mental retardation occurs; the degree of intellectual deficit is

Table 13–1. Treatment of Genetic Disease by Metabolic Manipulation

Type of Metabolic Intervention	Substance or Technique	Example
Avoidance	Antimalarial drugs Isoniazid	G6PD deficiency Slow acetylators
Dietary restriction	Phenylalanine Galactose	PKU Galactosemia
Replacement	Thyroxine Biotin	Congenital hypothyroidism Biotinidase deficiency
Diversion	Sodium benzoate Oral resins	Urea cycle disorders Familial hypercholesterolemia
Inhibition	Lovastatin	Familial hypercholesterolemia
Depletion	Plasma exchange therapy	Familial hypercholesterolemia

Modified from Rosenberg (1990).

directly related to the delay in the institution of the low-phenylalanine diet. The normal mental status of patients with benign hyperphenylalaninemia demonstrates that effective treatment of classic PKU can be achieved if the phenylalanine levels can be kept below about 0.7 mM. Without this guidance from nature, many clinical trials would have been required to establish a "safe" plasma phenylalanine level in the classic disease. It is now recommended that patients with PKU remain on a low phenylalanine diet for life because neurological and behavioral abnormalities develop in many (though not all) patients if the diet is stopped. However, even in patients who have been treated throughout life, it is now clear that even when the IQ is normal or near normal, there are neuropsychological deficits (e.g., in conceptual, visuospatial, and language skills), although treatment produces results vastly superior to the outcome without treatment.

Replacement

The provision of essential metabolites, cofactors, or hormones whose deficiency is due to a genetic disease is simple in concept and often in application. Some of the most successfully treated single-gene defects belong to this category. An important example is **congenital hypothyroidism,** which results from a variety of defects (10 to 15 percent of which are genetic) in the formation of the thyroid gland or of its major product, thyroxine. Because congenital hypothyroidism is common (about 1/4000 neonates) and treatment can prevent the associated mental retardation, neonatal screening is conducted in many countries, so that thyroxine administration may be initiated as soon as possible after birth to prevent the severe intellectual defects that are otherwise inevitable. In **biotinidase deficiency** (see Chapter 12), the enzymopathy prevents the recovery of biotin from biotinylated proteins and thus prevents recycling of this enzyme cofactor. The administration of large amounts of biotin is completely corrective if given before serious neurological sequelae develop.

Diversion

Diversion therapy is the enhanced use of alternative metabolic pathways to reduce the concentration of a harmful metabolite. The diversion strat-

egy has been successfully applied to the treatment of the **urea cycle disorders.** The function of the urea cycle is to convert ammonia, which is neurotoxic, to urea, which is a benign end product that is excreted. If the cycle is disrupted by an enzyme defect such as argininosuccinate synthetase or lyase deficiency, the consequent hyperammonemia can be only partially controlled by dietary protein restriction. The ammonia can be reduced to normal levels by diversion to metabolic pathways that are normally of minor significance, leading to synthesis of harmless compounds. For example, the administration of sodium benzoate forces its ligation with glycine to form hippurate, which is excreted in the urine (Fig. 13–3). Glycine synthesis is thereby increased, and for each mole of glycine formed, one mole of ammonia is consumed.

A similar approach has been successful in helping to reduce the cholesterol level in *heterozygotes* for **familial hypercholesterolemia** (reviewed in Chapter 12). The single normal low-density lipoprotein (LDL) receptor gene of these patients can be stimulated to produce more hepatic receptors for LDL-bound cholesterol by the diversion of an increased fraction of cholesterol to bile acid synthesis. Because 70 percent of all LDL-receptor mediated uptake of cholesterol is by the liver, a significant reduction in plasma cholesterol can be achieved (Goldstein and Brown, 1989). The increase in bile acid synthesis is obtained by the oral administration of nonabsorbable resins such as cholestyramine and colestipol, which bind bile acids in the intestine and increase their fecal excretion (Fig. 13–4). An important principle illustrated

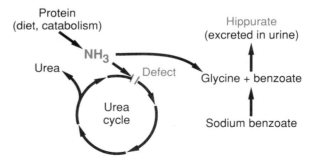

Figure 13–3. The strategy of metabolite diversion. In this example, ammonia cannot be removed by the urea cycle because of a genetic defect of a urea cycle enzyme. The administration of sodium benzoate diverts ammonia to glycine synthesis, and the nitrogen moiety is subsequently excreted as hippurate.

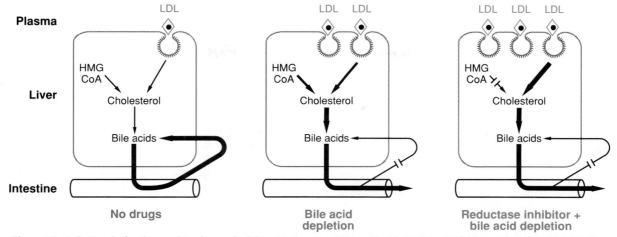

Figure 13–4. Rationale for the combined use of a bile acid–binding resin and an inhibitor of 3-hydroxy-3-methylglutaryl CoA reductase (HMG CoA reductase) in the treatment of familial hypercholesterolemia heterozygotes. (From Brown MS, Goldstein JL [1986] A receptor-mediated pathway for cholesterol homeostasis. Science 232:4. Copyright by the Nobel Foundation.)

by this example is that autosomal dominant diseases may sometimes be treated by increasing the expression of the normal allele.

Inhibition

The pharmacological inhibition of enzymes is sometimes used to modify the metabolic abnormalities of inborn errors. This principle is effectively exploited in the treatment of familial hypercholesterolemia. If methods are used to decrease the cholesterol load by diverting it to other compounds or by removing it with physical methods, as described in the next section, the liver tries to compensate for the cholesterol deficiency by up-regulating cholesterol synthesis (Goldstein and Brown, 1989). Consequently, the treatment of heterozygotes with familial hypercholesterolemia is more effective if hepatic cholesterol synthesis is simultaneously inhibited. The development of powerful competitive inhibitors of the rate-limiting enzyme of cholesterol synthesis, hydroxymethylglutaryl coenzyme A (HMG CoA) reductase, has allowed a rational combined approach that is highly effective. One inhibitor, lovastatin, effects a 50 to 60 percent decrease in plasma LDL cholesterol levels when used together with cholestyramine (Fig. 13–4). The long-term safety of this drug is presently being determined. Homozygotes with familial hypercholesterolemia can be treated by the methods used for heterozygotes if

there is some residual LDL receptor activity. For the remainder of homozygotes, however, these strategies are uniformly ineffective.

Depletion

Genetic diseases characterized by the accumulation of a harmful compound are sometimes treated by direct removal of the compound from the body. Homozygotes for familial hypercholesterolemia have been shown to respond to plasma exchange with 50 percent or greater reductions in LDL cholesterol. A modification of this approach involves the selective removal of plasma LDL by continuous extracorporeal passage of the plasma over columns that bind the protein component of LDL (see Fig. 12–7).

Treatment at the Level of the Protein

If a mutant protein has some residual function, it may be possible to enhance this activity by increasing the stability of the protein or by increasing the residual working capacity of each abnormal molecule. With enzymopathies, the improvement in function obtained by this approach is usually very small—on the order of a few percent—but this increment is often all that is required to restore biochemical homeostasis. It is obvious that mutations that prevent the synthesis of the protein (null alleles) are not amenable to this approach. On the other hand, most proteins do not interact with "corrective" ligands that can be given in large amounts, and in these cases treatment at the protein level can be achieved only by replacement of the protein.

Enhancement of the Function of the Mutant Protein

The biochemical abnormalities of a number of metabolic diseases may respond, sometimes dramatically, to the administration of large amounts of the vitamin cofactor of the enzyme impaired by the mutation (Table 13–2). In fact, the **vitamin-responsive inborn errors** are among the most successfully treated of all genetic diseases (Rosenberg, 1976). In biotinidase deficiency, alluded to earlier, the response occurs because the administered biotin replaces the biotin that fails to be recycled because of the defect. Various mechanisms explain the therapeutic effect in other responsive disorders. For example, in some conditions, in order to overcome reduced affinity of the mutant enzyme for the cofactor, the system is saturated with the cofactor (Fig. 13–5). The vitamins used are nontoxic, allowing the safe administration of doses that are 100 to 500 times greater than required for normal nutrition. For example, about 50 percent of patients with **homocystinuria** due to cystathionine synthase deficiency (see Fig. 12–22) respond to the administration of high doses of pyridoxine (vitamin B_6), and in most of these pa-

tients, homocystine disappears completely from the plasma. The increase in enzyme activity, as assessed in liver extracts of responsive patients, is only a fewfold: in one case, for example, from 1.5 to only 4.5 percent of control activity. The molecular basis of the pyridoxine response is uncertain; stabilization of the mutant enzyme by its pyridoxal phosphate cofactor is one possible mechanism. In any case, pyridoxine treatment substantially improves the clinical course of the disease in responsive patients. The molecular defects in nonresponsive patients are as yet undefined, but such patients generally have no residual activity.

Protein Replacement

The principal types of protein replacement used to date are summarized in Table 13–2. Protein replacement is part of the *routine* therapeutic repertoire in only a few diseases, all of which affect proteins whose principal site of action is in the plasma or extracellular fluid. The prevention or arrest of bleeding episodes in patients with hemophilia by the infusion of plasma fractions enriched for factor VIII is the prime example. The years of experience with this disease also indicate the problems that can be anticipated as new strategies, outlined below, encourage attempts at the replacement of other, particularly intracellular, polypeptides. The problems include the difficulty of procuring sufficient amounts of the protein to treat all patients at the optimal frequency (this problem is still a major one in the management of hemophilia), the need to administer the protein at a

Table 13–2. Treatment of Genetic Disease at the Level of the Mutant Protein

Strategy	Example	Status
Enhancement of Mutant Protein Function		
Cofactor administration to increase enzyme activity	Pyridoxine-responsive homocystinuria	Treatment of choice in the ~50% of patients who are responsive
Protein Replacement		
Replacement of an extracellular protein	Factor VIII in hemophilia A Alpha$_1$-antitrypsin in α_1-AT deficiency	Well established and quite effective Biochemically effective; long-term trial in progress
Extracellular replacement of an intracellular protein	Polyethylene glycol-modified adenosine deaminase (PEG-ADA) in ADA deficiency	Dramatic clinical improvement; long-term effects under study
Replacement of intracellular proteins: cell targeting	Modified glucocerebrosidase in Gaucher disease	Biochemically effective in a small number of patients; long-term trials in progress

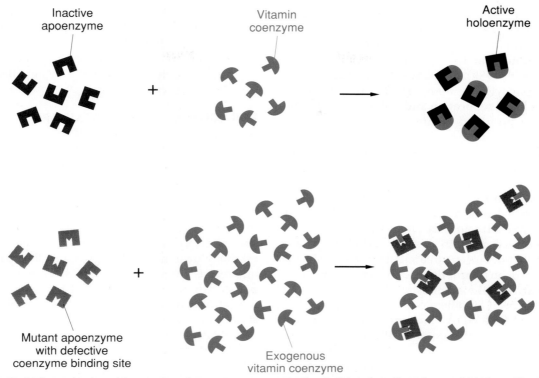

Inactive
apoenzyme

Vitamin
coenzyme

Active
holoenzyme

Mutant apoenzyme
with defective
coenzyme binding site

Exogenous
vitamin coenzyme

Figure 13 – 5. The mechanism of the response of a mutant apoenzyme to the administration of its cofactor at high doses. Vitamin-responsive enzyme defects are often due to mutations that reduce the normal affinity (top) of the enzyme protein (apoenzyme) for the cofactor needed to activate it. In the presence of the high concentrations of the cofactor that result from the administration of up to 500 times the normal daily requirement, the mutant enzyme acquires a small amount of activity sufficient to restore biochemical normalcy. (Redrawn from Valle D [1987] Genetic disease: An overview of current therapy. Hosp Pract 22(7):167–182.)

frequency consistent with its half-life (only 8 to 10 hours for factor VIII), the formation of neutralizing antibodies in some patients (5 percent of classic hemophiliacs), and the contamination of the protein with foreign agents, particularly viruses (hepatitis, human immunodeficiency virus) (Vehar et al., 1989).

REPLACEMENT OF AN EXTRACELLULAR PROTEIN: ALPHA₁-ANTITRYPSIN DEFICIENCY

As reviewed in Chapter 12, alpha$_1$-antitrypsin (α_1-AT) is the major inhibitor of neutrophil elastase, a destructive proteolytic enzyme stored in neutrophils. There are between 20,000 and 40,000 Z/Z homozygotes in North America alone; thus α_1-AT deficiency is a significant cause of premature death in the adult population (see Fig. 12 – 23). The object of therapy is to redress the imbalance between elastase and α_1-AT by delivering α_1-AT in adequate amounts to the pulmonary epi-

thelium and to the alveolar interstitial fluid. An important first step in this direction has been taken by Wewers and associates (1987), who demonstrated the biochemical efficacy of α_1-AT replacement therapy. Human α_1-AT can be infused intravenously into α_1-AT-deficient patients in doses sufficiently large to maintain the interstitial α_1-AT concentration at an effective inhibitory level for 1 month. More than 1000 patients worldwide are now receiving this treatment in order to ascertain whether, over a period of years, it is capable of arresting the pulmonary destruction (Crystal, 1990).

EXTRACELLULAR REPLACEMENT OF AN INTRACELLULAR ENZYME: ADENOSINE DEAMINASE DEFICIENCY

Adenosine deaminase (ADA) is a critical enzyme of purine metabolism that catalyzes the deamination of adenosine to inosine and of deoxyadenosine to deoxyinosine (see Fig. 12 – 2). The pathological effects of ADA deficiency, an autosomal recessive disease, result entirely from abnormalities in lymphocytes, in which the enzyme is normally found at its highest level (Kredich and Hershfield, 1989). Deoxyadenosine accumulation in lymphocytes has numerous adverse effects that impair DNA replication and cell division. The result is a profound failure of both cell-mediated (T-cell) and humoral (B-cell) immunity, making ADA deficiency one of the causes of severe combined immunodeficiency (SCID). Untreated patients die of infection within the first 2 years of life. Although an ADA-deficient patient is the subject of the first attempt at human gene transfer therapy (discussed later in this chapter), bone marrow transplantation from a fully HLA-compatible donor is the current treatment of choice. In the absence of an appropriate donor, a promising new alternative is the administration of bovine ADA that has been modified to be more effective.

Modified ADA. Numerous studies established that the infusion of normal red blood cells into patients with ADA deficiency reduces the levels of toxic metabolites, particularly deoxyadenosine. However, the response has not been uniformly good and is often unsustained. To circumvent these problems, Hershfield and colleagues (1987, 1991) modified bovine ADA by covalently attaching to it an inert polymer, polyethylene glycol (PEG). PEG-modified ADA has little immunogenicity and a strikingly long half-life of 3 to 6 days (in comparison with 30 minutes in the normal mouse). In more than a dozen patients, weekly PEG-ADA replacement therapy has almost completely corrected the metabolic abnormalities in purine metabolism; about half of the patients have recovered near-normal immune function, and the remainder have shown partial responses. More important, dramatic clinical improvement has occurred in virtually all patients. Although the effects of long-term administration of this modified protein remain to be determined, this approach represents a major new strategy for the treatment of genetic disease.

The general principles exemplified by the use of PEG-ADA are that (1) proteins can be chemically modified to improve their effectiveness as pharmacological reagents, without necessarily interfering with their biological activity and (2) an enzyme that is normally located inside the cell can be effective extracellularly if its substrate is in equilibrium with the extracellular fluid and if its product can be taken up by the cells that require it. As illustrated in the following section, the strategy of modification can be extended to proteins that can function only intracellularly, by targeting the protein to a specific cell type.

REPLACEMENT OF INTRACELLULAR PROTEINS: TARGETED ENZYMES

The feasibility of directing a polypeptide to a specific cell and a particular intracellular compartment has been demonstrated for **Gaucher disease,** the most prevalent lysosomal storage disorder. This autosomal recessive condition is due to a deficiency of the enzyme glucocerebrosidase. Its substrate, glucocerebroside, is a complex lipid normally degraded in the lysosome. The pathology results from glucocerebroside accumulation, particularly in the lysosomes of macrophages in the reticuloendothelial system. The macrophage storage process leads to gross enlargement of the liver and spleen. In addition, the bone marrow is slowly replaced by lipid-laden macrophages ("Gaucher cells") that ultimately compromise the production of erythrocytes and platelets, producing anemia and thrombocytopenia. Bone lesions cause episodic pain, osteonecrosis, and much morbidity. A minority of patients have progressive central nervous system degeneration.

Glucocerebrosidase replacement in Gaucher disease illustrates the problems of targeting the protein both to a particular type of cell and to a specific intracellular address, in this case the macrophage and the lysosome, respectively. Gaucher disease is a suitable model for several reasons. First, because in most patients the central nervous system is not involved, the enzyme must be delivered only to the peripheral reticuloendothelial system. Second, the only alternative therapy at present is bone marrow transplantation (to be discussed), so that there is a great need for treatment that entails less risk. Third, an abundant source of the human enzyme, the placenta, is readily available. Finally, the biology of the macrophage is sufficiently well understood to have suggested a strategy for targeting the enzyme to it.

In an encouraging initial report, Barton and coauthors (1990) demonstrated that the intravenous infusion of glucocerebrosidase into a patient with Gaucher disease had significant clinical benefits. The success depended on a critical modifica-

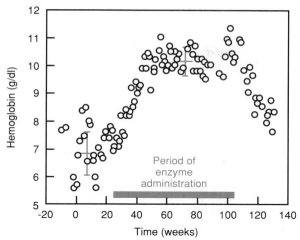

Figure 13-6. The effect of weekly intravenous infusions of modified glucocerebrosidase on the hemoglobin concentration of a child with Gaucher disease. The bar on the abcissa represents the period of enzyme administration. (Redrawn from Barton NW, Furbish FS, Murray GJ, et al. [1990] Therapeutic response to intravenous infusions of glucocerebrosidase in a patient with Gaucher disease. Proc Natl Acad Sci USA 87:1913–1916.)

therapy was accompanied by an increase in the hemoglobin to near-normal values (Fig. 13–6), an increased platelet count, and radiological improvement in the bony abnormalities. The hematological parameters returned to pretreatment levels when the infusions were stopped.

The long-term efficacy of this approach remains to be determined. However, this study demonstrates an important strategy and illustrates the feasibility of directing an intracellular enzyme to its physiologically relevant location to produce clinically significant effects. For many diseases, it should be possible to produce, using the cloned gene, large amounts of the protein in culture and to modify the structure of the polypeptide as required for specific cellular and intracellular targeting.

tion of the placental enzyme that allowed its targeting to the macrophage. The modified enzyme has terminal mannose sugars that are specifically bound by a protein on the macrophage plasma membrane. Once bound, the enzyme is internalized and delivered to the lysosome. Beginning at 4 years of age, a boy with Gaucher disease (without neurological involvement) received weekly injections of the enzyme over an 18-month period. The

Modulation of Gene Expression

As the vitamin-responsive inborn errors have demonstrated, even small increases in the function of a mutant protein may be advantageous if it has some residual function. Therapeutic effects have also been obtained, in at least one disorder (chronic granulomatous disease), by eliciting small increases in the amount of messenger RNA transcribed from the affected locus (Table 13–3). An alternative strategy, under study for sickle cell disease, is to increase the expression of normal genes that may be able to compensate for the mutation at

Table 13–3. Treatment by Modification of the Genome or Its Expression

Type of Modification	Example	Status
Pharmacological Modulation of Gene Expression	Hydroxyurea to stimulate γ globin (and thus Hb F) synthesis in sickle cell disease	Investigational; effective in short-term; long-term effects unknown
	IFN-γ to improve phagocytic function in chronic granulomatous disease	Same as above
Partial Modification of the Somatic Genotype		
By transplantation	Bone marrow transplantation in thalassemia	Curative with an HLA-matched donor; good results overall
	Bone marrow transplantation in lysosomal storage diseases	Encouraging results in some diseases, even if the brain is affected
	Liver transplantation in alpha₁-antitrypsin deficiency	~65% survival over 5 years for genetic liver disease
By gene transfer into somatic tissues	ADA deficiency: a pilot study in one patient	Investigational; in future, likely to be successful for many diseases

another locus. These examples illustrate concepts that are likely to be applicable to a variety of conditions. Their inclusion is not meant to suggest that they are established therapy.

Interferon Gamma Therapy in Chronic Granulomatous Disease. X-linked chronic granulomatous disease (CGD) is an uncommon disorder characterized by a defect in host defense that leads to severe, recurrent, and often fatal pyogenic infections beginning in early childhood. The phagocytes of affected boys ingest bacteria normally but cannot kill them efficiently because of an inability to generate superoxide (O_2^-), an oxygen metabolite that mediates the killing. The gene affected in this condition is very near the DMD gene on the X chromosome (see Fig. 8–6) and was cloned by one of the positional cloning strategies that led to the isolation of the DMD gene (see Chapter 8). The X-linked CGD locus encodes the heavy chain of cytochrome b, a component of the oxidase that generates superoxide in phagocytes.

Because interferon-γ (IFN-γ) was known to enhance the oxidase activity of normal phagocytes, Ezekowitz and his colleagues (1987, 1988) administered IFN-γ to four boys with X-linked CGD. Before treatment, the phagocytes of three of these patients had small but detectable bursts of oxidase activity (unlike those of severely affected patients), suggesting that increased activity might be obtained by greater production of cytochrome b from the affected locus. IFN-γ increased the cytochrome b content, superoxide production, and killing of *Staphylococcus aureus* in the granulocytes of all four patients. The IFN-γ effect was associated with small but definite increases in the abundance of the cytochrome b chain. Presumably, the cytochrome b polypeptide of these patients is partially functional, and increased expression of the residual function lessened the physiological defect. Alternatively, these patients may have a regulatory defect that is partially overcome by the IFN-γ.

Hydroxyurea in Sickle Cell Disease. The mutation in the β-globin gene that causes sickle cell disease has no effect on the expression of other non-α globins, including γ globin (see Chapter 11). Because Hb F ($\alpha_2\gamma_2$) is a perfectly adequate oxygen carrier in postnatal life, the induction of γ-globin gene expression would be advantageous to patients with sickle cell disease, particularly since

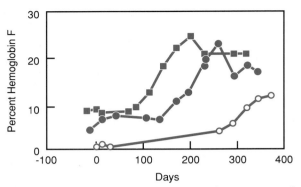

Figure 13–7. The effect of hydroxyurea on the percentage of hemoglobin F in three patients with sickle cell disease. (Adapted from Goldberg MA, Brugnara C, Dover GJ, et al. [1990] Treatment of sickle cell anemia with hydroxyurea and erythropoietin. N Engl J Med 323:366–372.)

Hb F inhibits the polymerization of deoxyhemoglobin S (Noguchi et al., 1988). Hydroxyurea is one of a group of antitumor agents that have been shown to stimulate the synthesis of γ-globin synthesis, and therefore of fetal hemoglobin (Hb F), although the mechanism by which it produces this effect is unclear. Two reports have suggested that the increased formation of Hb F has beneficial effects in patients with sickle cell disease, at least in the short term (Fig. 13–7; Rodgers et al., 1990; Goldberg et al., 1990). In studies lasting up to several months, a rise in the level of Hb F was accompanied by reduced hemolysis, probably reflecting a decrease in Hb S polymerization. Further study is required to establish the long-term benefits of this treatment and to identify side effects. At a minimum, these studies demonstrate that it is possible to increase the postnatal expression of genes to a therapeutically significant degree.

Modification of the Somatic Genome

Transplantation

Transplanted cells retain the genotype of the donor, and consequently transplantation can be regarded as a form of gene transfer therapy because it leads to a modification of the somatic genome. Because the genome of the recipient remains unchanged in all other cells, the recipient becomes in effect a chimera, not only at the locus of interest, but at many other loci as well. There are two general indications for the use of transplantation in the treatment of genetic disease. First, transplantation is done to provide the genes for a protein that is defective or absent in the recipient. This indication has the ironic consequence that a grossly normal organ is sometimes removed because its biochemical dysfunction is damaging another tissue. This is the case, for example, with liver transplantation for homozygous familial hypercholesterolemia. However, as experience with partial transplantation (for example, of liver cells to an ectopic location) grows, and if gene transfer therapy proves successful, whole organ transplants for this reason may become less frequent (Beaudet et al., 1989). The second and more common indication for transplantation is to replace a damaged organ (for example, a liver that has become cirrhotic in alpha$_1$-antitrypsin deficiency). Some examples of the uses of transplantation in genetic disease are provided in Table 13–3.

BONE MARROW TRANSPLANTATION IN NON–STORAGE DISEASES

Bone marrow transplantation is the treatment of choice for a variety of immune deficiency disorders, including severe combined immunodeficiency (SCID) of any type. Apart from a few other conditions with no other effective therapy, its role in the management of genetic disease in general is less certain and under careful evaluation. For example, conventional treatment of thalassemia by frequent transfusions and iron chelation has, in some centers, produced excellent results (Weatherall et al., 1989). On the other hand, very good outcomes have also been obtained in the treatment of *β*-thalassemia patients under 16 years of age with bone marrow transplantation (Lucarelli et al., 1990). Nearly all patients (94 percent) with normal liver function and a history of good chelation therapy had 3-year survivals that were event free, and none experienced recurrence of the disease. Before any decision can be made concerning the best mode of treatment (standard vs. bone marrow transplantation), long-term evaluation must be made of patients who were relatively healthy before the initiation of treatment and then were treated with one or the other approach.

BONE MARROW TRANSPLANTATION IN LYSOSOMAL STORAGE DISEASES

Mechanism of Effect. In the late 1980s, a cautiously encouraging picture began to emerge from animal and human studies of bone marrow transplantation in lysosomal storage diseases. In acting through the two mechanisms depicted in Figure 13–8, bone marrow transplants may prove to be effective in correcting lysosomal storage in many tissues and perhaps, in some cases, even the brain. First, the transplanted cells are a source of lysosomal enzymes that can be transferred to other cells through the extracellular fluid, as initially shown by the cocultivation experiments of Neufeld and colleagues with Hurler and Hunter syndrome cells (discussed in Chapter 12). Because bone marrow–derived cells constitute about 10 percent of the total cell mass of the body (Parkman, 1986), the quantitative impact of enzymes transferred from them may be significant. Second, the mononuclear-phagocyte system in most if not all tissues is derived from bone marrow stem cells (Gale et al., 1978; Parkman, 1986), so that, after bone marrow transplantation, this system is of donor origin throughout the body. Of special note are the brain perivascular microglial cells, whose marrow origin (Perry and Gordon, 1988) may account for the apparent effect of bone marrow transplantation on nervous system damage in some storage disorders.

It is now well established that bone marrow transplantation reduces the enlargement of the liver, the spleen, and sometimes the heart that occurs in certain storage diseases such as Hurler syndrome and Gaucher disease (Parkman, 1986; Barranger and Ginns, 1989; Krivit, 1989). The effects on the brain pathology in patients with Hurler syndrome are considerably less certain (Shull et al., 1987); long-term studies over years must be done before the outcome for the brain can be evaluated.

To date, the most promising result for a lysosomal storage disease affecting the central nervous system has been obtained in a single case of a patient with a disorder that leads to white matter degeneration: metachromatic leukodystrophy (Krivit et al., 1990). The result offers hope that early treatment might have some effect on the neurological manifestations of this and perhaps

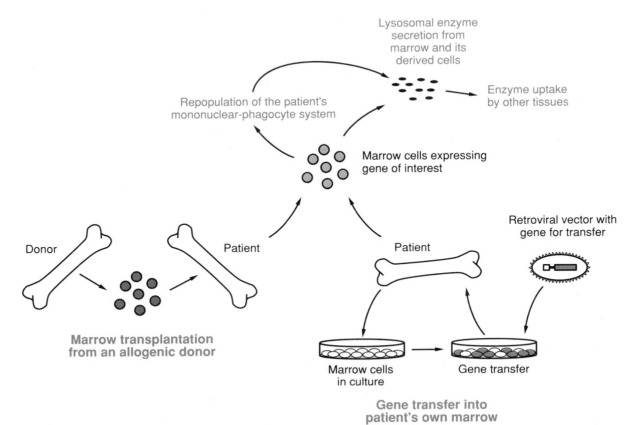

Figure 13–8. The two major mechanisms by which bone marrow transplantation or gene transfer into bone marrow may reduce the substrate accumulation in lysosomal storage diseases. The donor or transfected marrow expands to repopulate the monocyte macrophage system of the patient. In addition, lysosomal enzymes are transferred from the bone-marrow–derived cells to the enzyme-deficient cells.

other storage disorders. The success of bone marrow transplantation for storage diseases may be disease dependent and perhaps also dependent on when the procedure is performed in relation to the onset of symptoms. Presymptomatic children may have a better outcome (Krivit et al., 1990).

LIVER TRANSPLANTATION

For some metabolic liver diseases, liver transplantation is the treatment of choice because it is the only treatment that offers any hope (Esquivel et al., 1988; Starzl et al., 1989). For example, alpha$_1$-antitrypsin deficiency accounts for about half of the liver transplants done in the pediatric population and is the most common genetic disease for which liver transplantation is performed (Esquivel et al., 1988). Liver transplantation has now been performed for more than a dozen genetic diseases. At present, about two thirds of the recipients are

alive 5 years after surgery, and for almost all patients, the quality of life is generally much improved by the transplantation.

POSSIBLE TREATMENT OF DUCHENNE MUSCULAR DYSTROPHY (DMD) WITH MYOBLAST IMPLANTATION

The isolation and characterization of the DMD gene and its products offers the hope that it will soon be possible to understand the biological role of dystrophin; thus one might develop rational pharmacological therapy that addresses specifically the pathophysiological changes that lead to muscle cell death in DMD. A second therapeutic strategy would be to transfer a functional DMD gene into affected patients. Another proposed treatment is to transplant myoblasts from a normal donor into dystrophin-deficient muscle, where they are expected to fuse with and become part of the patient's muscle tissue. Preliminary myoblast transplantation studies in mice with mutations in dystrophin have been encouraging, but in human patients many difficulties are likely to be encountered with this approach (Partridge et al., 1989; Karpati et al., 1989). Limited trials of myoblast transplantation in DMD boys are being conducted to determine the tolerance and efficacy of the procedure in single muscles.

PROBLEMS WITH TRANSPLANTATION

The mortality following transplantation is significant, and the morbidity from superimposed infection and graft-versus-host disease is substantial. Posselt and colleagues (1990) found that the immunological rejection of transplanted pancreatic islet cells could be completely prevented by transplantation of the cells into the thymus, an immunologically privileged site. It appears that proteins present in the thymus at the time of T-cell maturation may not be recognized as foreign. Not only did the transplanted islet cells survive indefinitely, but the procedure also induced a state of donor-specific unresponsiveness in the recipient, so that a second graft from the same donor was tolerated at an extrathymic site. If this strategy proves to be generally applicable, it may allow transplantation without immunosuppression, an event that could transform the current therapeutic status of many genetic diseases.

A further problem is the finite supply of organs. For example, for all indications, between 4000 and 5000 liver transplants may be needed annually in the United States alone (Starzl et al., 1989). Finally, it remains to be demonstrated that transplanted organs are generally capable of functioning normally for a lifetime.

Gene Transfer Therapy

Recombinant DNA technology has made it possible to consider the correction of genetic disease at the most fundamental level, the gene (Belmont and Caskey, 1986; Culliton, 1989; Friedmann, 1989). By transferring functional copies of the relevant gene to the patient, permanent correction of the reversible features of the mutant phenotype may be possible. Although the first attempt at the *permanent* genetic cure of an inherited human disease has yet to be made, the first transfer of a gene into humans has been reported (Rosenberg et al.,

1990; Cournoyer and Caskey, 1990), the first gene transfer for the treatment of a patient with a genetic disease (ADA deficiency) has been approved and initiated, and preliminary studies in animals and humans suggest that gene therapy may ultimately be successful in many diseases. This section outlines the potential, methods, and probable limitations of gene transfer for the treatment of human genetic disease. The minimal requirements that must be met before the use of gene transfer can be considered for the treatment of a genetic disorder are listed in the box.

Minimal Requirements for Gene Transfer Therapy of a Genetic Disorder

1. Identification of the affected locus.
2. A complementary DNA (cDNA) clone of the gene.
3. A substantial disease burden and a favorable risk-benefit ratio in comparison with alternative therapy.
4. Sufficient knowledge of the biochemical basis of the disease to be confident that the gene transfer is likely to correct the biochemical pathology and to prevent or reverse critical phenotypic abnormalities.
5. An appropriate target cell with sufficiently defined biology and, ideally, a long half-life or good replicative potential in vivo.
6. Adequate data from cultured cell and animal studies to suggest that the vector, gene construct, and target cell are suitable.

GENE TRANSFER: GENERAL CONSIDERATIONS

The goal of gene transfer is to improve a patient's health by correction of the mutant phenotype. For this purpose, the delivery of the normal gene to appropriate *somatic* cells (as opposed to the germline) is required. Quite apart from the ethical and technical difficulties involved, it is neither necessary nor desirable to alter the germline of the patient being treated for a genetic disease. One risk is that any effort to integrate a normal copy of a gene into the germline (or into a fertilized egg) would carry a substantial risk of introducing new mutation.

In this discussion, the term "transferred gene" refers to any DNA construct that contains the coding sequences of the gene in question, under the control of appropriate regulatory elements. Most often, a transferred gene consists of a cDNA under the control of a promoter that may not necessarily be the natural promoter of the gene (Fig. 13–9). The regulatory elements must be chosen so that the gene is transcribed in the target cells at adequate levels and, if required, is responsive to essential regulatory signals.

For many diseases, the *addition* of the normal gene would suffice to correct a reversible phenotype, such as the increased phenylalanine level in PKU. In these conditions, it would generally not be important where in the genome of a cell the transferred gene inserts. Gene *replacement* or *correction* —the excision of the mutant gene (or part of it) and its substitution in the normal locus with a normal copy—is much more difficult and is not likely to be required for the management of many genetic disorders. In any case, such a feat is impossible at present for most tissues. However, in some situations it may eventually be possible to remove or ablate the relevant mutant cells (such as bone marrow) and to replace them with cells (pre-

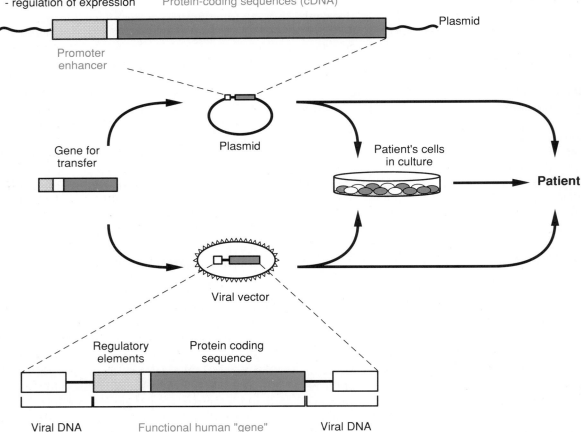

Figure 13–9. The two strategies that can be used to transfer a gene to a patient with a genetic disease, based on expression of a human "gene" modified for use in gene transfer (top) or based on a retroviral vector with a human cDNA for gene transfer (bottom). The viral components at the ends of the molecule are required for, among other functions, the integration of the vector into the host genome.

viously cultured from the patient) in which the mutant gene has been corrected. This approach is particularly desirable in disorders due to mutations in genes with large and complex regulatory elements, such as the globins (see Chapter 11). Also included in this group might be diseases in which the presence of the mutant gene product is detrimental and not easily overcome by increased production of the normal product from the transferred gene, such as patients with osteogenesis imperfecta due to dominant negative alleles in the proα1 chains of type I collagen (see Chapter 12).

THE TARGET CELL

One of the critical considerations in choosing an appropriate target cell is that it have either a long in vivo half life or significant replicative potential, so that the biological effect of the transfer can be of useful duration. Ideally, the target cells are the stem cells or progenitor cells that give rise to all the differentiated cells that constitute the mature tissue. Introduction of the gene into stem cells can result in the expression of the transferred gene in the large population of daughter cells. At present, bone marrow is the only tissue that meets these criteria and for which the culture and reimplantation steps are routine. Bone marrow transfer will be appropriate for diseases affecting blood cells, such as ADA deficiency, thalassemia, sickle cell disease, and chronic granulomatous disease. However, gene transfer into marrow stem cells may also be effective for other diseases that do not affect marrow per se (for example, PKU). In these instances, the blood circulation would deliver the substrate to the enzyme in the marrow and also remove the product. In addition, if the encouraging results of bone marrow transplantation in some storage diseases are confirmed, gene transfer into marrow may also be applicable to these conditions (Fig. 13–8).

With respect to cells that cannot divide extensively in culture and then be reimplanted in the patient, or that do not have identifiable stem or progenitor cells in the mature animal, other strategies must be developed. For example, hepatocytes can be briefly maintained in primary culture, transfected with the gene, and then returned to the animal. Alternatively, direct introduction of the gene into the target cells in vivo (by injection or other physical methods or, as explained later, by using retroviral vectors) has been demonstrated,

for example, with several cell types, including liver, muscle, and epithelial cells. Endothelial cells may prove to be particularly useful targets for gene transfer because they line the walls of blood vessels. The protein product of a gene expressed in endothelial cells can be designed to be released into the circulation, to produce a systemic effect. A logistical consideration that arises with all these approaches is that the number of cells into which the gene must be introduced may be very large. For example, the approximate number of liver cells into which a normally functioning gene would have to be transferred to correct a typical inborn error of metabolism, such as PKU, is about 5 percent of the hepatocyte mass, or approximately 10^{10} cells (Arias et al., 1982).

It should not be forgotten that the target cell must also provide any additional proteins or ligands required for the biological activity of the polypeptide (Table 12–9).

TRANSFER STRATEGIES

A gene may be transferred into appropriate cells by one of two general strategies (Fig. 13–9). First, however, it must be placed in a vector to carry it into the target cells. The vector can be a plasmid or viral DNA (see the next section). Introduction of the vector into the patient may then be achieved directly by injection into the target tissue. Alternatively, it may be possible to modify the virus so that it is taken up from the extracellular fluid by the target cell. The initial gene transfer studies, however, will probably involve culturing the target cells of the patient, introducing the gene into the cells in culture, and then returning the cells to the patient.

RETROVIRAL VECTORS

One of the most widely used classes of vectors for gene transfer studies is derived from retroviruses, simple RNA viruses with only three structural genes that can be removed and replaced with the gene to be transferred (Fig. 13–9) (Friedmann, 1989). A major advantage of viral vectors is that they are capable of entering virtually every cell in the target population. The present generation of retroviral vectors has been engineered to render them incapable of replication. Other qualities that make them suitable include the fact that they are nontoxic to the cell, that only a low number of copies of the viral DNA (with the transferred gene) integrate into the host genome, that the integrated DNA is stable, and that retroviral vectors can accommodate rather large segments of added DNA (up to 8 kb), commodious enough for many genes that might be transferred. A limitation of retroviral vectors is that the viral DNA does not integrate into the host DNA of nondividing cells, precluding the use of such vectors in many tissues.

CURRENT PROBLEMS IN USING GENE TRANSFER THERAPY

In addition to the minimal requirements outlined in the box, other objectives may have to be met to allow the use of gene transfer therapy in some diseases:

1. **The ability to maintain sufficiently high expression of the transferred gene in the target cells.** Although in some disorders as little as 2 to 5 percent of normal gene expression may be sufficient to prevent the pathology, diseases such as thalassemia will require much higher levels of expression of the transferred gene.

2. **Appropriate regulation of the gene.** Tight regulation is critical in some diseases and unimportant in others. In thalassemia, for example, overexpression of the transferred gene would cause a new imbalance of globin chains, whereas low levels of expression would be ineffective. In contrast, in some enzymopathies, abnormally high levels of expression may have no adverse effect.

3. **The ability to introduce the gene into nondividing cells, particularly the nervous system.** This is critical for the treatment of neurological disorders such as Tay-Sachs disease or Huntington disease.

4. **Development of the technology to deliver very large genes to the target cell.** An example is the coding region of dystrophin (11 kb), the gene affected in Duchenne muscular dystrophy.

RISKS OF GENE TRANSFER THERAPY

Comprehensive reviews of the possible risks of gene transfer therapy have been made by others, most recently Friedmann (1989). One major concern is that the transferred gene will integrate into the patient's DNA and activate a proto-oncogene or disrupt a tumor-suppressor gene, leading possibly to malignancy (Chapter 16). The illicit expression of an oncogene is less likely to occur with retroviral vectors that have been altered to mini-

mize the ability of their promoters to activate the expression of adjacent host genes (Friedmann, 1989). The inactivation of a tumor-suppressor gene (by insertion of the transferred DNA into it) is likely to be infrequent and, as such, is an acceptable risk in diseases for which there is no therapeutic alternative. The inactivation of other genes will in general be without significant effect, since lethal mutations are rare and kill only single cells. Because the integration site of a retrovirus or other DNA is more or less random, there is little chance that the same cellular gene will be disrupted by the integrating DNA in more than one cell.

ETHICAL CONSIDERATIONS

As with any new treatment, proposals for trials of gene transfer into patients must be subjected to rigorous scrutiny by regulatory agencies and hospital ethics committees. However, virtually all governmental and religious agencies that have examined proposals for human gene transfer for the treatment of genetic disease have agreed that it is an approach that should be pursued (Friedmann, 1989). In contrast to the transfer of genes into the germline, somatic gene transfer therapy raises few ethical issues that are not routinely considered when other novel therapy is evaluated (for example, a new anticancer drug). One problem is that a gene may be inadvertently introduced into the germline of a patient, where it may cause a mutation, depending on where it integrates in the genome. Although this is a real possibility, it is likely to be infrequent, and on this ground it seems difficult to justify withholding carefully planned and reviewed trials of gene transfer from patients who have no other recourse. In reality, however, the problem of germline modification is not confined to gene transfer therapy. For example, the chemotherapies used in the treatment of malignancy are known to be mutagenic, but this risk has been accepted because of the benefits of the therapy.

THE FIRST GENE TRANSFER IN HUMANS

All of the issues just discussed were carefully considered before approval was given, by the Recombinant DNA Advisory Committee of the National Institutes of Health, for the first gene transfer studies in patients. In conducting these studies, Rosenberg and his associates (1990) have begun the long and careful assessment of gene transfer for the management of human disease. Ironically, this first clinical application of gene transfer was not for the treatment of a single gene disorder but rather to evaluate the immunotherapy of melanoma in five patients, through the use of tumor-infiltrating lymphocytes. The lymphocytes were removed from each patient and transfected in vitro with a selectable marker gene in a retroviral vector. On reinjection into the patient, the lymphocytes expressed the marker gene, were present for as long as 2 months after administration, and were not associated with any side effects. These studies demonstrated the feasibility and safety of gene transfer in humans by means of retroviral vectors and suggested that lymphocytes may be appropriate cells for gene therapy of other diseases.

CANDIDATE DISEASES FOR GENE TRANSFER THERAPY

A number of single-gene disorders, many of which have been mentioned in the preceding discussion, are potential candidates for correction by gene transfer. These include hematopoietic conditions such as thalassemia and various forms of immunodeficiency, as well as disorders such as phenylketonuria, familial hypercholesterolemia, and alpha$_1$-antitrypsin deficiency, each affecting proteins made in the liver (Belmont and Caskey, 1986). Additional considerations relevant to the use of gene therapy for three important disorders are outlined below.

Adenosine Deaminase Deficiency. This condition, although rare, is one of the major candidate diseases for gene transfer therapy, and the first transfer of a gene for the correction of a genetic disease was performed in an ADA-deficient girl late in 1990. The minimal requirements listed in the box have been fulfilled, and low-level expression is likely to be corrective. In addition, the cures obtained by bone marrow transplantation indicate that transfer of the ADA gene into marrow stem cells will probably be effective, provided that the transferred gene sustains adequate levels of expression in a sufficient number of cells. Successful long-term expression of the human ADA gene after its transfer into the marrow of mice (Moore et al., 1990) suggests that permanent correction of the disease may be feasible by this approach. Using gene transfer of lymphocytes, in a strategy similar to that used for the patients with melanoma described earlier, scientists at the National Institutes of Health transferred an ADA-

containing retroviral vector into the T lymphocytes of a patient with ADA deficiency. The transfected cells were then returned to the patient. Although this approach cannot permanently correct the defect (because the life of these lymphocytes may not exceed 2 months), repeated use of this procedure may be effective, and it allows ongoing assessment of the safety of the procedure.

Cystic Fibrosis. Virus-mediated gene transfer has been used to successfully correct the cystic fibrosis (CF) defect in cultured cell lines derived from CF patients (Rich et al., 1990; Drumm et al., 1990). These studies represent a critical step toward the effective treatment of this otherwise lethal disease. One of the major problems, many of which have been mentioned in the preceding discussion, will be in introducing the gene into the target cells, the respiratory epithelium, whose dysfunction determines the mortality of the disease. The recent demonstration that genes in retroviral vectors can be transferred directly into the wall of arteries in vivo (Nabel et al., 1990) offers hope that a comparable approach might be effective in the respiratory tract in patients with CF.

Duchenne Muscular Dystrophy. A special problem in DMD is the size (11 kb) of the dystrophin cDNA that encodes the protein, too large to be accommodated by the present generation of retroviral vectors. However, the identification of a patient with Becker muscular dystrophy mild enough to allow him to drive his automobile at age 65 (England et al., 1990) suggests that it may not be necessary to use the whole dystrophin coding region for gene transfer. In this patient, the mutant allele (depicted in Fig. 12–11) lacks 46 percent of the coding region, so that highly repetitive sequences homologous to a cytoskeletal protein called spectrin have been deleted. The shortened dystrophin retains sufficient function to prevent the complete DMD phenotype. These findings emphasize the need for basic research to identify the critical functional domains of the protein, so that they can be retained in any therapeutic cDNA.

The direct injection of gene vectors into muscle is feasible (Wolff et al., 1990) and indicates a potential approach for placing a dystrophin gene into DMD patients. The major difficulty with any gene transfer therapy for DMD, however, is the requirement that the gene be put into a significant fraction of the skeletal muscle mass (and in some patients, into the cardiac muscle as well). At present, it is not possible to envision how this logistical barrier might be overcome.

General References

Beaudet AL, Scriver CR, Sly WS, Valle D (1989) Genetics and biochemistry of variant human phenotypes. *In* Scriver CR, Beaudet AL, Sly WS, Valle D (eds) The metabolic basis of inherited disease, 6th ed. McGraw-Hill, New York, pp. 3–53.

Belmont JW, Caskey CT (1986) Developments leading to human gene therapy. *In* Kucherlapati R (ed) Gene transfer. Plenum Press, New York, pp. 411–441.

Cournoyer D, Caskey CT (1990) Gene transfer into humans. N Engl J Med 323:601–602.

Culliton BJ (1989) Designing cells to deliver drugs. Science 246:746–751.

Desnick RJ (ed) (1991) Treatment of genetic diseases. Churchill Livingstone, New York.

Friedmann T (1989) Progress toward human gene therapy. Science 244:1275–1282.

Hirschhorn R (1987) Therapy of genetic disorders. N Engl J Med 316:623–624.

Parkman R (1986) The application of bone marrow transplantation to the treatment of genetic diseases. Science 232:1373–1378.

Rosenberg LE (1976) Vitamin responsive inherited metabolic disorders. Adv Hum Genet 6:1–74.

Rosenberg LE (1990) Treating genetic diseases: Lessons from three children. Pediat Res 27:S10–S16.

Starzl TE, Demetris AJ, Van Thiel D (1989) Liver transplantation. N Engl J Med 321:1014–1022.

Valle D (1987) Genetic disease: An overview of current therapy. Hosp Pract 22(7):167–182.

Problems

1. Describe the genetic differences that might account for the fact that the phagocytes of some patients with X-linked chronic granulomatous disease respond to IFN-γ in vitro and others do not.

2. Identify some of the restrictions on the types of proteins that can be considered for extracellular replacement therapy, as exemplified by PEG-ADA. What makes this approach inappropriate for phenylalanine hydroxylase deficiency? For Hurler syndrome? For Lesch-Nyhan syndrome? If Tay-Sachs disease caused only liver disease, would this strategy succeed? If not, why?

3. A 3-year-old girl, Rhonda, has familial hypercholesterolemia due to a deletion of the 5′ end of the gene. The mutation removed the promoter and the first two exons of each allele. (Rhonda's parents are second cousins.) You explain to the parents that she will require plasma exchange therapy every 1 to 2 weeks for years. At the clinic, however, they meet another family with a 5-year-old boy with the same disease. The boy has been treated with drugs with some success. Rhonda's parents want to know why she has not been offered similar pharmacological therapy. Explain.

4. What classes of mutations are likely to be found in homocystinuric patients who are not responsive to the administration of large doses (1000 mg/day) of pyridoxine (vitamin B_6)? How might you explain the fact that Tom is completely responsive whereas his first cousin Allan has only a partial reduction in plasma homocystine when given the same amount of vitamin B_6?

5. You have just cloned the gene for phenylalanine hydroxylase (PAH) and wish ultimately to introduce it into patients with PKU. Your approach will be to culture cells from the patient, introduce a functional version of the gene into the cells, and reintroduce the cells into the patient.
   a) What DNA components do you need to make a functional PAH protein in a gene transfer experiment?
   b) Which tissues would you choose in which to express the enzyme, and why? How does this choice affect your gene construct in (a)?
   c) You introduce your version of the gene into fibroblasts cultured from a skin biopsy from the patient. Northern (RNA) blot analysis shows that the messenger RNA is present in normal amounts and is the correct size. However, no PAH enzyme activity can be detected in the cells. What kinds of abnormalities in the transferred gene would explain this finding?
   d) You have corrected all the problems identified in (c). On introducing the new version of the gene into the cultured cells, you now find that the PAH protein is present in great abundance, and when you harvest the cells and assay the enzyme (in the presence of all the required components), normal activity is obtained. However, when you add ^{3}H-labeled phenylalanine to the cells in culture, no ^{3}H-labeled tyrosine is formed (in contrast, some cultured liver cells produce a large quantity of ^{3}H-labeled tyrosine in this situation). What are the most likely explanations for the failure to form ^{3}H-tyrosine? How does this result affect your gene therapy approach to patients?
   e) You have developed a method to introduce your functional version of the gene directly into a large proportion of the hepatocytes of patients with PAH deficiency. Unexpectedly, you find that much lower levels of PAH enzymatic activity are obtained in patients in whom significant amounts of the inactive PAH homodimer were detectable in hepatocytes before treatment than in patients who had no detectable PAH polypeptide before treatment. How can you explain this result? How might you overcome the problem?

CHAPTER 14

GENETICS OF THE IMMUNE SYSTEM

The genetic organization and control of the immune system demonstrates several genetic phenomena that are shown less clearly or not at all by other systems: extensive polymorphism, linkage disequilibrium, an obvious evolutionary relationship between its various components, and, especially, a unique system of encoding great diversity within relatively few loci. The genes of the immune system not only are clinically important in relation to transplantation, autoimmune disease, and response to infection and as causes of a number of single-gene disorders, but they also provide excellent models for the analysis of human variation and gene expression. The application of molecular techniques has greatly expanded the understanding of the immune response while at the same time revealing new layers of complexity that remain to be explored.

Higher organisms are unique in their ability to distinguish between "self" and "nonself" and to mount a reaction selectively against a very broad spectrum of foreign antigens. This reaction is mediated by the complex interactive network of cells and cellular cytokines of the immune system and is referred to as the **immune response.** Genetic factors play a key role not only in the generation of the normal immune response but also in the development of aberrant immune reactions and consequent immune-mediated disease. In this chapter we describe the genetic basis of the immune response and discuss a number of single-gene disorders of the immune system as well as diseases in which immune-related genes, such as those of the **major histocompatibility complex** (MHC), contribute to but do not exclusively encode disease susceptibility.

The discussion here is not intended to provide a comprehensive review of immunology or immunogenetics, for which the reader is directed to the General References listed at the end of the chapter. Rather, we introduce some of the gene systems that govern immune function, and we reinforce the concept that, with the exception of monozygotic twins (or other multiple births), each person is genetically unique. Much of human immunological uniqueness depends on the expression of the genes of the MHC, and thus in the discussion that follows we highlight this gene system, as well as two others within the same superfamily that encode additional key components of the immune response: **immunoglobulins** (Igs) and **T-cell antigen receptors** (TCRs).

THE MAJOR HISTOCOMPATIBILITY COMPLEX

The MHC is a complex locus, composed of a large cluster of genes located on the short arm of chromosome 6 (Fig. 14–1). On the basis of structural and functional differences, these genes are categorized into three classes, each of which is highly complex and polymorphic. Two of the three classes, class I and class II, correspond to the human leukocyte antigen (HLA) genes, originally discovered by virtue of their importance in tissue transplantation between unrelated individuals.

The class I genes (HLA-A, HLA-B, and HLA-C) encode antigens that are an integral part of the plasma membrane of nucleated cells. These antigens not only are involved in transplant rejection, but are also critical to immunocompetence and are intricately involved in antigen recognition, lymphocyte interactions, and the development of self-tolerance. A class I antigen consists of two polypeptide subunits, a heavy chain encoded within the MHC and a nonpolymorphic polypeptide, β_2-microglobulin, which is encoded by a gene outside the MHC, mapping to chromosome 15.

The class II locus is composed of several subregions that encode the HLA-DP, HLA-DQ, and HLA-DR antigens. These molecules are expressed primarily on B lymphocytes, macrophages, and activated T lymphocytes, but under certain conditions they may be expressed by other cell types as well. Each class II molecule is a heterodimer, composed of α and β subunits, both of which are encoded by the MHC. Like the class I antigens, they are integral to the cell membrane and to immune cellular interactions and function. The HLA class I and class II antigens play a critical role in the initiation of an immune response and specifically in the "presentation" of antigen to T lymphocytes, which cannot recognize and respond to antigen unless it is complexed with an HLA molecule.

The class III genes are not HLA genes but include genes for proteins such as properdin factors B, C2 and C4, which are part of the complement system, a series of polymorphic serum proteins and membrane receptors closely involved in immune function. Also in this region are genes that when defective cause single-gene diseases, such as the gene for 21-hydroxylase; deficiency of 21-hydroxylase is associated with one form of congenital adrenal hyperplasia (see Chapter 10). Thus class III genes appear to be functionally distinct from class I and class II genes, and they are not considered further here.

A number of other gene loci within the MHC are genetically linked to the HLA genes but are functionally unrelated to them. These include the genes for tumor necrosis factor and lymphotoxin, as well as other genes, more recently isolated, for which a function remains to be defined.

There is a striking similarity, both in organization and in DNA sequence, between HLA class I and class II genes and between the HLA genes and the immunoglobulin and T-cell receptor genes described in the following sections. The similarity among these genes and a number of others has led to their classification into a gene family designated the **immunoglobulin gene superfamily** (see later discussion). The members of the family appear to be evolutionarily related genes, whose products

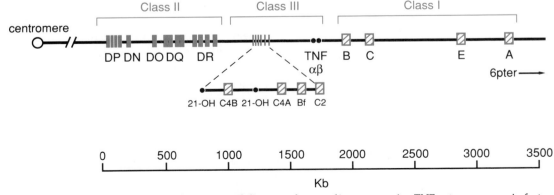

Figure 14–1. A schematic of the major histocompatibility complex on chromosome 6p. TNF = tumor necrosis factor; Bf = properdin factor B; C2,C4$_A$, C4B = complement components; 21-OH = 21-hydroxylase. (One of the 21-OH loci is a pseudogene.) For discussion, see text.

serve a wide variety of functions beyond the immunological role of HLA molecules and immunoglobulins.

Polymorphism and the Inheritance of HLA Haplotypes

The HLA system is highly polymorphic. Numerous distinct antigenic variants have already been recognized at each of HLA-A, HLA-B, HLA-C, HLA-DP, HLA-DQ, and HLA-DR. Table 14–1 indicates the complexity and extensive polymorphism of the system. Each person inherits one variant of each of the HLA subgroups from each parent. According to the current system of HLA nomenclature, not all these antigenic variants (specificities) are direct products of single genes; some, particularly variants of the HLA-DR and HLA-DQ subgroups, are localized to subregions of genes, to a particular chain or to an $\alpha\beta$ combination.

HLA typing, classically performed by using sera of multiparous females, has revealed considerable variation in the profile and frequency of HLA variants among different populations. HLA-A2, for example, is among the most frequent HLA-A specificities in all populations, whereas HLA-A24 is found in Caucasians but not in Blacks or Asians.

The HLA alleles on a given chromosome are so closely linked that they are transmitted together as a haplotype. The alleles are codominant; each parent has two haplotypes, expresses both, and, as shown in Figure 14–2, transmits one or the other to each child. As a result, parent and child share only one haplotype, and there is a 25 percent chance that two sibs inherit matching HLA haplotypes. Because acceptance of transplanted tissues largely correlates with the degree of similarity between donor and recipient HLA haplotypes (and ABO blood groups), the favored donor for bone marrow or organ transplantation is an ABO-compatible and HLA-compatible sibling of the recipient.

The HLA haplotypes show marked linkage disequilibrium (see Chapter 8). Certain haplotypes are much more frequent than expected, whereas others are exceptionally rare, and most of the 3×10^7 phenotypic combinations theoretically possible among Caucasians have never been observed. Sometimes the search for a suitable bone-marrow donor is unsuccessful in spite of a wide search. There is also a striking ethnic distribution

Table 14–1. Antigens of the HLA System

HLA-A	HLA-B	HLA-C	HLA-D	HLA-DR	HLA-DQ	HLA-DP
A1, A2	B5, B7	Cw1–Cw11	Dw1–Dw26	DR1–DR5	DQw1–DQw9	DPw1–DPw6
A3, A9	B8			DR7		
A10, A11	B12–B18			DR9		
A23–A26	B21			DRw6		
A28–A32	B27			DRw8		
Aw19	B35			DRw10–DRw18		
Aw33	B37–B40			DRw52		
Aw34	B44			DRw53		
Aw36	B45					
Aw43	B49					
Aw66	B51					
Aw68	Bw4, Bw6					
Aw69	Bw22, Bw41					
Aw74	Bw42					
	Bw46–Bw50					
	Bw52–Bw65					
	Bw67					
	Bw70–Bw73					
	Bw75–Bw77					

Data as of 1987. From Kostyu DD, Amos DB (1989) The HLA complex: Genetic polymorphism and disease susceptibility. *In* Scriver CR, Beaudet AL, Sly WS, Valle D (eds) The metabolic basis of inherited disease, 6th ed. McGraw-Hill, New York, pp. 225–249.

w ("workshop") indicates an antigen that is not completely established at this time. Many antigens are variants of previously recognized antigens.

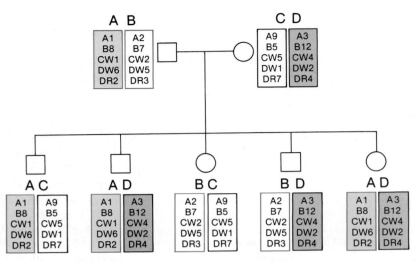

Figure 14-2. The inheritance of HLA haplotypes. Usually a haplotype is transmitted, as shown in this figure, as a unit. In extremely rare instances, a parent will transmit a recombinant haplotype to the child.

of haplotypes, in addition to the ethnic distribution of single HLA markers mentioned earlier.

HLA and Disease Association

With the increasing delineation of HLA alleles has come an appreciation of the association between certain diseases and specific HLA antigens or haplotypes. As is apparent from Table 14–2, most of these disorders are autoimmune—that is, associated with an immune response apparently directed against one or more self-antigens. The strongest HLA-disease association known is that between narcolepsy and HLA-DR2; almost 100 percent of narcolepsy patients express this class II antigen, in comparison with only about 16 percent of healthy controls. However, only a small percentage of persons with HLA-DR2 develop narcolepsy, and the relative risk of narcolepsy in those people, in comparison with people who do not have HLA-DR2, is only 34 (see footnote of Table 14–2). There is also a very strong association between HLA-B27 and ankylosing spondylitis, a chronic inflammatory disease of the spine and sacroiliac joints. Whereas only 5 percent of Caucasians in general are B27-positive, at least 90 percent of Caucasians with ankylosing spondylitis are B27-positive. The risk of developing ankylosing spondylitis is at least 90 times higher for people who have HLA-B27 than for those who do not. Similarly, Reiter disease and reactive arthritis,

conditions that closely resemble ankylosing spondylitis, are also strongly associated with the B27 antigen. A further example is the association of insulin-dependent diabetes mellitus with HLA-DR3 and HLA-DR4, especially with HLA-DR3/HLA-DR4 heterozygosity.

The etiological relevance of most of the HLA-disease associations remains obscure. In most cases, the association is related to the immune response and does not depend on physical proximity of a disease-causing gene to the HLA loci. Two exceptions, however, are the autosomal recessive disorders primary hemochromatosis and congenital adrenal hyperplasia due to 21-hydroxylase deficiency, in which the defective genes do lie within the MHC. Analysis of the various 21-hydroxylase mutations responsible for adrenal hyperplasia has revealed that different mutations at this locus originally occurred on different haplotype backgrounds and have remained in linkage disequilibrium with these specific haplotype markers. The hemochromatosis gene has not yet been isolated but is very closely linked to the HLA-A locus.

Even though the basis of most HLA-disease associations is unknown, the evidence to date suggests that the HLA genes are not solely responsible for susceptibility to specific diseases but do predispose to certain diseases, along with other genetic or environmental factors. As the HLA molecules are integral to T-cell antigen recognition, it is speculated that their role in disease pathogenesis may relate to differences in the capacity of these poly-

Table 14–2. Examples of Association Between HLA Antigens and Disease

Disease	HLA Antigen	Frequency of antigen(%)*		Relative Risk†	Comments
		Controls	*Patients*		
Narcolepsy	DR2	16	~100	30–100	Almost all patients have DR2
Ankylosing spondylitis	B27	3.4	>90	80–100	
Congenital adrenal hyperplasia (21-OH deficiency)	Bw47	0.2	25	80–150	Autosomal recessive; other congenital adrenal hyperplasia mutations show different associations
Celiac disease	DR3	12	60	10	Other HLA antigens also associated
	DR7	12	—		
Insulin-dependent diabetes mellitus	DR3	12	50	5–30	Relative risk highest in DR3/DR4 heterozygotes; other DR antigens also affect risk
	DR4	13	38		
Hemochromatosis	A3	13	75	20	Autosomal recessive, linked to HLA complex
Rheumatoid arthritis	DR4	13	—	5	Heterogeneous, other antigens also associated
Multiple sclerosis	DR2	16	55	4	Other associations also
Psoriasis	Cw6	9	>50	4	Ethnic variation
	DR7	12	—		
Myasthenia gravis	DR3	12	—	3	Ethnic variation
	DQw2	18	—		
Systemic lupus erythematosus	DR2	16	>70	3	
	DR3	12	—		

Adapted from Kostyu and Amos (1989) and Bell et al. (1989), with additional data from McKusick (1990).
* Frequency data are for Caucasian populations and are approximate.
† The relative risk is approximate and is calculated as follows: ad/bc, where a = number of patients with the antigen; b = number of controls with the antigen; c = number of patients without the antigen; d = number of controls without the antigen

morphic proteins to interact with antigen and the T-cell receptor in the initiation of an immune response (Fig. 14–3). This hypothesis, which implies a direct pathogenetic role for the HLA molecule, is supported by the finding, described in some detail in Chapter 15, that the association between HLA-DR4 and insulin-dependent diabetes mellitus is related to a single amino acid change in one of the external domains of the HLA-DQ β chain. However, the precise mechanism whereby this substitution confers disease susceptibility is still unknown.

IMMUNOGLOBULINS

Antibodies are immunoglobulins that are elicited in response to a stimulus by a foreign antigen and can recognize and bind that antigen and facilitate its elimination. They are mediators of the immune response in the HLA-related diseases just described, as well as in response to foreign antigens.

A number of genetic diseases are due to deficiencies of immunoglobulins (Table 14–3). However, the primary significance of immunoglobulins from the perspective of genetics is that they exhibit a unique property, **somatic rearrangement,** by which genes of the germline are rearranged in somatic cells to generate diversity.

Antibodies exist in two forms: a membrane-bound form, on B lymphocytes, and a soluble or secreted form. Secreted antibodies are produced by plasma cells, which are derived from B lymphocytes by proliferation and maturation. This process, known as B-cell activation, is initiated by interaction between a specific antigen and a suitable antibody molecule on the B-cell membrane. Such an interaction results in the clonal expansion and differentiation of the B cell, with consequent formation of both plasma cells, which secrete antibodies specific for the inciting antigens, and memory B cells capable of responding promptly and strongly to any later challenge by the same antigen.

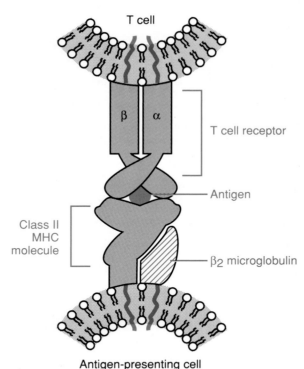

Figure 14-3. Schematic representation of the interaction between an MHC molecule, foreign protein, and T-cell receptor. (Adapted from Sinha AA, Lopez MT, McDevitt HO [1990] Autoimmune diseases: The failure of self tolerance. Science 248:1380-1387.)

Immunoglobulin Structure and Diversity

One of the most puzzling issues of immunogenetics used to be the mechanism whereby a seemingly infinite number of different antibodies could be encoded in the germline DNA of any one individual. It is estimated that each human being can generate a repertoire of about 10^8 different antibodies, yet the genome is composed of only 3×10^9 base pairs of DNA. This seeming disparity has been reconciled by the demonstration that antibodies are encoded in the germline by a relatively small number of genes that, during B-cell development, undergo a unique process of somatic rearrangement and recombination that allows for the generation of enormous diversity. The potential to create such huge numbers of different antibodies appears to have evolved as a mechanism for protection against the large array of environmental infectious organisms, toxic agents, and autologous malignant cells to which a person may be exposed.

Ig molecules are composed of four polypeptide chains, two identical heavy (H) chains and two identical light (L) chains, that are held together by interchain disulfide bonds (Fig. 14-4). Intrachain disulfide bonds subdivide each chain into a series of homologous domains. On the basis of structural differences at the carboxyl terminal portion, the H chains are subdivided into five classes or isotypes, γ, α, μ, δ, and ϵ, and the corre-

Table 14-3. Examples of Single-Gene Disorders of the Immune System

Disease	Inheritance*	Comments
Adenosine deaminase (ADA) deficiency	AR	Cause of one form of SCID, with dysfunction of B and T lymphocytes, impaired cellular immunity, decreased immunoglobulin production
Agammaglobulinemia, X-linked	XR	Heterogeneous; usual type marked by lack of plasma cells and susceptibility to bacterial but not viral infection; presumed basic defect in pathway of B-cell differentiation
Ataxia-telangiectasia (AT)	AR	Defect in DNA repair with chromosome breakage; immune defect and hypoplasia of thymus
Chronic granulomatous disease	XR	Neutrophils able to phagocytize bacteria but not to kill them; affects cytochrome that participates in cellular respiration; heterogeneous; has occurred as part of contiguous gene syndrome
Severe combined immunodeficiency disease (SCID)	AR, XR	Several different autosomal recessive and X-linked disorders can cause SCID (e.g., ADA deficiency); basic defect is in stem-cell differentiation
Wiskott-Aldrich syndrome	XR	Eczema, thrombocytopenia, immunodeficiency, bloody diarrhea; basic defect not known

* AR, autosomal recessive; XR, X-linked recessive

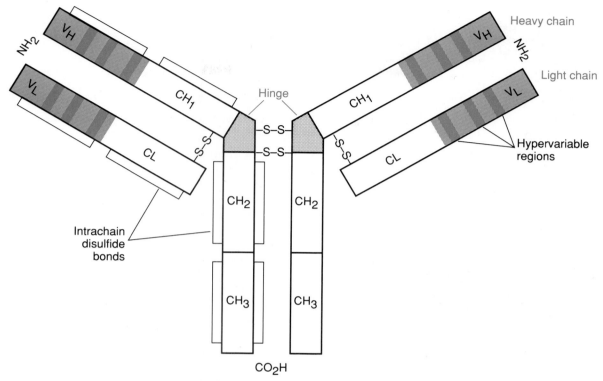

Figure 14-4. Basic structure of an immunoglobulin molecule, consisting of two identical light chains and two identical heavy chains. Each chain consists of a variable region (V) and a constant region (C). NH_2 = amino terminus. CO_2H = carboxyl terminus.

sponding Igs are accordingly named IgG, IgA, IgM, IgD, and IgE. As indicated in Table 14-4, the different Ig classes differ functionally as well as structurally. The L chains of immunoglobulin molecules may also be of two types, κ and λ, but not both in the same antibody. Therefore, the antibody produced by a single B cell contains only a single H-chain isotype and a single L-chain subtype. Moreover, unlike other autosomal loci, within a single cell only one of the pair of parental alleles for each H-chain is expressed: either the paternal or the maternal allele, but not both. The same is true for each L-chain. These phenomena, known as **isotypic exclusion** and **allelic exclusion**, respectively, are still not fully understood.

Each H and L chain of an Ig protein consists of two segments, the constant (C) and the variable (V) regions. The constant region, which determines the class of the Ig molecule, is located at the carboxyl terminus, and its amino acid sequence is relatively conserved among Igs of the same class. By contrast, the V region is located at the amino terminus and its amino acid sequence shows wide variation among different regions. The V regions of the H and L chains form the antigen-binding site and determine the antibody specificity.

The genes encoding the H and L chains are located in three unlinked chromosomal regions. The κ L-chain genes are on chromosome 2 at band 2p13, the λ L-chain genes are on chromosome 22 at band 22q11, and the H-chain genes, for all five isotypes, are on chromosome 14 at band 14q32. Each H and L chain is encoded by multiple segments that are widely separated in the germline. The L-chain V-region domain is encoded by V and joining (J) segments, whereas the H-chain V region is encoded by three gene segments: the V and J segments and a third unit, the diversity (D) segment (Fig. 14-5). In total, each cluster of Ig genes spans many millions of base pairs.

During B-cell differentiation, the DNA at the immunoglobulin loci undergoes somatic rearrangement. For the light chains, a single V segment and a single J segment are juxtaposed, with

Table 14–4. Immunoglobulin Classes and Their Functions

Ig Class	Percentage of Total	Light Chain	Heavy Chain	Function
IgG	80	κ or λ	γ (4 subclasses)	Responsible for combating infection; crosses placenta, thus gives passive immunity to fetus and newborn
IgM	6	κ or λ	μ (2 subclasses)	First antibody formed in response to antigen; more effective than IgG in fixing complement; forms rheumatoid factor
IgA	13	κ or λ	α (2 subclasses)	Especially important in secretions; protects body surfaces and defends gut against microorganisms
IgD	1	κ or λ	δ (2 subclasses)	Not clear
IgE	low	κ or λ	ϵ	Involved in allergic reactions and release of histamine; may combat intestinal parasites

loss of the intervening DNA, to form a complete variable region gene. For the heavy chains, a D segment and a J segment are juxtaposed and then combine with a V segment. Thus as shown schematically in Figure 14–6, generation of a κ light chain involves a recombination that juxtaposes one of the many V_κ segments to one of the J_κ regions. This rearranged segment is then transcribed, and the intervening sequences between the J_κ and C_κ segments are removed by RNA splicing to generate a mature mRNA for translation into a specific κ light chain. The λ light chain undergoes a similar process of rearrangement before transcription but has a somewhat different germline organization; there are fewer V segments, and the V and J segments are each associated with a different C_λ segment (Figs. 14–5 and 14–6). Even greater diversity can be generated at the H-chain gene locus because of the additional use of one of multiple D segments in the formation of the H-chain variable region (Fig. 14–5).

In addition to the diversification possibilities provided by the recombination of multiple germline gene segments, somatic point mutation within the V-region genes provides another important mechanism for great expansion of the potential repertoire of antibody specificities.

Antibody diversity can therefore be generated by several molecular mechanisms, including the following:

1. The recombinatorial assortment of different sets of gene elements.
2. The availability of multiple V, D, and J segments.
3. Junctional diversity, created by the imprecise joining of the various elements and the random insertion of nucleotides not encoded in the germline (so-called N sequences) between recombining V and D elements or D and J elements.
4. Somatic mutation within the V region segments.
5. The possibility of pairing between any of the H-chain isotypes and L-chain subtypes.

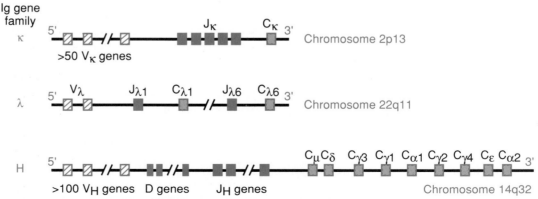

Figure 14–5. Structure of the immunoglobulin gene clusters. Coding and noncoding regions are not drawn to scale. The exact number of genes and the overall size of the gene clusters is not known.

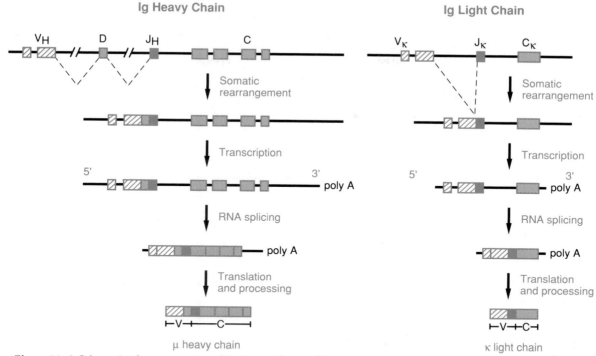

Ig Heavy Chain

Ig Light Chain

Figure 14-6. Schematic of rearrangement of the heavy chain and light chain immunoglobulin genes in antibody formation.

THE T-CELL ANTIGEN RECEPTOR

The mechanism of generation of diversity characteristic of the immunoglobulins is shared by another member of the immunoglobulin gene superfamily, the T-cell receptor (TCR). The TCR represents the T-cell analog of membrane-bound immunoglobulin on B cells (Fig. 14–3). The receptor is a transmembrane glycoprotein composed of either an α and a β chain (TCR α:β) or a γ and a δ chain (TCR γ:δ). Almost all T cells in the peripheral circulation bear the α:β receptor, which plays a key role in antigen recognition and in the genesis of T-cell helper or cytotoxic activity. The function of the TCR γ:δ receptor is not clear but appears related to T-cell ontogeny.

Unlike immunoglobulin, the TCR has no soluble form. However, the TCR resembles the Ig molecule structurally; all chains have both constant and variable sections, the variable sections being generated by an assortment of V, D, and J segments. Thus the TCR genes, which are encoded in three separate chromosomal regions (Fig. 14–7), appear to be members of the immunoglobulin gene superfamily, sharing ancestry with the immunoglobulin genes.

Just as for the Ig genes, the recombination of multiple germline elements, imprecision of joining, and the possibility of various α-chain:β-chain combinations create extensive diversity. The genesis of TCRs, however, unlike that of Igs, does not involve somatic mutation. A second and very significant difference between the two classes of antigen receptor is the prerequisite role for MHC molecules in T-cell antigen recognition. The T-cell receptor cannot recognize an antigen unless the antigen is presented as a processed peptide complexed with an MHC molecule (Fig. 14–3). Thus the T-cell receptor is specific for the combination of peptide and protein, a phenomenon known as **MHC restriction.**

THE IMMUNOGLOBULIN GENE SUPERFAMILY

A gene superfamily is defined as a series of genes that share evolutionary homology, but do not nec-

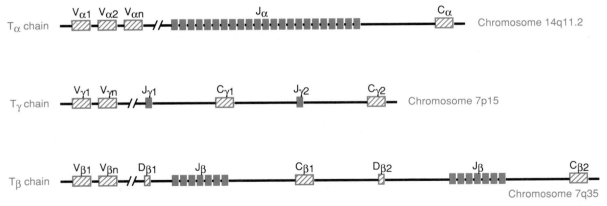

Figure 14–7. Germline arrangement of TCR genes. The β-chain gene cluster consists of multiple variable (V) gene segments and two sets of diversity (D), joining (J), and constant (C) region gene segments. The α-chain gene cluster contains many V gene segments, at least 40 J segments, and a single C gene segment. The γ-chain gene cluster has at least six V segments, along with two sets of J and C gene segments. The overall size of each gene cluster is not known.

essarily share function, genetic linkage, or coordinate regulation (Hood et al., 1985). The members of the Ig gene superfamily, although functionally distinct, share patterns of primary sequence and tertiary structure. As shown in the box, the group contains many kinds of genes, most of which encode proteins involved in either cell adhesion or binding on the cell surface.

The processes that favored the enormous diversification of this gene family require further clarification, which should eventually provide very important insights into the area of immune

and nonimmune cellular recognition and interaction.

SINGLE-GENE DISORDERS OF THE IMMUNE SYSTEM

The significance of the role played by the immune system in host defense becomes particularly evident when one or more components of the system are defective. The number and variety of single-gene disorders of the immune system, of which Table 14–3 gives examples, indicate that many aspects of immune function are under single-gene control.

The cellular level and molecular basis of most of the primary immunodeficiencies are currently unknown. One immunodeficiency gene that has already been cloned and characterized is a gene for X-linked **chronic granulomatous disease** (CGD), a disorder of neutrophils discussed in Chapter 13. The identification of the single genes encoding other inherited immunodeficiencies should yield very important insights pertaining to the genetic control of the immune response.

Isolation of the genes underlying the various primary immunodeficiency disorders also makes possible their potential treatment by somatic cell gene therapy. The immunodeficiency diseases are particularly appropriate candidates for this therapeutic approach, both because of their considerable morbidity and mortality and because the defects underlying the abnormal phenotypes are largely restricted to hematopoietic cells and could

---

Components of the Immunoglobulin Gene Superfamily

Genes involved in the immune response, including Igs, TCRs, MHC antigens, and T-cell glycoproteins CD3, CD4, and CD8

Nervous system molecules, such as N-CAM (neural cell adhesion molecule) and MAG (myelin-associated glycoprotein)

Growth factor receptors, such as PDGFR (receptor for platelet-derived growth factor)

Molecules found on both neural and lymphoid cells, such as Thy-1, the function of which is unknown at present

therefore be corrected by introduction of a normal gene into the patient's bone marrow cells as a replacement. As described in Chapter 13, adenosine deaminase deficiency, an autosomal recessive trait associated with severe combined immunodeficiency, was the first human disease treated by somatic gene therapy.

General References

Auffray C, Strominger JL (1986) Molecular genetics of the human major histocompatibility complex. Adv Hum Genet 15:197–247.

Bell JI, Todd JA, McDevitt HO (1989) The molecular basis of HLA-disease association. Adv Hum Genet 18:1–41.

Hunkapiller T, Hood L (1989) Diversity of the immunoglobulin gene superfamily. Adv Immunol 44:1–63.

Kostyu DD, Amos DB (1989) The HLA complex: Genetic polymorphism and disease susceptibility. *In* Scriver CR, Beaudet AL, Sly WS, Valle D (eds) The metabolic basis of inherited disease, 6th ed. McGraw-Hill, New York, pp. 225–249.

Litwin SD (ed) (1989) Human immunogenetics: Basic principles and clinical relevance. M Dekker, New York.

Roitt M, Brostoff J, Male DK (1989) Immunology, 6th ed. CV Mosby, St. Louis.

Williamson AR, Turner MW (1987) Essential immunogenetics. Blackwell Scientific, Oxford.

Problems

1. Ankylosing spondylitis and HLA-B27 are closely *associated*. The HLA-B locus and the locus for 21-hydroxylase (mutations at which lead to congenital adrenal hyperplasia) are closely *linked*. Distinguish between these two concepts.

2. a) Arrange the following family members in order of their probability of sharing two HLA haplotypes with the recipient and thus being suitable donors of tissues or organs: sib, father, MZ twin, DZ twin, half-sib, mother, unrelated person, first cousin.
   b) Why is an MZ twin of a recipient not necessarily the donor of choice?

3. How does somatic rearrangement of immunoglobulin and T-cell receptor genes differ from the splicing of introns and exons that is characteristic of most genes?

4. How does expression of immunoglobulin genes differ from the expression of most or all other autosomal loci?

5. For some X-linked immunodeficiencies, such as Wiskott-Aldrich syndrome, agammaglobulinemia, and severe combined immunodeficiency (SCID), certain cell populations in carrier females show nonrandom X inactivation; that is, all cells contain the X with the normal allele active, unlike other tissues that show random X inactivation in the same women. The affected cell population is characteristic of each disorder; that is, B cells in agammaglobulinemia, B and T cells in SCID, and T cells in Wiskott-Aldrich syndrome (Conley and Puck, 1988; Conley et al., 1988). Explain. Would you expect to find random or nonrandom X inactivation in cells from carriers of autosomal forms of immunodeficiency?

GENETICS OF DISORDERS WITH MULTIFACTORIAL INHERITANCE

The basis of many single-gene diseases has already been demonstrated at the protein and the DNA levels by the approaches of biochemical and molecular genetics. In addition, cytogenetics has revealed the chromosomal basis of a small but growing number of significant disorders. Among genetic phenotypes in general, however, single-gene or cytogenetic defects are greatly outnumbered by common disorders that appear to run in families but are neither single-gene nor chromosomal in origin. These disorders, which are still for the most part poorly understood genetically, are said to show **multifactorial inheritance,** indicating that they are caused by multiple factors, both genetic and, in many cases, environmental. Many congenital malformations show multifactorial inheritance. Other multifactorial disorders, in which the role of environment appears to be relatively large and the underlying etiology may be heterogeneous and complex, appear as common disorders of adult life.

Multifactorial inheritance is defined as inheritance by a combination of genetic factors and in some cases also nongenetic factors, each with only a relatively small effect. The term **polygenic**

inheritance has a more restricted meaning, assuming inheritance by a large number of genes with small, equal, additive effects, and in this formal sense it may not apply to any human disorder. Traits are sometimes loosely called polygenic when they are caused by multiple genes with no obvious environmental component, but in actual experience it is often hard to judge whether environment plays any causative role.

Multifactorial disorders recur within families, but they do not show any particular pedigree pattern in an individual family. Genetically, they have common characteristics that allow estimation of their multifactorial background and estimation of recurrence risks for relatives in collections of families; however, the recurrence risks are averages, and the actual risk for an individual family may be larger or smaller than the average.

In this chapter we consider the genetic aspects of three different classes of multifactorial traits:

1. Many normal characteristics have multifactorial inheritance and are characterized by **continuous variation.** For these characteristics, an "abnormal" phenotype is simply an extreme var-

iant of the normal range; examples include many cases of nonspecific mental retardation and of unusually tall or short stature.

2. A second group of multifactorial disorders is made up of common single congenital malformations, in which there appears to be underlying continuous variation in liability to a particular disorder, but there is no clinical effect until the patient's liability exceeds a "threshold" for the abnormal phenotype. These are usually known as **multifactorial threshold traits.**

3. The third group comprises the **common disorders of adult life** that make up a large part of clinical medicine, such as coronary artery disease, diabetes mellitus, hypertension, obesity, and most forms of cancer, as well as common psychiatric illnesses, such as manic-depressive psychosis and schizophrenia. Environmental factors are considered to play a large part in these disorders, even though the role of genetics in their etiology is undeniable. In a sense, common disorders of adult life can also be considered threshold traits, but because of the complexity of the risk factors that can lead to them, they are regarded instead as a separate class.

CONTINUOUS VARIATION

The Normal Distribution

The concept of multifactorial inheritance arose originally from genetic experiments with continuously variable, measurable traits (sometimes called quantitative traits) from which it could be shown that additive variation at just a few loci could produce a distribution approximating a normal (Gaussian) curve.

Many continuously variable human traits, such as stature, have a normal distribution in the population. As a rule, when a quantitative trait has a normal distribution in a population, measurements more than two standard deviations above or below the population mean are regarded as "abnormal." The interval between the mean and two standard deviations above and below it ($\bar{x} \pm 2\sigma$) includes more than 94 percent of all measurements. The concept of the normal range is fundamental to clinical medicine; for example, in pediatrics height, weight, head circumference, and other measurements are compared with the "normal" expected measurements for a child's sex and age.

Figure 15–1 shows a population distribution of stature. Both genetic and environmental factors are involved in the determination of adult stature, and the assumption is that the genetic factors are, for the most part, genes with individually small effects. Major genes and chromosome disorders that affect stature (e.g., achondroplasia, growth hormone deficiency, Marfan syndrome, or Klinefelter syndrome) are so rare that they have little if any observable effect on the distribution curve of the entire population.

Analysis of the inheritance of stature has shown that the mean stature of offspring is closer to the mean stature in the population than is the

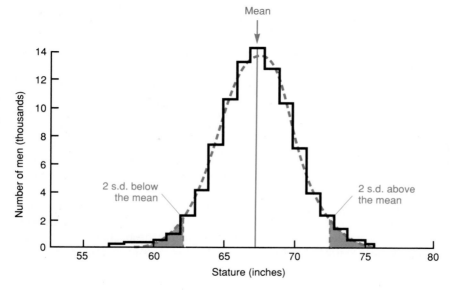

Figure 15–1. Distribution of stature in a sample of 91,163 young English males in 1939. The red line is a normal (Gaussian) curve with the same mean and standard deviation (s.d.) as the observed data. The shaded areas indicate persons of unusually tall or short stature (greater than two s.d. above or below the mean). (Adapted from Harrison GA, Weiner JS, Tanner JM, et al. [1977] Human Biology, 2nd ed. Oxford University Press, Oxford.)

Table 15–1. Degree of Relationship and Genes in Common

Relationship to Proband	Proportion of Genes in Common with Proband
Monozygotic twin	1
First-degree relative (parent, dizygotic twin or other sib, child)	1/2
Second-degree relative (grandparent, uncle or aunt, half-sib, nephew or niece, grandchild)	1/4
Third-degree relative (great-grandparent, great-grandchild, first cousin, etc.)	1/8

See Figure 4–2 for examples of degrees of relationship.

mean stature of their parents (the "midparent mean"). In other words, although tall parents tend to have tall children and short parents tend to have short children, the distribution of stature in the offspring is wide enough that a small proportion of offspring of tall parents are short and, similarly, a small proportion of offspring of short parents are tall. The statistical principle of regression to the mean, when applied to genetics, explains the finding that for quantitative traits, the offspring have, *on the average*, less extreme phenotypes than do their parents.

Correlation Between Relatives

For continuously variable traits such as stature, if mating is random and environmental factors are not involved, the theoretical correlation between first-degree relatives (parent-child or sib-sib) is .50. In more general terms, the correlation between relatives is proportional to their genes in common — that is, to the proportion of their genes that they have inherited from the same ancestral source. Relatives of the same degree have the same proportion of genes in common (Table 15–1). For analysis of continuously variable multifactorial traits, all relatives of the same degree are considered together, and the correlation coefficient is calculated for the combined group:

Often, however, the genetic background of a trait is more complex and the correlation is lower than observed here for stature. For example, there may be major genes as well as minor genes or significant environmental factors such as nutrition or infection. Genetic analysis then requires large samples and sophisticated data analysis.

Heritability

Many multifactorial traits are influenced both by genes and by environment, and the concept of **heritability** was developed in order to separate their relative roles. Heritability is a useful measure because even when the actual genetic basis of a trait is not known, the importance of genetic components in its causation is indicated by its heritability; the higher the heritability, the more important the genetic factors, and this information can eventually lead to a better understanding of the precise causes. By definition, heritability is the proportion of the *total phenotypic variance (V)* of a trait that is caused by additive *genetic variance*. Statistically, variance is a measure of how much an individual value is likely to vary from the mean of a group.

The phenotype of a multifactorial trait is taken as the sum of three values:

1. *g*, contribution of additive genetic factors, with variance *G*.

2. *b*, contribution of environment within the family, with variance *B*.

3. *e*, contribution of random environmental factors, with variance *E*.

Heritability (h^2), then is

$$\frac{G}{G+B+E} = \frac{G}{V}$$

Thus in general terms heritability is a measure of whether the role of genetic factors in determining a given phenotype (or liability to a phenotype) is large or small.

Variable	Parent–child	Sib–sib
Genes in common	.50	.50
Correlation coefficient for stature	.51	.56

One method of estimating the heritability of a trait is by comparison of data on concordance for the trait in monozygotic (MZ) twins (who share 100 percent of their genes) and dizygotic (DZ) twins (who share 50 percent of their genes). The formula then becomes

$$h^2 = \frac{\text{variance in DZ pairs} - \text{variance in MZ pairs}}{\text{variance in DZ pairs}}$$

If the trait is determined chiefly by environment, this ratio approaches 0; if determination is primarily genetic, MZ pairs show little variance, and the ratio approaches 1.

MULTIFACTORIAL THRESHOLD TRAITS

The concept of multifactorial inheritance becomes more complex when, instead of continuous variation, there is a sharp distinction between normal and abnormal phenotypes. One model proposed to explain the genetic basis of a number of common congenital malformations is that there is underlying continuous variation in **liability** to the malformation, with a **threshold** marking the point at which the liability is actually expressed as an abnormal phenotype (Fig. 15–2).

Several common congenital malformations that have a population frequency of the order of 1/1000, and that occur as isolated defects and not part of a syndrome, have been shown to conform reasonably well to the family patterns predicted by the multifactorial threshold model (Table 15–2). These multifactorial traits have certain common characteristics (summarized in the box) that distinguish them from Mendelian traits. These characteristics can be illustrated by the family distribution of a number of multifactorial threshold traits, including pyloric stenosis, neural tube defects, congenital heart defects, and possibly cleft lip and palate.

Pyloric Stenosis

Pyloric stenosis, as the name implies, is an anomaly of the pylorus in which hypertrophy and hyperplasia of the smooth muscle narrows the antrum of the stomach so that it easily becomes obstructed. Infants with pyloric stenosis have severe feeding problems, with projectile vomiting. The obstruction can be relieved surgically.

Pyloric stenosis is five times as common in boys as in girls (about 5 per 1000 male births and 1 per 1000 female births), but its family pattern is

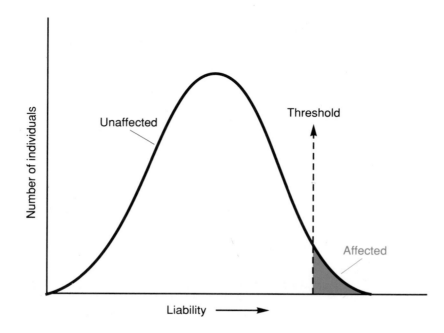

Figure 15–2. The multifactorial threshold model. Liability to a trait is distributed normally, with a threshold dividing the population into unaffected and affected classes.

Characteristics of Multifactorial Inheritance

1. **Although the disorder is obviously familial, there is no distinctive pattern of inheritance within a single family.**

2. **The risk to first-degree relatives, determined from family studies, is approximately the square root of the population risk.**

As a consequence, the lower the population incidence, the greater the *relative* increase in risk for first-degree relatives. However, only rather large differences in population frequency make an appreciable difference to the recurrence risk.

3. **The risk is sharply lower for second-degree than for first-degree relatives, but it declines less rapidly for more remote relatives.**

This characteristic distinguishes multifactorial inheritance from autosomal dominant inheritance, in which the risk drops by half with each step of more distant relationship. It is also different from the autosomal recessive pattern, in which virtually no relatives other than sibs are at risk.

4. **The recurrence risk is higher when more than one family member is affected.**

Multiple cases suggest that the liability is high in that particular family (illustrated in Table 15–4). In contrast, for single-gene traits the risk to the next child remains unchanged even after two, three, or more affected children have been born.

5. **The more severe the malformation, the greater the recurrence risk.**

More severely affected patients, and their relatives, have greater liability (see discussion of severity in cleft lip and palate).

6. **If a multifactorial trait is more frequent in one sex than in the other, the risk is higher for relatives of patients of the *less* susceptible sex.**

An affected person of the less susceptible sex is likely to have a higher liability, and thus any relative has a greater risk of being affected (see discussion of pyloric stenosis).

7. **If the concordance rate in DZ twins is less than half the rate in MZ twins, the trait cannot be autosomal dominant, and if it is less than a quarter of the MZ rate, it cannot be autosomal recessive.**

The concordance rate for non–insulin-dependent diabetes mellitus (NIDDM) is close to 100 percent in MZ twins but only about 10 percent in DZ pairs; at first glance the MZ data support a single-gene model with complete penetrance, but the low concordance rate in DZ twins contradicts this impression, and further studies have supported the conclusion that NIDDM has complex etiology.

8. **An increased recurrence risk when the parents are consanguineous suggests that multiple factors with additive effects may be involved.**

For multifactorial traits, the risk to subsequent sibs is increased when the parents are consanguineous. This is in contrast to autosomal recessive inheritance; although parental consanguinity usually indicates a high probability of autosomal recessive inheritance, the recurrence risk (1/4) is the same whether the parents are consanguineous or not.

distinctive: as measured in terms of multiples of the population risk, affected females are much more likely than affected males to have affected children, and among the children of both affected males and affected females, the sons are more likely than the daughters to be affected (Table 15–3). The inheritance obviously does not fit any Mendelian pattern.

Table 15–2. Some Common Congenital Malformations
with Multifactorial Inheritance

Malformation	Population Incidence (per 1000) (approximate)
Cleft lip with/without cleft palate	.4–1.7
Cleft palate	.4
Congenital dislocation of hip	2*
Congenital heart defects	4–8
Ventricular septal defect	1.7
Patent ductus arteriosus	.5
Atrial septal defect	1.0
Aortic stenosis	.5
Neural tube defects	2–10
Anencephaly	variable
Spina bifida	variable
Pyloric stenosis	1†
	5*

Note: Many of these disorders are heterogeneous and are usually but not invariably multifactorial. Data from Carter (1976), Nora (1968), and Lin and Garver (1988).
* Per 1000 males; †per 1000 females.

The model proposed by Carter (1976) to fit the observed family data is that pyloric stenosis is a multifactorial threshold trait, with the added feature that the threshold dividing children with normal phenotypes from those with pyloric stenosis is different for the two sexes (Fig. 15–3). Liability to the malformation is assumed to be continuously distributed in the population and to be determined by multiple factors, some genetic (in view of the fact that the disorder runs in families) and others possibly environmental. The underlying liability is separated into normal and abnormal phenotypes by a threshold that, in anatomical terms, marks the point of the maximal amount of abnormality of the pylorus compatible with normal function.

If the underlying liability to a trait is continuous but the threshold is lower in males than in females, affected females have, on the average, more extreme liability (that is, liability that is farther from the population mean in the distribution curve) than do affected males. Regression to the mean predicts that the more extreme the parent's liability is, the higher above the population mean is the mean of the offspring; in other words, offspring of affected females have a higher mean liability to pyloric stenosis than do offspring of affected males (Table 15–3). However, males have a lower liability threshold than females; thus, regardless of which parent is affected, the liability of male offspring is more likely to fall beyond the threshold, and males are therefore more likely than females to be affected. Sons of affected mothers are at the highest risk, about 20 percent. Similar risks apply to sibs of patients.

Table 15–3. Pyloric Stenosis in Offspring
of Index Patients

Relatives	Risk	Multiple of Population Risk
Sons of male patients	1/18	11
Daughters of male patients	1/42	24
Sons of female patients	1/5	40
Daughters of female patients	1/14	70

From Carter CO (1969) Genetics of common disorders. Br Med Bull 25:52–57.

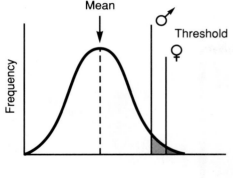

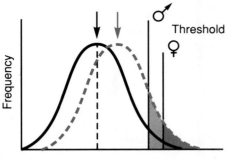

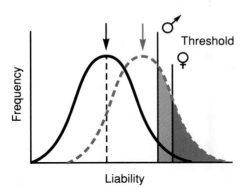

Figure 15-3. An interpretation of the sex ratio and familial distribution of pyloric stenosis in terms of the multifactorial threshold model. Liability to pyloric stenosis is distributed normally, with a more extreme threshold in females than in males. The distribution of genetic liability in relatives of male and female probands (red curve) is shifted in comparison with that of the general population (solid curve). (Based on Carter CO [1964] The genetics of common malformations. *In* Fishbein M [ed] Congenital malformations. International Medical Congress, New York.)

Neural Tube Defects

Anencephaly and **spina bifida** are neural tube defects (NTDs) that frequently occur together in families and are considered to have common pathogenesis (Fig. 15-4). In anencephaly, the forebrain, overlying meninges, vault of the skull, and skin are all absent. Many infants with anencephaly are stillborn, and those born alive survive a few hours at most. About two thirds of affected infants are female. In spina bifida, there is failure of fusion of the arches of the vertebrae, typically in the lumbar region. There are varying degrees of severity, ranging from spina bifida occulta, in which the defect is in the bony arch only, to spina bifida aperta, often associated with meningocele (protrusion of meninges) or meningomyelocele (protrusion of neural elements as well as meninges; Fig. 15-4). The incidence of spina bifida is a little higher in females than in males.

As a group, NTDs are a leading cause of stillbirth, death in early infancy, and handicap in surviving children. Their population incidence is variable, ranging from almost 1 percent in Ireland to 0.2 percent or less in the United States. There is considerable ethnic and geographic variation; for example, the incidence in Sikhs in British Columbia, Canada, is more than twice the overall popu-

DEFECTS IN CLOSURE OF NEURAL TUBE

Dorsal View of Normal Embryo of 23 Days

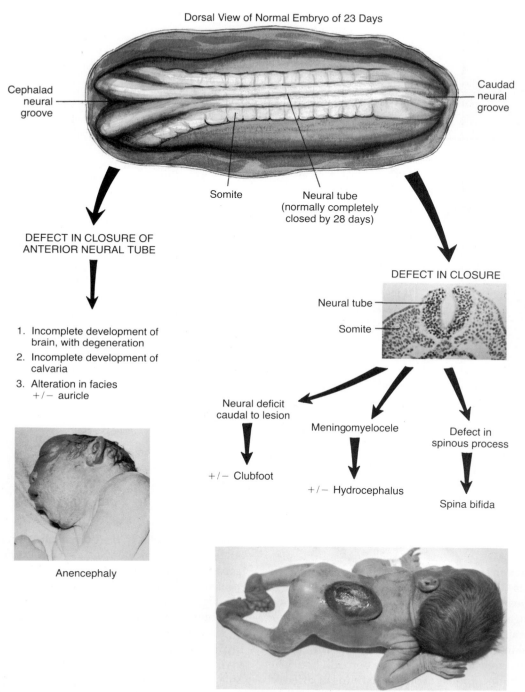

Cephalad neural groove

Caudad neural groove

Somite

Neural tube (normally completely closed by 28 days)

DEFECT IN CLOSURE OF ANTERIOR NEURAL TUBE

1. Incomplete development of brain, with degeneration
2. Incomplete development of calvaria
3. Alteration in facies +/− auricle

Anencephaly

DEFECT IN CLOSURE

Neural tube

Somite

Neural deficit caudal to lesion

Meningomyelocele

Defect in spinous process

+/− Clubfoot

+/− Hydrocephalus

Spina bifida

Meningomyelocele with partially epithelialized sac

Figure 15-4. The origin of the neural tube defects anencephaly and spina bifida. (From Jones KL [1988] Smith's Recognizable patterns of human malformation, 4th ed. WB Saunders, Philadelphia.)

Table 15–4. Recurrence Risks (%) for Cleft Lip with or without Cleft Palate
and for Neural Tube Malformations

Affected Relatives	Cleft Lip with/ without Cleft Palate	Anencephaly and Spina Bifida
No sibs		
Neither parent	0.1	0.3
One parent	3	4.5
Both parents	34	30
1 sib		
Neither parent	3	4
One parent	11	12
Both parents	40	38
2 sibs		
Neither parent	8	10
One parent	19	20
Both parents	45	43
1 sib and 1 second-degree relative		
Neither parent	6	7
One parent	16	18
Both parents	43	42
1 sib and 1 third-degree relative		
Neither parent	4	5.5
One parent	14	16
Both parents	44	42

From Bonaiti-Pellié C, Smith C (1974) Risk tables for genetic counselling in some common congenital malformations. J Med Genet 11:374–377.

lation rate, but less than half the rate for Sikhs in India. The frequency also appears to vary with social factors and season of birth, and oscillates widely over time (with a marked decrease in recent years).

It is believed that nutritional factors may account for at least part of the variation. This possibility, supported by a survey that showed that in at least one population the recurrence risk was reduced markedly by periconceptional vitamin supplementation (Smithells et al., 1980), led to extensive testing in other populations. Unfortunately, there is still no consensus that vitamin supplementation is helpful in preventing NTDs in most at-risk pregnancies.

A small proportion of NTDs have specific causes: for example, amniotic bands (fibrous connections between the amnion and fetus caused by early rupture of the amnion, which may disrupt structures during their embryological development), some single-gene defects with pleiotropic expression, some chromosome disorders, and some teratogens. Most NTDs, however, are isolated defects that are presumed to have multifactorial inheritance. The recurrence risks within families are given in Table 15–4. About 95 percent

of all patients with NTDs, however, are the first children in their extended families known to have this malformation.

NTDs rank high among the conditions for which prenatal diagnosis is possible. Anencephaly and most cases of open spina bifida can be identified prenatally by detection of excessive levels of alpha-fetoprotein in the amniotic fluid and maternal serum and by ultrasonographic scanning (see Chapter 19 for further discussion). In a few cases in which anencephaly has been diagnosed prenatally, the pregnancies have been allowed to continue in order to provide organs for other infants born with congenital defects, especially heart defects. Like all experimentation with fetal tissue, this is a highly controversial area at the present time.

Congenital Heart Defects

Congenital heart defects (CHDs) are very common, with a frequency of about 4 to 8 cases per 1000 births. They are a heterogeneous group, caused in some cases by single-gene or chromosomal mechanisms and in others by exposure to teratogens such as rubella infection or maternal diabetes. In most cases, however, the cause is unknown, and most are regarded as multifactorial.

There are many types of CHDs, with different population incidences and empiric risks. One prediction of the multifactorial threshold model is that the risk for first-degree relatives is equal to the square root of the population incidence of a multifactorial trait (see box). This relationship is not true for single-gene traits, in which the risk to sibs is largely *independent* of the population frequency. When the incidence of several common types of heart defect is compared with the recurrence risk in sibs, the figures are in reasonably close agreement with this prediction. For example:

Defect	Population Incidence (approximate)	Frequency in Sibs (%)	Square Root of Population Incidence (%)
Ventricular septal defect	1/575	4.3	4.2
Patent ductus arteriosus	1/1200	3.2	2.9
Atrial septal defect	1/1500	3.2	2.6
Aortic stenosis	1/2250	2.6	2.1

These figures come from a study by Nora (1968) in which the defects were classified anatomically. However, it is known that when heart defects recur in a family, the affected children do not necessarily have the same anatomical defect. When the classification is based on developmental mechanism rather than anatomy, five main groups of CHDs can be distinguished (Clark, 1986): flow lesions, abnormalities of cell migration, cell death, abnormalities in extracellular matrix, and defects in targeted growth. A familial pattern is found only in the group with flow lesions, a large category that includes hypoplastic left heart syndrome, coarctation of the aorta, atrial septal defect of the secundum type, pulmonary valve stenosis, a common type of ventricular septal defect, and other forms.

Are isolated congenital heart defects multifactorial? At present the family data are not really adequate to confirm or deny the hypothesis. Until more is known, the figures just given can be used as estimates of the recurrence risk in first-degree relatives, and a low risk (not much higher than the population risk) can be given to second- and third-degree relatives of index patients. By the same token, relatives of index patients with types of CHDs other than flow lesions can be offered reassurance. For further reassurance, many CHDs can now be assessed prenatally by ultrasonography (see Chapter 19).

Cleft Lip and Cleft Palate

Cleft lip with or without cleft palate, or CL(P), is one of the most common congenital malformations. CL(P), which is causally distinct from isolated cleft palate without cleft lip, originates as a failure of fusion of the frontal process with the maxillary process at about the 35th day of gestation. About 60 to 80 percent of those affected are males. CL(P) is heterogeneous and includes isolated single-gene forms, numerous single-gene syndromes, forms associated with chromosomal disorders (especially trisomy 13), cases resulting from teratogenic exposure (rubella embryopathy, thalidomide, or anticonvulsants), and forms that appear in nonfamilial syndromes. In the past, almost every conceivable mode of inheritance has been proposed for CL(P), even though it has many of the features of a classic multifactorial threshold trait (Fraser, 1989).

There is considerable variation in frequency in different racial groups: about 1.7 per 1000 in Japanese, 1.0 per 1000 in Caucasians, and 0.4 per 1000 in American Blacks. Relatively high rates are also seen in some North American populations of Asian descent—for example, in Indians of the southwest United States and the west coast of Canada. The concordance rate is about 30 percent in MZ twins and about 5 percent (the same as the risk for non-twin sibs) in DZ twins.

Severity and Recurrence Risk

One of the predictions of multifactorial inheritance used to distinguish it from single-gene inheritance is that more severe expression, because it indicates greater liability, would be associated with a higher recurrence risk (see box). In accordance with this prediction, family studies of CL(P) have shown an increase in recurrence risk as the severity increases from unilateral to bilateral and from cleft lip alone (CL) to cleft lip with cleft palate (CLP) (Melnick, 1980):

Phenotype of Proband	Incidence in Sibs (%)
Unilateral CL without CP	4.0
Unilateral CLP	4.9
Bilateral CL without CP	6.7
Bilateral CLP	8.0

Segregation Analysis of CL(P) Family Data

Complex segregation analysis of a large number of pedigrees of CL(P) has shown that in certain populations there might be a major gene for liability to CL(P) as well as multiple minor genes, contrary to expectations of the simple threshold model. In a Danish study, the data were consistent with multifactorial inheritance in only about two thirds of cases, suggesting in the remaining third the action of a major autosomal recessive gene with low penetrance; in contrast, data from a Japanese study fit the multifactorial threshold model without the hypothesis of a major liability gene. The firm identification of a putative liability gene would contribute to understanding of the molecular development of the lip and palate. Until better insight into the basis of the defect is gained, however, the empiric risk figures (Tables 15–4 and 15–5) are the only guidelines available for genetic counseling.

Genetic Counseling of Families of Patients with Multifactorial Traits

Genetic counseling for multifactorial disorders follows in general the principles outlined in the box. In brief review, the following points must be considered:

1. The recurrence risk is much higher for first-degree relatives of affected family members than for more distant relatives.

2. The best estimate of the recurrence risk is the **empiric risk,** which is simply the recurrence risk observed in similar families, for the same degree of relationship. It is often useful to state it as a multiple of the population risk of the defect.

The empiric risk is based entirely on past experience and does not imply that the genetic and environmental factors in the pathogenesis of the malformation are understood. An empiric risk is an average for the population and is not necessarily accurate for a specific family.

3. The recurrence risk is increased by:

  * the presence of more than one affected relative;
  * a severe form of the disorder;
  * an affected person of the sex *less* likely to be affected;
  * consanguineous parentage.

4. Two common errors in risk calculation should be avoided:

  * If the parent of a child with a multifactorial birth defect has another child by a different partner, the children are *second*-degree, not first-degree, relatives, and the

Table 15–5. Empiric Risks for Some Congenital Malformations

Population Affected	Cleft Lip with/without Cleft Palate	Pyloric Stenosis (Females Only)
General population	0.001	0.001
First-degree relatives	×40	×10
Second-degree relatives	×7	×5
Third-degree relatives	×3	×1.5

From Carter CO (1969) Genetics of common disorders. Br Med Bull 25:52–57. Risks to relatives are stated as multiples of the population risk.

empiric risk for the second child is much lower than if the children had both parents in common (usually, the risk is approximately 1 percent instead of approximately 5 percent).

• When an unaffected uncle or aunt of a child with a multifactorial defect inquires about the risk of the same defect in his or her own offspring, the relevant risk is not the risk to the consultand (a second-degree relative of the index patient) but the risk to the *offspring* of the consultand (third-degree relatives).

COMPLEX DISORDERS OF ADULT LIFE

The common chronic disorders that account for much of the morbidity and mortality in adult life have always been a problem to geneticists. Although they are definitely familial and in a broad sense they behave as multifactorial threshold traits, the effect of environment on their expression appears to be much greater than for other genetic diseases; in fact, the physician's role is often one of attempting to adjust the environment to normalize the phenotype.

One reason that these disorders have been so hard to analyze genetically is that their causes are usually heterogeneous. Until specific entities have been defined within broad disease categories, as familial hypercholesterolemia has been disentangled from other, genetically different causes of coronary artery disease, a full understanding of these disorders and their genetics cannot be expected. For now, population-based empiric risks, although often inadequate, are the only source available for genetic prediction.

Coronary Artery Disease

By any measure, coronary artery disease (CAD) is a major health problem, particularly in males aged 45 or more. Most cases appear to be multifactorial, with a marked effect of environment.

Familial hypercholesterolemia, an autosomal dominant defect of the low-density lipoprotein receptor discussed in Chapter 12, accounts for only about 5 percent of survivors of myocardial infarc-

tion, the chief clinical manifestation of CAD. Although there are other single-gene causes, the adverse risk factors associated with CAD include nongenetic as well as genetic factors, and most cases of CAD are therefore thought to show multifactorial inheritance:

Genetic Factors	Nongenetic Factors
Male sex	Increasing age
Family history of CAD	Smoking
Single-gene abnormalities of lipoproteins and lipids	Physical inactivity
Other disorders with genetic components:	Stress
• hypertension	
• obesity	
• diabetes mellitus	

The risk factors for CAD include several other multifactorial disorders with genetic components: hypertension, obesity, and diabetes mellitus. In this context, the abnormal phenotype associated with these disorders contributes to an environment that enhances the risk of CAD.

One feature of CAD that is consistent with multifactorial inheritance is that whereas males are at higher risk of death from myocardial infarction both in the population and within affected families, the recurrence risk in relatives is somewhat greater when the proband is female. The risks of death from ischemic heart disease among 35- to 55-year-old first-degree relatives of probands with ischemic heart disease (Slack and Evans, 1966) are as follows:

Relationship	Risk of Death
Male relative of male proband	1/12
Female relative of male proband	1/36
Male relative of female proband	1/10
Female relative of female proband	1/12

CAD is often an incidental finding in family histories of patients with other genetic diseases. In view of the high recurrence risk, physicians and genetic counselors may need to consider whether first-degree relatives of patients with CAD should be evaluated further and offered counseling, even when CAD is not the primary genetic problem for which the patient or relative has been referred.

Obesity

Large differences in body weight and fat distribution, even among people of the same sex and age, are due chiefly to genetic factors, although there is no question that environment (in the form of diet and exercise) also plays a role. Two recent studies of body weight in MZ twins demonstrate the twin method of assessing the relative importance of genes and environment in obesity.

As mentioned earlier in this chapter, comparison of MZ twins reared together or apart and of DZ twins reared together or apart is a classical way of measuring heritability of complex traits. A recent Swedish study of the body-mass index (weight in kilograms divided by square of the height in meters) of twins showed a high heritability value: that is, a strong influence of heredity on the body-mass index ($h^2 = .70$ to $.80$; Stunkard et al., 1990).

In another study, only MZ twin pairs were studied in order to measure the genetic component of the response to overfeeding (Bouchard et al., 1990). When the effect of overfeeding was compared within the twin pairs and in the total group, it was found that the members of a pair resembled one another much more closely in weight gain and fat distribution than they resembled others in the group, again demonstrating the importance of genetic factors in weight gain.

Diabetes Mellitus

The genetics of diabetes mellitus is notoriously complex, but there have been some recent developments suggesting that much of the complexity may soon be clarified. There are two main types of diabetes mellitus, **insulin-dependent (IDDM)** and **non-insulin-dependent (NIDDM)**, representing about 10 percent and 88 percent of all cases, respectively. Both forms "breed true" in families, and they differ in typical onset age, MZ twin concordances, and HLA associations:

Variable	IDDM	NIDDM
Onset age	Usually <40 years	Usually >40 years
MZ twin concordance	30%–50%	Close to 100%
HLA associations	Strong (see text)	None

Insulin-Dependent Diabetes Mellitus

IDDM has an incidence of about 1 in 200 Caucasians and usually manifests early in life. It results from destruction of the β cells of the pancreas, which normally produce insulin. The β cell destruction responsible for IDDM appears to be an autoimmune process, and HLA haplotypes DR3 and DR4 are strongly associated with liability to the disease.

About 95 percent of all IDDM patients (in comparison with about half the normal population) have HLA-DR3 or HLA-DR4; DR3/DR4 heterozygotes are particularly susceptible to IDDM. This is one of the strongest HLA-disease associations known (see Chapter 14). Family studies suggest that the HLA association accounts for more than half the heritability of IDDM.

A large international study has established the importance of the DR3 and DR4 association in IDDM (Thomson et al., 1988). From this study the following risk figures for siblings of index patients can be derived in relation to whether the patient and sib share two, one, or no parental haplotypes:

Average risk to sib of IDDM patient	6.0%
Risk if:	
Proband and sib both DR3/DR4	19.2%
Proband and sib share two haplotypes	12.9%
Proband and sib share one haplotype	4.7%
Proband and sib share no haplotype	1.8%

All these figures are well below the MZ twin concordance rate of 30 to 50 percent, suggesting that the HLA constitution alone does not fully explain the genetics of IDDM. There must be other genes, elsewhere in the genome, that also predispose to the development of IDDM.

Molecular Analysis. New insights into the basis of IDDM have come from molecular analysis of the HLA class II genes, which are responsible for immune responsiveness. Sequencing of the DQ_β alleles and their products shows that there is no specific allele for susceptibility to IDDM. Every allele found in diabetics is also found in nondiabetic controls. However, in the DR4 haplotype, the presence of aspartic acid (Asp) at position 57 of the DQ_β chain is closely associated with resistance to IDDM, whereas other amino acids at this position (alanine, valine, or serine) confer susceptibility

(Todd et al., 1987). About 90 percent of patients with IDDM are homozygous for DQ$_\beta$ genes that do *not* encode Asp at position 57.

The strength of an HLA-disease association is often measured by the **relative risk,** which may be calculated from the incidence of the specific HLA type in patients and controls as follows:

Relative risk $= ad/bc$, where

$a =$ number of patients with the antigen,
$b =$ number of controls with the antigen,
$c =$ number of patients without the antigen,
$d =$ number of controls without the antigen.

If the frequency of the trait in question (in our example, being 57Asp-negative) is the same in patients and controls, this value will be 1. According to Morel and colleagues (1988), the relative risk that 57Asp-negative individuals will develop IDDM is 107, strong evidence that the DQ molecule, especially amino acid 57 of its β chain, is responsible for the autoimmune response that destroys the insulin-producing cells of the pancreas. The amino acid at position 57 of the β chain may have an important role in peptide binding and thus in T-cell recognition (see also Chapter 14).

This finding represents a major step forward in the understanding of IDDM and of disease susceptibility in general. Although there are probably other susceptibility genes for IDDM, both within and outside the major histocompatibility complex, as well as predisposing nongenetic factors that are still poorly understood, we now have a molecular handle on IDDM that may contribute not only to further analysis of IDDM but to the analysis of other HLA-associated diseases as well.

disease will develop in an individual patient. Although in principle the methods of genetic linkage analysis (Chapter 8) can be applied to multifactorial or polygenic traits, in practice this will be quite difficult.

Efforts to map major genes for **manic-depressive psychosis,** for example, have led to confusing results; in different studies the responsible gene has been mapped tentatively to three different chromosome regions (6p, 11p, and Xq), while in other studies the proposed linkages to two of these (11p and Xq) have not been confirmed. At this time it is not clear whether manic-depressive psychosis is determined, at least in part, by genes at any or all of these loci.

For **schizophrenia,** there is some evidence for at least two genetic types, one of which appears to be localized to chromosome 5q (McGillivray et al., 1990); in other words, schizophrenia apparently *can* have a single-gene origin, although whether it usually does is not at all certain. In spite of the difficulties encountered in attempts to map genes playing a role in these disorders, an effort may eventually lead to the identification of candidate genes; manic-depressive psychosis and schizophrenia are so important clinically and so common in the population that they warrant the effort that will be required to come to terms with them. The successes of the molecular approach in coronary artery disease and diabetes mellitus, and the increasing power of computerized complex segregation analysis of large data sets, allow one to be optimistic about the longer term prospects of successfully dissecting the genetic causes of common adult diseases.

Other Complex Genetic Disorders

Earlier in this chapter, several other common, complex genetic disorders of adult life were listed: hypertension, cancer, manic-depressive psychosis, and schizophrenia. The genetic components of all of these have been difficult to identify. Most are heterogeneous, and a large part of their analysis will involve dissecting the heterogeneity, finding genes responsible for different genetic forms, and establishing risk factors, separate from the genetic background, that increase the probability that the

General References

Carter CO (1976) Genetics of common single malformations. Br Med Bull 32:21–26.

Emery AEH (1986) Methodology in medical genetics, 2nd ed. Churchill Livingstone, Edinburgh.

Field LL (1988) Invited editorial: Insulin-dependent diabetes mellitus: A model for the study of multifactorial diseases. Am J Hum Genet 43:793–798.

Fraser FC (1989) Mapping the cleft lip genes: The first fix? Am J Hum Genet 45:345–347.

Lin AE, Garver KL (1988) Genetic counseling for congenital heart defects. J Pediatr 113:1105–1109.

Marx J (1990) Dissecting the complex diseases. Science 247:1540–1542.

Todd JA, Bell JI, McDevitt HO (1988) A molecular basis for genetic susceptibility to insulin-dependent diabetes mellitus. Trends Genet 4:129–134.

Problems

1. For a certain malformation, the recurrence risk in sibs and offspring of affected persons is 10 percent, the risk in nieces and nephews is 5 percent, and the risk in first cousins is 2.5 percent.
   a) Is this more likely to be an autosomal dominant trait with reduced penetrance or a multifactorial trait? Explain.
   b) What other information might support your conclusion?

2. A large sex difference in affected persons is often a clue to X-linked inheritance. How would you establish that pyloric stenosis is multifactorial rather than X-linked?

3. A series of children with a particular congenital malformation includes both boys and girls. In all cases, the parents are normal. How would you determine whether the malformation is more likely to be multifactorial than autosomal recessive?

CHAPTER
16

GENETICS OF CANCER

Cancer is one of the most common and severe problems of clinical medicine. Statistics show that cancer in some form strikes more than one third of the population, accounts for more than 20 percent of all deaths, and, in developed countries, is responsible for more than 10 percent of the total cost of medical care.

Cancer is not a single disease but rather a name applied to a great variety of malignant tumors that are formed by the same basic process of uncontrolled growth. Cell proliferation results in a mass (neoplasm or tumor) that invades neighboring tissues (hence the name *cancer*, meaning crab) and may also metastasize to more distant sites. The growth is autonomous, increasingly malignant, and, if untreated, invariably fatal. Early diagnosis and early treatment are vital, and identification of persons at increased risk of cancer before its development is an important objective of cancer research.

A tumor is composed of a parenchyma of proliferating cells, with a stroma of connective tissue and blood vessels. There are three main forms: **sarcomas,** in which the tumor has arisen in mesenchymal tissue; **carcinomas,** which originate in epithelial tissue; and **hematopoietic** and **lymphoid malignancies** such as leukemias and lymphomas. Within the major groups, tumors are classified by site, tissue type, and degree of malignancy. Most cancers are disorders of later life, but some are characteristic of childhood or may exhibit a greater degree of malignancy if they occur in younger persons.

THE GENETIC NATURE OF CANCER

The concept of cancer as a genetic disease is relatively new. Perhaps 5 percent of all cancers appear to follow a familial pattern; in the great majority, however, inheritance seems to play little or no part. Nevertheless, many cancers, like other diseases that show features of multifactorial inheritance (see Chapter 15), have a significant genetic component in that certain people are more susceptible to developing a particular malignancy as a result of genetic defects that predispose to cancer. Furthermore, it has become apparent that essentially all cancer—even in the absence of any apparent inherited component—is the result of mutations in somatic cells and that its progression also involves the expression of a series of genes.

In the past, viruses and exposure to environmental agents such as ionizing radiation were blamed for most cancers. It is now recognized that the underlying cause is gene mutation and that when carcinogenic agents are involved, they operate by causing mutation. The mutations that lead to cancer affect genes responsible for cell proliferation, cell development, and other fundamental cellular activities. When normal regulation is al-

365

tered, uncontrolled growth is initiated and a malignant tumor develops.

The understanding of the genetic basis of cancer that has begun to emerge after many decades of investigation has come about largely through the application of molecular genetics to the analysis of various forms of malignant disease. As so often happens in medical genetics, the abnormal has provided insight into the normal: learning what goes wrong in cancer has also helped to clarify the genetic control of many aspects of normal cell growth.

The field of cancer genetics is one of the fastest moving in biology and medicine today, and our understanding of cancer mechanisms is increasing rapidly. Although much remains to be learned, the outlines of a unifying hypothesis are beginning to emerge. In this chapter we consider the current state of knowledge of the genetic basis of cancer, including the role of specific genes in causing both inherited and sporadic cancers.

The Clonal Nature of Cancer

There is strong evidence that a tumor is a clone of cells derived from a single ancestral cell in which the initiating event (a somatic mutation) has taken place. The clonal nature of tumors has been recognized for many years. The original evidence came from the study of tumors in women heterozygous for the X-linked enzyme glucose-6-phosphate dehydrogenase (G6PD). As previously discussed, because of X inactivation, only one of a pair of X-linked alleles in a female heterozygote is expressed in a somatic cell. Cell lines derived from tumors in these women expressed one or the other G6PD allele but not both, indicating that each tumor had grown from a single cell. The characteristic chromosomal rearrangements in many types of cancer, such as the translocations seen in Burkitt lymphoma and in chronic myelogenous leukemia (to be described later), also indicate that these malignancies are of single-cell origin.

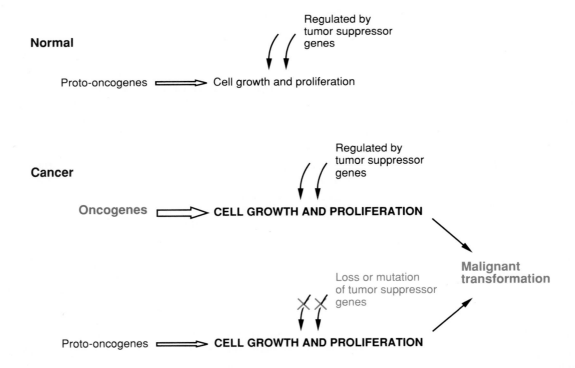

Figure 16–1. General scheme for mechanisms of oncogenesis by proto-oncogene activation and mutation or loss of tumor suppressor genes. Cell growth and proliferation is stimulated by the products of proto-oncogenes and is under the negative control of tumor-suppressor genes that prevent overgrowth. Action of oncogenes is dominant and requires only a single mutation, leading to uncontrolled cell growth. Action of tumor-suppressor genes is recessive; when both alleles are mutated or lost, cell growth is unregulated and leads to tumor formation. See text for discussion.

TWO KINDS OF CANCER GENES

Genes that cause cancer are of two distinct types: **oncogenes** and **tumor-suppressor genes.** The two types have opposite effects in carcinogenesis. Oncogenes facilitate malignant transformation, whereas tumor-suppressor genes, as the name implies, block tumor development by regulating genes involved in cell growth (Fig. 16–1).

Oncogenes

Oncogenes are genes that affect normal cell growth and development. If an oncogene is altered or overexpressed, either as a result of a mutation in the gene itself or by altered external control, the cell in which the change occurred can undergo uncontrolled growth, eventually becoming malignant. Most oncogenes are mutated ("activated") forms of normal genes, called **proto-oncogenes,** that are involved in the control of cell proliferation and differentiation (Miller et al., 1990).

Oncogenes can be identified experimentally in DNA transfer studies by their ability to transform a nontumorigenic mouse cell line in culture to generate foci of cells with tumorigenic properties. To date, more than 50 human oncogenes (and

thus their normal proto-oncogenes) have been identified, largely on the basis of DNA transfection studies with genomic DNA from human tumors. Examples of some of these oncogenes are given in Table 16–1.

It is noteworthy that many (but not all) of the oncogenes identified in human tumors have turned out to be related to viral oncogenes previously isolated from RNA tumor viruses. The demonstration that genetic information from a virus could change a normal cell into a malignant one established that genes could act as central controllers of malignant conversion. RNA viruses known as **retroviruses** have the unique property of transcribing RNA into DNA, using the enzyme reverse transcriptase. The viral DNA can then be integrated into the chromosomal DNA of the host and expressed. When the so-called *src* oncogene (transforming sequences from the Rous sarcoma virus) was characterized, it was found to be not a true viral gene but a host gene that had been picked up by an ancestor of the virus through a process termed **transduction.** The equivalent host gene was the first proto-oncogene to be recognized; now, as mentioned before, it is recognized that many proto-oncogenes are related to specific RNA tumor viruses (Table 16–1). (Unlike the oncogenes of retroviruses, the oncogenes of DNA tumor viruses, such as Simian virus 40 [SV40] and

Table 16–1. Selected Examples of Oncogenes

Oncogene	Source	Map Location of Proto-Oncogene	Biochemical Property
Signal Transduction Proteins			
abl	Abelson murine leukemia virus	9q34	Protein kinase
src	Rous sarcoma virus (chicken)	20q12–13	Protein kinase
trk	Human colon carcinoma	1q32	Protein kinase
H-*ras*	Harvey rat sarcoma virus	11p15.5	GTPase
N-*ras*	Various human tumors (neuroblastomas)	1p13	GTPase
Nuclear DNA-Binding Proteins			
myc	Chicken sarcoma	8q24	Binds DNA
N-*myc*	Human neuroblastoma	2p24	Unknown
Secreted Growth Factors			
sis	Simian sarcoma virus	22q12.3–13.1	β-chain of platelet-derived growth factor (PDGF)
Growth Factor Cell Surface Receptors			
erbA	Avian erythroblastosis	17q21–22	Steroid receptor

Based on Park M, Van de Woude GF (1989) Oncogenes: Genes associated with neoplastic disease. *In* Scriver CR, Beaudet AL, Sly WS, Valle D (eds). The metabolic basis of inherited disease, 6th ed. McGraw-Hill, New York, pp. 251–276.

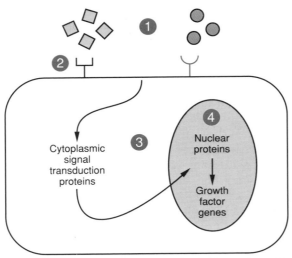

Figure 16–2. Signal transduction and growth regulation by products of proto-oncogenes, classified by their location and function in the cell. Deregulation of a proto-oncogene can lead to malignant transformation. 1. Secreted growth factors, such as EGF (embryonic growth factor) and PDGF (platelet-derived growth factor). 2. Specific receptors for the secreted growth factors. 3. Cytoplasmic signal transduction proteins such as *ras, src,* and *abl,* which are protein kinases and GTP-binding proteins. 4. Nuclear proteins such as *myc* interact with genes by DNA binding.

polyoma virus, are not transduced proto-oncogenes but are viral genes.) Proto-oncogenes have remained highly conserved in evolution; for example, the proto-oncogene H—*ras* (so named because it was originally identified in the Harvey rat sarcoma virus) and its corresponding protein have been found in organisms as far apart in the evolutionary scale as humans and yeast, suggesting that these proteins have essential biological roles. The various roles of several classes of proto-oncogene in growth regulation are illustrated in Figure 16–2.

Proto-Oncogene Activation

An important early finding related to proto-oncogenes came from the molecular analysis of a *ras* oncogene derived from a bladder carcinoma cell line. The oncogene and its counterpart proto-oncogene differed in only a single base pair. The alteration, a **point mutation** in a somatic cell of the tumor, led to synthesis of an abnormal gene product, which was able to stimulate the growth of the cell line, changing it into a tumor. Oncogenes have a dominant effect at the cellular level; that is, when activated, a single mutant allele is sufficient to change the phenotype of a cell from normal to malignant. *Ras* point mutations are observed in many tumors, and the *ras* genes have been shown experimentally to be the target of known carcinogens, a finding that supports a role for mutated *ras* genes in the development of many cancers.

Structural mutation is only one of several mechanisms that can induce activation of proto-oncogenes (Table 16–2). **Chromosomal translocations** are a common mechanism for proto-oncogene activation in a variety of cancers (Table 16–3). In chronic myelogenous leukemia (CML), which is discussed in more detail later, increased expression and malignant transformation are related to the translocation of the *abl* proto-oncogene from its normal position on chromosome 9 to the breakpoint in chromosome 22 in a hematopoietic stem cell. The 9;22 translocation directly contributes to the development of the malignant phenotype and is also a strong diagnostic indicator of CML, as other characteristic translocations are in other specific types of cancer (Table 16–3).

Cytogenetic changes are hallmarks of cancer and are much more common in later and more malignant or invasive stages than in earlier stages of tumor development (Mitelman, 1988). So far,

Table 16–2. Mechanisms of Activation of Proto-Oncogenes

Mechanism	Type of Gene Activated	Result
Regulatory mutation	Growth factor genes	Increased expression or secretion
Structural mutation	Growth factor receptors, signal transducing proteins	Allows autonomy of expression
Translocation, retroviral insertion, gene amplification	Nuclear oncogenes	Overexpression

From Miller DM, Blume S, Borst M, et al. (1990) Oncogenes, malignant transformation, and modern medicine. Am J Med Sci 300: 59–69.

Table 16–3. Characteristic Chromosome Translocations in
Selected Human Malignancies

Neoplasm	Chromosome Translocation	% of Cases	Proto-Oncogene Affected
Burkitt lymphoma	t(8;14)(q24;q32)	80%	*myc*
	t(8;22)(q24;q11)	15%	
	t(2;8)(q11;q24)	5%	
Chronic myelogenous leukemia	t(9;22)(q34;q11)	90%–95%	BCR-*abl*
Acute lymphocytic leukemia	t(9;22)(q34;q11)	10%–15%	BCR-*abl*
Acute lymphoblastic leukemia	t(1;19)(q23;p13)		*prl* homeobox gene
Acute promyelocytic leukemia	t(15;17)(q22;q11)		retinoic acid receptor
Chronic lymphocytic leukemia	t(11;14)(q13;q32)	10%–30%	*bcl-1*
Follicular lymphoma	t(14;18)(q32;q21)		*bcl-2*

Based on Croce (1987); Park and Van de Woude (1989); Nourse et al. (1990); Borrow et al. (1990).

most of the cytogenetic studies of tumor progression have been concerned with leukemias. In CML, for example, at the blast crisis stage, there may be several additional cytogenetic abnormalities, including numerical or structural changes, such as a second copy of the 9;22 translocation chromosome or an isochromosome for 17q. In advanced stages of other forms of leukemia, translocations are common. A focus of cancer research is the cytogenetic and molecular definition of these abnormalities, many of which are already known to be related to proto-oncogenes and presumably allow enhanced proto-oncogene expression (see discussion later in this chapter; Mitelman and Heim, 1988).

Another important mechanism for overexpression is **gene amplification,** a process that is rare or nonexistent in normal cells but sometimes common in cancer cells. Amplified segments of DNA are often detected as two types of cytogenetic change, **double minutes** (very small accessory chromosomes) and **homogeneously staining regions** (HSRs), that do not band normally and contain multiple, amplified copies of a particular DNA segment. How and why double minutes and HSRs occur is poorly understood, but amplified regions are known to include extra copies of proto-oncogenes with effects on cell growth. For example, the N-*myc* proto-oncogene is amplified

up to 200 times in 40 percent of neuroblastomas. The phenomenon is thought to be related to tumor progression.

Requirement for More Than One Activated Gene. An important aspect of the initiation and promotion of carcinogenesis by activated proto-oncogenes is that mutation of a single gene alone seems unable to achieve transformation; rather, separate genes with complementary effects seem to be required. Although the details of the experiments demonstrating that normal cells require cooperation between different activated oncogenes in order to undergo transformation are not described here, the conclusion is an important one: malignant transformation is a multi-event process, not to be achieved by a single step.

Tumor-Suppressor Genes

Whereas the products of proto-oncogenes promote growth, the products of tumor-suppressor genes normally block abnormal growth and malignant transformation, and contribute to malignancy only when the function of both alleles is lost. In other words, in contrast to mutations in proto-oncogenes, which are dominant in their action, mutations in tumor-suppressor genes are recessive (Fig. 16–1).

The Two-Hit Origin of Cancer

The existence of recessive mutations leading to cancer was originally suggested in the 1960s by DeMars. He made the prescient suggestion that some forms of cancer might be initiated when a cell in a person heterozygous for a recessive germ-line mutation undergoes a second, somatic mutation, thus rendering the cell homozygous, giving rise to a tumor. This "two-hit" hypothesis was expanded by Knudson (1971), who proposed that forms of cancer such as **retinoblastoma,** which occur in both hereditary and sporadic forms, could be explained on the basis that in the hereditary form the first mutation is carried in the germline, whereas in the sporadic form both mutations are somatic, occurring in the same somatic cell. The normal genes are now known as tumor-suppressor genes, which play regulatory roles in cell proliferation, differentiation, and other basic cellular functions. Inactivation of tumor-suppressor genes by mutation or some other mechanism leads to loss of regulation and therefore is oncogenic (Fig. 16–1).

Tumor-Suppressor Genes in Many Forms of Cancer

As described in detail later, tumor-suppressor genes have been implicated in several Mendelian forms of cancer, including retinoblastoma; Wilms tumor; familial polyposis coli; neurofibromatosis, type 1; and the rare form of familial cancer known as Li-Fraumeni syndrome. Although in each of these disorders autosomal dominant inheritance is either the rule or at least seen in a proportion of cases, loss or alteration of *both* copies of the responsible tumor-suppressor gene is required for tumor development. The explanation of this seeming paradox is that a single functional copy of a tumor-suppressor gene is enough to provide a normal cellular phenotype; however, a cell in which one copy is already altered or lost, by either germline or somatic mutation, will lose its ability to suppress tumor development if by chance it acquires a somatic mutation at the remaining allele. Because tumors are clonal by nature, this event can cause a tumor even if it happens in only one of the numerous cells of a tissue.

The significance of tumor-suppressor genes is not limited to autosomal dominant forms of cancer. As described later, tumor-suppressor genes are also involved in the progression of several common, nonheritable forms of cancer, such as colorectal cancer.

Tumor Progression by Clonal Evolution

The scheme just outlined, whereby the development of malignancy requires only the activation of a proto-oncogene or loss of function of both alleles of a tumor-suppressor gene, is grossly oversimplified. Instead, tumor formation is a multistep process involving a succession of genetic changes in the evolving tumor cell population.

One of the surprising findings about tumor progression is that loss or inactivation of the same gene may contribute to the development of several different common cancers. For example, the p53 gene on the short arm of chromosome 17 is missing or abnormal in cells of sporadic lung and breast cancers. The retinoblastoma gene is missing or defective in nearly all cases of small-cell carcinoma of the lung and in many other cases of lung cancer, but not in cancers such as colon cancer. Although the full picture of secondary genetic changes and their role in tumor progression is not yet clear, it is already obvious that several mutations at different loci are required if a tumor is to reach its full malignant potential.

The products of several tumor-suppressor genes have been isolated (Table 16–4). Because tumor-suppressor genes and their products are by nature protective against cancer, it is hoped that their understanding will eventually lead to improved methods of anticancer therapy.

Tumor-Suppressor Genes in Colon Cancer

Figure 16–3 shows the stepwise series of genetic changes proposed to take place in the development of a common malignancy, **colon cancer,** as it evolves from the normal phenotype through adenoma and carcinoma to metastasis. The initial change, even in the common nonheritable form of colon cancer, which affects more than 150,000 individuals per year in the United States alone, involves alteration in a gene on chromosome 5, which may be the same tumor-suppressor gene

Table 16–4. Products of Selected Tumor-Suppressor Genes

Tumor-Suppressor Gene	Gene Product and Possible Functions	Disorders in Which Gene Affected	
		Familial	*Sporadic*
RB1	p110, cell cycle regulation	Retinoblastoma	Small-cell lung carcinomas; lung cancers
WT1	zinc finger protein, DNA binding	Wilms tumor	Lung cancer
TP53	p53, cell cycle regulation	Li-Fraumeni syndrome	Lung cancer; breast cancer
NF1	GTPase activating protein	Neurofibromatosis, type 1	Unknown
DCC	Protein involved in cell-surface interactions	Unknown	Colorectal cancer

that is mutated in the rare familial forms of colon cancer, familial polyposis coli and Gardner syndrome (see later section). The gene on chromosome 5 that is mutated in colorectal cancers, called MCC (for "mutated in colon cancer"), has been cloned and somatic mutations have been identified in tumors from three individuals with sporadic colorectal carcinoma (Kinzler et al., 1991). MCC is thus a candidate for the putative tumor-suppressor gene responsible for the first event in initiation of colon cancer (Fig. 16–3). Several subsequent changes also involve loss of other chromosomes or chromosomal segments, which presumably indicates loss of a tumor-suppressor allele from those chromosomes.

One of these tumor suppressors, from chromosome 18q21, is mutated or missing in more than 70 percent of cases of colorectal carcinoma (Fearon et al., 1990). Because this gene, called DCC (for "deleted in colon cancer"), is only one of several mutations that must accumulate before a colon cell becomes cancerous, attempts to identify the precancerous state should have important health consequences. At-risk individuals identified on the basis of loss or mutation of the MCC or

DCC genes could then be monitored closely. In addition, early detection of colon cancer should allow successful surgical intervention in a greater proportion of cases.

FAMILIAL CANCER

Many forms of cancer have a higher incidence in relatives of patients than in the general population, and, as mentioned earlier, some show Mendelian inheritance. Familial cancers, whether Mendelian or not, tend to be specific in terms of site, tissue involved, and histological characteristics of the tumor. Extensive epidemiological studies have shown an increased incidence of non-Mendelian forms of cancer, in the 2 percent range, in first-degree relatives of probands. It is also known that some families have an above-average risk of cancer, whereas other families have a below-average risk. In many studies it is impossible to know whether the altered risk level results from genetic or environmental factors; in either case, however, a family history of cancer in a first-

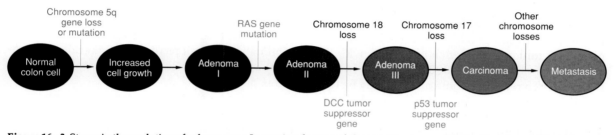

Figure 16–3. Stages in the evolution of colon cancer. Increasing degrees of abnormality are associated with sequential loss of tumor suppressor genes from several chromosomes, and activation of the *ras* proto-oncogene. The order of events is usually but not always as shown here. (Based on Stanbridge EA [1990] Identifying tumor suppressor genes in human colorectal cancer. Science 247:12–13.)

degree or second-degree relative of a patient should arouse the physician's suspicion.

Although individuals genetically predisposed to cancer represent probably less than 5 percent of all cancer patients, the genetic basis for their disease has great significance. The familial cases of cancer provide strong confirmation that germline, as well as somatic, mutations can contribute to cancer. The significance of this observation can be best appreciated in light of the information presented in the previous section. If a series of 5 to 10 mutations is required for a malignancy to develop (Fig. 16–3), an inherited mutation at any one of the critical genes would be expected to have a dramatic impact on the predisposition of carriers to cancer, and could account for a substantial portion of all cancers, including the vast majority that are not recognized as "familial" (Ponder, 1990). In addition, the familial cases of cancer provide the best opportunity to identify and isolate the genes mutated in the common cancers.

Mendelian Forms of Cancer

There are more than 50 Mendelian disorders in which the risk of cancer is very high, in some cases close to 100 percent, and other cancers that are only rarely inherited even though they result from a defect in a single pair of alleles. Some (and perhaps many) forms of cancer occur in both heritable and sporadic forms. A striking feature of heritable cancer is that there may be multiple primary tumors, whereas in sporadic cancer the occurrence of more than one primary tumor is rare. The Mendelian disorders discussed in this section have been particularly helpful in understanding the origin of cancer.

Retinoblastoma

Retinoblastoma, the prototype of diseases caused by mutation in tumor-suppressor genes, is a rare malignant tumor of the retina in infants, with an incidence of about 1 in 20,000 births (Fig. 16–4). Diagnosis of a retinoblastoma must usually be followed by removal of the affected eye, although smaller tumors, diagnosed at an early stage, can be treated by local therapy so that vision can be preserved.

About 40 percent of cases of retinoblastoma are of the heritable form, in which the child in-

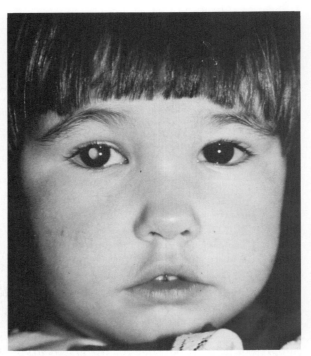

Figure 16–4. Retinoblastoma in a young girl, showing as a white reflex in the affected eye when light reflects directly off the tumor surface. (Photograph courtesy of B. L. Gallie, The Hospital for Sick Children, Toronto.)

herits one mutant allele at the retinoblastoma locus (RB1) through the germline, and a somatic mutation in a single retinal cell has caused loss of function of the remaining normal allele, thus initiating development of the tumor (Fig. 16–5). There are often multiple tumors, and both eyes are usually affected. The disorder is inherited as a dominant trait, since the likelihood of a somatic mutation occurring in at least one of the more than 10^6 retinoblasts is extremely high, and thus heterozygotes for the disorder are likely to be affected. Nevertheless, the penetrance of retinoblastoma, although high, is not complete, since the occurrence of the second mutation is a matter of chance. Nonmalignant lesions of the retina (called retinomas) are present in the eyes of some relatives of index patients.

The other 60 percent of cases of retinoblastoma are nonheritable (sporadic); in these cases both RB1 alleles in a single retinal cell have been inactivated by somatic mutation. Because this is a rare event, there is usually only a single tumor (the retinoblastoma is unilateral), and the average

Mendelian   **Sporadic**

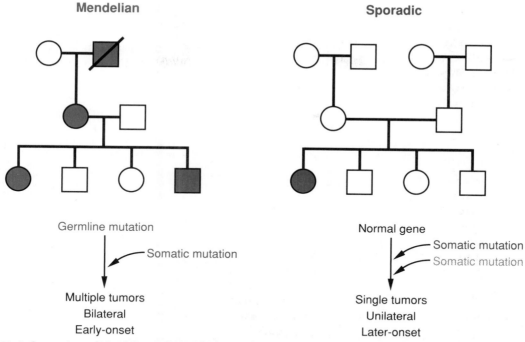

Figure 16-5. Comparison of Mendelian and sporadic forms of cancers such as retinoblastoma, the WAGR syndrome, and familial polyposis of the colon. Mechanisms of somatic mutation are presented in Figure 16-6. See text of discussion.

onset age is later than in infants with the heritable form (Fig. 16-5). For genetic counseling, an important further point is that 15 percent of patients with unilateral retinoblastoma have the heritable type but by chance develop a tumor in only one eye.

Infants with heritable retinoblastoma have a greatly increased (400-fold) risk of developing mesenchymal tumors such as osteogenic sarcomas, fibrosarcomas, and melanomas in early adult life. The risk is much higher if the child has received radiation therapy. The relative risk of developing leukemia, however, is not increased.

The RB1 gene has been mapped to chromosome 13, in band 13q14. The inherited mutation in a few percent of retinoblastoma patients is due to deletion or translocation of this portion of chromosome 13, a finding that was instrumental in assigning the RB1 gene to this location. Such chromosomal changes, if they involve adjacent DNA segments, may lead to dysmorphic features in addition to retinoblastoma. Other chromosome abnormalities, such as an isochromosome of chromosome 6p, are found only in retinoblastoma tumors and not in other patient tissues.

The RB1 gene is expressed in many tissues other than retina, although it initiates tumors only in the retina and a small number of secondary sites (leading to osteogenic sarcoma, fibrosarcoma, and melanoma). As noted earlier, the gene product, described as p110 RB1 (a protein 110 kilodaltons in size), is also absent or mutant in a number of cell lines derived from certain other tumors during their progression (Table 16-4).

Loss of Heterozygosity. Analysis of DNA polymorphisms in the region close to the RB1 locus in tumors from both heritable and sporadic retinoblastoma patients led to an unusual but highly significant genetic discovery. Whereas individuals from whom the tumors were taken were heterozygous at many loci, the tumors were *homozygous* at the same loci. Thus the tumor DNA samples contained alleles from only one of the two chromosome 13 homologs, revealing a loss of heterozygosity for stretches of 13q in the region of the gene. In familial cases, the retained chromosome 13 is the one inherited from the affected parent—that is, the one with the abnormal RB1 allele. Loss of heterozygosity may occur by structural deletion, but there are other mechanisms, such as mitotic

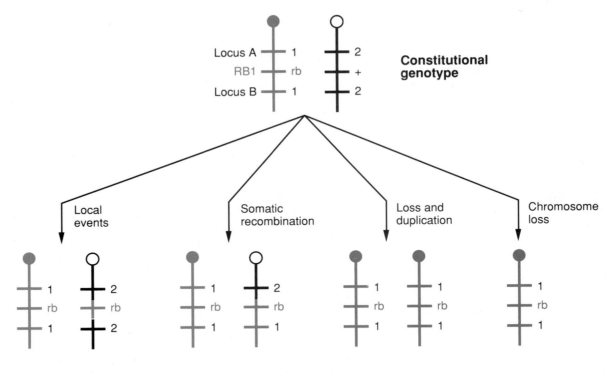

Figure 16-6. Chromosomal mechanisms that could lead to loss of heterozygosity for DNA markers at or near a tumor-suppressor gene in an individual heterozygous for a germline mutation, illustrated in the case of the retinoblastoma gene on chromosome 13q.

recombination or nondisjunction (Fig. 16-6). It is the most common mutational mechanism by which the remaining normal RB1 allele is lost in heterozygotes. Loss of heterozygosity is also a feature of Wilms tumor, as well as a number of other tumors, both heritable and sporadic, and is often considered evidence for the existence of a tumor-suppressor gene (Table 16-5).

Wilms Tumor

Wilms tumor, an embryonic kidney tumor, is in some ways analogous to retinoblastoma in that it is a Mendelian disorder involving a tumor-suppressor gene, although it is less commonly observed in a heritable form. It is sometimes associated with a cytogenetically visible aberration at 11p13, and if

Table 16-5. Examples of Chromosomal Regions That Show Loss of Heterozygosity in Tumors

Chromosomal Region	Disorder(s)	Associated Tumor-Suppressor Gene
1q	Breast carcinoma	Unknown
3p	Small-cell lung carcinoma	Unknown
5q	Familial polyposis coli; colorectal carcinoma	MCC
11p	Wilms tumor; rhabdomyosarcoma	WT1
13q	Retinoblastoma; breast carcinoma; osteosarcomas	RB1
17p	Colorectal carcinoma; breast cancer	TP53
18q	Colorectal carcinoma	DCC
22	Neurofibromatosis, type 2	Unknown

Adapted from Sager (1989) and Weinberg (1990), with updates.

so it forms part of the **WAGR syndrome** (high risk of **W**ilms tumor, **a**niridia, **g**enitourinary anomalies, and mental **r**etardation), a contiguous gene syndrome involving a series of genes that map to this region. Loss of heterozygosity is a feature of the syndrome.

A gene encoding a zinc finger protein has been cloned from the 11p13 region missing in Wilms tumor patients and is likely to be the affected locus in at least some cases (Call et al., 1990; Huang et al., 1990). However, this may not be the only gene predisposing to Wilms tumor, because there are multiple genes expressed in the kidney from this region of chromosome 11 and because in some Wilms tumor families the predisposing locus maps to 11p15, and in others, the map position is unknown.

Familial Polyposis Coli

Colon cancer is one of the most common forms of cancer, accounting for about 15 percent of all cancer; as mentioned previously, a small proportion of colon cancer cases are due to autosomal dominant conditions such as familial polyposis coli or Gardner syndrome.

Familial polyposis coli (also known as familial adenomatous polyposis) is relatively common, with an incidence of about 1 in 10,000. In heterozygotes, numerous polyps, which themselves are benign growths, develop in the colon during the first two decades of life. In almost all cases, one or more of the polyps become malignant. Surgical removal of the colon (colectomy) prevents the development of malignancy. Because this disorder is autosomal dominant, relatives of affected persons must be examined periodically by colonoscopy. The responsible gene has been located on chromosome 5q, both by genetic linkage studies in affected families (as described in Chapter 8) and by demonstration of loss of heterozygosity in colon tumors. As with other mapped Mendelian disorders, linkage studies can now be used to identify the genetically susceptible family members. One candidate for the gene responsible for familial polyposis coli is the MCC gene from chromosome 5q21 that is mutated somatically in at least some sporadic colorectal carcinomas.

There are several other genetic forms of colon cancer, at least one of which, Gardner syndrome, is determined by a gene that maps to the same region of chromosome 5q and is probably allelic to the gene predisposing to familial polyposis coli. Patients with Gardner syndrome have additional anomalies, including osteomas of the jaw, and desmoids, which are tumors arising in the muscle of the abdominal wall.

Neurofibromatosis Type 1 (NF1)

As introduced in Chapter 4, NF1 is a relatively common autosomal dominant disorder that primarily affects the peripheral nervous system and is often characterized by large numbers of neurofibromas. Although these growths are benign, a minority of NF1 patients also show an increased incidence of malignancy. The abnormal cell growth observed in NF1 suggests that the normal gene may function in the regulation of cell growth in nerve tissue.

The NF1 gene was mapped to the proximal long arm of chromosome 17 by family linkage studies and was subsequently cloned by application of several of the positional cloning strategies presented in Chapter 8. Analysis of individual meiotic crossovers in family studies, as well as discovery of de novo translocations involving this region of chromosome 17 in two NF1 patients, refined the localization of the gene to 17q11.2. Detailed long-range mapping and cloning eventually led to isolation of a large gene that was interrupted by the two translocation breakpoints (Wallace et al., 1990; Viskochil et al., 1990). In addition, several single nucleotide substitutions were discovered in NF1 patients, thus establishing the identity of the gene and its involvement in NF1 (Cawthon et al., 1990).

Inspection of the sequence of the NF1 gene and its protein product demonstrated significant homology to proteins that activate the GTPase activity of the *ras* oncogene product (Fig. 16–2). This finding strongly suggests that the normal NF1 product interacts with *ras* to regulate growth-stimulating activity in normal cells. The mutant NF1 gene, then, may fail to regulate growth in the normal cells from which neurofibromas are derived, leading to inappropriate growth and tumor formation (Xu et al., 1990).

This model suggests that NF1 is a tumor-suppressor gene. By analogy with other domi-

nantly inherited tumor-suppressor gene mutations, loss or inactivation of the remaining normal
allele at the NF1 locus would be required to explain growth of either neurofibromas or other
solid tumors in NF1 patients. Alternatively, it may
be that multiple mutations in other genes have
additive effects and stimulate unregulated cell
growth, as seen in the clonal progression of colon
cancer (Fig. 16–3).

Li-Fraumeni Syndrome

There are rare "cancer families" in which there is a
striking history of a *variety* of forms of cancer (including several kinds of sarcoma, breast cancer,
and other neoplasms), affecting a number of family members at an unusually early age, in an autosomal dominant pedigree pattern (Fig. 16–7; Li,
1988). This highly variable phenotype is known as
the Li-Fraumeni syndrome (LFS). Because the
tumor-suppressor gene p53 is inactivated in the
sporadic forms of many of the cancers found in
LFS, p53 was considered a candidate for the gene

defective in LFS. DNA analysis of several LFS
families has now confirmed this hypothesis; affected members in LFS families carry a mutant
form of the p53 gene as a germline mutation (Malkin et al., 1990). Thus LFS is an extreme form of a
group of cancers that occur in both a sporadic and
a familial form; as seen also in retinoblastoma, in
the familial form one of the two mutations necessary to inactivate the p53 gene is present in the
germline, but in the sporadic form both mutations
are somatic events.

Familial Breast Cancer

Breast cancer has long been recognized to have a
strong genetic component. Population-based epi-
demological studies have shown that up to 10 percent of all women in North America will develop
breast cancer in their lifetime. Furthermore, a
woman's risk of developing breast cancer is increased up to threefold if one first-degree relative
is affected and up to tenfold if more than one first-

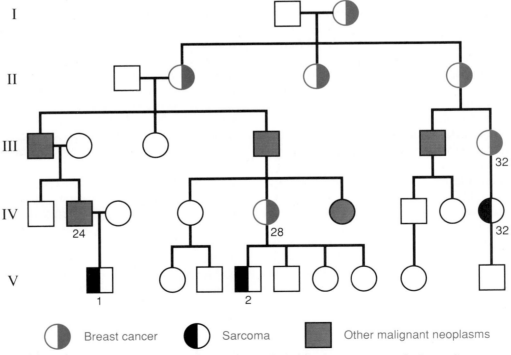

Figure 16-7. A pedigree of the Li-Fraumeni syndrome, in which breast cancer, sarcomas, and other malignant tumors have occurred. Ages at diagnosis are shown. (Redrawn from Li FP [1988] Cancer families: Human models of susceptibility to neoplasia — the Richard and Hinda Rosenthal Foundation award lecture. Cancer Res 48:5381–5386.)

degree relative is affected. These familial risks are increased even more if the onset of disease in the proband is at 40 years of age or less (Claus et al., 1990). Although as much as 20 percent of all breast cancer cases may have a significant genetic component as part of a polygenic or multifactorial mode of inheritance (see Chapter 15), a small proportion of cases appear to be due to a dominantly inherited Mendelian predisposition to breast cancer. These families share characteristic features of familial (as opposed to sporadic) cancer: multiple affected women, earlier age of onset, frequent bilateral disease, and an increased incidence of breast cancer in males.

Population studies have indicated that 2 to 5 percent of cases of breast cancer are due to inheritance of a major susceptibility gene (Claus et al., 1991). Genetic linkage studies in families with early-onset familial breast cancer have localized a dominant gene for increased susceptibility to breast cancer to the long arm of chromosome 17 (Hall et al., 1990). This susceptibility allele has an estimated frequency of .003. Thus the frequency of carrier females can be estimated to be nearly 1 percent. These studies also indicated that susceptibility to breast cancer is genetically heterogeneous; one or more other genes must be involved in later-onset familial breast cancer, since these families did *not* show linkage to the locus on chromosome 17q. Presymptomatic detection of women at risk for developing breast cancer as a result of any of these susceptibility genes is an important aim of current research, both in familial cases and in the larger number of sporadic cases.

Comparison of breast tumor tissue with normal tissue from the same women has shown loss of heterozygosity from a number of chromosomal regions, including 1p, 3p, 11p, 13q, 16q, and 17p, suggesting that there may be a number of genes important for breast tumor progression. Although the gene on chromosome 17p is likely the p53 tumor-suppressor gene shown to be defective in Li-Fraumeni syndrome, the other genes have not been identified.

Chromosome Instability Syndromes

The four rare autosomal recessive chromosome instability syndromes mentioned in Chapter 9 — **ataxia telangiectasia, Fanconi anemia, Bloom syndrome,** and **xeroderma pigmentosum** — are all associated with an increased risk of malignancy, particularly leukemia (see Table 9–7). The combination of chromosome breakage, susceptibility to chromosome damage by X-irradiation or ultraviolet light and certain chemical agents, and susceptibility to malignancy seen in these syndromes is not fully explained because the products of the various genes concerned have not been completely defined. One important conclusion to be drawn from the study of patients with chromosome breakage syndromes is that there is extensive variation in inborn resistance to damage to DNA by environmental agents. Clinically, radiography must be used with extreme caution if at all in ataxia telangiectasia, Fanconi anemia, and Bloom syndrome. Furthermore, prolonged exposure to sunlight must be avoided in xeroderma pigmentosum.

The genes that are defective in the chromosome instability syndromes may be viewed as cancer genes. Chromosome instability is a hallmark of cancer. The enzymes defective in these syndromes must be intimately involved in DNA repair and the maintenance of chromosome integrity. The genes for two of these defects (two forms of xeroderma pigmentosum) have been isolated. However, the precise involvement of the predicted gene products in DNA repair is still unknown.

Heterozygotes for these disorders may also be at an increased risk of malignancy. Relatives of ataxia telangiectasia homozygotes appear to have an increased risk of breast cancer; up to 7.5 percent of all breast cancer in young women may occur in ataxia telangiectasia heterozygotes (Swift et al., 1987). Thus cloning of the ataxia telangiectasia gene or genes (one of which has been mapped by family linkage studies to chromosome 11q; see Chapter 8) may allow preclinical identification of a class of individuals with a dramatic genetic predisposition to at least one of the common cancers.

CANCER CYTOGENETICS

Chromosome Translocations and Oncogenesis

A striking finding that unites the cytogenetics and molecular genetics of cancer is that in some instances, a proto-oncogene is activated by a chromosome translocation (Table 16–3). Two well-known examples, which were the first two in which the translocation breakpoints were cloned, are the translocation between chromosomes 8 and 14 in Burkitt lymphoma and the translocation between chromosomes 9 and 22 that is seen in chronic myelogenous leukemia.

Burkitt Lymphoma

Burkitt lymphoma is a B-cell tumor of the jaw that has an unusual geographical distribution: it is the most common tumor of children in equatorial Africa but is rare elsewhere. In most tumors of this type, the *myc* proto-oncogene is translocated from its normal chromosomal position at 8q24 to a position distal to the immunoglobulin heavy-chain locus at 14q32. Cytogenetically, this is seen as an apparently balanced 8;14 translocation. The exact mechanism by which the translocation allows activation of the *myc* gene and initiates the tumor is still not completely understood. The translocation presumably juxtaposes enhancer or other transcriptional activating sequences, normally associated with the immunoglobulin gene, near the *myc* gene. Supporting this hypothesis is the finding that other translocations observed in a smaller proportion of Burkitt lymphoma cases also involve immunoglobulin light-chain genes on chromosomes 22 or 2 (Table 16–3). Whatever the mechanism, these translocations clearly have an important effect on the *myc* gene, allowing its unregulated expression.

Chronic Myelogenous Leukemia (CML)

Originally, the cytogenetic abnormality observed in CML was described as a deletion of the long arm of chromosome 22, which is characteristic of the malignant cells of almost all patients with CML. After chromosome banding came into use, this so-called Philadelphia chromosome (Ph[1]) was identified by Rowley (1973) as the product of a translocation between chromosomes 9 and 22, the segment missing from chromosome 22 being translocated to chromosome 9 rather than deleted (Fig. 16–8). The translocation moves the proto-oncogene *abl* from its normal position on chromosome 9q to the "breakpoint cluster region" (BCR), a gene of unknown function on chromosome 22q. The juxtaposition of BCR sequences and *abl* sequences

allows the synthesis of a chimeric protein that is longer than the normal abl protein and has increased tyrosine kinase activity. Although the function of the normal abl and BCR proteins is not yet clear, the chimeric gene is assumed to change the expression and function of the abl protein in the malignant hematopoietic cells. Indeed, when a retroviral construct containing the chimeric gene was introduced into the bone marrow of healthy mice (by methods described in Chapter 13), the infected mice developed hematologic malignancies, including CML; this result suggests that the Philadelphia chromosome itself causes the malignancy (Daley et al., 1990).

Heritable Fragile Sites and Oncogenes

There are at least 17 sites on human chromosomes at which there is an inherited predisposition to breakage. Ten of these sites are at or near regions involved in chromosome aberrations in leukemias or lymphomas (acute nonlymphocytic leukemia and non-Hodgkin lymphoma), and some of the ten are at or near the sites of proto-oncogenes. So far, however, these observations are curiosities, and the possible association of hereditary fragile sites with predisposition to cancer remains unproved.

CANCER AND THE ENVIRONMENT

The risk of cancer shows significant variation among different populations and in the same population in different environments. For example, gastric cancer is almost three times as common among Japanese in Japan as among Japanese living in Hawaii or Los Angeles. Thus it seems that a considerable proportion of the risk must depend on exposure to carcinogens in the environment. The nature of environmental carcinogens, assessment of the additional risk associated with exposure, and ways of protecting the population from such hazards are matters of strong public concern.

The theme of this chapter is that cancer is a genetic disease, but there is no contradiction in considering the role of environment in carcinogenesis. Environmental agents act as mutagens that cause somatic mutations; the somatic mutations, in turn, are responsible for carcinogenesis.

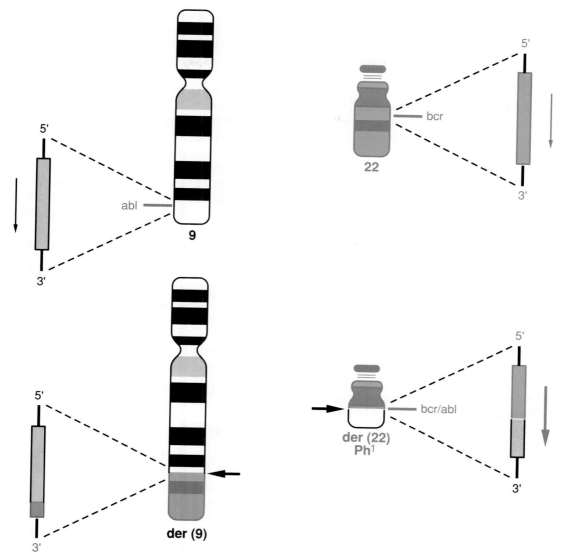

Figure 16–8. The Philadelphia chromosome translocation, t(9q34;22q11). The Philadelphia chromosome (Ph¹) is the derivative chromosome 22, which has exchanged part of its long arm for a segment of material from chromosome 9q that contains the *abl* oncogene. Formation of the chimeric *bcr-abl* gene on the Ph¹ chromosome is the critical genetic event in the development of chronic myelogenous leukemia.

According to some estimates based chiefly on data from the aftermath of the atomic bombings of Hiroshima and Nagasaki, as much as 75 percent of the risk of cancer may be environmental in origin.

Radiation

Ionizing radiation is known to cause an increased risk of cancer. The data for survivors of the Hiroshima and Nagasaki atomic bombings, and other exposed populations, show that there is a long latency period, in the 5-year range for leukemia but up to 40 years for some tumors. The risk is age-dependent, being greatest for children under 10 years of age and for the elderly. As noted earlier, radiation is much more damaging to people with inborn defects of DNA repair than to the general population. Everyone is exposed to some degree of ionizing radiation through background radiation (which varies greatly from place to place), medical exposure, and nuclear energy. Unfortunately, there are still large areas of uncertainty about the magnitude of the effects of radiation, especially low-level radiation, on cancer risks.

Chemical Carcinogens

Interest in the carcinogenic effect of chemicals dates back at least to the 18th century, when the high incidence of scrotal cancer in young chimney sweeps was noticed. Today there is concern about many possible chemical carcinogens, especially components of the diet, industrial carcinogens, and toxic wastes. Documentation of the risk of exposure is often difficult, but the level of concern is such that all clinicians should have a working knowledge of the subject and be able to distinguish between well-established facts and areas of uncertainty and debate.

A class of drug-metabolizing enzymes, encoded by the family of **cytochrome P450** genes (of which there are dozens and perhaps even hundreds in the human genome), are responsible for the detoxification of foreign chemicals. A number of the cytochrome P450 genes are polymorphic and underlie variation in drug metabolism (see discussion of pharmacogenetics in Chapter 12). One well-studied genetic polymorphism has been associated with susceptibility to lung cancer. The cytochrome P450 enzyme **aryl hydrocarbon hydroxylase** (AHH) is an inducible protein involved in the metabolism of polycyclic hydrocarbons, such as those found in cigarette smoke. AHH converts hydrocarbons into an epoxide form that is more easily excreted by the body but that happens to be carcinogenic. The extent of hydrocarbon metabolism is genetically controlled and shows polymorphic variation in the normal population. People who carry a "high-inducibility" allele, particularly those who are smokers, appear to be at an increased risk of lung cancer. Data indicate that cigarette smoke itself induces the CYP1A1 gene (which is responsible for AHH activity), even in normal lung tissue in people with high activity (McLemore et al., 1990). On the other hand, homozygotes for the recessive "low-inducibility" allele appear to be less likely to develop lung cancer, possibly because their AHH is less effective at converting the hydrocarbons to highly reactive carcinogens.

A second cytochrome P450 enzyme polymorphism, controlling the ability to metabolize the compound debrisoquin (a beta-adrenergic blocking agent), has also been associated with an increased susceptibility to lung cancer. A small proportion of people are "poor metabolizers" of debrisoquin and are homozygous for a recessive allele at the CYP2D6 cytochrome P450 gene on chromosome 22. These people appear to be more resistant to the potential carcinogenic effects of cigarette smoke or occupational lung carcinogens (such as asbestos or polycyclic aromatic hydrocarbons). "Extensive metabolizers" (homozygotes for a fully functional CYP2D6 allele) have a fourfold greater risk for lung cancer than do "poor metabolizers." This risk increases to eighteenfold among people exposed routinely to lung carcinogens (Caporaso et al., 1989). A similar association has been reported for bladder cancer.

Although the precise genetic and biochemical basis for the apparent differences in cancer susceptibility within the normal population remains to be determined, these associations could have significant public health consequences and may point eventually to a way of identifying people who are genetically predisposed to developing cancer.

CONCLUSION

Cancer is a genetic disorder in which the normal control of cell growth is lost. The basic mechanism in all cancers is mutation, either in the germline or, much more frequently, in somatic cells. Much remains to be learned about the genetic processes of carcinogenesis and about the environmental factors that can alter DNA and thus lead to malignancy. It is likely that new insights into the fundamental role of DNA changes in carcinogenesis will lead in the near future to improved and more specific ways of prevention and treatment of malignant disease.

General References

Bishop JM (1987) The molecular genetics of cancer. Science 235:308–311.
Marx J (1989) Many gene changes found in cancer. Science 24:1386–1388.
Knudson AG (1986) Genetics of human cancer. Ann Rev Genet 20:231–251.

Miller DM, Blume S, Borst M, et al (1990) Oncogenes, malignant transformation, and modern medicine. Am J Med Sci 300:59–69.

Mitelman F (1988) Catalogue of chromosome aberrations in cancer, 3rd ed. AR Liss, New York.

Nowell PC (1990) Cytogenetics of tumor progression. Cancer 65:2172–2177.

Ponder B (1988) Gene losses in human tumors. Nature 335: 400–402.

Ponder B (1990) Inherited predisposition to cancer. Trends Genet 6:213–218.

Rowley JD (1990) The Philadelphia chromosome translocation: A paradigm for understanding leukemia. Cancer 65:2178–2184.

Sager R (1990) Tumor suppressor genes: the puzzle and the promise. Science 246: 1406–1412.

Weinberg RA (1990) The genetic basis of cancer. Arch Surg 125:257–260.

Problems

1. A patient with retinoblastoma has a single tumor in one eye; the other eye is free of tumors. What steps would you take to try to determine whether this was sporadic or heritable retinoblastoma? What genetic counseling would you provide? What information should the parents have before a subsequent pregnancy?

2. Discuss possible reasons why colorectal cancer is an adult cancer, whereas retinoblastoma affects children.

3. Many tumor types are characterized by the presence of an isochromosome for the long arm of chromosome 17. Provide an explanation for this finding.

4. Many children with Fanconi anemia have limb defects. If an affected child requires surgery for the abnormal limb, what special considerations arise?

5. In some children with the mutant RB1 gene, nonmalignant retinomas appear in the eye. Explain why.

6. Wanda, whose sister has premenopausal bilateral breast cancer, has a greater risk of developing breast cancer herself (30 to 50 percent) than does Wilma, whose sister has premenopausal breast cancer in only one breast (10 to 15 percent). Both Wanda and Wilma, however, have a greater risk than does Winnie, who has a completely negative family history (about 5 percent). Considering the information in this chapter and in Chapter 15, provide an explanation for these empiric risk figures.

CHAPTER 17

GENETIC ASPECTS OF DEVELOPMENT

A central question of biology today is the nature of the regulation of gene expression that allows a fertilized ovum to develop into a mature organism. Genes differ in their expression both in time and in space. The early stages of development are concerned with the establishment and differentiation of the morphological structures of the body. Despite its clinical relevance and the extensive descriptive information available about the morphology of the human embryo (Moore, 1988), knowledge of the genes that control the process is still sparse. For many practical and ethical reasons, research on human embryos is limited, and almost all our information about these processes has come from studies in other organisms, most often the fruit fly *Drosophila*. Many of the genetic manipulations used with *Drosophila* have now become possible with the mouse, raising the prospect of rapid progress and new insights in the genetic analysis of mammalian development.

Not infrequently, the process of human development goes wrong. The most abnormal embryos and fetuses, of course, are not born alive but are aborted spontaneously at some stage between

fertilization and viability. Still, a significant proportion of pregnancies end with the birth of a child with some congenital anomaly or are selectively terminated because an anomaly has been identified in the fetus. The identification and delineation of syndromes of congenital abnormalities constitutes the field of **dysmorphology,** one of the most rapidly advancing specialties within clinical genetics.

This chapter is not intended to cover all aspects of human development, for which the reader is referred to textbooks listed in the General References at the end of the chapter. Rather, we briefly outline some directions in research on the molecular genetics of development that may ultimately lead to identification of the genes critical to human development and maldevelopment. We also review the biology of twinning and twins, a topic that is important both to the theme of early human development and to research into the relative roles of nature and nurture in normal development and genetic disease. Finally, we return to the topic of congenital anomalies, some of which have already been discussed in other contexts.

MOLECULAR GENETICS OF MAMMALIAN DEVELOPMENT

Early Stages of Mammalian Development

In the mouse and, by extension, in other mammals, the major events of very early development are the specification of cell lineage, segmentation, and regional specialization along the body axis.

A **cell lineage** is a clone of cells derived by sequential mitoses from a single original cell. An entire cell lineage, of course, extends from the fertilized egg to the differentiated adult form, but within it there are many distinct lineages of cells committed to a particular pathway of development. The expression of developmental control genes within some cell lineages has been analyzed in the mouse by molecular approaches. In the human, there is little direct information, but the evolutionary conservation of developmental control genes (Fig. 17–1) indicates that the same or very similar patterns of expression exist.

In the mouse embryo, during the preimplantation stage, two distinct extraembryonic cell lineages have been defined within the trophoblast: the trophoectoderm, which gives rise to the fetal components of the placenta, and the primitive endoderm, which gives rise to the endoderm layers of the yolk sac. At this stage the primitive ectoderm or inner cell mass, a group of centrally located cells that give rise to the fetus itself, remains undiffer-

entiated. Although in the mouse the extraembryonic lineages have been well characterized in terms of their origin and fate, it has been more difficult to analyze the developing embryo, and much less is known about the definition of cell lineages that occurs within it.

After implantation, additional cell lineages within the embryo are defined, and the embryo begins to undergo morphogenesis along its anteroposterior axis. In the human embryo, gastrulation (the process of converting the inner cell mass into an embryo with three primary germ layers) is completed in the third week. The anteroposterior axis is established within the primitive ectoderm by the formation of the primitive streak at the caudal end of the embryo. The neural tube is formed by the fusion of paired neural folds (see Fig. 15–4), and some cells of the crests of each neural fold separate and form the neural crest. The neural crest cells migrate into the future head and neck region, where they give rise to pigment cells, the branchial apparatus, and other structures. Meanwhile segmentation begins, with the appearance of paired mesodermal somites on each side of the developing neural tube.

In the anterior region of the neural tube itself, segmental structures called neuromeres appear. Studies in the chick embryo have shown that in the hindbrain, the neuromeres (known as rhombomeres in this region) define the later segmental arrangement of neurons and their axons. The rhombomeres derive from cell lineages analogous

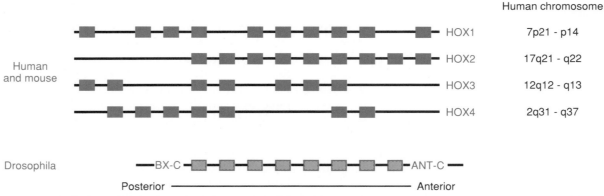

Figure 17–1. Schematic of the homeobox gene clusters in *Drosophila* and the mouse and human genomes. Both the mouse and human genomes contain these four clusters of homeobox genes. In both *Drosophila* and mammals (at least murine Hox-2), there is strict colinearity between the gene order on the chromosome and the sequence in which the genes are expressed; genes at the 5′ end (left) of the cluster are expressed in the posterior part of the nervous system and those at the 3′ end are expressed anteriorly. The molecular organization of the homeobox genes is still incompletely characterized, and the nomenclature is subject to change. (Sources: Graham et al., 1989; Kessel and Gruss, 1990; McKusick, 1990.)

to the "compartments" seen in developing insects: clones of cells derived from a few original cells programmed to express specific developmental genes (Fraser et al., 1990). Regional specialization proceeds down the body axis of the embryo, in both segmental and non-segmental tissue. Some of the genes that regulate this process have been characterized, and their functions defined.

Developmental Control Genes

The search for genes that control mammalian embryogenesis makes use of several approaches. In the most common strategy, putative developmental genes are sought on the basis of homologies to genes known to regulate development in *Drosophila*, mice, or other experimental organisms (Table 17–1). Only one family of developmental control genes is described here: the **homeobox genes,** so named because **homeotic mutations** in *Drosophila*, which change the identity of body segments, occur in genes that share a characteristic sequence, the homeobox.

Homeobox Genes

All homeobox genes contain a region (the homeobox) that encodes a 60 amino acid DNA-binding domain. Homeobox-containing proteins regulate gene action in development or act as tissue-specific transcription factors. Homeobox genes were first recognized as the sites of mutations in developmental mutants of *Drosophila*. The *Drosophila* mutation *Antennapedia*, which allows a second leg to develop in place of an antenna, is the prototype of homeotic mutations.

The majority of known homeobox genes of the mouse and humans are organized in four gene clusters on different chromosomes, each composed of a series of linked genes (Fig. 17–1). Presumably they have evolved, like the globin genes, by repeated gene duplication and divergence. As shown, this arrangement of genes is very similar to the sequence of linked genes found in *Drosophila*, strengthening the impression that the homeobox genes in humans, like their counterparts in the fruit fly, are critical for normal development.

Many homeobox genes begin to be transcribed in early gastrulation and continue to be expressed through midgestation in segmented tissues. Most are expressed in the central nervous system; many are also expressed in somites and their derivatives, and some are expressed in limb buds and elsewhere. At least in the HOX2 cluster (Fig. 17–1), and possibly in the others, the domain of expression of any one homeobox gene correlates with its chromosomal location, each successive gene being expressed in a zone with a boundary closer to the anterior end of the developing embryo.

The W Locus

The series of alleles at the W locus in the mouse has been intensively studied as a model of a genetically controlled developmental system and provides an example of a developmental problem due to mutation in a proto-oncogene. Mutations at this locus, in mice with homozygous or compound genotypes, produce animals deficient in the proliferation and differentiation of hematopoietic stem cells, primordial germ cells, and melanoblasts. The normal allele at this locus, the *c-kit* proto-oncogene, codes for a plasma membrane tyrosine kinase receptor, one of a family of genes that includes the receptor for platelet-derived growth factor (Chabot et al., 1988).

Transgenic Mice in Developmental Genetics

Transgenic mice, in which a segment of DNA (usually a single gene) from a different organism has been introduced into the germline, are widely used in the study of the complex processes of developmental genetics. Transgenic mice can be generated by direct microinjection of multiple copies of a specific cloned gene into the male pronucleus of a fertilized ovum (Fig. 17–2). The fertilized eggs

Table 17–1. Examples of Developmental Control Genes

Gene	Example
Genes containing homeoboxes	HOX1,2,3,4 clusters (see text)
Zinc-finger protein genes	ZFY (see Chapter 10)
Genes for growth factors and their receptors	Insulinlike growth factor II (see text)
Retinoic acid receptors	See text
Proto-oncogenes	W locus (see text)

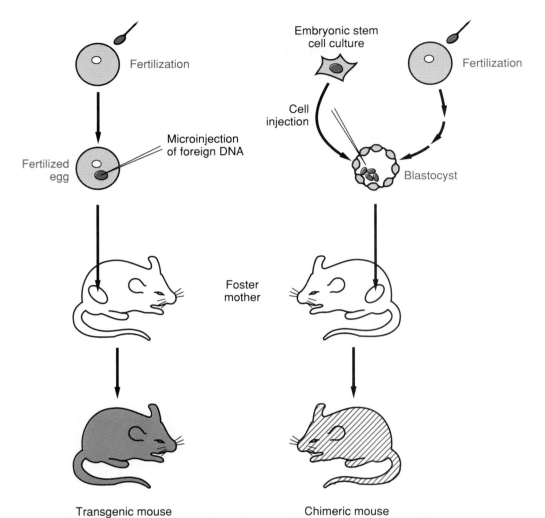

Figure 17–2. Methods for producing transgenic or chimeric mice for developmental studies. Left: DNA is directly microinjected into the male pronucleus of a fertilized ovum. The injected egg can then be surgically implanted into the oviduct of a pseudopregnant foster mother. A proportion of the offspring will be transgenic, containing the transferred DNA in all cells. Right: In a different scheme, the genome of pluripotent cells in culture can be altered by DNA transfer experiments, after which cells containing the new gene can be introduced into blastocysts. The mosaic blastocysts are then transferred to the uterus of a foster mother, which results in the birth of chimeric mice containing both normal and altered cells.

are then surgically implanted into the oviduct of a foster mother to continue development. In a small percentage of the offspring, the injected gene is incorporated into random locations in the recipient's genome, and at least some of these genes can be expressed, as shown by the presence of the gene product in somatic cells. Offspring of the original generation of transgenic mice can also express the transgenes if the genes were incorporated into the germline. The transgenic mouse system provides a

way of systematically evaluating the effects of different gene mutations on early development. Many human genes have been expressed in transgenic mice, where they can be analyzed for their expression in an in vivo context that is far more amenable to study and manipulation than is the human organism.

Figure 17–3 demonstrates the results of a classic experiment in which the gene for human growth hormone (ordinarily expressed only in the anterior pituitary gland) was combined with the promoter of the metallothionein gene and used to make transgenic mice, which, because of the broad specificity of the promoter, expressed the gene in many tissues and grew to giant size.

Another use of transgenic mice is to create mouse models of human genetic disease by experimentally disrupting a normal copy of a mouse gene in vitro and then injecting cells containing the newly mutated gene into host blastocysts (Fig. 17–2). Chimeric mice made in this way can then be directly examined to view the effects on early development of a particular gene mutation. A direct demonstration of the effect of a growth-factor gene on embryonic growth comes from an experiment in which the gene for insulin-like growth factor II was disrupted experimentally in this

manner. After construction of chimeric mice carrying the mutation, heterozygous progeny expressed a dominant form of marked growth deficiency (Fig. 17–4) but were otherwise normal (De Chiara et al., 1990).

NEW REPRODUCTIVE TECHNOLOGIES: IN VITRO FERTILIZATION AND EMBRYO TRANSFER

Beginning with the birth of the first "test tube baby" in 1978, fertilization of human ova in vitro and implantation to allow the fertilized ova to continue development have been widely used, with other reproductive technologies, as a means

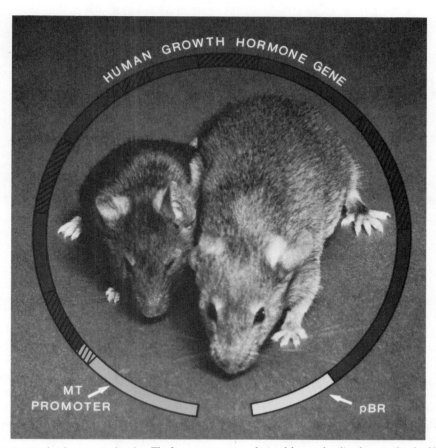

Figure 17–3. Gene expression in transgenic mice. The larger mouse was derived from a fertilized ovum that had been microinjected with human growth hormone (GH) genes fused to the promoter of the mouse metallothionein (MT) gene, so that growth hormone was overproduced. (Photograph courtesy of R. L. Brinster and R. E. Hammer, School of Veterinary Medicine, University of Pennsylvania, based on research described in Palmiter et al., 1983.)

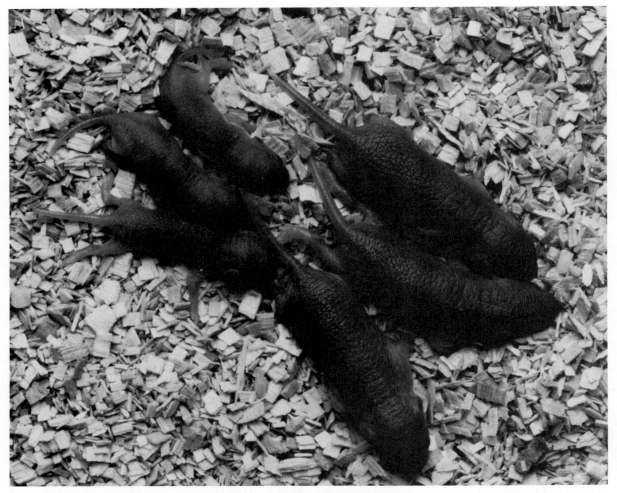

Figure 17–4. The smaller mice were derived from a transgenic mouse experiment in which the normal murine insulin-like growth factor II gene was experimentally mutated. Heterozygous mutant transgenic mice express a dominantly inherited growth deficiency. (Photograph courtesy of A. Efstratiadis, Columbia University, based on research described in DeChiara et al., 1990.)

of allowing infertile couples to have children. The procedure also opens another possibility, that of characterizing or even manipulating the zygote before implantation.

Preimplantation Diagnosis

With currently available techniques of micromanipulation and DNA amplification, a zygote known to be at risk for a specific genetic disorder could theoretically be diagnosed even before implantation. Molecular analysis of the DNA in a single cell with the polymerase chain reaction could be used to examine a specific gene known to con-

tain a particular mutation in the family being studied.

One practical application of this technology has already been made. Sex can be determined from a single cell, taken from a six- to eight-cell embryo and analyzed by DNA amplification of sequences from the Y chromosome, without killing the embryo; this procedure has already been used to identify female embryos for transfer, in cases in which a male would be at risk for a serious X-linked disorder (Handyside et al., 1990). Preimplantation diagnosis, when perfected, could become an option for many families at risk for genetic defects.

TWINS AND OTHER MULTIPLE BIRTHS

In human beings, twinning is an unusual event of early development. There are two types of twins, **monozygotic** (MZ) and **dizygotic** (DZ), or, in common terms, identical and fraternal. For a particular trait, a twin pair may be concordant (alike) or discordant (different). Comparison of concordance rate in MZ and DZ twins is a standard method used in medical genetics for comparison of the effects of genes and environment. If MZ pairs are not completely concordant for a given trait, genetic factors alone cannot account for the trait.

Comparison of concordance rates in MZ and DZ twins is used to measure the "heritability" of complex traits (see Chapter 15). Other types of twin comparisons can also be useful in the assessment of the role of genetics in determining certain characteristics. For example, the difference between the members of MZ pairs in response to some environmental factor can be compared with differences between unrelated persons (see discussion of twin study of response to overfeeding in Chapter 15).

Twins raised together or apart (that is, within the same or different environments) have been studied to analyze the relative effects of heredity and environment in the causation of a number of complex human traits.

Monozygotic Twins

MZ twins arise from a single zygote that divides into two separate embryos at an early stage, within the first 8 days after fertilization and perhaps as early as 3 days in some cases. The incidence of MZ twinning is much the same in all populations, about 1 in 260 births, and there is probably no familial tendency to MZ twinning. MZ twins are always of the same sex and have identical genetic markers, but are not necessarily phenotypically identical in all respects.

MZ twins may sometimes be discordant for a variety of congenital defects and genetic disorders, despite their origin from a single zygote. In addition to environmental differences and chance variation, the following reasons for discordance are recognized:

1. Mechanisms of embryological development, such as vascular abnormalities, that can lead to discordance for malformations.

2. Postzygotic changes such as somatic mutation leading to discordance for cancer, or somatic rearrangement of immunoglobulin or T-cell receptor genes.

3. Chromosome abnormalities originating in one zygote after the twinning event.

4. Uneven X inactivation between female MZ twins, with the result that one twin preferentially expresses the paternal X, the other the maternal X.

An important example of uneven X inactivation is the expression of Duchenne muscular dystrophy in twins heterozygous for this X-linked mutation. There have been several pairs of female MZ twins in which one was a manifesting carrier of DMD and the other, although also a carrier, did not show any manifestations of the mutant gene. Other X-linked disorders that have been found to be expressed in only one of a pair of female MZ twins include hemophilia A, glucose-6-phosphate dehydrogenase deficiency, and color blindness. The alternative situation, in which both members of the pair are manifesting or both are nonmanifesting, has not been reported (Richards et al., 1990).

Apart from their clinical significance, MZ twins discordant for X-linked disorders may help clarify the timing in early development of both MZ twinning and X inactivation. The discordant expression suggests that X inactivation precedes the twinning process, at least in discordant female MZ pairs if not in all female MZ pairs.

Malformations in Monozygotic Twins

For reasons that are not clear, the malformation rate is high in twins and is generally believed to be about twice as high in MZ as in DZ twins. About two thirds of all MZ twins have a single chorion with common circulation (Table 17–2). This allows vascular shunts between the twins, which may have serious consequences, including disruption of developing organs. Deformations (discussed later) due to constraint in the uterus are also seen.

Table 17–2. Frequency of Types of Placentas and Fetal Membranes in Twins

| Zygosity | Single Chorion | | Two Chorions | |
	Single Amnion	*Two Amnions*	*Single Placenta**	*Two Placentas*
MZ	Rare	65%	25%	10%
DZ	—	—	40%	60%

* Results from secondary fusion.

Dizygotic Twins

DZ twins result from the fertilization of two ova, shed in the same menstrual cycle, by separate sperm. They are as closely related as other sib pairs and may be either of the same sex or of different sexes.

The incidence of DZ twinning shows considerable variation, being about 1 in 500 in Asians, 1 in 125 in Caucasians, and as high as 1 in 20 in some African populations. The rate may be related to the maternal level of pituitary follicle-stimulating hormone (FSH). Unlike MZ twinning, which seems to be a chance event, a tendency to DZ twinning is familial, with a recurrence risk in families that is about triple the general population risk. Increasing maternal age and parity also slightly increase the chance of DZ twinning.

Genetically, the tendency to multiple ovulation that accounts for DZ twins can be viewed as an inherited trait expressed only in females; in other words, a twin pregnancy is something caused by the mother's physiology rather than the twins'. A female DZ twin has an increased risk of twin offspring, but her male co-twin does not, although his daughters do (White and Wyshak, 1964).

Higher multiple births (triplets, quadruplets, and so forth) may be identical sets, fraternal sets, or a mixture of both types. The use of ovulatory agents such as clomiphene citrate has increased the frequency of multiple ovulation, and there has been a corresponding increase in the frequency of twins and higher order multiple births. All the members of such sets, of course, originate from different zygotes.

Diagnosis of Twin Zygosity

It is often useful, for genetic prognosis in a twin of a patient with a genetic disease, for research pur-

poses, or even just to gratify normal curiosity, to know the zygosity of a twin pair. This information is essential if a medical procedure such as a life-saving bone marrow transplant depends on the diagnosis. Twin zygosity used to be determined by examination of fetal membranes at the time of birth (Table 17–2) or by painstaking comparison of genetic markers and dermatoglyphics. Today, however, molecular diagnosis is the method of choice because any two individuals who are *not* MZ twins are virtually certain to show differences in some of the large number of DNA markers that can be tested (see Fig. 6–10).

Limitations of Twin Studies

Although the twin method has contributed to the analysis of many complex human traits that have otherwise been difficult to interpret genetically, it is not without limitations. The chief drawback is that although a twin study can give information about the strength of the genetic predisposition to a disorder, it gives no insight into the genes concerned, their pattern of inheritance, or their mode of action.

A second problem with the method is that although postnatal environmental differences are assumed to be the same for both types of twins, this may be an oversimplification. MZ twins, because of their similarity, may seek the same environment and develop along much the same path. DZ pairs, especially male-female pairs, probably have more different environments than do MZ pairs. Consequently, for many research projects it is more appropriate to compare same-sexed DZ pairs with their MZ counterparts.

Perhaps the most important limitation relates to bias of ascertainment. MZ twin pairs who are concordant for a disease draw more than their share of attention, whereas discordant MZ pairs or DZ pairs are less likely to be reported.

Curiosities

Conjoined Twins. Conjoined twins, who may present severe problems in management if they survive, are MZ twins in whom the division into two separate zygotes has been late and incomplete. The recurrence risk of this rare accident of development, which occurs in about 1 percent of all MZ twin births, is not increased above the population risk. In a twin pregnancy, ultrasonography can usually reassure the parents and obstetrician that the twins are not conjoined.

The Disappearing Twin. Because ultrasonographic examination has become a routine part of prenatal care, it has become apparent that twin pregnancy is more common than once thought and that early loss and resorption of one member of a twin pair is not unusual. Errors in prenatal diagnosis may arise if extraembryonic tissues from the lost twin are sampled for prenatal diagnosis. Disappearance of one member of a twin pair may be responsible for some otherwise confusing discrepancies between prenatal cytogenetic findings and the karyotype of the newborn.

DZ Twins With Different Fathers. Twins of this type are theoretically possible and their existence was actually confirmed by genetic markers at least once (Terasaki et al., 1978).

Heterokaryotypic Twins. MZ twins with different karyotypes have been reported, although they are rare. Examples include pairs discordant for Down syndrome and unlike-sexed pairs in which the female had a 45,X karyotype. These cases arise postzygotically and are akin to chromosomal mosaics, in whom there are at least two cell lines derived from a single zygote.

DYSMORPHOLOGY

Congenital anomalies represent a significant proportion of the clinically significant disorders seen in newborns and older children. In a major study of almost 70,000 infants, liveborn or stillborn, it was found that 2.3 percent had at least one major structural malformation (Nelson and Holmes, 1989). After birth, additional anomalies can be recognized; thus the incidence reaches about 6 percent in 2-year-olds and 8 percent in 5-year-olds.

Dysmorphology is the area of clinical genetics concerned with the diagnosis and interpretation of patterns of structural defects. The diagnosis of a malformation syndrome is made on the basis of the overall pattern of anomalies in a patient; however, problems in interpretation may arise because the characteristic abnormalities of any syndrome vary to some extent from patient to patient.

Dysmorphologists give very precise meanings to the terms that they use to describe defects (Spranger et al., 1982). An **anomaly** is a structural abnormality of any type. Four types of clinically significant anomalies are defined:

1. A **malformation** is a morphological defect resulting from an intrinsically abnormal developmental process. Many malformation syndromes have been mentioned in earlier chapters. Chromosome disorders are in this category, as are single-gene malformations such as achondroplasia and Marfan syndrome.

2. A **disruption** is a morphological defect resulting from breakdown of, or interference with, an originally normal developmental process. Examples include abnormalities resulting from amniotic bands (fibrous bands that may form between the fetus and amnion) or limb reduction defects caused by vascular anomalies.

3. A **deformation** is an abnormality in form or position of a body part caused by a nondisruptive mechanical force. Deformations may be due to mechanical constraint in the uterus or to defects (neurological, myopathic, or connective tissue defects, for example) in the fetus itself.

4. **Dysplasia** is an abnormal organization of cells into tissues and its morphological consequence. There are many examples, including ectodermal dysplasia, a group of disorders in which there is dysplasia of tissues derived from ectoderm (skin, teeth, nails hair, and exocrine and sebaceous glands).

Sometimes either a structural defect or a mechanical factor can lead to multiple secondary effects. The total picture is then termed a **sequence,** to distinguish it from a **syndrome,** in which the multiple anomalies are thought to be independent rather than sequential although they have a single basic cause. For example, if a fetus has renal agenesis or some other defect that reduces the quantity of urine formed, oligohydramnios (deficiency of amniotic fluid) can cause compression of the fetus, with the characteristic Potter facies, pulmonary hypoplasia, and defects of limb positioning. A similar sequence follows loss of amniotic fluid by leakage from the amnion.

Not all anomalies are clinically significant, but even minor ones can be important as indicators of some serious problems in morphogenesis, especially when several minor anomalies are seen in an infant. It is important to keep in mind, however, that morphological variation is common and that not all variants are anomalies.

At present we have little information about the role of developmental genes in dysmorphology, but as knowledge increases, our ability to interpret the characteristic constellations of abnormal features seen in dysmorphic syndromes should follow. As one example, a mutation causing vertebral malformations in the mouse has been traced to a point mutation in a developmental gene Pax-1; this suggests that the normal Pax-1 gene functions in the development of the spinal column (Balling et al., 1988).

TERATOGENS

A teratogen is any agent that can produce a malformation or raise the population incidence of a malformation. Most known teratogens are infectious agents, radiation, or drugs (Table 17–3).

Table 17–3. Selected Teratogenic Agents

Infections
Cytomegalovirus
Rubella
Toxoplasmosis

Maternal Disorders
Insulin-dependent diabetes mellitus
Phenylketonuria

Drugs
Alcohol
Anticonvulsants
Chemotherapeutic agents
Cocaine
Coumadin
Isotretinoin
Streptomycin
Tetracyclines
Thalidomide
Valproic acid

Ionizing Radiation

Note: This is not a complete list. Source: Shepard TH (1989) Catalog of teratologic agents, 6th ed. Johns Hopkins University Press, Baltimore.

Undoubtedly the most notorious teratogen is **thalidomide**, a drug that was used for a short period in the early 1960s as a tranquilizer and antiemetic in early pregnancy. Virtually all the mothers who received this drug at a "sensitive stage" of early pregnancy produced babies with some degree of phocomelia (literally, "seal limbs"). Thus it appears that susceptibility to the teratogenic effect of thalidomide is a common human trait that unfortunately is not shared by the experimental animals used to test the drug.

Thalidomide remains the only example in which the introduction of a drug led to a dramatic rise in the incidence of a specific type of malformation, and withdrawal of the drug was immediately followed by a nearly complete drop in the incidence of the malformation. Of the many other teratogens that have been examined, or suspected, in "epidemics" of malformations, none has been shown to have a definite cause-and-effect relationship with a given type of abnormality, or an effect on all fetuses exposed at a sensitive stage. Failure to demonstrate such a relationship, however, cannot be regarded as proof that no causal connection exists; consequently the general public and the medical profession remain highly concerned about the possible role of a wide variety of environmental factors in teratogenesis.

Retinoic acid, a biologically active form of vitamin A that is highly effective in the treatment of acne, is a known teratogen and appears to affect all exposed human fetuses. Many physicians refuse to prescribe retinoic acid to women of childbearing age who are sexually active and not using contraceptives. In the frog *Xenopus*, retinoic acid has been identified as a morphogen, an endogenous signal molecule that specifies the anteroposterior axis during limb development and may also specify the anteroposterior axis of the central nervous system (Durston, 1989). In the mouse, its action is similar to that of homeobox gene products in that it is able to act as a potential morphogen in the limb bud (Kessel and Gruss, 1990).

Factors in Teratogenicity

In the analysis of teratogenicity, four important factors are recognized:

1. **Time of exposure to the teratogen.** Teratogens exert their effect when differentiation and

morphogenesis are at their peak. In rubella embryopathy, in which a maternal rubella infection is transmitted to the embryo or fetus, the malformations produced at an early stage (before the 8th week of pregnancy) are much more severe than those produced after the 14th week.

2. **Dosage.** There is little information on dosage in human studies, but animal research has shown the expected dose-response relationship. The dose affecting the fetus is of course partly determined by the mother's ability to metabolize the toxic substance, which is in turn influenced by her own genotype. **Maternal diabetes** is associated with a pronounced increase in the risk of major malformations of the fetal cardiovascular system and central nervous system (Becerra et al., 1990). Infants of mothers with gestational diabetes who require insulin during the third trimester of pregnancy are also at increased risk. There appears to be a dose-response effect, in that the better the glycemic control during the first trimester of pregnancy, the lower the risk of birth defects.

3. **Genotype of the fetus.** There are many proven examples in experimental animals, and a number of suspected human examples, of genetic differences in response to a teratogen. The anticonvulsant medication **phenytoin** is teratogenic, inducing a syndrome of craniofacial anomalies, prenatal and postnatal growth retardation, mental retardation, and limb defects known as the **fetal hydantoin syndrome** (Fig. 17–5). About 5 to 10 percent of exposed infants have the full-blown syndrome, whereas about one third have some deleterious effects and more than half are unaffected. The teratogenicity is associated with an elevated level of oxidative metabolites that are normally eliminated by the enzyme epoxide hydrolase, which appears to be a polymorphic enzyme with low-activity and high-activity alleles. In one report, low activity was associated with fetal hydantoin syndrome, and high activity with normal findings (Buehler et al., 1990). If confirmed, these findings could lead to a method of detecting fetuses at risk of fetal hydantoin syndrome.

4. **Maternal genotype.** At present, the teratogenic effect of the maternal genotype to children exposed in utero has been little studied. Any such effect would result from the abnormal metabolic consequences of a maternal genetic defect. An example is the increased risk of microcephaly and

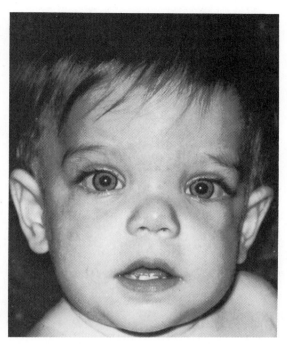

Figure 17–5. Fetal hydantoin syndrome, facial appearance. Note the low nasal bridge, small nose, hypertelorism, and bowed upper lip. Further details in text. (From Jones KL [1988] Smith's Recognizable patterns of human malformation, 4th ed. WB Saunders, Philadelphia.)

congenital heart defects in offspring of mothers with phenylketonuria (see Chapter 12).

Fetal Alcohol Syndrome

The damaging effects of alcohol on the developing fetus have been known for at least 20 years, and maternal alcohol consumption is recognized as perhaps *the* major cause of mental retardation. The consequences of alcohol exposure also include growth retardation both prenatally and postnatally, characteristic facies (Fig. 17–6), skeletal defects (including joint anomalies), and heart defects. There is an obvious dose-response effect; infants whose mothers drink more heavily have a more severe phenotype. Possible differences in risk related to genetic variation in alcohol metabolism have not been documented. Unlike those of other teratogens, the harmful effects of maternal alcohol ingestion are not restricted to a sensitive period of early pregnancy but extend throughout gestation.

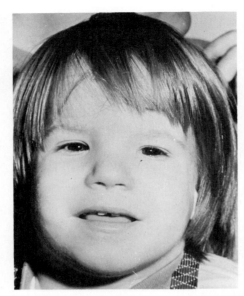

Figure 17–6. Fetal alcohol syndrome, facial features. Note the short palpebral fissures and mid-face hypoplasia. Further discussion in text. (From Jones KL [1988] Smith's Recognizable patterns of human malformation, 4th ed. WB Saunders, Philadelphia.)

CONCLUSION

Although developmental genetics is one of the most productive fields of molecular biology today and dysmorphology is one of the most rapidly advancing area in clinical genetics, there is still a great gap between what is known at the molecular level and what is seen clinically in the dysmorphic child. Bridging this gap and learning to interpret dysmorphic syndromes in terms of gene expression is one of the future challenges of medical genetics.

General References

Gorlin RJ, Cohen MM Jr, Levin LS (1990) Syndromes of the head and neck, 3rd ed. Oxford University Press, New York.
Graham JM Jr (1991) Smith's Recognizable patterns of human deformation, 2nd ed. WB Saunders, Philadelphia.
Jones KL (1988) Smith's Recognizable patterns of human malformation, 4th ed. WB Saunders, Philadelphia.
Kessel M, Gruss P (1990) Murine developmental control genes. Science 249:375–379.
MacGillivray I, Campbell DM, Thompson B (eds) (1988) Twinning and twins. John Wiley and Sons, Chichester.
Moore KL (1988) The developing human: Clinically oriented embryology, 4th ed. WB Saunders, Philadelphia.
Rossant J, Joyner AL (1989) Toward a molecular genetic analysis of mammalian development. Trends Genet 5:277–283.
Shepard TH (1989) Catalog of teratogenic agents, 6th ed. Johns Hopkins University Press, Baltimore.
Spranger J, Benirschke K, Hall JG, Lenz W, Lowry RB, Opitz JM, Pinsky L, Schwartzaden HG, Smith DW (1982) Errors of morphogenesis: Concepts and terms. Recommendations of an international working group. J Pediatr 100:160–165.

Problems

1. a) In a study of multiple sclerosis in twins, Ebers et al. found 70 twin pairs of which 27 were MZ, 20 were same-sex DZ, and 23 were male-female DZ. Overall, in the population studied, about 30 percent of twin pairs are MZ. Statistically, do these data suggest that ascertainment was biased or unbiased?

    b) Seven MZ pairs and one DZ pair were concordant for multiple sclerosis. What conclusion would you draw about the genetic basis of multiple sclerosis?

2. a) Suppose every family stopped reproduction after the birth of a son; what would be the effect on the sex ratio in the population?

    b) Suppose that sex selection became possible and 60 percent of newborn infants were male. What might the effects be on the birth rate in the next generation?

3. Are the following statements true or false? If true, what is the significance of the statement?

    _____ Homeobox genes have been strongly conserved in evolution.

    _____ Homeobox genes are found only in mammals.

    _____ A transgenic mouse is formed by fusion of genetically different embryos at an early developmental stage.

    _____ A proto-oncogene is a gene that directs the first step in oncogenesis.

    _____ Susceptibility to specific teratogens differs in different species.

    _____ There may be individual differences in sensitivity to specific teratogens.

    _____ Hydantoin causes birth defects in all fetuses exposed at a sensitive stage of early development.

    _____ When female MZ twins are heterozygous for an X-linked disorder, both twins are manifesting heterozygotes.

    _____ Many MZ twins have common placental circulation, but mixing of blood in DZ twins in utero is rare.

    _____ The recurrence risk for both kinds of twinning (MZ and DZ) is about 5 percent.

CHAPTER
18

GENETIC COUNSELING

Medical genetics is distinguished from other clinical specialties by its extension beyond the immediate patient to the family. When any clinical disorder is diagnosed, the affected person and family members often need help to understand and come to terms with the nature and consequences of the disorder and the means available to modify its consequences. If the disorder is heritable, there is an added dimension: the need to know the genetic risk and the means available to prevent its transmission. Genetic counseling, a core activity in medical genetics, is the process of providing such information. In this chapter, the general principles and procedures basic to genetic counseling are reviewed; the use of Bayesian statistical methodology and DNA analysis to refine estimates of the recurrence risk is described; and genetic screening, a public health activity in which genetic counseling plays a significant part, is discussed.

GENETIC COUNSELING IN CLINICAL GENETICS

Just as the unique feature of genetic disease is its tendency to recur within families, the unique aspect of genetic counseling is its focus, not just on the original patient, but also on members of the patient's family, both present and future. Genetic counseling may be provided by a physician as an integral part of clinical management, but as the body of genetic knowledge and the extent and sophistication of laboratory investigations have expanded, specialty genetics clinics have developed, and many physicians now prefer to refer patients with genetic disorders or family histories of genetic disorders to these clinics. The delivery of high-quality genetic services, both cognitive and laboratory based, is time consuming and labor intensive and thus expensive. However, the benefits to individual families, as well as the wider effects of genetic services on the reduction of genetic diseases in the population as a whole, can justify the costs.

Professional Responsibility in Genetic Counseling

The physician has a professional responsibility to ensure that genetic counseling is provided in appropriate cases and that it is accurate within currently accepted standards of practice. The responsibility, however, does not extend beyond the person seeking genetic advice (the **consultand**) to other family members; on the contrary, it is generally accepted that the consultand is entitled to confidentiality and that this confidentiality cannot be broken without the consultand's consent, regardless of the consequences for other at-risk family members. A quandary can arise when relatives at

395

high risk of a serious disease are not informed about the risk or possible ways of combating it, because the original consultand refuses consent. This is one of the serious ethical issues of medical genetics and one for which there is no easy solution.

The courts have upheld the principle of the physician's responsibility. In one legal case, the parents of a child with Down syndrome won a suit against their physician, claiming negligence because the mother had not been referred for prenatal diagnosis. In another case, parents who had been tested for carrier status with respect to Tay-Sachs disease were informed that they were both noncarriers (thus not at risk) but later had an affected child; the court upheld the claim of "wrongful life," a contention on behalf of the child that it should not have been allowed to be born.

From these and other examples, it is clear that in the United States and elsewhere, established standards of medical care require a physician to obtain a history that includes family and ethnic information, to advise parents of their genetic risks, and to offer prenatal diagnosis when indicated. Moreover, centralized quality control of the laboratories engaged in screening tests is expected.

Common Genetic Counseling Problems

Table 18–1 lists some of the most common problems that lead to genetic counseling. Often, the persons seeking genetic counseling are the parents of a child with one of the conditions listed, but the consultand may be an adult with an abnormality or a family history of an abnormality. Genetic counseling is an integral aspect of prenatal diag-

Table 18–1. Common Genetic Counseling Problems

Single-gene disorders, known or suspected
Multifactorial disorders, known or suspected
Chromosomal disorders, diagnosed in the consultand or a family member
An abnormal trait or carrier state, identified by genetic screening
Prenatal diagnosis for late maternal age or other causes
Consanguinity
Teratogen exposure
Repeated pregnancy loss or infertility

nosis (see Chapter 19). Typical problems encountered in genetic counseling have already been discussed in previous chapters in the context of the underlying genetic basis of the problem.

The Process of Genetic Counseling

As noted earlier, clinical genetics in comparison with other clinical fields requires extensive preparation and follow-up in addition to direct patient contact (Table 18–2). Typically, more than half the time required for a family referred for genetic services occurs before and after the clinic visit. Many precounseling and postcounseling functions, as well as a large part of the service provided at the clinic visit, are performed by nonphysician genetic counselors (as described later).

The stages defined in Table 18–2 are somewhat arbitrary; some families with genetic disorders are seen in genetics clinics repeatedly over a period of many years, even generations, for reassessment, whereas others appear for only a single appointment.

Determining Genetic Risks

The family member whose risk of a genetic disorder is to be determined is usually a first-degree relative of a proband, such as a subsequent sib of an affected child or a living or future child of an affected adult. In some families, especially for some autosomal dominant and X-linked traits, it may also be necessary to estimate the risk for more remote relatives. The risk may be easy to calculate if the condition is accurately diagnosed and the pattern of inheritance is known. On the other hand, it is not so easy to determine if questions of reduced penetrance or variability of expression must be considered or if new mutation occurs frequently at a particular locus. Laboratory tests that give equivocal results can add further complications.

When Mendelian risk figures are not available, reliance must be placed on empiric risk figures, which simply allow one to make an estimate on the basis of previous experience. This is all very well if there are good empiric risk figures and if the phenotype is not heterogeneous. However, when

Table 18–2. **Stages in Clinical Genetic Services**

Preassessment	Reason for referral
	Collection of family history information
	Clinical examination and laboratory tests of relatives if indicated
Clinical diagnosis and management	Consultand, possibly other family members
Recurrence risk estimation	Based on diagnosis, pedigree analysis, test results
Genetic counseling	Nature and consequences of disorder
	Recurrence risk
	Means of modification of consequences
	Means of prevention of recurrence (prenatal diagnosis and counseling)
Follow-up care	Referral to appropriate clinical specialists, health agencies, support groups, as required
	Continuing clinical assessment if indicated
	Continuing support by genetic counselor if indicated

a particular phenotype has an undetermined risk or can result from a variety of causes with different frequencies and with widely different risks, estimation of the recurrence risk is hazardous at best. In a later section, the estimation of recurrence risk in some typical clinical situations, both straightforward and more complicated, is considered.

Prevention of Recurrence

For many families seeking genetic counseling, one of the major goals is to prevent recurrence of the particular genetic disorder in question. Although prenatal diagnosis is one approach that can often be offered to families, it is by no means a universal solution to the risk of genetic problems in offspring. There are many disorders for which prenatal diagnosis is not feasible, and for many parents it is not acceptable even if available. Alternative measures available for prevention of recurrence include the following:

1. Genetic laboratory tests (karyotyping, biochemical analysis, or DNA analysis) will sometimes reassure couples with a family history of a genetic disorder that they themselves are not at increased risk of having a child with a specific genetic disease. In other cases such tests will indicate the need for preventive measures.

2. If the parents plan to have no children at all or any more children, *contraception* or *sterilization* may be their choice, and they may need information about the possible procedures or an appropriate referral.

3. For parents who want a child or more children, *adoption* is a possibility, but at present the number of children available for adoption does not meet the demand.

4. *Artificial insemination* may be appropriate if the father has a gene for an autosomal dominant or X-linked defect or has a heritable chromosome defect, but it is obviously not indicated if it is the mother who has such a defect. Artificial insemination is also useful if both parents are carriers of an autosomal recessive disorder. If it is used, genetic counseling and appropriate genetic tests of the sperm donor should be part of the process.

5. Use of the polymerase chain reaction allows DNA analysis of embryos in the preimplantation stage, even though this procedure is still experimental (see Chapter 17). For some parents, a decision not to implant an embryo found to be abnormal would be much more acceptable than abortion at a later stage.

If the parents decide to terminate a pregnancy, provision of information and support is an appropriate part of genetic counseling.

Psychological Aspects

Genetic disorders can lead to serious personal and family problems. Although this is also true of nongenetic disorders, the concern generated by knowledge that the condition might recur, the guilt felt by some individuals, and the need for reproductive decisions can give rise to severe distress. Many people have the strength to deal personally with such problems; they prefer receiving even bad news to remaining uninformed, and they make their own decisions on the basis of the most complete and accurate information they can obtain. Other people require much more support and may even need referral for psychotherapy. The psychological aspects of genetic counseling are beyond the scope of this book, but several books cited in the General References at the end of this chapter give an introduction to this important field.

Collaboration Between Genetics Centers

A striking feature of the development of genetic services has been the growth of a national and international network of collaboration. Although each disorder is rare, there are numerous different ones, and the research expertise to deal with any one of them tends to become clustered in one or a few genetics centers. Collaboration is a logical development, and sharing of experience improves the accuracy of genetic diagnosis and counseling.

Often the parents of a handicapped child are desperate to obtain help for the child and tend to look for that help outside their usual referral centers, often at great expense and not always from ethical sources. Obviously the parents are entitled to a second opinion, but the physician can sometimes prevent additional distress by pointing out that the medical community is worldwide and that there is rarely any advantage to be gained by self-referral to programs elsewhere.

Support Organizations

Organizations devoted to self-help are used by many families. These organizations, usually focused on a single disease or a group of diseases, can help those concerned to share their experience with others facing the same problem, to learn how to deal with the day-to-day problems caused by the disorder, to hear of new developments in therapy or prevention, and to promote research into the condition. Referral to support groups is often undertaken by genetics centers. A coalition known as the Alliance of Genetics Support Groups has

been formed to coordinate the activities of the many individual groups.

The Role and Training of Genetic Counselors

In genetics clinics, much time and effort must be expended on aspects that require specialized knowledge and skills other than clinical diagnosis and laboratory investigation. The qualified health professionals who perform these functions are usually known as **genetic counselors.** Programs designed to train genetic counselors for their role in the delivery of genetic services exist in several universities in North America and elsewhere, and genetic counseling has become recognized as a profession within the health sciences.

Typically, genetic counselors are graduates of a specialized program in medical genetics and counseling, usually of 2 years' duration and leading to a master's degree. In the United States, after satisfactorily completing the course, they are eligible to take the certification examination of the American Board of Medical Genetics.

Genetic counselors play an essential role in genetics clinics, participating in many aspects of the investigation and management of genetic problems. The genetic counselor is often the first point of contact with the clinic, provides genetic counseling directly to the consultands in many cases, and continues in a supportive role and as a source of information after the clinical investigation and formal counseling have been completed. Many genetic counselors engage in educational activities and research related to medical genetics. DNA analysis has opened a new field in which their special expertise can be applied because this novel and complex type of testing requires advanced knowledge of medical genetics and close liaison among referring physicians, DNA diagnostic laboratories, and the families themselves.

Currently, genetic counseling is evolving toward the status of a self-regulating health profession. In most areas, however, it has not yet achieved the legal status of licensure, which has been granted to some other health professions of longer standing, such as physiotherapy and clinical psychology. In a review of the state regulation of genetic counseling in the United States, Hochstetter and colleagues (1989) found that in at least one state, even the use of the term "counselor" is strictly controlled, under regulations that would not apply to most genetic counselors. There is obviously a need for improved recognition of the status of genetic counselors and definition of their role and legal responsibilities, in view of the essential part they play in the delivery of genetic services.

DETERMINING RECURRENCE RISKS

The estimation of recurrence risks is the central problem in genetic counseling. Ideally, it is based on knowledge of the genetic nature of the disorder in question and on the pedigree of the particular family being counseled. For most chromosomal disorders and for multifactorial traits, as discussed in previous chapters, recurrence risk estimates are empiric (Fig. 18–1). When a disorder is known to have single-gene inheritance, its recurrence risk for specific family members can usually be determined from the Mendelian principles discussed at length in Chapter 4 (Fig. 18–2). However, in particular circumstances, especially for those disorders that are characterized by a high frequency of new mutation, by a late age of onset, or by incomplete penetrance or variable expressivity, these calculations may be less than straightfor-

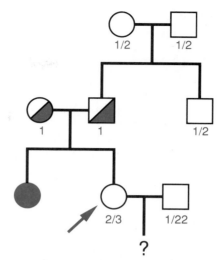

Figure 18–2. Mendelian risk estimates in genetic counseling. The consultand's sister is affected with an autosomal recessive condition, in this example cystic fibrosis (CF). The risk of other family members' being carriers can be determined through Mendelian principles and is indicated in the pedigree. The risk of the consultand's having an affected child is $2/3 \times 1/22 \times 1/4$, or less than 1 percent.

ward. Mendelian risk estimates can sometimes be modified by means of Bayesian analysis of the pedigree, which takes into account information about the family that may increase or decrease the prior Mendelian risk.

Bayesian Analysis in Risk Estimation

Bayes' theorem, first published in 1763, is a method of assessing the relative probability of two alternative possibilities, usually (in the context of genetic counseling) that an individual does or does not carry a particular allele. It has been widely applied in clinical decision making as well as in genetic pedigree analysis. Some examples of its use in pedigree analysis are examined in this section.

X-Linked Pedigrees

To illustrate the value of Bayesian analysis, consider the pedigrees shown in Figure 18–3. In Family A, the mother is an obligate carrier for hemophilia A, since her father was affected. Her risk of

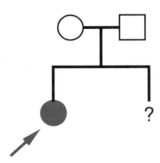

Figure 18–1. Empiric risk estimates in genetic counseling. A family with no other positive family history has one child affected with a disorder known to be multifactorial or chromosomal. What is the recurrence risk? If the child is affected with spina bifida, the empiric risk to a subsequent child is approximately 4 percent (see Chapter 15). If the child has Down syndrome, the empiric risk of recurrence would be approximately 1 percent if the karyotype were trisomy 21, but it might be substantially higher if one of the parents were a carrier of a Robertsonian translocation involving chromosome 21 (see Chapter 9).

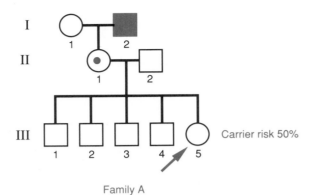

Family A

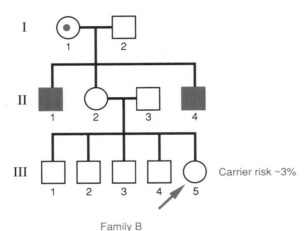

Family B

Figure 18–3. Modified risk estimates in genetic counseling. The consultands in the two families are at risk for having a son with hemophilia A. In Family A, the consultand's mother is an obligate heterozygote; in Family B, the consultand's mother may or may not be a carrier. Application of Bayesian analysis reduces the risk of being a carrier to only approximately 3 percent for the consultand in Family B, but not the consultand in Family A. See text for derivation of the modified risk.

transmitting the hemophilia gene is ½, and the fact that she has already had four unaffected sons does *not* reduce this risk. Thus the risk that the consultand (III-5) is a carrier is ½, and the overall risk of her having an affected child is ½ (the risk of being a carrier) $\times$ ¼ (the risk of transmitting the gene to an affected son), or ⅛. In Family B, however, the mother of the consultand may or may not be a carrier, and the consultand's Mendelian risk of being a carrier is therefore ¼. However, in this case, the fact that she has four unaffected brothers is relevant; one begins to suspect that maybe her mother is not a carrier. Bayesian analysis allows one to take this information into account in modi-

fying her risk of being a carrier and thus her risk of having an affected child. Indeed, overall, the consultand's risk of being a carrier of the hemophilia gene is only about 3 percent, and thus her risk of having an affected child is less than 1 percent.

How did we arrive at this figure? Before calculating the modified risk for the consultand (III-5), we must first determine the risk that her mother (II-2) is a carrier. II-2 is the daughter of an obligate carrier of the hemophilia A gene. Thus the Mendelian risk that she is a carrier (called the **prior probability**) is ½; the prior probability that she is *not* a carrier is, of course, also ½. II-2 has four normal sons. We now consider the probabilities that all four sons would or would not inherit a normal allele at the X-linked factor VIII locus from their mother under two conditions, that she *is* a carrier and that she is *not* a carrier; these are called the **conditional probabilities.** If II-2 is a carrier, the chance that all four sons would be unaffected is $(½)^4$, or ¹⁄₁₆. If, on the other hand, she is not a carrier, the probability that her sons would be unaffected is essentially 1.

We next consider the **joint probability,** which is the product of the prior and conditional risks. The joint probability that II-2 is a carrier with four normal sons is ½ (her prior risk of being a carrier) $\times$ ¹⁄₁₆ (the conditional risk of having four normal sons in such a case), or ¹⁄₃₂. The joint probability that II-2 is *not* a carrier is ½ $\times$ 1, or ½.

Now we can calculate the **posterior probability** that II-2 is a carrier. Given that her four sons are normal, there is a ¹⁄₃₂ chance that she is a carrier and a ½ chance that she is not; therefore, the posterior probability (expressed as a ratio) that she is a carrier is ¹⁄₃₂ : ½, or 1 : 16. Expressed as a fraction, the final probability that II-2 is a carrier is ¹⁄₁₇, and the final probability that she is not a carrier is ¹⁶⁄₁₇.

In summary:

	II-2 Is a Carrier	II-2 Is Not a Carrier
Prior probability	1/2	1/2
Conditional probability	1/16	1
Joint probability	1/32	1/2
Posterior probability	1/17	16/17

Finally, then, the consultand's risk of being a carrier is half her mother's risk, which is ½ $\times$ ¹⁄₁₇ =

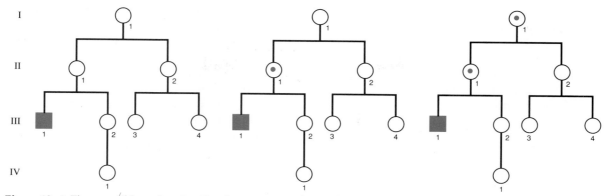

Figure 18-4. Three possible explanations for the occurrence of an isolated case of Duchenne muscular dystrophy (DMD): the affected boy might have a new mutant gene (left); his mother might be a carrier but actually have a new mutant gene (center); or both his mother and his grandmother might be carriers (right). Determination of which explanation is correct has significant implications for estimating risks for the boy's other relatives.

$\frac{1}{34}$, or approximately 3 percent. Thus application of Bayes' theorem to modify the Mendelian risk has reduced the consultand's prior risk of 25 percent to a final risk of only 3 percent.

This may seem like a lot of statistical maneuvering. However, the analysis allows genetic counselors to quantify what seemed intuitively likely from inspection of the pedigree: the fact that the consultand had four unaffected brothers raised a suspicion that she was less likely to be a carrier. The analysis having been performed, the final risk that III-5 is a carrier can be applied to genetic counseling. The risk that her first child will have hemophilia A is $\frac{1}{34} \times \frac{1}{4}$, or less than 1 percent. This is appreciably below the prior probability estimated without the genetic evidence provided by her brothers.

Isolated Cases of X-Linked Disorders. Perhaps the chief use of Bayesian analysis is in the estimation of carrier risks in X-linked lethal traits such as Duchenne muscular dystrophy (DMD) or ornithine transcarbamylase (OTC) deficiency. Because many cases of such disorders (theoretically up to one third of the total) represent new gene mutations, and another third occur in sons of women who carry new gene mutations, the simple Mendelian recurrence risks seen in less severe X-linked traits such as color blindness do not always apply. Instead, we combine the theoretical probability with a woman's own reproductive history to estimate the chance that she is a carrier.

Consider the family at risk for Duchenne muscular dystrophy shown in Figure 18-4. There are three possible explanations for this isolated

case of DMD, each with dramatically different risk estimates for the family:

1. III-1's condition may be the result of a new mutation. In this case, and if the possibility of gonadal mosaicism (see Chapter 4) is ignored, none of his female relatives will be at significant risk of being a carrier.

2. His mother, II-1, is a carrier, but her condition is the result of a new mutation. In this case, her daughter has a ½ risk of being a carrier, and her

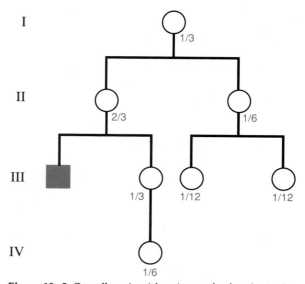

Figure 18-5. Overall carrier risk estimates for females in the family depicted in Figure 18-4. These risk estimates, based on genetic principles, can be further modified by considering information obtained from family history, carrier detection testing, or molecular genetic methods for direct detection of the mutation in the affected boy, using Bayesian calculations.

granddaughter (IV-1), has a ¼ risk. However, none of the other female relatives would be at significant risk.

3. His mother inherited a mutant allele from her mother (I-1), who is also a carrier. In this case, all of the female relatives have either a ½ or a ¼ risk of being carriers.

The prior probability of each of these three possibilities can be calculated to be ⅓. This is derived from first principles (as shown in the following box) or from Haldane's formula for calculating the proportion of new mutant genes (see Chapter 7). The prior risks for females in this family, as calculated from Bayesian analysis, are shown in Figure 18–5. As illustrated later, these risk estimates can be dramatically modified when additional information derived from carrier detection tests is available for genetic counseling.

If a carrier test is available, the results can be included to provide more accurate estimates of risk. Returning to the DMD pedigree in Figure 18–4, assume that the sister (III-2) of the affected boy is given a carrier test, serum creatine kinase (CK) determination, and is found to have a normal CK value. Extensive experience has shown that only about two thirds of obligate carriers have elevated CK values and one third have CK values in the normal range. The final probability for III-2 can now be revised:

	III-2 Is a Carrier	III-2 Is Not a Carrier
Prior probability	1/3	2/3
Conditional probability of normal CK	1/3	1
Joint probability	1/9	2/3
Posterior probability	1/7	6/7

Bayesian Calculations for Isolated Cases of X-Linked Lethal Disorders

For individual II-1 in Figure 18–4 (just as for any female in the general population), the prior risk that she is a DMD carrier is the chance that she inherited a mutant allele from her mother *plus* that chance that she received a newly mutated gene from her mother *plus* the chance that she received a newly mutated gene from her father. If the mutation rate is the same in males and females, the last two factors are each equivalent to the mutation rate, μ, and the prior risk then becomes the chance that she inherited a mutant allele from her mother *plus* 2μ. The chance that she inherited a mutant allele from her mother is ½ × the chance that her mother is a carrier. Because the prior chance that her mother is a carrier is the same as the prior risk that she herself is a carrier (just as it is the same for all females in the general population), the risk that she is a carrier becomes equal to ½ × the chance that she is a carrier *plus* 2μ. When the common terms are canceled out, the risk that any female in the population is a carrier must be 4μ.

Now, Bayesian analysis can be applied as in the example in the main text:

	II-1 Is a Carrier	II-1 Is Not a Carrier
Prior probability	4μ	$1 - 4\mu = 1$
Conditional probability of one affected son	1/2	μ
Joint probability	$4\mu \times 1/2 = 2\mu$	μ
Posterior probability	$2\mu/(2\mu + \mu) = 2/3$	1/3

Thus, the final probability that the mother of an isolated case of DMD is a carrier is ⅔, and the corresponding probability that the patient represents a new mutation must be ⅓. The final probability that the maternal grandmother of an isolated case (e.g., I-1 in Fig. 18–4) is a carrier can be calculated in a similar way: substituting a conditional probability of her having one affected grandson. The joint probabilities become μ that I-1 is a carrier and 2μ that she is not; therefore, the final risk that the grandmother is a carrier is ⅓ (Fig. 18–5).

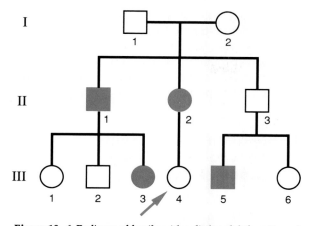

Figure 18–6. Pedigree of family with split-hand deformity and lack of penetrance. The consultand's risk of having a clinically affected child can be calculated to be approximately 8 percent. For discussion, see text.

Given this new information from the carrier test, the final risk that III-2 is a DMD carrier is ¹/₇, and the chance that she will have an affected son is ¹/₂₈.

Disorders With Incomplete Penetrance

To estimate the recurrence risk of disorders with incomplete penetrance, the probability that an apparently normal person actually carries the gene concerned must be considered.

Figure 18–6 shows a pedigree of split-hand deformity, an autosomal dominant abnormality with incomplete penetrance discussed in Chapter 4. An estimate of penetrance can be made from a single pedigree if it is large enough, or from a review of published pedigrees; we use 70 percent in our example.

The pedigree shows several people who must carry the gene but do not express it (i.e., in whom the defect is not penetrant): I-1 or I-2, and II-3. The other unaffected family members may or may not carry the gene.

If III-4 is the consultand, her risk of having a child with split-hand deformity can be estimated by either of the following methods:

	Heterozygous	Homozygous Normal
Prior probability of III-4's genotype	1/2	1/2
Conditional probability of her normal phenotype	3/10	1
Joint probability	3/20	1/2
Posterior probability of III-4's genotype	3/13	10/13
Prior probabilities of her child's genotype	$1/2 \times 3/13$ $= 3/26$	$10/13 + 3/26$ $= 23/26$
Joint probability that child's phenotype will be:		
abnormal	$7/10 \times 3/26$ $= 21/260$	0
normal	$3/10 \times 3/26$ $= 9/260$	23/26

Overall, then, the final risk that III-4 will have a child affected with the split-hand deformity is ²¹/₂₆₀, or approximately 8 percent.

A second way of illustrating this problem, which many people find easier to understand, is shown by the diagram below.

According to the branches in this diagram,

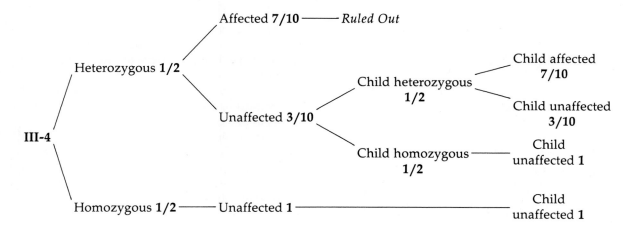

the joint probability of having an affected child is $\frac{1}{2} \times \frac{3}{10} \times \frac{1}{2} \times \frac{7}{10}$ or $\frac{21}{400}$. Similarly, the joint probability of an unaffected child is $(\frac{1}{2} \times \frac{3}{10} \times \frac{1}{2} \times \frac{3}{10}) + (\frac{1}{2} \times \frac{3}{10} \times \frac{1}{2} \times 1) + (\frac{1}{2} \times 1)$, or $\frac{239}{400}$. Overall, the final probability that III-4 will have an affected child is $\frac{21}{(21 + 239)} = \frac{21}{260}$, or approximately 8 percent.

Disorders With Late Age of Onset

Many autosomal dominant conditions characteristically show a late age of onset, beyond the age of reproduction. Thus it is not uncommon in genetic counseling to ask whether a person of reproductive age who is at risk for a particular autosomal dominant disorder carries the gene or not. The classical example of such a disorder is Huntington disease (HD; see box, Chapter 4).

Consider the HD pedigree in Figure 18–7, in which the consultand, an asymptomatic 30-year-old man, wishes to know the risk that he will pass on the HD gene to his offspring. His prior risk of having inherited the HD gene from his affected grandmother is $\frac{1}{4}$. Considering that only about 20 percent of persons with HD show symptoms at his age (see Fig. 4–4), Bayesian analysis results in a final risk estimate of approximately $\frac{1}{5}$ that he carries the gene, only marginally below the prior risk. However, the more significant aspect of the pedigree is that the consultand's father is also asymptomatic at age 55, an age by which approximately 80 percent of persons with HD show symptoms. According to Bayesian analysis of the *father's* risk of carrying the HD gene, his final risk, considering

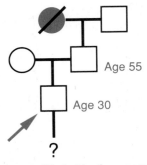

Figure 18–7. Age-modified risks for genetic counseling in Huntington disease. The fact that the consultand's father is asymptomatic at age 55 reduces the consultand's final risk of carrying the gene to approximately 1/15. (See Fig. 4–4 for age of onset graph.)

that he is asymptomatic, is $\frac{1}{6}$. Using this information, we now estimate the consultand's prior risk to be $\frac{1}{2} \times \frac{1}{6}$, or $\frac{1}{12}$, and his final risk is calculated to be approximately $\frac{1}{15}$. Thus the consultand has only about a 3 percent risk of transmitting the HD gene to his offspring.

Application of Molecular Genetics to Determining Recurrence Risks

Many disease genes can now be detected directly in carriers and affected persons by means of DNA analysis. This represents a major improvement in carrier detection and prenatal diagnosis, in many cases allowing determination of the presence or absence of a particular gene with essentially 100 percent accuracy.

There are two chief approaches to risk estimation by DNA analysis. The first is the conventional method, described in Chapter 8, of using **closely linked markers**, preferably markers flanking the gene. This method is indirect, but it works well if its relatively rigid requirements can be met:

1. There is close linkage between the mutation and the marker, so that recombination is unlikely.
2. The family is "informative"; that is, crucial family members are available for the study and are heterozygous for the markers as well as for the mutation.
3. The linkage phase is known or can be reasonably inferred.
4. No recombination has occurred between the markers being followed and the disease gene.

In favorable cases, at least some information can be obtained to modify the prior risk of certain family members' being carriers of the mutation in question.

The second method is by **direct detection of the mutation**, using gene, cDNA, or synthetic probes to detect a mutation in a patient's or other family member's genomic DNA. As described in Chapters 5 and 6, such methods are quick, accurate, and relatively noninvasive. Obviously, direct tests can be used only when the mutation or mutations responsible for a particular disorder are known.

Linkage Analysis in Duchenne Muscular Dystrophy

The hypothetical DMD pedigree shown in Figure 18–8 illustrates the use of linked markers to detect a carrier and to diagnose a fetus prenatally. In this family, the maternal grandmother is clearly a carrier, since she has had two affected sons. She is informative for DNA markers that flank the DMD gene (and that are known to have about a 5 percent chance of recombination) and for a marker within this large gene. The linkage phase in the maternal grandmother can be inferred from her two living sons because any phase other than that indicated in Figure 18–8 would require two recombination events (i.e., in the meioses leading to her two living sons). The consultand has inherited the same maternal haplotype as her affected brother and has an elevated creatine kinase level, indicating that she is almost certainly a carrier. The markers of her father are known, and she herself is informative at all four loci. Her linkage phase is known with certainty, and thus her risk of transmitting the affected haplotype to her offspring can be deter-

mined. The risk of a double recombination occurring in a meiosis in the consultand, which would have allowed her to transmit her mother's DMD gene with her father's flanking markers, is less than 1 percent, and so the probability that the fetus is unaffected is greater than 99 percent. Moreover, because the consultand's husband's markers are known, it can be predicted that her daughter has inherited the DMD gene and is a carrier.

Deletion Analysis in DMD With cDNA Probes

About 60 percent of DMD patients have deletions within the gene, and many of these deletions can be detected with a series of cDNA probes (see Figs. 12–11, 12–12). In the pedigree shown in Figure 18–8, if the DMD patient (II-4) had an identifiable deletion, the linkage analysis just described would be unnecessary. DNA from the fetus (obtained by methods described in Chapter 19) could be examined directly for the presence or absence of the deletion, and a diagnosis could be made with certainty.

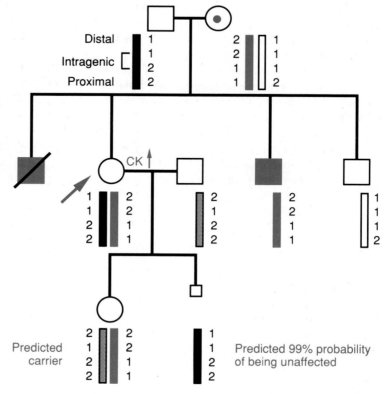

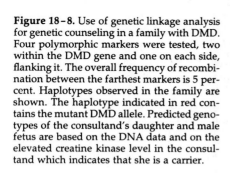

Figure 18–8. Use of genetic linkage analysis for genetic counseling in a family with DMD. Four polymorphic markers were tested, two within the DMD gene and one on each side, flanking it. The overall frequency of recombination between the farthest markers is 5 percent. Haplotypes observed in the family are shown. The haplotype indicated in red contains the mutant DMD allele. Predicted genotypes of the consultand's daughter and male fetus are based on the DNA data and on the elevated creatine kinase level in the consultand which indicates that she is a carrier.

At the present time, detection of a deletion in a heterozygous female is not completely reliable in most cases, although technology is improving. Identification of the mutant gene in female family members still normally requires the use of linked markers.

Detection of Mutations in Cystic Fibrosis (CF)

Carrier detection and prenatal diagnosis in CF makes use of the fact that in individuals of North European descent, about 70 percent of the CF mutations are due to the 3 base-pair deletion that removes the phenylalanine at position 508 (ΔF508; see Chapters 6 and 12). The polymerase chain reaction and hybridization with allele-specific oligonucleotides can be used easily and rapidly to identify carriers of the deletion and fetuses homozygous for it (see Fig. 6–22). The test is fully informative in about 50 percent of families of an affected child and partially informative in over 40 percent more. It can be helpful even when there is no DNA sample from an affected family member (Lemna et al., 1990). The limitation of the method is that 30 percent of CF mutations are not of this type and are not identifiable by this test. However, as additional mutations in different patients are identified (see Chapter 12), similar direct tests for these mutations are being developed.

Because DNA markers very closely linked to the CF locus are available, linkage analysis can be performed for almost all families in which detection of the mutation itself is not yet possible. Moreover, as described in Chapter 8, there is considerable linkage disequilibrium between particular CF mutations and the haplotypes of the closely linked markers, and haplotype analysis can help to refine risk estimates, even when the specific mutation in a particular family has not been identified.

Risk Estimates When a Gene Has Not Been Cloned

The examples just given have stressed two relatively common conditions for which the responsible gene has been cloned and extensively characterized. In these conditions, many mutations have been directly analyzed, and many DNA polymorphisms are available for performing linkage analy-

ses when direct detection is not possible. However, in most disorders, the gene for which a given family is at risk has not yet been cloned. In these cases, the role of DNA diagnostic services is somewhat more complicated and expensive. Even when the location of a gene is known with some precision because of successful linkage studies (see Chapter 8), there may be considerable uncertainty about the exact genetic distances between the disease gene and linked DNA markers used for diagnosis. Determination of risk estimates for the purpose of providing accurate genetic counseling may involve extensive studies of many family members with many different DNA probes to attempt to collect definitive information about location, phase, and the presence of possible recombination events.

As an example, consider the pedigree, shown in Figure 18–9, of a family with Marfan syndrome, an autosomal dominant connective tissue disorder characterized by long, thin extremities, arachnodactyly (long, spiderlike fingers), skeletal deformities, dislocated lenses, and sometimes severe heart complications that can result in sudden death (see Fig. 4–24). Because of markedly variable expressivity, many affected persons are overlooked or, conversely, unaffected (usually tall and slender) persons receive incorrect diagnoses because of one or more suggestive clinical findings. Because the Marfan syndrome gene has been mapped by linkage analysis to the long arm of chromosome 15, DNA diagnosis can assist in refining risk estimates for family members of uncertain genotype. A chromosome 15 DNA marker shows approximately 10 percent recombination with the Marfan gene; thus, genotypic information obtained at the marker locus can be used to predict the presence or absence of the Marfan gene.

In the family shown in Figure 18–9, individual III-3's prior risk of carrying the Marfan gene is ½. Furthermore, she has inherited the same allele at the DNA marker locus from her affected mother as did her unaffected brother. However, because of the possibility of recombination between the Marfan locus and the marker locus in one or more of the meioses in this family, a diagnosis cannot be reached with certainty. III-3's final risk of carrying the Marfan gene can be calculated to be 10 percent.

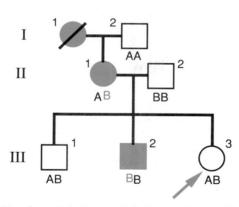

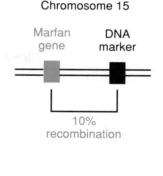

Chromosome 15

Figure 18–9. Use of genetic linkage analysis for genetic counseling in a family with Marfan syndrome. According to the pedigree, allele B at the DNA marker locus on chromosome 15 marks the maternal chromosome carrying the Marfan gene. The consultand did not receive this allele from her mother; her risk of carrying the gene is thus determined by the frequency of meiotic crossovers previously reported between this marker and the Marfan gene (10 percent).

POPULATION SCREENING FOR GENETIC DISEASE

In the examples just given, we considered examining relatives of a proband within a specific family for the presence or absence of particular genetic traits. **Genetic screening,** in contrast, is the search *in a population* for persons with certain genotypes that are known to be associated with a genetic disease, or predisposition to a genetic disease, in themselves or their descendants. Genetic screening is an important public health activity; it becomes more significant as more and better screening tests for genetic diseases become available. Screening at the population level (sometimes called nonproband screening) is not to be confused with screening for affected persons or carriers within families that are identified because of family history. Rather, it refers to programs in which the objective is to screen all members of a designated population, regardless of family history.

Screening of Newborns

The original objective of population screening of newborns was to identify infants with genetic disorders for which early treatment could prevent, or at least ameliorate, the consequences. Only three conditions are usually screened for in most populations:

1. Phenylketonuria (PKU).
2. Galactosemia.
3. Congenital hypothyroidism.

The prototype of such disorders is PKU (see box in Chapter 4); routine neonatal screening for PKU is provided in almost all developed countries. Galactosemia screening is less common. Screening for congenital hypothyroidism, which is not usually genetic but is treatable (see Chapter 13), is also given routinely in many countries. A number of other disorders are less commonly part of neonatal screening programs, including sickle cell anemia, biotinidase deficiency, and various aminoacidopathies. Many other conditions for which screening is feasible are not screened for because of low frequency or lack of a method of treatment.

The principles to be followed in neonatal screening programs are given in Table 18–3. The validity of test results is particularly important; false-positive results cause unnecessary concern to the parents, whereas false-negative results vitiate the whole objective of the program.

The original premise of neonatal screening was that if cases of a given disease were found early, treatment to avoid or ameliorate its effects could be instituted. Not everyone agrees that screening should be performed only for treatable conditions; for example, in the case of DMD, which so far is not treatable and is not usually diagnosed before the age of 2 years, it can be ar-

Table 18-3. Principles of Neonatal Screening
Programs

Disease	Clearly defined, treatable, reasonably high population incidence
Test	Large-scale, rapid, inexpensive Few false positives, ideally no false negatives
Follow-up requirements	Prompt, definitive diagnosis Prompt initiation of treatment Genetic counseling

gued that early identification is needed to ensure prompt genetic counseling and prevention of the birth of more affected children. Early diagnosis with genetic counseling can be helpful to the parents in planning their future pregnancies and can explain the rather nonspecific early manifestations of the disease (slowness in walking and mild retardation in some patients).

Heterozygote Screening

The principles of heterozygote screening are outlined in Table 18-4. There are three classes of heterozygotes for whom screening on a population basis might be considered, now or in the foreseeable future:

1. Carriers of autosomal recessive diseases with high incidence, at least in some ethnic group (e.g., Tay-Sachs disease, sickle cell anemia, β-thalassemia, and, possibly, CF).

2. Carriers of relatively common X-linked disorders.

3. Carriers of autosomal dominant disorders at a presymptomatic stage (e.g., Huntington disease, myotonic dystrophy).

Of the disorders listed, heterozygote screening has so far been used routinely only for Tay-Sachs disease in the Ashkenazi Jewish population (the prototype of carrier screening), sickle cell anemia in the Black population of North America, and β-thalassemia in high-incidence areas, especially

Table 18-4. Criteria for Heterozygote Screening
Programs

High frequency of carriers, at least in a specific population
Suitability of test for mass screening
Availability of genetic counseling
Availability of prenatal diagnosis

in Cyprus and Sardinia or among emigrants from those areas.

The impact of carrier screening in lowering the incidence of disease can be dramatic. Carrier screening for Tay-Sachs disease, carried out on a massive scale since 1969 and followed by prenatal diagnosis when indicated, has already lowered the incidence of Tay-Sachs disease by 65 to 85 percent in the Ashkenazi population. Prevention of β-thalassemia by carrier detection and prenatal diagnosis has brought about a similar drop in the incidence of the disease in Cyprus and Sardinia. In contrast, attempts to screen for carriers of sickle cell disease in the Black community of the United States have been less effective and so far have had little impact on the incidence of the disease. The success of carrier screening programs for Tay-Sachs disease and β-thalassemia, as well as the relative failure for sickle cell anemia, underscores the importance of community consultation and education and availability of genetic counseling and prenatal diagnosis as requirements for an effective program.

The feasibility of direct detection of the common CF mutation has led to serious consideration of the possibility of population-based heterozygote screening for CF. At present, because the $\Delta F508$ mutation accounts for nearly 70 percent of all CF mutations, about half the couples at risk (those in which both partners are heterozygous for the $\Delta F508$ mutation) could be identified; however, other couples at risk, in which only one member or neither has the $\Delta F508$ mutation, would be indistinguishable from other couples in the population (see Chapter 12).

In the total Caucasian population, if the frequency of all CF mutations is 0.022 (i.e., $\sqrt{1/2000}$), then the overall frequency of the $\Delta F508$ mutation is 0.022 × 0.70, or 0.015, and the combined frequency of other mutations about 0.007. In other words, in the general population, almost 1 of every hundred persons tested would have an undetected CF mutation. This is an uncomfortably high false-negative rate. (These calculations are true only for a population with the disease incidence and mutation characteristics mentioned earlier and are not true for other populations. For instance, in Ashkenazi Jewish couples, in whom the frequency of the $\Delta F508$ mutation appears to be low, only 9 percent of couples could be detected by screening at this time.)

The prospect of population screening for CF heterozygotes has been widely discussed, and the present consensus is that it would be premature. Many medical geneticists, however, disagree with this view and believe that heterozygote testing should begin now. A number of pilot programs will probably soon be set up, and over time, as experience is gained and additional mutations are identified, screening for CF heterozygotes may become standard practice. Heterozygote testing both of persons with a family history of CF and of their partners is already widely used.

Prenatal Screening

The test most commonly used for population screening in fetal life is chromosome analysis for late maternal age. This topic is discussed in the context of prenatal diagnosis in Chapter 19.

Negative Implications of Screening Programs

Although the ultimate objective of genetic screening is to improve the public health, negative aspects have been pointed out, including the following:

    1. Possible inaccuracy of test results.

    2. Invasion of privacy.

    3. Possible stigmatization on the basis of an abnormal finding.

    4. Failure to obtain informed consent and possible exercise of compulsion, overt or implied.

    5. The "right not to know" about one's deleterious genes.

    6. Possible lack of confidentiality of the data banks in which the findings are stored.

Obviously, these matters must be taken into consideration in the planning of screening programs. Today, however, few programs are initiated without an ethical review to ensure that such concerns are addressed.

CONCLUSION

In the future, as the knowledge base of medical genetics expands, the scope of genetic counseling will increase proportionately. For physicians, the challenge is to appreciate the importance of genetic counseling in medical practice and to under-stand its scientific basis, but to be aware of the limitations of our knowledge. To quote Sir William Osler, who wrote in a clinical context but could well have been discussing genetic risks, "Errors of judgment are bound to occur in the practice of an art that consists largely in balancing probabilities."

General References

Burnard P (1989) Counselling skills for health professionals. Chapman and Hall Ltd., London.

Emery AEH, Pullen I (eds) (1984) Psychological aspects of genetic counselling. Academic Press, London.

Gardner RJM, Sutherland GR (1989) Chromosome abnormalities and genetic counselling. Oxford University Press, Oxford.

Harper PS (1988) Practical genetic counselling, 3rd ed. Wright, London.

Kelly TE (1986) Clinical genetics and genetic counseling, 2nd ed. Year Book Medical Publishers, Chicago.

Murphy EA, Chase GA (1975) Principles of genetic counseling. Year Book Medical Publishers, Chicago.

Problems

1. You are consulted by a couple, Dorothy and David, who tell the following story: Dorothy's maternal grandfather Bruce had congenital stationary night blindness, which also affected Bruce's maternal uncle, Arthur; in other words, the family history appears to fit the X-linked pattern. (There is also an autosomal dominant form.) Dorothy and David have three unaffected children: a daughter, Elsie, and two sons, Edward and Eliot. Elsie is planning to have children in the near future. Dorothy wonders whether she should warn Elsie about the risk that she might be a carrier of a serious eye disorder. Sketch the pedigree and answer the following:
   a) What is the chance that Elsie is heterozygous?
   b) An ophthalmologist traces the family history in further detail and finds evidence that in this pedigree the disorder is not X-linked but autosomal dominant. There is no evidence that Dorothy's mother Cecile was affected. On this basis, what is the chance that Elsie is heterozygous?

2. A deceased boy, Nathan, was the only member of his family with DMD. He is survived by two sisters, Norma (who has a daughter, Olive) and Nancy (who has a daughter, Odette). His mother Molly has two sisters, Maud and Martha. Martha has two unaffected sons and two daughters, Nora and Nellie. Maud has one daughter, Naomi. No carrier tests are possible.

a) Sketch the pedigree, and calculate the posterior risks for all these females, using information provided in this chapter.

b) In many Molecular Diagnosis laboratories, prenatal diagnosis by DNA analysis is available only to women with greater than a 2 percent risk that a pregnancy will result in a son with DMD. Which of these women would not qualify?

3. In a village in Wales in 1984, 13 boys were born in succession before a girl was born. What is the probability of 13 successive male births? The probability of 13 successive births of a single sex?

4. Hemophilia A has an estimated fitness (f) of .70; in other words, hemophiliacs have 70 percent as many offspring as do controls. Emery (1986) noted that the incidence of hemophilia A in males (I) equals the chance of receiving a new mutation from the mother (μ) plus half the frequency of heterozygous females ($1/2H$); the incidence of carrier females is the same *plus* the chance of receiving the gene from an affected father, which is the incidence of affected males (I) multiplied by the fitness factor (f). In brief: $I = \mu + 1/2H$ and $H = 2\mu + 1/2H + If$.

a) For hemophilia A, what is the incidence of affected males? of carrier females? [Answer parts a) and b) in terms of multiples of the mutation rate.] If a woman has a son with an isolated case of hemophilia A, what is the relative risk that she is a carrier? What is the chance that her next son will be affected?

b) For DMD, $f = 0$. What is the population frequency of affected males? of carrier females?

c) Color blindness is thought to have normal fitness ($f = 1$). What is the incidence of carrier females if the frequency of color-blind males is 8 percent?

5. Match terms in section **B** with explanations or definitions in section **A**.

A

1. The probability that any woman in the population is a carrier of DMD.

2. Possible only if the exact mutation is known.

3. Used with DNA markers as an approach to risk estimation.

4. Prototype of newborn screening.

5. The Mendelian risk that a person is a carrier of a certain disorder.

6. The person seeking or receiving genetic counseling.

7. A person who on the basis of family history must be a heterozygote.

8. The probability that the mother of a child with an isolated case of DMD is a carrier.

9. A family in which markers linked to a locus of interest allow a mutation to be traced through a family.

10. Parent, full sib, or offspring (but not an MZ twin).

B

_____ Consultand
_____ 2/3
_____ Obligate heterozygote
_____ Prior probability
_____ Phenylketonuria
_____ Direct detection of a mutation
_____ Informative family
_____ 4μ
_____ First-degree relative
_____ Linkage analysis

6. Ira and Margie each have a sibling affected with cystic fibrosis. They have had three unaffected children and now wish to know their risk of having an affected child.

a) What are their prior risks of being carriers?

b) What is the risk of their having an affected child in *any* pregnancy?

c) Using Bayesian analysis to take into consideration the fact that they have already had three unaffected children, calculate the chance that their next child will be affected.

7. A 30-year-old woman with myotonic dystrophy comes in for counseling. Her son, age 8, shows no symptoms, but she wishes to know whether he will be affected with this autosomal dominant condition later in life. Approximately half of individuals carrying the mutant gene are asymptomatic before age 14 years. What is the risk that the son will eventually develop myotonic dystrophy?

8. A couple arrives in your clinic with their 7-month-old son, who has been moderately developmentally delayed from birth. The couple is contemplating having additional children, and you are asked whether this could be a genetic disorder.

a) Is this possible and, if so, what pattern or patterns of inheritance would fit this story?

b) Upon taking a detailed family history, you learn that both parents' families were originally from the same small village in northern Italy. How might this fact alter your assessment of the case?

c) You next learn that the mother has two sisters and five brothers. Both sisters have developmentally delayed children. How might this alter your assessment of the case?

9. You are addressing a Neurofibromatosis Association parents' meeting. A severely affected woman, 32 years old, comments that she is not at risk of passing on the disorder because her parents are not affected and her NF, therefore, is due to a new mutation. Comment.

CHAPTER 19

PRENATAL DIAGNOSIS

Prenatal diagnosis had its beginning in 1966, when Steele and Breg showed that the chromosome constitution of a fetus could be determined by analysis of cultured cells from the amniotic fluid. Because the association between late maternal age and an increased risk of Down syndrome was already well known, their report led directly to the development of prenatal diagnosis as a medical service. Prenatal diagnosis has already been referred to in the context of many specific genetic disorders, and in this chapter its scope, methodology, and limitations are considered in further detail.

The purpose of prenatal diagnosis is not simply to detect abnormalities in fetal life and allow termination of pregnancy when the fetus is found to have a defect. Rather, it has the following objectives:

1. To provide a range of informed choice to parents at risk of having a child with an abnormality.

2. To provide reassurance and reduce anxiety, especially among high-risk groups.

3. To allow couples at risk of a child with a specific defect, who might otherwise forgo having children, to begin a pregnancy with the knowledge that the presence or absence of the disorder in the fetus can be confirmed by testing.

Unfortunately, in a small proportion of cases the fetus is found to have a serious defect. Because effective prenatal therapy is not available for most disorders, the parents may then choose to terminate the pregnancy.

Some pregnant women who would not consider termination nevertheless request prenatal diagnosis in order to reduce anxiety or prepare for the birth of an abnormal child. The question then is whether the request is justified if invasive techniques with an associated risk of fetal loss would be required. In practice the use of prenatal diagnosis by invasive techniques, even when termination of pregnancy is not an option, appears to be on the increase because the risks are low and because many believe that parents are entitled to the information.

Few issues today are as hotly debated as elective abortion, but despite legal restrictions in some areas, elective abortion is widely used. Among all elective abortions, those performed because of prenatal diagnosis of an abnormality in the fetus account for only a very small proportion, less than 2 percent. Without a means of legal termination of pregnancy, prenatal diagnosis would not have developed into the accepted procedure that it has become. Nonetheless, it is important to stress that, in greater than 98 percent of cases, the findings in prenatal diagnosis are normal, and parents are reassured that their baby will be unaffected by the condition in question. Among all prenatal diagnoses, the proportion culminating in abortion is thus very small.

Prenatal diagnosis requires the collaboration of a number of disciplines: obstetrics; ultrasonography; clinical genetics, including assessment, diagnosis, and genetic counseling; and laboratory sciences, including cytogenetics, biochemistry, and DNA analysis. Because of the complexity of integrating these functions, prenatal diagnosis is usually arranged by referral to a multidisciplinary program, in which genetics plays an essential part.

In North America, about 8 percent of all pregnancies meet the criteria for prenatal diagnosis by amniocentesis or chorionic villus sampling (CVS). Both amniocentesis and CVS are invasive procedures associated with a small risk of fetal loss. Whereas amniocentesis or CVS is available to only a small percentage of pregnant women, a combination of maternal serum alpha-fetoprotein (MSAFP) assay and ultrasonographic scanning can be used for fetal evaluation in low-risk as well as high-risk pregnancies because both are noninvasive and without risk to the fetus. MSAFP assay can help to identify fetuses at increased risk of neural tube defects and other disorders, as described later in this chapter. Ultrasonography, in addition to its function in assessment of gestational age and fetal growth, enables geneticists and obstetricians to diagnose a number of morphological abnormalities, many of which are genetic in origin, at early gestational ages.

INDICATIONS FOR PRENATAL DIAGNOSIS

By far the leading indication for prenatal diagnosis is late maternal age. In North America and western Europe, according to statistical data for maternal age at birth in comparison with the number of prenatal diagnoses, at least half of all pregnant women over 35 years of age present for amniocentesis. In the United States, courts have considered a physician to be negligent if he or she fails to suggest prenatal diagnosis to older mothers.

The chief condition for which pregnant women of advanced age are at risk is, of course, Down syndrome (Fig. 19–1). Despite the widespread application of prenatal diagnosis to older women, many fetuses with Down syndrome are not identified prenatally because their mothers are under 35 years of age and thus too young to be eligible for amniocentesis or CVS. New diagnostic

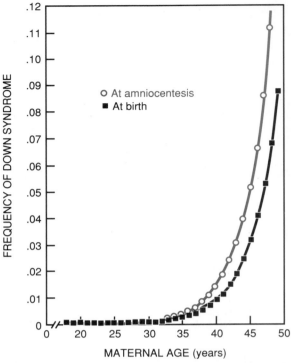

Figure 19–1. Maternal age dependence of incidence of trisomy 21 at birth and at time of amniocentesis. See also Chapter 9. (Data from Hook EB, Cross PK, Schreinemachers DM [1983] Chromosomal abnormality rates at amniocentesis and in liveborn infants. JAMA 249: 2034–2038.)

methods may help to identify a larger proportion of the fetuses at risk. The use of MSAFP assay and other tests on maternal serum, together with ultrasonographic examination, to improve the detection of fetuses with Down syndrome and other chromosome abnormalities is described later.

Prenatal diagnosis cannot be used to rule out all possible fetal defects. It is limited to determining whether the fetus has (or probably has) a designated condition for which the family history indicates an increased risk. If amniocentesis is performed for any reason, both the amniotic fluid alpha-fetoprotein (AFAFP) level and the karyotype are determined. Otherwise, tests are performed only for specific indications.

Guidelines

The generally accepted guidelines for eligibility of pregnant women for prenatal diagnosis by amniocentesis or CVS are based on evidence that the risk that the fetus is abnormal is at least as great as the risk of miscarriage from the procedure itself. As the scope of prenatal diagnosis expands and technology improves, the guidelines are sure to change, but at present the chief criteria are the following:

1. **Advanced maternal age (often at least 35 years at the expected date of confinement):** If there is no previous history of a chromosome abnormality, it is only in the advanced maternal age range that the risk of a chromosomally abnormal fetus exceeds the risk of miscarriage due to the procedure itself (see Table 9–4 for maternal age–specific risk of a fetus with a chromosome abnormality). The age cutoff used varies somewhat among different prenatal genetics centers but is usually at least 31 to 32 years of age.

2. **Previous child with a de novo chromosome abnormality:** If the parents of a child with a chromosome abnormality have normal chromosomes themselves, there may nevertheless be a risk of the same abnormality in a subsequent child. For example, if a woman under 30 years of age has a child with Down syndrome, the recurrence risk is about 1/100, in comparison with a general population risk of about 1/800. Parental mosaicism is a possible explanation of the increased risk.

3. **Presence of structural chromosome abnormality in one of the parents:** Here the risk of an abnormal child is usually 20 percent or less, but it may be higher. In the worst case, the risk of Down syndrome is 100 percent if either parent has a 21q21q Robertsonian translocation or isochromosome (see Chapter 9).

4. **Family history of some genetic defect that may be diagnosed or ruled out by biochemical or DNA analysis:** Most of these disorders are caused by single-gene defects and have risks of 25 percent or 50 percent in sibs of affected children. Cases in which the parents have been diagnosed as carriers after a population screening test rather than after the birth of an affected child are also in this category. Even before DNA analysis entered the picture, numerous biochemical disorders could be identified prenatally, and DNA analysis has greatly increased the number. Table 19–1 provides a list of some relatively common single-gene disorders for which prenatal diagnosis can be performed by DNA analysis, but it is by no means complete. Some of the diseases listed cannot be

Table 19–1. Selected Single-Gene Disorders for Which Prenatal Diagnosis by DNA Analysis Is Possible in Many Families

Cystic fibrosis	AR
Duchenne and Becker muscular dystrophy	X-linked
Fragile X syndrome (mental retardation)	X-linked
Hemophilia A and B	X-linked
Huntington disease	AD
Myotonic dystrophy	AD
Neurofibromatosis, type 1	AD
Ornithine transcarbamylase deficiency	X-linked
Phenylketonuria	AR
Retinoblastoma	AD
Sickle cell disease	AR
Tay-Sachs disease	AR
α- and β-thalassemias	AR

AR = autosomal recessive; AD = autosomal dominant.

detected by biochemical tests for enzymes or other gene products because the relevant gene product is not expressed in the fetal tissues sampled (chorionic villi or amniotic fluid cells). Many other disorders not included in Table 19–1 can be diagnosed prenatally by linkage analysis with DNA markers.

5. **Family history of an X-linked disorder for which there is no specific prenatal diagnostic test:** When there is no alternative method, the parents may use fetal sex determination to help them decide whether to continue or terminate the pregnancy. With the development of DNA analysis for prenatal diagnosis of X-linked disorders such as Duchenne muscular dystrophy and hemophilia A and B, first the fetal sex is determined, and then DNA analysis is performed if the fetus is male. The method of determining the sex of very early embryos by DNA analysis, described in Chapter 17, may eventually prove useful, but is still experimental.

6. **Risk of a neural tube defect (NTD):** Only first- and second-degree relatives of NTD patients are eligible for amniocentesis because of a significantly increased risk of having a child with an NTD, but many fetuses with open NTDs can now be detected by other tests, as described later.

PRELIMINARIES TO PRENATAL DIAGNOSIS

Prospective parents considering prenatal diagnosis need information that will allow them to understand their situation and to give or withhold consent for the procedure. In addition, the professional staff of the prenatal diagnosis program (physician and genetic counselor) need to assess the situation, determine the genetic risk, and learn whether other genetic problems should also be considered (for example, a possible risk of Tay-Sachs disease in the fetus of an Ashkenazi Jewish couple referred because of late maternal age). Ethnic background or family history may indicate the need for carrier tests of the parents in advance.

Preliminary genetic counseling of candidates for prenatal diagnosis usually deals with the following points: the risk that the fetus will be affected; the nature and probable consequences of the specific problem; the risks and limitations of the procedures to be used; the time required before a report can be issued; and the possible need for a repeat procedure in the event of a failed attempt or inconclusive finding. The parents need to be advised that a result may be difficult to interpret and that further tests and consultation may be required and that even then the results may not necessarily be definitive. Finally, although the great majority of prenatal diagnoses end in reassurance, the parents may in some cases want to consider termination of the pregnancy, and the time available for that decision is limited.

Numerous diseases cannot yet be diagnosed prenatally, but many others, including some of major significance, have moved from the impossible to the possible category, and the list is growing month by month. Keeping up with the rapid changes and serving as a central source of information about the current status of prenatal testing is one of the contributions of genetics clinics to medical practice in general.

PROCEDURES FOR OBTAINING FETAL TISSUE

Amniocentesis

Amniocentesis (tapping of the amnion) refers to the procedure of removing a sample of amniotic fluid transabdominally by syringe (Fig. 19–2A). The amniotic fluid contains cells of fetal origin that can be cultured for diagnostic tests. Ultrasonographic scanning facilitates the procedure by confirming the gestational age in advance and by outlining the position of the fetus and placenta. Amniocentesis is usually performed on an outpatient basis at about the 16th week after the last menstrual period; because of improvements in ultrasonographic scanning, however, the procedure can now be performed at a much earlier stage in pregnancy.

The complications associated with amniocentesis are relatively minor. There is a small risk of inducing miscarriage, estimated to be approximately 0.5 percent. Maternal infection is a rare complication. To prevent Rh immunization of the

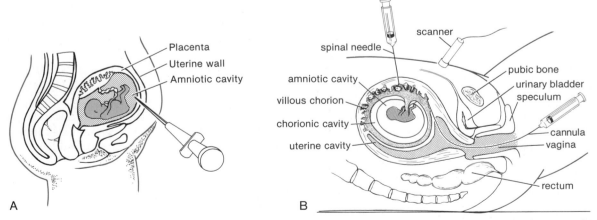

Figure 19–2. A. Amniocentesis. A needle is inserted transabdominally into the amniotic cavity, and a sample of amniotic fluid (usually about 20 ml) is withdrawn by syringe for diagnostic studies (e.g., chromosome studies, enzyme measurements, or DNA analysis). B. Chorionic villus sampling. Two alternative approaches are drawn: transcervical (by means of a flexible cannula) and transabdominal (with a spinal needle). In both approaches, success and safety depends on use of ultrasound imaging (scanner). (From Moore KL [1988] The developing human: Clinically oriented embryology, 4th ed. WB Saunders, Philadelphia.)

mother, administration of Rh immune globulin is routine for Rh-negative women. Many mothers express concern that the fetus might be injured by needle puncture, but serious abnormalities definitely related to needle puncture are extremely rare.

Chorionic Villus Sampling (CVS)

In CVS, fetal trophoblast tissue is aspirated from the villous area of the chorion transcervically or transabdominally as early as the 9th week of pregnancy (Fig. 19–2B). The rate of fetal loss due to CVS, when the fetus is viable at 9 to 12 weeks' gestation, is approximately 1 percent. This rate of loss is slightly more than the risk from amniocentesis (Canadian Collaborative Survey, 1989; Rhoads et al., 1989), although it may be decreasing with experience. The success of chromosome analysis, however, appears to be somewhat lower than with amniocentesis. A small proportion of CVS procedures fail or yield ambiguous results, and follow-up amniocentesis is required. Again, an improved success rate is expected with increasing experience.

CVS is still a limited service in many centers. Its major advantage over amniocentesis is that it allows the results of diagnostic procedures to be available at an early stage of pregnancy, thus reducing the period of uncertainty and allowing termination, if elected, to be performed on an outpatient basis, in the first trimester. A disadvantage is that AFAFP measurement cannot be performed at this stage and must be done later.

Embryological Development of the Chorionic Villi

A brief review of the early development of the chorionic villi helps to clarify some of the problems with the CVS technique (Fig. 19–3). The villi are derived from the trophoblast, the extraembryonic part of the blastocyst. During implantation, the trophoblast differentiates into the cytotrophoblast and the syncytiotrophoblast. The syncytiotrophoblast invades the uterine wall and eventually forms lacunae in which maternal blood is pooled. At the end of the second week, the **primary chorionic villi** are formed as proliferations of the cytotrophoblast that protrude into the syncytiotrophoblast. The villi soon begin to branch, and mesenchyme grows into them to form a core; the formation of a core characterizes the **secondary villi.** Networks of capillaries develop in the mesenchymal core, and circulation is established; the villi are then **tertiary villi.** The tertiary villi branch profusely, and by the end of the 8th week

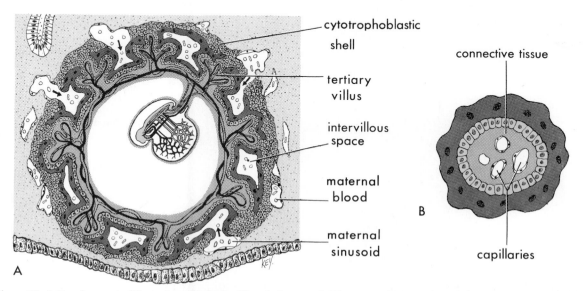

Figure 19–3. Development of the tertiary chorionic villi and placenta. A. Diagrammatic cross-section of an implanted embryo and placenta at about 21 days. B. Cross-section of a tertiary villus showing establishment of circulation in mesenchymal core, cytotrophoblast, and syncytiotrophoblast. (From Moore KL [1988] The developing human: Clinically oriented embryology, 4th ed. WB Saunders, Philadelphia.)

they cover the entire surface of the chorionic sac as the **chorion frondosum**, although part of the chorion subsequently becomes the **smooth chorion (chorion laeve)** as the villi in that area degenerate. The villi that are sampled for prenatal diagnosis are tertiary villi from the chorion frondosum and are composed of mesechymal core, cytotrophoblast, and an outer layer of syncytiotrophoblast.

Cordocentesis

Cordocentesis is a procedure used to obtain a sample of fetal blood directly from the umbilical cord with ultrasonographic guidance. The fetal blood sample requires only a few days in culture to provide cells suitable for chromosome analysis or

hematological studies. Cordocentesis is used to give a quick result when ultrasonographic examination has shown some fetal abnormality, when culture of amniotic fluid cells has failed, or when DNA diagnosis is not possible for a disorder that can be identified by biochemical tests of fetal plasma or blood cells.

ULTRASONOGRAPHY

Real-time scanning, a major improvement over static scanning in ultrasonographic technology, is increasingly important in prenatal diagnosis for fetal assessment and for the detection of morphological anomalies (Fig. 19–4). It permits accurate determination of fetal age, identifies multiple

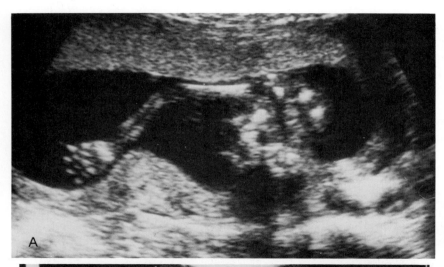
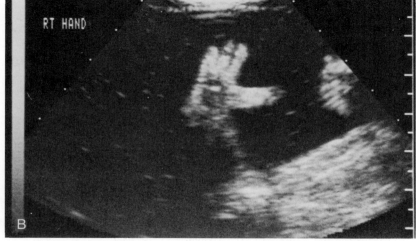

Figure 19–4. Ultrasonogram of hand of normal fetus (*A*) and fetus with Holt-Oram syndrome, an autosomal dominant defect with variable limb and heart abnormalities (*B*). (Photographs courtesy of A. Toi, Toronto General Hospital.)

pregnancies, and verifies fetal viability. It can even be used in midtrimester to identify fetal sex with a high degree of accuracy. The equipment and techniques used by ultrasonographers have improved so greatly that some malformations are now detectable in the first instance by routine ultrasonography early in midtrimester, even without a family history to indicate an increased risk. Although the possibility of associated risk to the fetus has been carefully assessed, there is no evidence that ultrasonography causes any fetal damage.

When a fetus is at risk for a single-gene disorder, detailed ultrasonography can sometimes detect the disorder or rule it out. Thus diagnostic ultrasonography is appropriate even if the risk is minimal. For example, achondroplasia in a child of unaffected parents is usually due to a new mutation, but very rarely it is the consequence of germ-

line mosaicism in one parent. In that case it is associated with an elevated recurrence risk (see Chapter 4); thus diagnostic ultrasonography is indicated for mothers who have had a previous achondroplastic child, even though the risk of having another affected child is small. The finding of a normal fetus can be very reassuring, while the identification of a fetus with achondroplasia can guide the remainder of the pregnancy and the delivery.

A number of isolated defects that tend to recur in families and are thought to have multifactorial inheritance can also be identified by ultrasonography, including congenital heart defects, neural tube malformations (Fig. 19–5), and cleft lip and palate. Table 19–2 lists some abnormalities in which the diagnosis can be made by ultrasonographic scanning. This procedure can also be

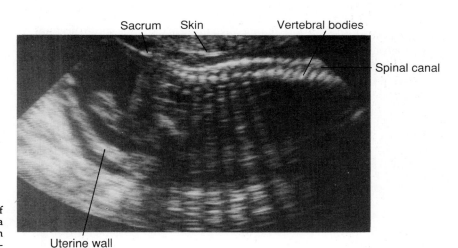

Figure 19–5. Ultrasonograms of spinal canal and neural tube in a normal fetus (top) and a fetus with a neural tube defect (bottom). Ultrasound clearly shows the meningomyelocele sac protruding through the skin. Compare with Figure 15–4. (Photographs courtesy of A. Toi, Toronto General Hospital.)

Table 19–2. Selected Defects That Can Be Diagnosed Prenatally or Ruled Out by Diagnostic Ultrasonographic Scanning

Single-gene disorders
Polycystic kidney disease
Skeletal dysplasias

Disorders usually thought of as multifactorial
Cleft lip and palate
Congenital heart defects
Neural tube defects

Anomalies that may indicate a syndrome
Abnormal facies
Abnormal genitalia
Cystic hygroma
Polydactyly

used to visualize anatomical defects suggestive of chromosome abnormalities. When the suspicion of a chromosome defect has been raised, it can be confirmed or ruled out by chromosome analysis.

Many malformations identified by ultrasonographic scanning are not detected until relatively late in gestation, when abortion is no longer an option. Even so, the karyotype is important for evaluation of the prognosis and management of the pregnancy and delivery, as well as for genetic counseling with respect to future pregnancies.

LABORATORY STUDIES

Cytogenetics

Either amniocentesis or CVS can provide fetal cells for karyotyping, as well as for biochemical or DNA analysis. Preparation and analysis of chromosomes from cultured amniotic fluid cells or cultured chorionic villi require at least 2 weeks.

Chorionic villi can be used for karyotyping after either short-term incubation or long-term culture. Short-term incubation, although providing a result more quickly, yields poor-quality preparations in which the banding resolution is inadequate for detailed analysis. Most laboratories use both techniques, but if only one is used, long-term culture of the cells of the mesenchymal core is the technique of choice at present.

Because molecular cytogenetic techniques for evaluating chromosome number are becoming available, it may be possible to screen interphase nuclei in fetal cells immediately after amniocentesis or CVS for the common aneuploidies of chromosomes 13, 18, 21, X, and Y. Such approaches for rapid prenatal cytogenetic assessment are currently under evaluation.

Chromosome Analysis After Ultrasonography

Because some defects detectable by ultrasonography are associated with chromosome abnormalities, karyotyping of either amniotic fluid cells or fetal blood cells obtained by cordocentesis may be performed after ultrasonographic detection of an abnormality. High rates of chromosome abnormalities have been found in cases referred because of cystic hygroma, limb abnormalities, omphalocele, duodenal stenosis, hydrocephalus, and malformations of the face. Chromosome disorders are more frequently found when multiple rather than isolated malformations are detected; in one study, almost 30 percent of fetuses karyotyped because of multiple malformations had chromosome abnormalities (Eydoux et al., 1989).

The karyotypes most often seen in fetuses ascertained by abnormal ultrasonographic findings are the common autosomal trisomies (21, 18, and 13), 45,X (Turner syndrome), and unbalanced structural abnormalities. A cervical hygroma frequently indicates a 45,X karyotype, but they can also occur in Down syndrome and trisomy 18, as well as in fetuses with normal karyotypes.

Problems in Prenatal Chromosome Analysis

Mosaicism. When mosaicism is found in cultured fetal cells, there may be problems in interpretation, both as to whether the fetus is truly mosaic and as to the clinical significance of the observation.

In amniotic fluid cell cultures, cytogeneticists distinguish three levels of mosaicism: a single unusual cell, which can usually be disregarded as **pseudomosaicism;** mosaicism involving several cells or colonies of cells in a single primary culture, which is difficult to interpret but considered likely to be pseudomosaicism that has arisen in culture; and **true mosaicism,** detected in multiple colonies from several different primary cultures. Postnatal studies have confirmed that true mosaicism in culture is associated with a high risk that mosaicism is truly present in the fetus. However, the probability varies with different situations; mosaicism for structural aberrations, for example, is hardly ever confirmed.

Maternal cell contamination is a possible explanation of some cases of apparent mosaicism with XX and XY cell lines. It is more common in long-term CVS cultures than in amniotic fluid cell cultures, as a consequence of the intimate association between the chorionic villi and the maternal tissue. To minimize the risk of maternal cell contamination, any maternal decidua present in a chorionic villus sample are carefully dissected and removed. When maternal cell contamination is suspected and cannot be disproved (for example, by comparison of chromosome heteromorphisms in the maternal and fetal cells), amniocentesis is usually performed later to allow a second chromosome study.

In CVS studies, discrepancies between the karyotypes found in cytotrophoblast, villous stroma, and fetus have been reported in about 2 percent of pregnancies studied at 10 to 11 weeks' gestation. Mosaicism in the placenta but not present in the fetus (confined placental mosaicism) is quite common. Placental mosaicism with a normal cell line and a trisomic cell line has also been reported when a liveborn infant or fetus has nonmosaic trisomy 13 or trisomy 18, the percentage of placental cells with a normal karyotype ranging from 12 to 100 percent (Kalousek et al., 1989). This finding implies that when the zygote is trisomic, a normal cell line established by postzygotic loss of the additional chromosome in a progenitor cell of the cytotrophoblast can improve the probability of intrauterine survival of a trisomic fetus.

The difficulty of confirming and interpreting mosaicism is perhaps the most serious problem in genetic counseling for prenatal diagnosis because there is inadequate follow-up information on the numerous possible types and extents of mosaicism. Further studies (amniocentesis that follows CVS, or cordocentesis that follows amniocentesis) and the medical literature may provide some guidance, but sometimes the interpretation remains uncertain. Ultrasonographic scanning may provide some reassurance if there is normal growth and if no congenital anomalies can be demonstrated.

The parents are usually warned in advance of the possibility that mosaicism may be found and of the uncertainty of interpreting such a finding. An effort is made to verify any abnormal chromosome findings after birth or, in the case of termination, in fetal tissues.

Culture Failure. If couples are to have an opportunity to consider termination of a pregnancy when an abnormality is found in the fetus, they need to be provided with the information at the earliest possible time. Because prenatal diagnosis is always a race against time, the rate of culture failure is a major concern. When a CVS culture fails, there is time to repeat the chromosome study with amniocentesis. If an amniotic fluid cell culture fails and there is no time to repeat the procedure, cordocentesis and culture of fetal blood is a useful alternative.

Unexpected Adverse Findings. Occasionally, prenatal chromosome analysis done primarily to rule out trisomy 21 reveals some other unusual chromosome finding: for example, a normal chromosome number but a common variant, a rare rearrangement, or a marker chromosome. In such a case, because the significance of the finding in the fetus cannot be assessed until the parental karyotypes are known, both parents are karyotyped in order to determine whether the variant seen in the fetus is de novo or inherited. If the same variant is seen in a normal parent, it is probably a normal variant without untoward consequences. On the other hand, if one parent is found to be a carrier of a structural rearrangement seen in unbalanced form in the fetus, the consequences for the fetus may be serious.

Biochemical Assays for Metabolic Diseases

More than 100 metabolic disorders can be diagnosed prenatally in chorionic villus tissue or cultured amniotic fluid cells, and a few rare conditions can even be identified directly by assay of a substance in amniotic fluid (Table 19–3). Most metabolic disorders are rare in the general population but have a high recurrence risk (usually 25 percent within sibships, since most are autosomal recessive conditions). Because each condition is rare, the experience of the laboratory performing the prenatal diagnostic testing is very important; thus referral to specialized centers is often desirable.

Table 19–3. Examples of Metabolic Disorders Diagnosed by Enzyme Assay in Chorionic Villi or Cultured Amniotic Fluid Cells

Carbohydrate disorders
Galactosemia
Glycogen storage disease, types II, III, and IV

Amino acid disorders
Citrullinemia
Maple syrup urine disease

Organic acidemias
Methylmalonic acidemias

Purine and pyrimidine disorders
Adenosine deaminase deficiency

Lysosomal disorders
Tay-Sachs disease

Disorders of hormone synthesis
Steroid sulfatase deficiency

Disorders of connective tissue
Hypophosphatasia

Biochemical tests have one significant advantage over DNA analysis in some cases: whereas DNA analysis by direct detection of a mutation is accurate only for that mutation and not for other alleles at the locus, biochemical testing can detect abnormalities caused by any mutant allele that has a significant effect on the function of the protein. This advantage is particularly significant for disorders characterized by a high degree of allelic heterogeneity or by a high proportion of new mutations (i.e., X-linked recessive lethals).

DNA Analysis

Numerous disorders, many of which were not previously detectable prenatally, can now be diagnosed by DNA analysis (Table 19–1). DNA analysis can be performed either by means of closely linked markers or by direct detection of the mutation. Many techniques can be used for direct mutation screening (Table 19–4). This is a rapidly growing area in prenatal diagnosis. The number of disorders that can be diagnosed and the precision and efficiency of analysis are increasing weekly as new approaches are developed, as new mutations are characterized, and as additional genetic diseases are mapped by genetic linkage studies.

When possible, direct methods of detecting a particular mutation are preferred (Fig. 19–6).

Table 19–4. Prenatal Diagnosis by DNA Analysis

Direct Methods

Southern Blotting to Detect Gene Deletions or Rearrangements
Example: 60% of Duchenne muscular dystrophy mutations are deletions (Chapter 12)

Southern Blotting and Restriction Enzyme Analysis to Detect Point Mutations That Alter Restriction Sites
Examples: *Mst*II site in sickle cell anemia (Chapter 11); *Taq*I site in hemophilia A (Chapter 6); *Taq*I site in X-linked ornithine transcarbamylase deficiency (Fig. 19–6)

Allele-Specific Oligonucleotides to Detect Previously Characterized Mutations
Examples: 3-bp deletion in cystic fibrosis (Fig. 6–22); Z mutation in alpha$_1$-antitrypsin deficiency (Chapter 12)

Polymerase Chain Reaction Amplification to Detect Deletions or Previously Characterized Mutations
Examples: deletions in Duchenne muscular dystrophy or Lesch-Nyhan syndrome (Fig. 6–21); specific mutations in Tay-Sachs disease (Chapter 6) or cystic fibrosis

Indirect Methods

DNA Polymorphisms Within or Near Disease Loci to Detect Mutations in a Particular Gene
Examples: polymorphisms within the phenylalanine hydroxylase gene for prenatal diagnosis of phenylketonuria; polymorphisms near factor VIII gene for prenatal diagnosis of hemophilia A (Fig. 19–7)

DNA Polymorphisms Linked to Disease Loci to Diagnose Unknown Mutations in a Particular Gene Whose Map Position Is Known
Examples: numerous disorders that have been mapped to a chromosomal region by family linkage studies, but that have not yet been cloned (see Chapter 8)

However, because the spectrum of mutations varies from disorder to disorder, and often between racial and ethnic groups within a particular disorder, the application of DNA analysis to prenatal diagnosis remains highly specialized, and specific diagnostic laboratories develop particular expertise for the subset of genetic disorders most often presenting in their practice or research. The degree of certainty of the diagnosis approaches 100 percent when direct detection of a mutation is possible, although, as noted earlier, if the disorder in the patient in actually due to a different mutation from the one that is being sought, DNA analysis may fail to detect it.

When application of direct methods of diagnosis is impossible or impractical, the indirect approach of genetic linkage analysis can be used (Fig. 19–7). However, if linked DNA markers are used, the accuracy of diagnosis depends on how closely linked the markers are to the mutation and on

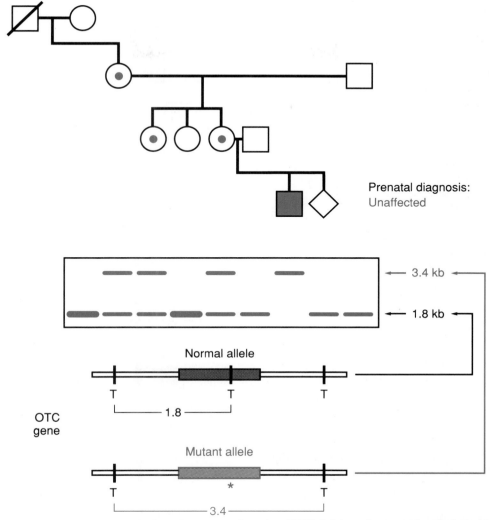

Figure 19-6. Prenatal exclusion of X-linked ornithine transcarbamylase (OTC) deficiency in an at-risk male fetus, by using direct methods of DNA analysis. Mutation in the OTC gene destroys a *Taq*I restriction site (T) in a coding exon, resulting in a 3.4-kb *Taq*I fragment rather than the normal 1.8-kb fragment. Because the presence or absence of the 3.4-kb fragment is a direct marker for the mutation, it can be used in prenatal diagnosis to predict that a male fetus will be unaffected. DNA was prepared from cultured amniotic fluid cells obtained by amniocentesis. Direct detection of the OTC mutation also demonstrates that a new mutation occurred in the germline of one of the great grandparents: the maternal grandmother carries the mutation, but her mother (and presumably her father) did not. (Data from Nussbaum RL, Boggs BA, Beaudet AL, et al [1986] New mutation and prenatal diagnosis in ornithine transcarbamylase deficiency. Am J Hum Genet 38: 149–158.)

whether appropriate family studies can be performed and are informative (see Chapters 8 and 18).

Alpha-Fetoprotein Assay

Alpha-fetoprotein can be assayed either in amniotic fluid or in maternal serum. Both assays are extremely useful in prenatal diagnosis, chiefly for

assessing the risk of an open neural tube defect but also for other reasons, outlined as follows.

Amniotic Fluid Alpha-Fetoprotein (AFAFP)

Alpha-fetoprotein concentration is measured by immunoassay, a relatively simple and inexpensive method that can be applied to all amniotic fluid

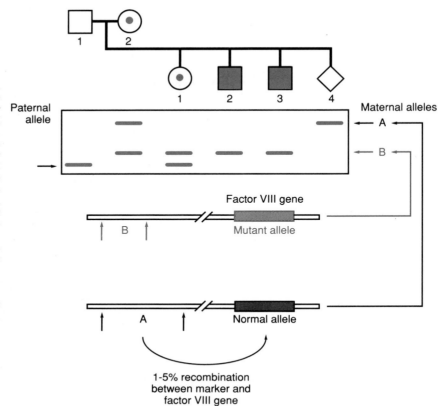

Figure 19–7. Prenatal diagnosis in a family with hemophilia A, made with a polymorphic DNA marker closely linked to the factor VIII gene. In affected boys II-2 and II-3, the B allele at the linked marker is associated with the mutant factor VIII allele. The father has allele C at the linked marker locus. A male fetus has inherited allele A and is predicted to be unaffected with hemophilia A. The polymorphic marker and the factor VIII gene are separated by a genetic distance of 1 to 5 percent recombination. Thus the fetus has a 1 to 5 percent chance of being affected and a 95 to 99 percent chance of being unaffected. (Modified from Antonarakis SE [1989] Diagnosis of genetic disorders at the DNA level. N Engl J Med 320:153–163.)

samples regardless of the specific indication for the amniocentesis. When the AFAFP assay is used in conjunction with ultrasonographic scanning at 18 to 19 weeks' gestation, about 99 percent of fetuses with open spina bifida and virtually all fetuses with anencephaly can be identified. To interpret the findings, the normal range must be established in relation to gestational age and to the factors other than an open neural tube defect (NTD) that can affect the AFAFP level. Abnormally low values are rare, but abnormally high concentrations can result from several conditions other than the presence of an open neural tube defect:

1. Underestimation of gestational age. The concentration is higher at about the 12th to the 14th week than at the 16th week, when amniocentesis is most often performed.
2. Fetal blood contamination.
3. Fetal death.
4. Twin pregnancy.
5. Fetal abnormalities (omphalocele, at least

one form of congenital nephrosis, other rare problems).
6. Genetic variation in the normal concentration.

These causes of an elevated AFAFP level can be identified by ultrasonographic examination.

Although AFAFP concentration is more reliable than MSAFP concentration (discussed next) for diagnosis of open NTDs, MSAFP assay and detailed diagnostic ultrasonography may in some cases be useful alternatives because they do not require amniocentesis. In many prenatal diagnosis programs, second-degree or more remote relatives of patients usually receive only MSAFP assay as a first step.

Maternal Serum Alpha-Fetoprotein (MSAFP)

When the fetus has an open NTD, the concentration of alpha-fetoprotein is likely to be higher than normal in the maternal serum as well as in the

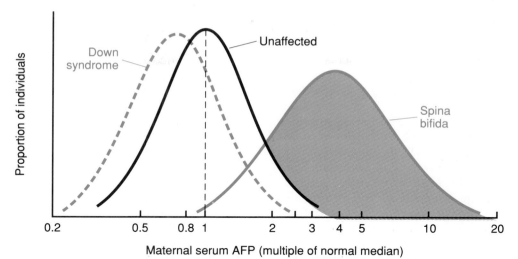

Figure 19-8. Maternal serum alpha-fetoprotein (AFP) concentration, expressed as multiples of the median, in normal fetuses, fetuses with open neural tube defects, and fetuses with Down syndrome. (Redrawn from Wald NJ, Cuckle HS [1987] Recent advances in screening for neural tube defects and Down syndrome. *In* Rodeck C [ed]: Prenatal diagnosis. Baillière Tindall, London, pp. 649–676.)

amniotic fluid. This observation is the basis for the use of MSAFP measurement as a test for open NTDs. Because an estimated 95 percent of infants with NTDs are born into families with no known history of this malformation, a relatively simple test that can be followed up by more specific tests constitutes a significant advance. As shown in Figure 19–8, there is considerable overlap between the normal range for MSAFP and the range of concentration found when the fetus has an open NTD. If an elevated concentration is defined as two multiples of the median, one can estimate that 20 percent of fetuses with open NTDs remain undetected.

Low MSAFP concentration also gives cause for concern. The report that MSAFP tends to be low when the fetus has Down syndrome or other chromosome defects (Merkatz et al., 1984) has led to attempts to take both maternal age and alpha-fetoprotein levels into account in calculating "35-year-equivalent-risk" values: that is, the risk estimates for MSAFP values that, combined with risk estimates for maternal age, yield estimates of a risk of having a fetus with Down syndrome that are equivalent to such a risk for a 35-year-old woman without MSAFP testing (Table 19–5).

In clinical practice, MSAFP assay is likely to become a standard test in all pregnancies; thus it is

even more closely related to the everyday concerns of primary physicians than are the rare abnormalities or even the common genetic defects that form so much of the subject matter of medical genetics. Physicians need to be able to interpret high or low concentrations and to know which further tests should be considered in each situation.

Other Tests in Maternal Serum. The concentrations of two other substances in maternal

Table 19–5. MSAFP Levels That Make the Risk of Having a Down Syndrome Fetus in Women Younger than 35 Years Equivalent to the Risk in a Woman Aged 35 (1/380)

Maternal Age	MSAFP Concentration*
35	1.00
34	.84
33	.72
32	.64
31	.59
30	.58
25–29	.51–.56
20–24	.43–.49

Source: Milunsky A (1986) Genetic disorders of the fetus, 2nd ed. Plenum Press, New York.
* In multiples of the median.

serum, unconjugated estriol and human chorionic gonadotrophin (HCG), have also been found to be unusual when the fetus has Down syndrome. The level of unconjugated estriol is *reduced*, with a median value of approximately 0.79 multiples of the median, in comparison with controls. (By definition, the control multiple of the median is 1.0.) Unconjugated estriol concentration is also reduced in women who are smokers and in general in cases of fetal immaturity. HCG in maternal serum is significantly *higher* than normal, with a median of 2 multiples of the median, when the fetus has Down syndrome. Maternal age and measurement of alpha-fetoprotein, unconjugated estriol, and HCG in maternal serum can be used together to improve the rate of detection of pregnancies with a high risk of a chromosomally abnormal fetus, which can then be specifically diagnosed by amniocentesis (Wald et al., 1988). Rigorous evaluation of the ability of these maternal serum tests to accurately predict high-risk pregnancies is eagerly awaited; if confirmed and found to be reliable, these prenatal tests might be offered to all pregnant women, regardless of age, and would therefore be expected to have a significant impact on the diagnosis and birth incidence of Down syndrome.

CONCLUDING COMMENTS

Prenatal diagnosis is a constantly changing field, with expanding knowledge and new technologies; thus any attempt to define the state of the art rapidly becomes outdated. Physicians need to be aware of the likelihood of changes and the importance of obtaining access to the latest information, which should be available to them through prenatal diagnosis programs or genetic clinics. By the same token, genetic clinics must accept the responsibility of keeping current with new developments and the practicalities of obtaining access to them. Families who may use prenatal diagnosis should also be made aware of the importance of obtaining the latest information before undertaking a pregnancy or before making an irrevocable decision not to reproduce. Many couples at risk of having a child with a severe genetic disorder have been able to have healthy children because of prenatal diagnosis.

The Effect of Prenatal Diagnosis on the Prevention of Inherited Disease

At the population level, diagnosis combined with elective abortion has led to a major decline in the incidence of a few serious disorders in designated population groups, namely Tay-Sachs disease and β-thalassemia. However, prenatal diagnosis cannot reduce the gene frequency of these disorders because it is usually the heterozygotes who propagate the genes. In fact, there is a possibility that the frequency of some deleterious genes will increase if couples compensate for the loss of homozygotes by having additional children, who have a two-thirds risk of being heterozygotes.

The advantage of prenatal diagnosis is not to the population but to the immediate family. Parents at risk of having a child with a serious abnormality can undertake pregnancies that they may otherwise not have risked, with the knowledge that they can learn early in a pregnancy whether their child has the abnormality.

People involved in prenatal diagnosis, parents and health professionals alike, must give consideration to its ethical aspects. New reproductive technologies have added to the ethical concerns. The difficulty, as always, is to balance the benefits to individuals against the benefits to society as a whole. To deal with the future and its unknown possibilities, health professionals and the families with whom they work need to be aware of developments in both applied and basic genetic research. Indeed, the application of genetic knowledge to the improvement of human health is the ultimate goal of genetics in medicine.

General References

Boehm CS (1988) Prenatal diagnosis and carrier detection by DNA analysis. Prog Med Genet 7:143–179.
Goldberg JD, Golbus MS (1988) Chorionic villus sampling. Adv Hum Genet 17:1–25.
Milunsky A (ed) (1986) Genetic disorders and the fetus: Diagnosis, prevention, and treatment, 2nd ed. Plenum Press, New York.
Simpson JL, Elias S (1989) Prenatal diagnosis of genetic disorders. *In* Creasy RK, Resnik R (eds) Maternal-fetal medicine. WB Saunders, Philadelphia, pp. 78–107.

Problems

1. Match the term in the top section with the appropriate comment in the bottom section.
   - (a) Rh immune globulin
   - (b) 9th week of pregnancy
   - (c) Cordocentesis
   - (d) Mosaicism
   - (e) 16th week of pregnancy
   - (f) Alpha-fetoprotein in maternal serum
   - (g) Aneuploidy
   - (h) Cystic hygroma
   - (i) Chorionic villi
   - (j) Amniotic fluid

   _____ Method of obtaining fetal blood for karyotyping
   _____ Usual time at which amniocentesis is performed
   _____ Reduced level when fetus has Down syndrome
   _____ Contains fetal cells viable in culture
   _____ Major cytogenetic problem in prenatal diagnosis
   _____ Ultrasonographic diagnosis indicates possible Turner syndrome
   _____ Risk increases with maternal age
   _____ Usual time at which CVS is performed
   _____ Derived from extraembryonic tissue
   _____ Used to prevent immunization of Rh-negative women

2. A couple has a child with Down syndrome, who has a 21q21q translocation inherited from the mother. Could prenatal diagnosis be helpful in the couple's next pregnancy? Explain.

3. Cultured cells from a chorionic villus sample show two cell lines: 46,XX and 46,XY. Does this necessarily mean the fetus is abnormal? Explain.

4. What two chief types of information about a fetus can be indicated (though not proved) by assay of alpha-fetoprotein in maternal serum?

5. If all fetuses with the following disorders could be identified and the pregnancies were terminated, what would be the effect on the population frequency of the disease? On the population frequency of mutant alleles at the locus?
   - a) PKU
   - b) Neurofibromatosis, type 1
   - c) Huntington disease

6. A couple has had a first-trimester spontaneous abortion in their first pregnancy and requests counseling.
   - a) What proportion of all pregnancies abort in the first trimester?
   - b) What is the most common genetic abnormality found in such cases?
   - c) Assuming that there are no other indications, should this couple be offered prenatal diagnosis for their next pregnancy?

7. A couple has a boy with galactosemia, an autosomal recessive disorder, and requests prenatal diagnosis. The Molecular Diagnostic Laboratory at your hospital uses a complementary DNA probe for the GALT gene and Southern blotting and finds that the family is informative for a restriction fragment length polymorphism (RFLP) with two alleles. Both parents are heterozygous and their affected child is homozygous for allele 1. His unaffected sister is homozygous for allele 2. The fetus is heterozygous.
   - a) Which allele in each parent is in coupling with the mutant galactosemia allele?
   - b) What diagnosis would you give the family regarding the fetus?
   - c) What is the sister's likely genotype?
   - d) Should the laboratory consider the possibility of recombination between the mutation and the linked RFLP? Explain.

8. Discuss the relative advantages and disadvantages of the following diagnostic procedures and cite types of disorders in which they are indicated or not indicated: biochemical assays of enzyme activity; Southern blotting for linkage analysis; allele-specific testing with allele-specific oligonucleotides or the polymerase chain reaction.

GLOSSARY

Acceptor splice site The boundary between the 3′ end of an intron and the 5′ end of the adjacent exon.

Acentric A chromosome fragment lacking a centromere.

Acrocentric A chromosome with the centromere near one end; in humans the acrocentric chromosomes (13, 14, 15, 21, and 22) have satellited short arms that carry genes for ribosomal RNA.

Allele One of the alternative versions of a gene that may occupy a given locus.

Allelic heterogeneity The situation in which there are different mutant alleles at the same locus, each capable of producing an abnormal phenotype.

Allogenic In transplantation, denotes individuals (or tissues) of the same species, but having different antigens.

***Alu* repeat sequence** In the human genome, one of a set of about 300,000 dispersed, related sequences each about 300 base pairs long, so named because they have an *Alu* I cleavage site near the middle of the sequence.

Amino acids The building blocks of protein, for which DNA carries the genetic code. The amino acids are listed in Table 3–3.

Amniocentesis A procedure used in prenatal diagnosis to obtain amniotic fluid. Amniotic fluid is withdrawn from the amniotic sac by syringe after insertion of a hollow needle into the amnion through the abdominal wall and uterine wall.

Amplification In molecular biology, the production of multiple copies of a sequence of DNA.

Anaphase The phase of mitosis or meiosis at which the chromosomes leave the equatorial plate and pass to the poles of the cell.

Aneuploid Any chromosome number that is not an exact multiple of the haploid number. Also, an individual with an aneuploid chromosome number. The common forms of aneuploidy in humans are trisomy (the presence of an extra chromosome) or monosomy (the absence of a single chromosome).

Anticipation The term used to denote the progressively earlier appearance and increased severity of a disease in successive generations. It is thought to result from bias of ascertainment.

Antisense strand of DNA The noncoding DNA strand, which is complementary to mRNA and serves as the template for RNA synthesis. Also called *the transcribed strand.*

Ascertainment The method of selection of individuals for inclusion in a genetic study.

Association The occurrence together in a population of two or more phenotypic characteristics more often than expected by chance. Not to be confused with *linkage.*

Assortative mating Selection of a mate with preference for a particular genotype; that is, nonrandom mating. May be positive (preference for a mate of the same genotype) or negative (preference for a mate of a different genotype).

Assortment The random distribution of different combinations of the parental chromosomes to the gametes. Nonallelic genes assort independently to the gametes, unless they are linked.

Autosome Any nuclear chromosome other than the sex chromosomes; 22 pairs in the human karyotype.

Bacteriophage A virus that infects bacteria, used in molecular biology as a vector for cloning.

Banding A technique of staining chromosomes in a characteristic pattern of lateral bands. See *G bands, Q bands*.

Barr body The sex chromatin, as seen in female somatic cells, representing an inactive X chromosome. Named for Murray Barr.

Base pair (bp) A pair of complementary nucleotide bases, as in double-stranded DNA. Used as the unit of measurement of the length of a DNA sequence.

Bayesian analysis A mathematical method widely used in genetic counseling to calculate recurrence risks. The method combines information from several sources (genetics, pedigree information, and test results) to determine the probability that a specific individual might develop or transmit a certain disorder.

Benign trait A variant trait with no clinical significance.

Bivalent A pair of homologous chromosomes in association as seen at metaphase of the first meiotic division.

Blood group A genetically determined antigen on a red cell. The antigens formed by a set of allelic genes make up a blood group system.

Candidate gene In a search for a disease gene, a candidate gene is a gene known to be located in the region of interest whose product has biochemical or other properties suggesting that it may prove to be the disease gene being sought.

Cap A modified nucleotide added to the 5′ end of a growing mRNA chain, apparently required for normal processing, stability, and translation of mRNA.

Cap site The site of initiation of transcription.

Carrier An individual heterozygous for a particular (often mutant) allele. The term is used for heterozygotes for autosomal recessive alleles, for females heterozygous for X-linked alleles, or, less commonly, for an individual heterozygous for an autosomal dominant allele but not expressing it (e.g., a heterozygote for the Huntington disease allele in the presymptomatic stage).

CCAAT box A DNA sequence found about 75 to 80 base pairs upstream from the transcription initiation site of many genes, important in transcription.

cDNA Complementary DNA or copy DNA, synthetic DNA transcribed from a specific RNA through the action of the enzyme reverse transcriptase. To be distinguished from *genomic DNA*.

CentiMorgan (cM) The unit of linkage, named for Thomas Hunt Morgan. Two loci are 1 cM apart if recombination is detected between them in 1 percent of meioses.

Centromere The primary constriction along the chromosome, a region at which the sister chromatids are held together and at which the kinetochore is formed.

Chain termination mutation A mutation that generates a stop codon, thus preventing further synthesis of the polypeptide chain.

Chiasma Literally, a cross. The term refers to the crossing of chromatid strands of homologous chromosomes, seen at the diplotene of the first meiotic division. Chiasmata are thought to be evidence of interchange of chromosomal material (crossovers) between members of a chromosome pair.

Chimera An individual composed of cells from two different zygotes. In humans, *blood group chimeras* result from exchange of hematopoietic stem cells by dizygotic twins in utero; *dispermic chimeras*, which are very rare, result from fusion of two zygotes into one individual. In mice, chimeras can be generated experimentally by gene transfer studies.

Chorionic villus sampling (CVS) A procedure used for prenatal diagnosis at 8 to 10 weeks' gestation. Fetal tissue for analysis is withdrawn from the villous area of the chorion either transcervically or transabdominally, under ultrasonographic guidance.

Chromatid In a dividing cell, after DNA synthesis, a chromosome is seen to be composed of two identical parallel strands, the sister chromatids, connected at the centromere. At anaphase, the chromatids separate, each becoming a chromosome of a daughter cell. At the subsequent S phase, the chromosome is replicated and again is made up of paired chromatids.

Chromatin The association of DNA and proteins of which chromosomes are composed.

Chromomere A densely coiled region of chromatin on a chromosome. Chromomeres give the extended chromosome a beaded appearance, especially obvious in meiotic prophase.

Chromosomal disorder A clinical condition caused by an abnormal chromosome constitution in which there is extra or missing chromosome material (either a whole chromosome or a chromosome segment).

Chromosomal satellite A small mass of chromatin at the end of the short arm of each chromatid of an acrocentric chromosome. Not to be confused with *satellite DNA*.

Chromosome jumping A method of molecular cloning that allows the cloning of DNA sequences up to 100 kb away from a starting clone.

Chromosome walking A method of molecular cloning that involves the sequential isolation of clones carrying overlapping sequences of DNA, eventually allowing long sequences of DNA to be cloned. The standard method of trying to locate a specific gene within a defined region.

Clinical heterogeneity The production of clinically different phenotypes from mutations in the same gene.

Clone A cell line derived by mitosis from a single ancestral diploid cell. In molecular biology, a copy of DNA sequences created by recombinant DNA techniques.

Coding strand In double-stranded DNA, the strand that has the same 5'-to-3' sense (and sequence, except that T substitutes for U in mRNA) as does mRNA. The coding strand is the strand that is *not* transcribed by RNA polymerase. Also called the *sense strand*.

Codominant If both alleles of a pair are expressed in the heterozygous state, then the alleles (or the traits determined by them, or both) are codominant.

Codon A triplet of three bases in a DNA or RNA molecule, specifying a single amino acid.

Coefficient of inbreeding (F) The probability that an individual has received both alleles of a pair from an identical ancestral source. Also, the proportion of loci at which an individual is homozygous by descent.

Cofactor-responsive disease A genetic disease in which a specific biochemical abnormality affecting a single mutant protein (usually an enzyme) is corrected by the administration of pharmacological amounts of the specific cofactor of the mutant protein (e.g., vitamin B_6-responsive homocystinuria).

Colinearity The parallel relationship between the base sequence of the DNA of a gene (or the RNA transcribed from it) and the amino acid sequence of the corresponding polypeptide.

Complementarity The complementary nature of base pairing in DNA.

Complementary DNA (cDNA) DNA synthesized from a messenger RNA template, through the enzyme reverse transcriptase. See *genomic DNA* for comparison.

Complementation In genetics, the ability of two different genetic defects to correct for one another, thus demonstrating that the defects are not identical.

Compound (compound heterozygote) An individual, or a genotype, with two different mutant alleles at the same locus.

Concordant In human genetics, a twin pair in which both members exhibit a certain trait.

Conditional probability In Bayesian analysis, this is the chance of an observed outcome given the prior probability of the consultand's genotype. The product of the prior and conditional probabilities is the joint probability.

Congenital Present at birth; not necessarily genetic.

Consanguinity Relationship by descent from a common ancestor.

Consensus sequence In genes or proteins, an idealized sequence in which each base or amino acid residue represents the one most frequently found at that position when many actual sequences are compared. For example, the consensus sequence for splice donor or acceptor sites.

Consultand The individual requesting genetic counseling.

Contact inhibition The property of normal cells in culture that cease to grow when they come into contact with one another. This property is lost by malignant cells.

Contiguous gene syndrome A syndrome resulting from a microdeletion of chromosomal DNA extending over two or more contiguous loci. Also called *segmental aneusomy*.

CRM Cross-reacting material. A protein produced by a mutant gene that reacts antigenically with antibody against the unaltered protein.

Crossover or crossing over The reciprocal exchange of segments between chromatids of homologous chromosomes, a characteristic of prophase of the first meiotic division. See also *recombination*.

Cryptic splice site A DNA sequence similar to the consensus splice site but not normally used. Used when the normal splice site is altered by mutation or when a mutation in the cryptic site increases its use by the splicing apparatus. May be in a coding or a noncoding sequence.

Cytogenetics The study of the relationship of the microscopic appearance of chromosomes and their behavior during cell division to the genotype and phenotype of the individual. More generally, the study of human chromosomes and their abnormalities.

Cytotrophoblast The fetal cells of the chorionic villi that are sampled for karyotyping and DNA analysis.

Degeneracy of the code The genetic code is described as degenerate because most of the 20 amino acids are specified by more than one of the 64 codons.

Deletion The loss of a sequence of DNA from a chromosome. The deleted DNA may be of any length from a single base to a large part of a chromosome.

Denaturation The conversion of DNA from the double-stranded to the single-stranded state, usually accomplished by heating to destroy chemical bonds involved in base pairing.

Deoxyribonucleic acid See *DNA.*

Dermatoglyphics The patterns of the ridged skin of the digits, palms, and soles, which are useful in the diagnosis of Down syndrome and some other disorders.

Dicentric A structurally abnormal chromosome with two centromeres.

Dictyotene The stage of the first meiotic division in which a human oocyte remains from late fetal life until ovulation.

Diploid The number of chromosomes in most somatic cells, which is double the number found in the gametes. In humans, the diploid chromosome number is 46.

Discordant In human genetics, a twin pair of which one member shows a certain trait and the other does not. See *concordant*.

Dizygotic (DZ) twins Twins produced by two separate ova, separately fertilized. Also called *fraternal twins*.

DNA (deoxyribonucleic acid) The molecule that encodes the genes responsible for the structure and function of living organisms and allows the transmission of genetic information from generation to generation.

DNA methylation Addition of a methyl residue to a cytosine base in the DNA molecule to form 5-methylcytosine. C bases are methylated chiefly when they are in a CpG sequence and base paired with a previously methylated sequence; thus a methylation pattern can be maintained throughout a series of cell divisions. Plays an important but not completely understood role in gene expression.

DNA polymerase An enzyme that can synthesize a new DNA strand, using a previously synthesized DNA strand as a template.

Domain A region of the amino acid sequence of a protein that can be equated with a particular function, or a corresponding segment of a gene.

Dominant A trait is dominant if it is phenotypically expressed in heterozygotes. Modifications of this definition are discussed in the text.

Dominant negative mutation A mutation in a polypeptide that disrupts the function of the wild-type allele in the same cell.

Donor splice site The boundary between the 3′ end of an exon and the 5′ end of the next intron.

Dosage compensation As a consequence of X inactivation, the amount of product formed by the two copies of an X-lined gene in females is equivalent to the amount formed by the single gene in males. See *X inactivation*.

Double heterozygote An individual who is heterozygous at each of two different loci. Contrast with *compound heterozygote*.

Dysmorphism Morphological developmental abnormalities, as seen in many syndromes of genetic or environmental origin.

Ecogenetic disorder A disorder resulting from the interaction of a genetic predisposition to a specific disease with an environmental factor.

Empiric risk The probability that a trait will occur or recur in a family, based on past experience rather than on knowledge of the causative mechanism.

Enhancer A DNA sequence that acts in *cis* (i.e., on the same chromosome) to increase transcription of a nearby gene. The enhancer may be upstream or downstream to the gene and may be in the same or the reverse orientation.

Enzymopathy A metabolic disorder resulting from deficiency or abnormality of a specific enzyme.

Epigenetic The term that refers to any factor that can affect the phenotype without change in the genotype.

Euchromatin The chromatin that shows the staining characteristics of the chromosome arms and the majority of the chromosome complement, decondensing and becoming light-staining during interphase. Contrast with *heterochromatin*.

Eukaryote A unicellular or multicellular organism in which the cells have a nucleus with a nuclear membrane and other specialized characteristics. See also *prokaryote*.

Euploid Any chromosome number that is an exact multiple of the number in a haploid gamete (n). Most somatic cells are diploid (2n). Contrast with *aneuploid*.

Exon A transcribed region of a gene that is present in mature messenger RNA.

Expressivity The extent to which a genetic defect is expressed. If there is variable expressivity, the trait may vary in expression from mild to severe but is never completely unexpressed in individuals who have the corresponding genotype.

F See *coefficient of inbreeding.*

F_1 ("F one") The first-generation progeny of a mating.

Familial Any trait that is more common in relatives of an affected individual than in the general population, whether the cause is genetic, environmental, or both.

Fetoscopy A technique for direct visualization of the fetus.

Fitness (f) The probability of transmitting one's genes to the next generation and of their survival in that generation to be passed on to the next, in relation to the average probability for the population.

Flanking sequence A region of a gene preceding or following the transcribed region.

Founder effect A high frequency of a mutant gene in a population founded by a small ancestral group when one or more of the founders was a carrier of the mutant gene.

Frameshift mutation A mutation involving a deletion or insertion that is not an exact multiple of 3 base pairs and thus changes the reading frame of the gene. The stop codon thus formed will not be the normal one, and in almost all cases a truncated or elongated protein will be made.

G bands The dark and light cross-bands seen in chromosomes after treatment with trypsin and Giemsa stain.

Gamete A reproductive cell (ovum or sperm) with the haploid chromosome number.

Gene A hereditary unit; in molecular terms, a sequence of chromosomal DNA that is required for production of a functional product.

Gene dosage The number of copies of a particular gene in the genome.

Gene family A set of genes containing related exons, indicating that the genes have evolved from an ancestral gene by duplication and subsequent divergence.

Gene flow Gradual diffusion of genes from one population to another by migration and mating.

Gene map A representation of chromosomal locations of mapped genes.

Gene pool All the genes present at a given locus in the population.

Genes in common Those genes inherited by two individuals from a common ancestral source.

Genetic Determined by genes. Not to be confused with *congenital.*

Genetic code The base triplets that specify the 20 amino acids found in proteins. (See Table 3–3.)

Genetic compound A genotype, or an individual, with two different mutant alleles at the same locus. Not to be confused with a *homozygote,* in whom the mutant alleles are identical.

Genetic counseling The provision of information to affected individuals or family members at risk of a disorder that may be genetic, concerning the consequences of the disorder, the probability of developing or transmitting it, and the ways in which it may be prevented or ameliorated.

Genetic drift Random fluctuation of gene frequencies in small populations.

Genetic heterogeneity The occurrence of the same or similar phenotypes from different genetic mechanisms. See *allelic heterogeneity, clinical heterogeneity, locus heterogeneity.*

Genetic lethal A gene or genetically determined trait that leads to failure to reproduce, although not necessarily to early death.

Genetic load The sum total of death and defect caused by mutant genes.

Genetic marker A locus that has readily classifiable alleles and can be used in genetic studies. It may be a gene or a restriction enzyme site, or any characteristic of DNA that allows different versions of a locus (or its product) to be distinguished from each other and followed through families. See *polymorphism.*

Genetic screening Testing on a population basis to identify individuals at risk of having or of transmitting a specific disorder.

Genome The complete DNA sequence, containing the entire genetic information, of a gamete, an individual, a population, or a species.

Genomic DNA The chromosomal DNA sequence of a gene or segment of a gene, including the DNA sequence of noncoding as well as coding regions. Also, DNA that has been isolated directly from cells or chromosomes or the cloned copies of all or part of such DNA.

Genotype (1) The genetic constitution (genome). (2) More specifically, the alleles present at one locus.

Germline The cell line from which gametes are derived.

Germline mosaicism In an individual, the presence of two or more genetically different types of germline cells, resulting from mutation during the proliferation and differentiation of the germline.

Giemsa banding Treatment of human chromosomes with trypsin and Giemsa stain to produce a characteristic pattern of transverse dark and light bands (G bands).

Haploid The chromosome number of a normal gamete, with only one member of each chromosome pair. In humans, the haploid number is 23.

Haplotype (1) A group of alleles from closely linked loci, usually inherited as a unit. (2) A set of restriction fragment lengths closely linked to one another and to a gene of interest.

Hardy-Weinberg law The law that relates gene frequency to genotype frequency, used in clinical genetics to determine allele frequency and heterozygote frequency when the incidence of a disorder is known.

Hemizygous A term that describes the genotype of an individual who has only one representative of a chromosome or chromosome segment, rather than the usual two; refers especially to X-linked genes in the male but also applies to genes on any chromosome segment that is deleted on the homologous chromosome.

Heritability A statistical measure of the degree to which a trait is genetically determined.

Heterochromatin Chromatin that stains darkly throughout the cell cycle, even in interphase. Generally thought to be late replicating and genetically inactive. Composed of satellite DNA in regions such as centromeres, acrocentric short arms, and 1qh, 9qh, 16qh, and Yqh (*constitutive heterochromatin*). The inactive X chromosome is sometimes also referred to as *facultative heterochromatin.*

Heterogeneity See *allelic heterogeneity, clinical heterogeneity, genetic heterogeneity, locus heterogeneity.*

Heterokaryon A cell with two separate nuclei, formed by fusion of two genetically different cells.

Heteromorphism A normal morphological or staining variant of a chromosome.

Heteroploid Any chromosome number other than the normal.

Heterozygote (heterozygous) An individual or genotype with two different alleles at a given locus on a pair of homologous chromosomes. Typically, one allele is the normal form, and the other is mutant, but the term is also used to refer to heterozygosity for different normal alleles.

Histocompatibility A host will accept a particular graft only if it is histocompatible — that is, if the graft contains no antigens that the host lacks.

Histones Proteins associated with DNA in the chromosomes, rich in basic amino acids (lysine or arginine) and virtually invariant throughout eukaryote evolution.

Holandric A pattern of inheritance of genes on the Y chromosomes from a father to all his sons but none of his daughters.

Holoenzyme The functional compound formed by the binding of an apoenzyme and its appropriate coenzyme.

Homeobox gene A gene that contains a conserved 180 base pair coding region termed a *homeobox*. The 60 amino acid residues of the homeobox encode a DNA binding domain, which is consistent with the role of homeobox genes in regulating gene expression, particularly in development.

Homologous chromosomes (homologs) A pair of chromosomes of one type, one inherited from each parent, having the same gene loci in the same order. (Exception: see *uniparental disomy.*)

Homozygote (homozygous) An individual or genotype with identical alleles at a given locus on a pair of homologous chromosomes.

Housekeeping genes Genes expressed in most or all cells because their products provide basic functions.

Human Genome Project A major current research project, international in scope, that aims to map and sequence the entire human genome.

Hybrid cell A cell formed by fusion of two cells of different origin in which the two nuclei have merged into one. Can be cloned to produce hybrid cell lines.

Hybridization In molecular biology, complementary pairing of an RNA and a DNA strand or of two different DNA strands (reannealing). In somatic cell genetics, fusion of two somatic cells, often from different organisms, to form a hybrid cell containing the genetic information of both parental cell types.

Immunoblot See *Western blot.*

Imprinting The differential expression of genetic material, at either a chromosomal or an allelic level, depending on whether the genetic material has been inherited from the male or female parent.

Inborn error of metabolism A genetically determined biochemical disorder in which a specific protein defect produces a metabolic block that may have pathological consequences.

Inbreeding The mating of closely related individuals. The progeny of close relatives are said to be *inbred.*

Index case An affected family member who first draws attention to a pedigree of a genetic disorder. See *proband.*

Insertion A chromosomal abnormality in which a DNA segment from one chromosome is inserted into a nonhomologous chromosome.

In situ hybridization Mapping a gene by molecular hybridization of a cloned DNA sequence, labeled by radioactivity or fluorescence, to a chromosome spread on a slide.

Intergenic DNA The untranscribed DNA of unknown function that makes up a large proportion of the total DNA.

Interphase The part of the cell cycle between two successive mitoses.

Intervening sequence See *intron.*

Intron A segment of a gene that is initially transcribed but is then removed from within the primary RNA transcript by splicing together the sequences (exons) on either side of it.

Inversion A chromosomal rearrangement in which a segment of a chromosome is reversed end to end. If the centromere is included in the inversion, the inversion is *pericentric;* if not, it is *paracentric.*

Isochromosome An abnormal chromosome in which one arm is duplicated (forming two arms of equal length, with the same loci in reverse sequence), and the other arm is deleted.

Isolate A subpopulation in which matings take place exclusively or usually with other members of the same subpopulation.

Isolated case An individual who is the only member of his or her kindred affected by a genetic disorder, either by chance or by new mutation. See also *sporadic*.

Karyotype The chromosome constitution of an individual. The term is also used for a photomicrograph of the chromosomes of an individual arranged in the standard classification and for the process of preparing such a photomicrograph.

kb (kilobase) A unit of 1000 bases in a DNA or RNA sequence. In double-stranded DNA, kilobase pairs.

Kindred An extended family.

Kinetochore A structure at the centromere to which the spindle fibers are attached.

L1 repeat sequence A family of moderately repetitive DNA composed of many thousands of copies of long (approximately 1 to 6 kb) interspersed sequences.

Linkage Genes on the same chromosome show linkage if they have a tendency to be transmitted together through meiosis. Contrast with *synteny*.

Linkage disequilibrium The tendency of specific combinations of alleles at two or more linked loci to occur together on the same chromosome more frequently than would be expected by chance.

Linkage map A chromosome map showing the relative positions of genes and other DNA markers on the chromosomes, as determined by linkage studies.

Locus The position of a gene on a chromosome. Different forms of the gene (alleles) may occupy the locus.

Locus heterogeneity The situation in which mutations at two or more distinct loci can produce the same or closely similar phenotypes.

Lod score A statistical method that tests genetic marker data in families to determine whether two loci are linked. The lod score is the logarithm to base 10 of the odds in favor of linkage. By convention, a lod score of 3 (odds of 1000:1 in favor) is taken as proof of linkage, and a lod score of -2 (100:1 against) as proof that the loci are unlinked. (See Appendix III.)

Lyonization A term used for the phenomenon of X inactivation, which was first proposed by the geneticist Mary Lyon.

Major histocompatibility complex (MHC) The complex locus on chromosome 6p that includes the highly polymorphic human leukocyte antigen (HLA) genes.

Manifesting heterozygote A female heterozygous for an X-linked disorder in whom, because of nonrandom X inactivation, the trait is expressed clinically with approximately the same degree of severity as in hemizygous affected males.

Meiosis The special type of cell division occurring in the germ cells by which gametes containing the haploid chromosome number are produced from diploid cells. Two meiotic divisions occur: meiosis I and meiosis II. Reduction in number takes place during meiosis I. Not to be confused with *mitosis*.

Messenger RNA (mRNA) An RNA, transcribed from the DNA of a gene, that directs the sequence of amino acids of the encoded polypeptide.

Metaphase The stage of mitosis or meiosis in which the chromosomes have reached their maximal condensation and are lined up on the equatorial plane of the cell, attached to the spindle fibers. This is the stage at which chromosomes are most easily studied.

Methemoglobin The oxidized form of hemoglobin, containing iron in the ferric rather than the ferrous state, and incapable of binding oxygen.

Microdeletion A chromosomal deletion too small to be seen under the microscope. See also *contiguous gene syndrome.*

Missense mutation Mutation that changes a codon specific for one amino acid to specify another amino acid.

Mitochondrial DNA The DNA in the circular chromosome of the mitochondria, which are cytoplasmic organelles that possess their own unique DNA. Mitochondrial DNA is present in many copies per cell, is maternally inherited, and evolves 5 to 10 times as rapidly as genomic DNA.

Mitochondrial inheritance The inheritance of a disorder encoded in the mitochondrial genome.

Mitosis The process of ordinary cell division, resulting in the formation of two cells genetically identical to the parent cell. Not to be confused with *meiosis.*

Monosomy A chromosome constitution in which one member of a chromosome pair is missing, as in 45,X Turner syndrome.

Monozygotic (MZ) twins Twins derived from a single zygote and thus genetically identical.

Mosaic An individual or tissue with at least two cell lines differing in genotype or karyotype, derived from a single zygote. Not to be confused with *chimera.*

Mosaicism In an individual or in one or more tissues, the condition in which there are two or more cell lines, derived from a single zygote but differing genetically because of postzygotic mutation or nondisjunction.

Multifactorial inheritance The type of inheritance shown by traits that are determined by a combination of multiple factors, genetic and possibly also environmental.

Multiplex Refers to a pedigree in which there is more than one case of a particular disorder.

Mutagen An agent that increases the spontaneous mutation rate by causing changes in DNA.

Mutant A gene that has been altered by mutation; an individual carrying a mutant gene.

Mutation Any permanent heritable change in the sequence of genomic DNA.

Mutation rate (μ) The frequency of mutation at a given locus, expressed as mutations per locus per gamete (or per generation, which is the same).

Noncoding strand See *antisense strand.*

Nondisjunction The failure of two members of a chromosome pair to disjoin during meiosis I, or two chromatids of a chromosome to disjoin during meiosis II or mitosis, so that both pass to one daughter cell and the other daughter cell receives neither.

Nonsense mutation A single-base substitution in DNA resulting in a chain-termination codon.

Northern blot A blotting technique, named for its analogy to Southern blotting, for detection of RNA molecules by hybridization to a complementary DNA probe.

Nucleosome The primary structural unit of chromatin, consisting of 146 base pairs of DNA wrapped twice around a core of eight histone molecules.

Nucleotide A molecule composed of a nitrogenous base, a 5-carbon sugar, and a phosphate group. A nucleic acid is a polymer of many nucleotides.

Null mutation An allele that results either in the absence of the gene product or absence of any function at the phenotypic level.

Obligate heterozygote An individual who may be clinically unaffected but on the basis of pedigree analysis must carry a mutant allele.

Oligonucleotide A short DNA molecule (usually 8 to 50 base pairs), synthesized for use as a probe.

Oncogene A dominantly acting gene involved in unregulated cell growth and proliferation, responsible for tumor development. Mutation, overexpression, or amplification of oncogenes in somatic cells may lead to neoplastic transformation. Contrast with *proto-oncogene* and with *tumor-suppressor gene*.

Ontogeny The developmental history of an organism.

p In cytogenetics, the short arm of a chromosome (from the French *petit*). In population genetics, the frequency of the more common allele of a pair. In biochemistry, abbreviation of *protein* (e.g., p53 is a protein 53 kilodaltons in size).

Palindrome In molecular biology, a nucleotide sequence in which the 5' to 3' sequence of one strand of a segment of DNA is the same as that of its complementary strand. The sites of many restriction enzymes are palindromes.

PCR See *polymerase chain reaction*.

Pedigree In medical genetics, a diagram of a family history indicating the family members, their relationship to the proband, and their status with respect to a particular hereditary condition.

Penetrance Concept referring to the all-or-none expression of a mutant genotype. Usually refers to dominant traits in heterozygotes. If a condition is expressed in less than 100 percent of persons who carry the responsible allele, it is said to have *reduced penetrance*; if, for example, only 70 percent of persons with the allele express the trait, it is 70 percent penetrant. Contrast with *expressivity*.

Pharmacogenetics The area of biochemical genetics concerned with drug responses and their genetically controlled variations.

Phenocopy A mimic of a phenotype that is usually determined by a specific genotype, produced instead by the interaction of some environmental factor with a different genotype.

Phenotype The observed biochemical, physiological, and morphological characteristics of an individual, as determined by his or her genotype and the environment in which it is expressed. Also, in a more limited sense, the expression of some particular gene or genes.

Philadelphia chromosome (Ph¹) The structurally abnormal chromosome 22 that typically occurs in a proportion of the bone marrow cells in most patients with chronic myelogenous leukemia. The abnormality is a reciprocal translocation between the distal portion of the long arm of chromosome 22 and the distal portion of the long arm of chromosome 9.

PIC See *polymorphism information content*.

Plasmid Independently replicating, extrachromosomal circular DNA molecules in bacteria, used in molecular biology as vectors for cloned segments of DNA.

Pleiotropy Multiple phenotypic effects of a single gene or gene pair. The term is used particularly when the effects are ordinarily thought to be unrelated.

Point mutation A single nucleotide base pair change in DNA.

Polyadenylation site In the synthesis of mature mRNA, a site at which a sequence of 20 to 200 adenosine residues (the polyA tail) is added to the 3' end of an RNA transcript, aiding its transport out of the nucleus and usually its stability.

Polygenic Inheritance determined by many genes at different loci, with small additive effects. Also termed *quantitative*. Not to be confused with *multifactorial*, in which environmental as well as genetic factors may be involved.

Polymerase chain reaction (PCR) A technique in which a short DNA or RNA sequence can be amplified $> 10^6$ times, by means of two flanking oligonucleotide primers and repeated cycles of amplification with DNA polymerase. Permits analysis of a short sequence from very small quantities of DNA or RNA without the necessity of cloning it first.

Polymorphism The occurrence together in a population of two or more alternative genotypes, each at a frequency greater than that which could be maintained by recurrent mutation alone. A locus is arbitrarily considered to be polymorphic if the rarer allele has a frequency of .01, so that the heterozygote frequency is at least .02.

Polymorphism information content (PIC) A measure of the degree of informativeness of a genetic marker. Depends on the number of alleles at the marker locus and their relative frequencies. The higher the PIC value, the more useful the marker. Formally, the chance that any offspring of any couple will be informative at a particular locus.

Polypeptide A chain of amino acids, held together by peptide bonds between the amino group of one and the carboxyl group of an adjoining one. A protein molecule may be composed of a single polypeptide chain or of two or more identical or different polypeptides.

Polyploid Any multiple of the basic haploid chromosome number other than the diploid number; thus 3n, 4n, and so forth.

Positional cloning The molecular cloning of a gene on the basis of knowledge of its map position, without prior knowledge of the gene product. Sometimes called *reverse genetics*.

Primary constriction See *centromere*.

Primary transcript The first RNA transcript of a gene, containing introns as well as exons.

Private mutation A very rare mutation, perhaps known in only a single family or single population.

Proband The family member through whom the family is ascertained. If affected, may be called the *index case*.

Probe In molecular genetics, a labeled DNA or RNA sequence used to detect the presence of a complementary sequence by molecular hybridization; or a reagent capable of recognizing a desired clone in a mixture of many DNA or RNA sequences.

Prokaryote A simple unicellular organism, such as a bacterium, lacking a separate nucleus and simpler than eukaryotic cells in other ways. See *eukaryote*.

Promoter DNA sequences located in the 5' end of a gene that determine the site of initiation of transcription and the quantity and sometimes the tissue distribution of mRNA.

Prophase The first stage of cell division, during which the chromosomes become visible as discrete structures and subsequently thicken and shorten. Prophase of the first meiotic division is further characterized by pairing (synapsis) of homologous chromosomes.

Propositus See *proband*.

Proto-oncogene A normal gene, involved in some aspect of cell division or proliferation, that if activated by a mutational event is capable of becoming an oncogene. See *oncogene*.

Pseudodominant See *quasidominant*.

Pseudogene An inactive gene within a gene family, derived by mutation of an ancestral active gene. An evolutionary relic.

Pulsed field gel electrophoresis An electrophoretic technique that allows the separation of relatively long sequences of DNA, up to >5000 kb.

q In cytogenetics, the long arm of a chromosome; in population genetics, the frequency of the less common allele of a pair.

Q bands The pattern of bright and dim fluorescent cross-bands seen on chromosomes under ultraviolet light after quinacrine staining.

Quasidominant The pattern of inheritance of an autosomal recessive trait produced by the mating of a homozygous affected person with a heterozygote for the same disorder, so that recessively affected members appear in two or more successive generations.

Random mating Selection of a mate without regard to the genotype of the mate. In a randomly mating population, the frequencies of the various matings are determined solely by the frequencies of the genes concerned.

Reading frame One of three possible ways of reading a nucleotide sequence as a series of triplets. An open reading frame contains no termination codons and thus is potentially translatable into protein.

Recessive A trait or gene that is expressed only in homozygotes or hemizygotes.

Reciprocal translocation Chromosomal rearrangement involving exchange of segments between nonhomologous chromosomes.

Recombinant An individual who has a new combination of genes not found together in either parent. Usually applied to linkage analysis.

Recombinant chromosome A chromosome that results from exchange of reciprocal segments by crossing over in a homologous pair of parental chromosomes during meiosis.

Recombinant DNA A DNA molecule constructed from segments from more than one parental DNA molecule.

Recombination The formation of new combinations of linked genes by crossing over between their loci.

Recurrence risk The probability that a genetic disorder present in one or more members of a family will recur in another member of the same or a subsequent generation.

Reduction division The first meiotic division, so called because at this stage the chromosome number per cell is reduced from diploid to haploid.

Regulatory gene A gene that codes for an RNA or protein molecule that regulates the expression of other genes.

Repetitive DNA DNA sequences that are present in multiple copies in the genome.

Restriction endonuclease An enzyme, derived from bacteria, that can recognize a specific sequence of DNA and cut the (usually double-stranded) DNA molecule within the recognition site or at some nearby site.

Restriction fragment length polymorphism (RFLP) A polymorphic difference in DNA sequence between individuals that can be recognized by restriction endonucleases. See *polymorphism.*

Restriction map A linear array of sites on DNA cleaved by various restriction endonucleases.

Restriction site A short sequence in DNA that can be recognized and cut by a specific restriction endonuclease.

Retrovirus A virus, with an RNA genome, that propagates by conversion of the RNA into DNA by the enzyme reverse transcriptase.

Reverse genetics The molecular approach to identifying genes on the basis of their location in the genome, without knowledge of the gene product. See *positional cloning.*

Reverse transcriptase An enzyme that catalyzes the synthesis of DNA on an RNA template.

RFLP See *restriction fragment length polymorphism.*

Ribonucleic acid See *RNA.*

Ribosomes Cytoplasmic organelles composed of ribosomal RNA and protein, on which polypeptide synthesis from messenger RNA occurs.

Ring chromosome A structurally abnormal chromosome in which the end of each chromosome arm has been deleted and the broken arms have reunited in ring formation.

RNA (ribonucleic acid) A nucleic acid formed upon a DNA template, containing ribose instead of deoxyribose. Messenger RNA (mRNA) is the template on which polypeptides are synthesized. Transfer RNA (tRNA), in cooperation with the ribosomes, brings activated amino acids into position along the mRNA template. Ribosomal RNA (rRNA), a component of the ribosomes, functions as a nonspecific site of polypeptide synthesis. See text for further details.

RNA polymerase An enzyme that synthesizes RNA on a DNA template.

Robertsonian translocation A translocation between two acrocentric chromosomes by fusion at or near the centromere, with loss of the short arms.

Satellite DNA DNA containing many tandem repeats of a short basic repeating unit. Not to be confused with *chromosomal satellite.*

Scaffold The nuclear structure observed when histones are experimentally removed from chromosomes. Thought to represent a structural component of the nucleus and of chromosomes.

Segmental aneusomy Loss of a small segment from one chromosome of a pair, resulting in hemizygosity for genes in that segment on the homologous chromosome. See also *contiguous gene syndrome.*

Segregation In genetics, the separation of alleles at meiosis. Because alleles occupy the same locus on homologous chromosomes, they pass to different gametes; that is, they segregate.

Selection In population genetics, the operation of forces that determine the relative fitness of a genotype in the population, thus affecting the frequency of the gene concerned.

Sense strand See *coding strand.*

Sex chromatin See *Barr body.*

Sex chromosomes Chromosomes responsible for sex determination. In humans, XX in female, XY in male.

Sex-influenced A trait that is not X-linked in its pattern of inheritance but is expressed differently, either in degree or in frequency, in males and females.

Sex-limited A trait that is expressed in only one sex, although the gene that determines the trait is not X-linked.

Sex-linked Old term for X-linked, now little used because formally it fails to distinguish between X- and Y-linkage.

Sib, sibling A brother or a sister. *Sibling* specifically refers to a younger *sib.*

Sibship All the sibs in a family.

Silent allele A mutant gene that has no detectable phenotypic effect.

Simplex In human genetics, the term used to describe a family history with only one member affected by a genetic disorder.

Single-gene disorder A disorder due to one or more mutant alleles at a single locus.

Sister chromatid exchange The exchange of segments of DNA between sister chromatids. Occurs with particularly high frequency in patients with Bloom syndrome.

Somatic cell genetics The study of genetic phenomena in cultured somatic cells.

Somatic cell hybrid See *hybrid cell.*

Somatic mutation A mutation occurring in a somatic cell rather than in the germline.

Southern blot A technique, devised by Ed Southern, for transferring DNA fragments that have been separated by agarose gel electrophoresis to a nitrocellulose filter, on which specific DNA fragments can then be detected by their hybridization to radioactive probes.

Splicing The splicing out of introns and splicing together of exons in the generation of mature mRNA from the primary transcript.

Sporadic In medical genetics, a case of a disease caused by a new mutation.

Stop codon See *termination codon*.

Structural gene A gene coding for any RNA or protein product.

Structural protein A protein that serves a structural role in the body, such as collagen.

Synapsis Close pairing of homologous chromosomes in prophase of the first meiotic division.

Syndrome A characteristic overall pattern of anomalies, presumed to be causally related.

Synteny The physical presence together on the same chromosome of two or more gene loci, whether or not they are close enough together for linkage to be demonstrated.

Tandem repeats Two or more copies of the same (or very similar) DNA sequence arranged in a direct head-to-tail succession along a chromosome.

TATA box A consensus sequence in the promoter region of many genes that is located about 25 base pairs upstream from the start site of transcription and that determines the start site.

Telomere The end of each chromosome arm. Human telomeres end with tandem copies of the sequence $(TTAGGG)_n$, which is required for the proper replication of chromosome ends.

Telophase The stage of cell division that begins when the daughter chromosomes reach the poles of the dividing cell and that lasts until the two daughter cells take on the appearance of interphase cells.

Teratogen An agent that produces or raises the incidence of congenital malformations.

Termination codon One of the three codons (UAG, UAA and UGA) that terminate synthesis of a polypeptide. Also called a *stop codon*. (See Table 3–3.)

Transcription The synthesis of a single-stranded RNA molecule from a DNA template in the cell nucleus, catalyzed by RNA polymerase.

Transfection Transfer of a gene, or cDNA (next to a promoter), into a cell, enabling the transfected cell to form a new gene product.

Transgenic mice Mice that carry a foreign gene (''transgene'') in their genome, produced by injection of oocytes with the foreign DNA. DNA that is integrated into the mouse genome may be expressed. If the transgene has been incorporated into the germline, it may also be transmitted to the progeny.

Transition A mutation in which one purine is substituted for the other (A for G or G for A) or one pyrimidine is substituted for the other (C for T or T for C). See *transversion*.

Translation The synthesis of a polypeptide from its mRNA template.

Translocation The transfer of a segment of one chromosome to another chromosome. If two nonhomologous chromosomes exchange pieces, the translocation is reciprocal. See also *Robertsonian translocation*.

Transversion A mutation in which either purine is substituted for either pyrimidine or vice versa. See *transition*.

Triploid A cell with three copies of each chromosome, or an individual made up of such cells.

Trisomy The state of having three representatives of a given chromosome instead of the usual pair, as in trisomy 21 (Down syndrome).

Tumor-suppressor gene A normal gene involved in the regulation of cell growth. Recessive mutations can lead to tumor development, as in the retinoblastoma gene or the p53 gene. Contrast with *oncogene*.

Ultrasonography A technique in which high-frequency sound waves are used to examine internal body structures, useful in prenatal diagnosis.

Unequal crossing over Crossing over between similar DNA sequences that are mis-aligned, resulting in sequences with deletion or duplication of DNA segments. A cause of a number of genetic variants.

Uniparental disomy The presence in a karyotype of two chromosomes of a pair both inherited from one parent, with no representative of that chromosome from the other parent.

Vector In cloning, the plasmid or phage used to carry a cloned DNA segment.

VNTR (variable number of tandem repeats) A type of DNA polymorphism created by a tandem arrangement of multiple copies of short DNA sequences. Highly polymorphic, used in linkage studies and in DNA "fingerprinting" for paternity testing and forensic medicine.

Western blot Technique analogous to Southern blotting, used for detection of proteins, usually by immunological methods.

Wild type Term used to indicate the normal allele (often symbolized as +) or the normal phenotype.

X;autosome translocation Reciprocal translocation between an X chromosome and an autosome. Of particular medical interest because this type of translocation allows the expression of an X-linked disease in a female if the breakpoint in the X chromosome disrupts a gene.

X inactivation Inactivation of genes on one X chromosome in somatic cells of female mammals, occurring early in embryonic life, at about the time of implantation.

X linkage Genes on the X chromosome, or traits determined by such genes, are X-linked.

Y linkage Genes on the Y chromosome, or traits determined by such genes, are Y-linked.

Zygosity Twins may be either monozygotic (MZ) or dizygotic (DZ). To determine whether a certain twin pair is MZ or DZ is to determine their zygosity.

LITERATURE CITED

(See also General References at the end of each chapter.)

A

Allderdice PW, Browne N, Murphy DP (1975) Chromosome 3 deletion q21 → qter duplication p25 → pter syndrome in children of carriers of a pericentric inversion inv(3) (p25q21). Am J Hum Genet 27:699–718.

Anderson MP, Rich DP, Gregory RJ, et al (1991) Generation of cAMP-activated chloride currents by expression of CFTR. Science 251:679–682.

Antonarakis SE (1988) Molecular genetics of hemophilia A and B. Adv Hum Genet 17:27–59.

Antonarakis SE (1989) Diagnosis of genetic disorders at the DNA level. N Engl J Med 320:153–163.

Antonarakis SE, the Down Syndrome Collaborative Group (1991) Parental origin of the extra chromosome in trisomy 21 as indicated by analysis of DNA polymorphisms. N Engl J Med 324:872–876.

Arias IM, Popper H, Schachter D, Shafritz DA (eds) (1982) The liver: Biology and pathology. Raven Press, New York.

B

Baird PA, Anderson TW, Newcombe HB, Lowry RB (1988) Genetic disorders in children and young adults: A population study. Am J Hum Genet 42:677–693.

Baird PA, Sadovnick AD (1988) Causes of death to age 30 in Down syndrome. Am J Hum Genet 43:239–248.

Baird PA, Sadovnick AD (1989) Life tables for Down syndrome. Hum Genet 82:291–292.

Bakker E, Veenema H, Den Dunnen JT, et al (1989) Germinal mosaicism increases the recurrence risk for "new" Duchenne muscular dystrophy mutations. J Med Genet 26:553–559.

Balling R, Deutsch U, Gruss P (1988) *undulated,* a mutation affecting the development of the mouse skeleton, has a point mutation in the paired box of *Pax 1.* Cell 55:531–535.

Barker D, Hostikka SK, Zhou J, et al (1990) Identification of mutations in the COL4A5 collagen gene in Alport syndrome. Science 248:1224–1226.

Barker D, Wright E, Nguyen K, et al (1987) Gene for von Recklinghausen's neurofibromatosis is in the pericentromeric region of chromosome 17. Science 236:1100–1102.

Barr ML (1960) Sexual dimorphism in interphase nuclei. Am J Hum Genet 12:118–127.

Barr ML, Bertram EG (1949) A morphological distinction between neurons of the male and female, and the behavior of the nucleolar satellite during accelerated nucleoprotein synthesis. Nature 163:676–677.

Barranger JA, Ginns EI (1989) Glucoceramide lipidoses. *In* Scriver CR, Beaudet AL, Sly WS, Valle D (eds) The metabolic basis of inherited disease, 6th ed. McGraw-Hill, New York, pp. 1677–1698.

Barton NW, Furbish FS, Murray GJ et al (1990) Therapeutic response to intravenous infusions of glucocerebrosidase in a patient with Gaucher disease. Proc Natl Acad Sci USA 87:1913–1916.

Beaudet AL, Scriver CR, Sly WS, et al (1989) Genetics and biochemistry of variant human phenotypes. *In* Scriver CR, Beaudet AL, Sly WS, Valle D (eds) The metabolic basis of inherited disease, 6th ed. McGraw-Hill, New York, pp. 3–53.

Beaudet AL, Feldman GL, Fernbach SD, et al (1989) Linkage disequilibrium, cystic fibrosis, and genetic counseling. Am J Hum Genet 44:319–326.

Becerra JE, Khoury MJ, Cordero JF, Erickson JD (1990) Diabetes mellitus during pregnancy and the risks for specific birth defects: A population-based case-control study. Pediatrics 85:1–9.

Bell JI, Todd JA, McDevitt HO (1989) The molecular basis of HLA-disease association. Adv Hum Genet 18:1–41.

Berg P (1981) Dissections and reconstructions of genes and chromosomes. Science 213:296–303.

Bernardi G (1989) The isochore organization of the human genome. Ann Rev Genet 23:637–661.

Berta P, Hawkins JR, Sinclair AH, et al (1990) Genetic evidence equating *SRY* and the testis-determining factor. Nature 348:448–450.

Bickmore WA, Sumner AT (1989) Mammalian chromosome banding—An expression of genome organization. Trends Genet 5:144–149.

Boat TF, Welsh MJ, Beaudet AL (1989) Cystic fibrosis. *In* Scriver CR, Beaudet AL, Sly WS, Valle D (eds) The metabolic basis of inherited disease, 6th ed. McGraw-Hill, New York, pp. 2649–2680.

Bonaiti-Pellié C, Smith C (1974) Risk tables for genetic counselling in some common congenital malformations. J Med Genet 11:374–377.

Borgaonkar DS (1989) Chromosomal variation in man: A catalog of chromosomal variants and anomalies, 5th ed. Alan R. Liss, New York.

Borrow J, Goddard AD, Sheer D, Solomon E (1990) Molecular analysis of acute promyelocytic leukemia breakpoint cluster region on chromosome 17. Science 249:1577–1580.

Botstein D (1990) 1989 Allen award address. Am J Hum Genet 47:887–891.

Botstein D, White RL, Skolnick M, Davis RW (1980) Construction of a genetic linkage map using restriction fragment length polymorphisms. Am J Hum Genet 32:314–331.

Bouchard C, Tremblay A, Desprès J-P, et al (1990) The response to long-term overfeeding in identical twins. N Engl J Med 322:1477–1482.

Boué A, Boué J, Gropp A (1985) Cytogenetics of pregnancy wastage. Ann Rev Genet 14:1–57.

Brown CJ, Ballabio A, Rupert J, et al (1991) A gene from the region of the human X inactivation center is expressed exclusively from the inactive X chromosome. Nature 349:38–44.

Brown CJ, Willard HF (1990) Localization of a gene that escapes inactivation to the X chromosome proximal short arm: Implications for X inactivation. Am J Hum Genet 45:273–279.

Buehler BA, Delimont D, van Waes M, Finnell RH (1990) Prenatal prediction of risk of the fetal hydantoin syndrome. N Engl J Med 322:1567–1572.

Bunn FH (1987) Human hemoglobins: Normal and abnormal. In Nathan DG, Oski FA (eds) Hematology of infancy and childhood, 3rd ed. WB Saunders, Philadelphia, pp. 613–640.

Burgoyne PS (1989) Thumbs down for zinc finger? Nature 342:860–862.

Burke DT, Carle CF, Olson MV (1987) Cloning of large segments of exogenous DNA into yeast by means of artificial chromosome vectors. Science 236:806–812.

Butler MG, Palmer CG (1983) Parental origin of chromosome 15 deletion in Prader-Willi syndrome. Lancet 1:1285–1286.

Byers PH (1989) Disorders of collagen biosynthesis and structure. In Scriver CR, Beaudet AL, Sly WS, Valle D (eds) The metabolic basis of inherited disease, 6th ed. McGraw-Hill, New York, pp. 2805–2842.

Byers PH (1990) Brittle bones–fragile molecules: Disorders of collagen gene structure and expression. Trends Genet 6:293–300.

C

Call KM, Glaser T, Ito CY, et al (1990) Isolation and characterization of a zinc finger polypeptide gene at the human chromosome 11 Wilms tumor locus. Cell 60:509–520.

Canadian Collaborative CVS-Amniocentesis Clinical Trial Group (1989) Multicentre randomised clinical trial of chorion villus sampling and amniocentesis: First report. Lancet 1:1–6.

Caporaso N, Hayes RB, Dosemeci M, et al (1989) Lung cancer risk, occupational exposure, and the debrisoquine metabolic phenotype. Cancer Res 49:3675–3679.

Carson NAJ, Cusworth DC, Dent CE, et al (1963) Homocystinuria: A new inborn error of metabolism associated with mental deficiency. Arch Dis Child 38:425–436.

Carter CO (1964) Genetics of common malformations. In Fishbein M (ed) Congenital malformations. International Medical Congress, New York, pp. 306–313.

Carter CO (1969) Genetics of common disorders. Br Med Bull 25:52–57.

Carter CO (1976) Genetics of common single malformations. Br Med Bull 32:21–26.

Cavalli-Sforza LL, Bodmer W (1971) The genetics of human populations. WH Freeman, San Francisco.

Cawthon RM, Weiss R, Xu G, et al (1990) A major segment of the neurofibromatosis type 1 gene: cDNA sequence, genomic structure, and point mutations. Cell 62:193–201.

Chabot B, Stephenson DA, Chapman VM, et al (1988) The proto-oncogene c-kit encoding a transmembrane tyrosine kinase receptor maps to the mouse W locus. Nature 335:88–89.

Chakraborty R, Lidsky AS, Daiger SP, et al (1987) Polymorphic DNA haplotypes at the human phenylalanine hydroxylase locus and their relationship with phenylketonuria. Hum Genet 76:40–46.

Chang JC, Kan YW (1982) A sensitive new prenatal test for sickle-cell anemia. N Engl J Med 307:30–32.

Cherif-Zahar B, Bloy C, le Van Kim C, et al (1990) Molecular cloning and protein structure of a human blood group Rh polypeptide. Proc Natl Acad Sci USA 87:6243–6247.

Childs B (1982) Genetics in the medical curriculum. Am J Med Genet 13:319–324.

Clark DWJ (1985) Genetically determined variability in acetylation and oxidation. Drugs 29:342–375.

Clark EB (1987) Pathogenesis of cardiac malformations. In Pierpont ME, Moller JH (eds) Genetics in cardiovascular disease. Martinus Nyhoff, Norwell, MA, pp. 3–11.

Claus EB, Risch NJ, Thompson WD (1990) Age at onset as an indicator of familial risk of breast cancer. Am J Epidemiol 131:961–972.

Claus EB, Risch NJ, Thompson WD (1991) Genetic analysis of breast cancer in the cancer and steroid hormone study. Am J Hum Genet 48:232–242.

Cohn DH, Starman BJ, Blumberg B, Byers PH (1990) Recurrence of lethal osteogenesis imperfecta due to parental mosaicism for a dominant mutation in a human type 1 collagen gene (COL1A1). Am J Hum Genet 46:591–601.

Conley ME, Lavoie A, Briggs C, et al (1988) Non-random X chromosome inactivation in B cells from carriers of X-linked severe combined immunodeficiency. Proc Natl Acad Sci USA 85:3090–3094.

Conley ME, Puck JM (1988) Carrier detection in typical and atypical X-linked agammaglobulinemia. J Pediatr 112:688–694.

Conneally PM, Wallace MR, Gusella JF, Wexler NS (1984) Huntington disease: Estimation of heterozygote status using linked genetic markers. Genet Epidemiol 1:81–88.

Cooper DN, Krawczak M (1990) The mutational spectrum of single basepair substitutions causing human genetic disease: Patterns and predictions. Hum Genet 85:55–74.

Cooper DN, Smith BA, Cooke HJ, et al (1985) An estimate of unique DNA sequence heterozygosity in the human genome. Hum Genet 69:201–205.

Costa T, Scriver CR, Childs B (1985) The effect of Mendelian disease on human health: A measurement. Am J Med Genet 21:231–242.

Cox DW (1989) α_1-antitrypsin deficiency. In Scriver CR, Beaudet AL, Sly WS, Valle D (eds) The metabolic basis of inherited disease, 6th ed. McGraw-Hill, New York, pp. 2409–2437.

Croce CM (1987) Role of chromosome translocations in human neoplasia. Cell 49:155–156.

Crossley M, Brownlee GG (1990) Disruption of a C/EBP site in the factor IX promoter is associated with hemophilia B. Nature 345:444–446.

Crystal RG (1990) α_1-antitrypsin deficiency, emphysema, and liver disease. J Clin Invest 85:1343–1352.

Crystal RG, Brantly ML, Hubbard RC, et al (1989) The alpha$_1$-antitrypsin gene and its mutations. Chest 95:196–208.

Cutting GR, Kasch LM, Rosenstein BJ, et al (1990) A cluster of cystic fibrosis mutations in the first nucleotide-binding fold of the cystic fibrosis conductance regulator protein. Nature 346:366–368.

Cutting GR, Kasch LM, Rosenstein BJ, et al (1990) Two cystic fibrosis patients with mild pulmonary disease and nonsense mutations in each CFTR gene. N Engl J Med 323:1685–1689.

Cystic Fibrosis Genetic Analysis Consortium (1990) Worldwide survey of the ΔF508 mutation. Am J Hum Genet 47:354–359.

D

Daley GQ, Van Etten RA, Baltimore D (1990) Induction of chronic myelogenous leukemia in mice by the P210[bcr/abl] gene of the Philadelphia chromosome. Science 247:824–830.

Davidson RG, Nitowsky HM, Childs B (1963) Demonstration of two populations of cells in the human female heterozygous for glucose-6-phosphate dehydrogenase variants. Proc Natl Acad Sci USA 50:481–485.

Davies KE (1990) Complementary endeavors. Nature 348:110–111.

Dean M, White MB, Amos J, et al (1990) Multiple mutations in highly conserved residues are found in mildly affected cystic fibrosis patients. Cell 61:863–870.

DeChiara TM, Efstratiadis A, Robertson EJ (1990) A growth-deficiency phenotype in heterozygous mice carrying an insulin-like growth factor II gene disrupted by targeting. Nature 345:78–80.

de la Chapelle A (1988) The complicated issue of human sex determination. Am J Hum Genet 43:1–3.

Diamond JM, Rotter JI (1987) Observing the founder effect in human evolution. Nature 329:105–106.

Drumm ML, Pope HA, Cliff WH, et al (1990) Correction of the cystic fibrosis defect in vitro by retrovirus-mediated gene transfer. Cell 62:1227–1233.

Drummond-Borg M, Deeb SS, Motulsky AG (1989) Molecular patterns of X chromosome-linked color vision genes among 134 men of European ancestry. Proc Natl Acad Sci USA 86:983–987.

Dryja TP, McGee TL, Reichel E, et al (1990) A point mutation of the rhodopsin gene in one form of retinitis pigmentosa. Nature 343:364–366.

Dulbecco R (1986) A turning point in cancer research: Sequencing the human genome. Science 231:1055–1056.

Durston AJ, Timmermans JP, Hage WJ, et al (1989) Retinoic acid causes an anteroposterior transformation in the developing nervous system. Nature 340:140–144.

E

Ebers GC, Bulman DE, Sadovnick AD, et al (1986) A population-based study of multiple sclerosis in twins. N Engl J Med 315:1638–1642.

Edwards J (1956) Antenatal detection of hereditary disorders. Lancet 270:579.

Eiberg H, Mohr J, Schmiegelow K, et al (1985) Linkage relationships of paraoxonase (PON) with other markers: Indication of PON-cystic fibrosis synteny. Clin Genet 28:265–271.

Emery AEH (1986) Methodology in medical genetics, 2nd ed. Churchill Livingstone, Edinburgh.

England SB, Nicholson LVB, Johnson MA, et al (1990) Very mild muscular dystrophy associated with the deletion of 46% of dystrophin. Nature 343:180–182.

Enver T, Raich N, Ebens AJ, et al (1990) Developmental regulation of human fetal-to-adult globin gene switching in transgenic mice. Nature 344:309–313.

Epstein CJ (1986) The consequences of chromosome imbalance: Principles, mechanisms, and models. Cambridge University Press, New York.

Epstein CJ (1989) Down syndrome. In Scriver CJ, Beaudet AL, Sly W, Valle D (eds) The metabolic basis of inherited disease, 6th ed. McGraw-Hill, New York, pp. 291–326.

Esquivel CO, Marino IR, Fioravanti V, Van Thiel DH (1988) Liver transplantation for metabolic disease of the liver. Gastroenterol Clin North Am 17:167–175.

Evans DAP (1989) N-acetyltransferase. Pharmacol Ther 42:157–234.

Eydoux P, Choiset A, LePorrier N, et al (1989) Chromosomal prenatal diagnosis: Study of 936 cases of intrauterine abnormalities after ultrasound assessment. Prenat Diagn 9:255–269.

Ezekowitz RAB, Dinauer MC, Jaffe HS, et al (1988) Partial correction of the phagocyte defect in patients with X-linked chronic granulomatous disease by subcutaneous interferon gamma. N Engl J Med 319:146–152.

Ezekowitz RAB, Orkin SH, Newburger PE (1987) Recombinant interferon gamma augments phagocyte superoxide production and X-chronic granulomatous disease gene expression in X-linked variant chronic granulomatous disease. J Clin Invest 80:1009–1016.

F

Fearon ER, Cho ER, Nigro JM et al (1990) Identification of a chromosome 18q gene that is altered in colorectal cancers. Science 247:49–56.

Ferguson-Smith MA (1966) X-Y chromosomal interchange in the aetiology of true hermaphroditism and of XX Klinefelter's syndrome. Lancet 2:495–496.

Fisher EMC, Beer-Romero P, Brown LG, et al (1990) Homologous ribosomal protein genes on the human X and Y chromosomes: Escape from X inactivation and implications for Turner syndrome. Cell 61:1205–1218.

Fölling A (1934) Über Ausscheidung von Phenylbrenztraubensäure in den Harn als Stoffwechselanomalie in Verbindung mit Imbezillität. Hoppe-Seyler's Z Physiol Chem 227:169–176.

Ford CE, Jones K, Polani P, et al (1959) A sex chromosome anomaly in a case of gonadal dysgenesis (Turner syndrome). Lancet 1:711–713.

Fraser FC (1989) Invited editorial: Mapping the cleft lip genes: The first fix? Am J Hum Genet 45:345–347.

Fraser S, Keynes R, Lumsden A (1990) Segmentation in the chick embryo hindbrain is defined by cell lineage restrictions. Nature 344:431–435.

Fritsch EF, Maniatis T (1987) Methods of molecular genetics. In Stamatoyannopoulos G, Nienhuis AW, Leder P, Majerus PW (eds) The molecular basis of blood diseases. WB Saunders, Philadelphia, pp. 1–27.

G

Gahl WA, Renlund M, Thoene JG (1989) Lysosomal transport disorders: Cystinosis and sialic acid storage disorders. In Scriver CR, Beaudet AL, Sly WS, Valle D (eds) The metabolic basis of inherited disease, 6th ed. McGraw-Hill, New York, pp. 2619–2647.

Gale RP, Sparkes RS, Gold DW (1978) Bone marrow origin of hepatic macrophages (Kupffer cells) in humans. Science 201:937–938.

Gardner RJM, Sutherland GR (1989) Chromosome abnormalities and genetic counseling. Oxford University Press, New York.

Gibbs RA, Nguyen PN, Edwards A, et al (1990) Multiplex DNA deletion detection and exon sequencing of the hypoxanthine phosphoribosyltransferase gene in Lesch-Nyhan families. Genomics 7:235–244.

Giblett ER (1983) Erythrocyte antigens and antibodies. In Williams WJ, Beutler E, Erslev AJ, Lichtman MA (eds) Hematology, 3rd ed. McGraw-Hill, New York, pp. 1491–1505.

Gilbert W (1985) Genes-in-pieces revisited. Science 228:823.

Gillard EF, Chamberlain JS, Murphy EG, et al (1989) Molecular and phenotypic analysis of patients with deletions within the deletion-rich region of the Duchenne muscular dystrophy (DMD) gene. Am J Hum Genet 45:507–520.

Gitschier J, Levinson B, Lehesjoki AE, de la Chapelle A (1989) Mosaicism and sporadic hemophilia: Implications for carrier determination. Lancet 1:273–274.

Gitschier J, Wood WI, Goralka TM, et al (1984) Characterization of the human factor VIII gene. Nature 312:326–336.

Goldberg MA, Brugnara C, Dover GJ, et al (1990) Treatment of sickle cell anemia with hydroxyurea and erythropoietin. N Engl J Med 323:366–372.

Goldstein JL, Brown MS (1989) Familial hypercholesterolemia. *In* Scriver CR, Beaudet AL, Sly WS, and Valle D (eds) The metabolic basis of inherited disease, 6th ed. McGraw-Hill, New York, pp. 1215–1250.

Graham A, Papalopulu N, Krumlauf R (1989) The murine and Drosophila homeobox gene complexes have common features of organization and expression. Cell 57:367–378.

Grant DM, Mörike K, Eichelbaum E, Meyer UA (1990) Acetylation pharmacogenetics: The slow acetylator phenotype is caused by decreased or absent arylamine N-acetyltransferase in human liver. J Clin Invest 85:968–972.

Grant DM, Spielberg SP (1991) Genetic regulation of drug metabolism. *In* Polin RA, Fox WW (eds) Developmental pharmacology and pharmacokinetics. WB Saunders, Philadelphia, Chap. 14.

Gusella JF, Wexler NS, Conneally PM, et al (1983) A polymorphic DNA marker genetically linked to Huntington's disease. Nature 306:234–238.

H

Haldane JBS, Smith CAB (1947) A new estimate of the linkage between the genes for color-blindness and hemophilia in man. Ann Eugen 14:10–31.

Hall JG (1988) Somatic mosaicism: Observations related to clinical genetics. Am J Hum Genet 43:355–363.

Hall JM, Lee MK, Newman B, et al (1990) Linkage of early-onset familial breast cancer to chromosome 17q21. Science 250:1684–1689.

Handyside AH, Kontogianni EH, Hardy K, Winston RML (1990) Pregnancies from biopsied human preimplantation embryos sexed by Y-specific DNA amplification. Nature 344:768–770.

Harper PS (1989) The muscular dystrophies. *In* Scriver CR, Beaudet AL, Sly WS, Valle D (eds) The metabolic basis of inherited disease, 6th ed. McGraw-Hill, New York, pp. 2869–2902.

Harper PS (1989) Myotonic dystrophy, 2nd ed. WB Saunders, Philadelphia.

Harper PS, Frezal J, Ferguson-Smith MA, et al (1989) Report of the committee on clinical disorders and chromosomal deletion syndromes. Human Gene Mapping 10: Tenth international workshop on human gene mapping. Cytogenet Cell Genet 51:563–611.

Harris H (1980) The principles of human biochemical genetics, 3rd ed. Elsevier/North-Holland Press, Amsterdam.

Harrison GA, Weiner JS, Tanner JM, et al (1977) Human biology, 3rd ed. Oxford University Press, Oxford, England.

Harrison MR, Adzick NS, Longaker MT, et al (1990) Successful repair in utero of a fetal diaphragmatic hernia after removal of herniated viscera from the left thorax. N Engl J Med 322:1582–1584.

Hassold T, Jacobs PA (1984) Trisomy in man. Ann Rev Genet 18:69–97.

Hassold TJ, Jacobs PA, Leppert M, Sheldon M (1987) Cytogenetic and molecular studies of trisomy 13. J Med Genet 24:725–732.

Hayes A, Costa T, Scriver CR, Childs B (1985) The effect of Mendelian disease on human health. II: Response to treatment. Am J Med Genet 21:243–255.

Hershfield MS, Buckley RH, Greenberg ML, et al (1987) Treat-

ment of adenosine deaminase deficiency with polyethylene glycol-modified adenosine deaminase. N Engl J Med 316:589–596.

Hershfield MS, Chaffee S (in press) PEG-enzyme replacement therapy for adenosine deaminase deficiency. *In* Desnick RJ (ed) Treatment of genetic diseases. Churchill Livingstone, New York.

Hickman S, Neufeld EF (1972) A hypothesis for I-cell disease: Defective hydrolases that do not enter lysosomes. Biochem Biophys Res Commun 49:922–999.

Hirschhorn K (1987) Chromosomes and their abnormalities. *In* Behrman RE, Vaughan VC (eds) Nelson textbook of pediatrics, 13th ed. WB Saunders, Philadelphia, pp. 247–267.

Hobbs HH, Russell DW, Brown MS, Goldstein JL (1990) The LDL receptor locus in familial hypercholesterolemia. Ann Rev Genet 24:133–170.

Hoechstetter L, Warren N, Neidich K (1989) State regulation of the practice of counseling — A national review. Am J Hum Genet 45:A122.

Holmquist GP (1987) Role of replication time in the control of tissue-specific gene expression. Am J Hum Genet 40:151–173.

Hood LE, Kronenberg M, Hunkapiller T (1985) T-cell antigen receptors and the immunoglobulin supergene family. Cell 40:225–229.

Hook EB (1986) The impact of aneuploidy upon public health. *In* Dellarco VL, Voytek PE, Hollaender A (eds) Aneuploidy: Etiology and mechanisms. Plenum Press, New York, pp. 7–34.

Hook EB (1989) Maternal age-specific rates of chromosome abnormalities at chorionic villus study: A revision. Am J Hum Genet 45:474–477.

Hook EB, Cross PK (1987) Rates of mutant and inherited structural cytogenetic abnormalities detected at amniocentesis: Results on about 63,000 fetuses. Ann Hum Genet 51:27–55.

Hook EB, Cross PK, Jackson L, et al (1988) Maternal age-specific rates of 47,+21 and other cytogenetic abnormalities diagnosed in the first trimester of pregnancy in chorionic villus biopsy specimens: Comparison with rates expected from observations at amniocentesis. Am J Hum Genet 42:797–807.

Hook EB, Cross PK, Schreinemachers DM (1983) Chromosomal abnormality rates at amniocentesis and in live-born infants. JAMA 249:2034–2038.

Hook EB, Hamerton JL (1977) The frequency of chromosome abnormalities detected in consecutive newborn studies, differences between studies, results by sex and by severity of phenotypic involvement. *In* Hook EB, Porter IH (eds) Population cytogenetics, studies in humans. Academic Press, New York, pp. 63–79.

Hook EB, Porter IH (1977) Population cytogenetics: Studies in humans. Academic Press, New York.

Hook EB, Warburton D (1983) The distribution of chromosomal genotypes associated with Turner syndrome: Live-birth prevalence rates and evidence for diminished fetal mortality and severity in genotypes associated with structural X abnormalities or mosaicism. Hum Genet 64:24–27.

Huang A, Campbell CE, Bonetta L, et al (1990) Tissue, developmental, and tumor-specific expression of divergent transcripts in Wilms tumor. Science 250:991–994.

Huggins M, Bloch M, Kanani S, et al (1990) Ethical and legal dilemmas arising during predictive testing for adult-onset disease: The experience of Huntington disease. Am J Hum Genet 47:4–12.

Hunkapiller T, Hood L (1989) Diversity of the immunoglobulin gene superfamily. Adv Immunol 44:1–63.

Hyde SC, Emsley P, Hartshorn MJ, et al (1990) Structural

model of ATP-binding proteins associated with cystic fibrosis, multidrug resistance and bacterial transport. Nature 346:362–365.

I

Ingram VM (1956) Specific chemical difference between the globins of normal human and sickle-cell anemia hemoglobin. Nature 178:792–794.

Ingram VM (1986) Sickle cell disease—molecular and cellular pathogenesis. In Bunn HF, Forget BG (eds) Hemoglobin: Molecular, genetic, and clinical aspects. WB Saunders, Philadelphia, pp. 453–501.

J

Jacobs PA, Hassold TJ, Whittington E, et al (1988) Klinefelter's syndrome: An analysis of the origin of the additional sex chromosome using molecular probes. Ann Hum Genet 52:93–109.

Jacobs PA, Hunt PA, Mayer M, Bart RD (1981) Duchenne muscular dystrophy in a female with an X/autosome translocation: Further evidence that the DMD locus is at Xp21. Am J Hum Genet 33:513–518.

Jacobs PA, Price WH, Court-Brown WM, et al (1968) Chromosome studies on men in a maximum security hospital. Ann Hum Genet 31:339–358.

Jacobs PA, Strong JA (1959) A case of human sexuality having a possible XXY sex determining mechanism. Nature 183:302–303.

Jager RJ, Anvret M, Hall K, Scherer G (1990) A human XY female with a frame shift mutation in the candidate testis-determining gene SRY. Nature 348:452–454.

Jeffreys AJ (1979) DNA sequence variants in the γ, δ, and β globin genes of man. Cell 18:1–10.

Jeffreys AJ, Wilson V, Thein SL (1985) Hypervariable 'minisatellite' regions in human DNA. Nature 314:67–73.

Jones KL (1988) Smith's Recognizable patterns of human malformation, 4th ed. WB Saunders, Philadelphia.

Jorgensen AL, Deeb SS, Motulsky AG (1990) Molecular genetics of X chromosome-linked color vision among populations of African and Japanese ancestry: High frequency of a shortened red pigment gene among Afro-Americans. Proc Natl Acad Sci USA 87:6512–6516.

Journel H, Melki J, Turleau C, et al (1990) Rett phenotype with X/autosome translocation: Possible mapping to the short arm of chromosome X. Am J Med Genet 35:142–147.

K

Kalousek DK, Barrett IJ, McGillivray BC (1989) Placental mosaicism and intrauterine survival of trisomies 13 and 18. Am J Hum Genet 44:338–343.

Kan YW (1978) Hemoglobin abnormalities: Molecular and evolutionary studies. The Harvey Lectures, series 76. Academic Press, New York, pp. 75–93.

Kan YW, Dozy AM (1978) Polymorphism of DNA sequence adjacent to human β-globin structural gene: Relationship to sickle mutation. Proc Natl Acad Sci USA 75:5631–5635.

Kappas A, Sassa S, Galbraith RA, Nordmann Y (1989) The porphyrias. In Scriver CR, Beaudet AL, Sly WS, Valle D (eds) The metabolic basis of inherited disease, 6th ed. McGraw-Hill, New York, pp. 1305–1365.

Kark JA, Posey DM, Schumacher HR, Ruehle CJ (1987) Sickle-cell trait as a risk factor for sudden death in physical training. N Engl J Med 317:781–787.

Karpati G, Pouliot Y, Zubrzycka-Gaarn E, et al (1989) Dystrophin is expressed in mdx skeletal muscle fibres after normal myoblast transplantation. Am J Pathol 135:27–32.

Kartner N, Hanrahan JW, Jensen TJ, et al (1991) Expression of the cystic fibrosis gene in non-epithelial invertebrate cells produces a regulated anion conductance. Cell 64:681–691.

Kazazian HH Jr (1990) The thalassemia syndromes: Molecular basis and prenatal diagnosis in 1990. In Miescher LA, Jaffe ER (eds) Seminars in hematology. WB Saunders, Philadelphia, pp. 209–228.

Kazazian HH Jr, Boehm CD (1988) Molecular basis and prenatal diagnosis of beta-thalassemia. Blood 72:1107–1116.

Kazazian HH, Wong C, Youssoufian H, et al (1988) Hemophilia A resulting from de novo insertion of L1 sequences represents a novel mechanism for mutation in man. Nature 332:164–166.

Kelikian H (1974) Congenital deformities of the hand and forearm. WB Saunders, Philadelphia.

Kerem B-S, Rommens JR, Buchanan JA, et al (1989) Identification of the cystic fibrosis gene: Genetic analysis. Science 245:1073–1078.

Kerem B-S, Zielenski J, Markiewicz D, et al (1990a) Identification of mutations in regions corresponding to the two putative nucleotide (ATP)-binding folds of the cystic fibrosis gene. Proc Natl Acad Sci USA 87:8447–8451.

Kerem E, Corey M, Kerem B-S, et al (1990b) The relationship between genotype and phenotype in cystic fibrosis: analysis of the most common mutation (ΔF508). N Engl J Med 323:1517–1522.

Kessel M, Gruss P (1990) Murine developmental control genes. Science 249:375–379.

Kidd KK, Bowcock AM, Schmidtke J, et al (1989) Report of the DNA committee and catalogs of cloned and mapped genes and DNA polymorphisms. Human Gene Mapping 10: Tenth international workshop on human gene mapping. Cytogenet Cell Genet 51:622–947.

Kimberling MJ, Fain PR, Kenyon JB, et al (1988) Linkage heterogeneity of autosomal dominant polycystic kidney disease. N Engl J Med 319:913–918.

Kinzler KW, Nilbert MC, Vogelstein B, et al (1991) Identification of a gene located at chromosome 5q21 that is mutated in colorectal cancers. Science 251:1366–1370.

Kioussis D, Vanin E, deLange T, et al (1983) β-globin gene inactivation by DNA translocation in $\gamma\beta$-thalassaemia. Nature 306:662–666.

Knoll JH, Nichols RD, Magenis RE, et al (1989) Angelman and Prader-Willi syndromes share a common chromosome 15 deletion but differ in parental origin of the deletion. Am J Med Genet 32:285–290.

Knudson AG (1971) Mutation and cancer: Statistical study of retinoblastoma. Proc Natl Acad Sci USA 68:820–823.

Koopman P, Gubbay J, Collignon J, Lovell-Badge R (1989) Zfy gene expression patterns are not compatible with a primary role in mouse sex determination. Nature 342:940–942.

Korenberg J, Rykowski M (1988) Human genome organization: Alu, Lines, and the molecular structure of metaphase chromosome bands. Cell 53:391–400.

Korenberg JR, Kawashima H, Pulst SM, et al (1990) Molecular definition of a region of chromosome 21 that causes features of the Down syndrome phenotype. Am J Hum Genet 47:236–246.

Kostyu DD, Amos DB (1989) The HLA complex: Genetic polymorphism and disease susceptibility. In Scriver CR, Beaudet AL, Sly WS, Valle D (eds) The metabolic basis of inherited disease, 6th ed. McGraw-Hill, New York, pp. 225–249.

Kouri RE, McKinney CE, Slomiany DJ, et al (1982) Positive correlation between high aryl hydrocarbon hydroxylase activity and primary lung cancer as analyzed in cryopreserved lymphocytes. Cancer Res 42:5030–5037.

Kredich NM, Hershfield MS (1989) Immunodeficiency diseases caused by adenosine deaminase deficiency and purine nucleoside phosphorylase deficiency. *In* Scriver CR, Beaudet AL, Sly WS, Valle D (eds) The metabolic basis of inherited disease, 6th ed. McGraw-Hill, New York, pp. 1045–1075.

Krivit W (1989) A summary of 75 patients with storage disease treated by bone marrow transplantation. *In* Hobbs JR (ed) Correction of certain genetic diseases by transplantation. Westminster Medical School Research Trust, London, pp. 179–186.

Krivit W, Shapiro E, Kennedy W, et al (1990) Treatment of late infantile metachromatic leukodystrophy by bone marrow transplantation. N Engl J Med 322:28–32.

Kunkel LM, Monaco AP, Middlesworth W, et al (1985) Specific cloning of DNA fragments absent from the DNA of a male patient with an X chromosome deletion. Proc Natl Acad Sci USA 82:4778–4782.

Kwok SCM, Ledley FD, Dilella AG, et al (1985) Nucleotide sequence of a full-length complementary DNA clone and amino acid sequence of human phenylalanine hydroxylase. Biochemistry 24:556–561.

L

Laberge C (1969) Hereditary tyrosinemia in a French Canadian isolate. Am J Hum Genet 21:36–45.

La Du BN, Barteels CF, Nogueira CP, et al (1990) Phenotypic and molecular biological analysis of human serum cholinesterase variants. Clin Biochem 23:423–431.

Larsson C (1978) Natural history and life expectancy in severe alpha$_1$-antitrypsin deficiency, Pi Z. Acta Med Scand 204:345–351.

Latt SA, Willard HF, Gerald PS (1976) BrdU-33258 Hoechst analysis of DNA replication in human lymphocytes with supernumerary or structurally abnormal X chromosomes. Chromosoma 57:135–153.

Lawn RM, Efstratiadis A, O'Connell C, et al (1980) The nucleotide sequence of the human β-globin gene. Cell 21:647–651.

Lawn RM, Fritsch EF, Parker RC, et al (1978) The isolation and characterization of linked δ and β globin genes from a cloned library of human DNA. Cell 15:1157–1174.

Lawrence PA (1990) Compartments in vertebrates. Nature 344:382–383.

Lazarow PB, Moser HW (1989) Disorders of peroxisome biogenesis. *In* Scriver CR, Beaudet AL, Sly WS, Valle D (eds) The metabolic basis of inherited disease, 6th ed. McGraw-Hill, New York, pp. 1479–1509.

Ledbetter DH, Cavenee WK (1989) Molecular cytogenetics: Interface of cytogenetics and monogenic disorders. *In* Scriver CJ, Beaudet AL, Sly W, Valle D (eds) The metabolic basis of inherited disease, 6th ed. McGraw-Hill, New York, pp. 343–371.

Ledley FD, Jansen R, Nham SU, et al (1990) Mutation eliminating mitochondrial leader sequence of methylmalonyl-CoA mutase causes *mut°* methylmalonic acidemia. Proc Natl Acad Sci USA 87:3147–3150.

Lehrman LE, Goldstein JL, Russell DW, Brown MS (1987) Duplication of seven exons in the LDL receptor gene caused by Alu-Alu recombination in a subject with familial hypercholesterolemia. Cell 48:827–835.

Lejeune J, Gautier M, Turpin R (1959) Etude des chromosomes somatiques de neuf enfants mongoliens. CR Acad Sci Paris 248:1721–1722.

Lemna WK, Feldman GL, Kerem B, et al (1990) Mutation analysis for heterozygote detection and the prenatal diagnosis of cystic fibrosis. N Engl J Med 322:291–296.

Lenke RR, Levy HL (1980) Maternal phenylketonuria and hyperphenylalaninemia. An international study of untreated and treated pregnancies. N Engl J Med 303:1202–1208.

Levilliers J, Quack B, Weissenbach J, et al (1989) Exchange of terminal portions of X- and Y- chromosomal short arms in human XY females. Proc Natl Acad Sci USA 86:2296–2300.

Li FP (1988) Cancer families: Human models of susceptibility to neoplasia—The Richard and Hinda Rosenthal Foundation award lecture. Cancer Res 48:5381–5386.

Lin AE, Garver KL (1988) Genetic counselling for congenital heart defects. J Pediatr 113:1105–1109.

Lubsen NH, Renwick JH, Tsui LC, et al (1987) A locus for a human hereditary cataract is closely linked to the γ-crystallin gene family. Proc Natl Acad Sci USA 84:489–492.

Lucarelli G, Galimberti M, Polchi P, et al (1990) Bone marrow transplantation in patients with thalassemia. N Engl J Med 322:417–421.

Luzzatto L, Mehta A (1989) Glucose-6-phosphate dehydrogenase deficiency. *In* Scriver CR, Beaudet AL, Sly WS, Valle D (eds) The metabolic basis of inherited disease, 6th ed. McGraw-Hill, New York, pp. 2237–2265.

Lyon MF (1961) Gene action in the X-chromosome of the mouse (*Mus musculus L.*). Nature 190:372–373.

Lyon MF (1962) Sex chromatin and gene action in the mammalian X-chromosome. Am J Hum Genet 14:135–148.

M

MacLennan DH, Duff C, Zorzato F, et al (1990) Ryanodine receptor gene is a candidate for predisposition to malignant hyperthermia. Nature 343:559–561.

Maddalena A, Sosnoski DM, Berry GT, Nussbaum RL (1988) Mosaicism for an intragenic deletion in a boy with mild ornithine transcarbamylase deficiency. N Engl J Med 319:999–1003.

Magenis RE, Toth-Fejel S, Allen LJ, et al (1990) Comparison of the 15q deletions in Prader-Willi and Angelman syndromes: Specific regions, extent of deletions, parental origin, and clinical consequences. Am J Med Genet 35:333–349.

Malkin D, Li FP, Strong LC, et al (1990) Germ line p53 mutations in a familial syndrome of breast cancer, sarcomas, and other neoplasms. Science 250:1233–1238.

Mandel JL, Willard HF, Nussbaum RL, et al (1989) Report of the committee on the genetic constitution of the X chromosome. Human Gene Mapping 10: Tenth international workshop on human gene mapping. Cytogenet Cell Genet 51:384–437.

Martin RH (1989) Segregation analysis of translocations by the study of human sperm chromosome complements. Am J Hum Genet 44:461–463.

May KK, Jacobs PA, Lee M, et al (1990) The parental origin of the extra chromosome in 47,XXX females. Am J Hum Genet 46:754–761.

McCarthy TV, Healy SJM, Heffron JJA, et al (1990) Localization of the malignant hyperthermia susceptibility locus to human chromosome 19q12-13.2. Nature 343:562–564.

McFadden DE, Kalousek DK (1988) Triploid phenotypes in embryos and fetuses. Lab Invest 58(1):6P.

McGillivray BC, Bassett AS, Langlois S, et al (1990) Familial 5q11.2-q13.3 segmental duplication cosegregating with multiple anomalies, including schizophrenia. Am J Med Genet 35:10–13.

McGuire MC, Nogueira CP, Bartels CF, et al (1989) Identification of the structural mutation responsible for the dibucaine-resistant (atypical) variant form of human serum cholinesterase. Proc Natl Acad Sci USA 86:953–957.

McKusick VA (1990) Mendelian inheritance in man: Catalogs of autosomal dominant, autosomal recessive, and X-linked phenotypes, 9th ed. Johns Hopkins University Press, Baltimore.

McLemore TL, Adelberg S, Liu MC, et al (1990) Expression of CYP1A1 gene in patients with lung cancer: Evidence for cigarette smoke-induced gene expression in normal lung tissue and for altered gene regulation in primary pulmonary carcinomas. J Natl Cancer Inst 82:1333–1339.

McWilliam P, Farrar GJ, Kenna P, et al (1989) Autosomal dominant retinitis pigmentosa (ADRP): Localization of an ADRP gene to the long arm of chromosome 3. Genomics 5:619–622.

Melnick M, Bixler D, Fogh-Andersen P, et al (1980) Cleft lip +/− cleft palate: An overview of the literature and an analysis of Danish cases born between 1941 and 1968. Am J Med Genet 6:83–97.

Merkatz IR, Nitowsky HM, Macri JN, et al (1984) An association between low maternal serum alpha-fetoprotein and fetal chromosome abnormalities. Am J Obstet Gynecol 148:886–894.

Miller DA, Choi YC, Miller OJ (1983) Chromosome localization of highly repetitive human DNAs and amplified ribosomal DNA with restriction enzymes. Science 219:395–397.

Miller DM, Blume S, Borst M, et al (1990) Oncogenes, malignant transformation, and modern medicine. Am J Med Sci 300:59–69.

Milunsky A (1986) Genetic disorders of the fetus, 2nd ed. Plenum Press, New York.

Mitchell GA, Brody LC, Sipila I, et al (1989) At least two mutant alleles of ornithine-δ-aminotransferase cause gyrate atrophy of the choroid and retina in Finns. Proc Natl Acad Sci USA 86:197–201.

Mitelman F (1988) Catalogue of chromosome aberrations in cancer, 3rd ed. Alan R. Liss, New York.

Mitelman F, Heim S (1988) Consistent involvement of only 71 of the 329 chromosomal bands of the human genome in primary neoplasia-associated rearrangements. Cancer Res 48:7115–7119.

Monaco AP, Bertelson CJ, Liechti-Gallati S, et al (1988) An explanation for the phenotypic differences between patients bearing partial deletions of the DMD locus. Genomics 2:90–95.

Moore KA, Fletcher FA, Villalon DK, et al (1990) Human adenosine deaminase expression in mice. Blood 75:2085 2092.

Moore KL, Barr ML (1955) Smears from the oral mucosa in the determination of chromosomal sex. Lancet 2:57–58.

Morel PA, Dorman JS, Todd JA, et al (1988) Aspartic acid at position 57 of the HLA-DQ beta chain protects against type I diabetes: A family study. Proc Natl Acad Sci USA 85:8111–8115.

Mourant AE (1983) Blood relations: Blood groups and anthropology. Oxford University Press, Oxford, England.

Mudd SH, Levy HL, Skovby F (1989) Disorders of transsulfuration. In Scriver CR, Beaudet AL, Sly WS, Vale D (eds) The metabolic basis of inherited disease, 6th ed. McGraw-Hill, New York, pp. 693–734.

N

Nabel EG, Plautz G, Nabel GJ (1990) Site-specific gene expression in vivo by direct gene transfer into the arterial wall. Science 249:1285–1288.

Nathans J, Davenport CM, Maumenee IH, et al (1989) Molecular genetics of human blue cone monochromacy. Science 245:831–838.

Nathans J, Thomas D, Hogness DS (1986) Molecular genetics of human color vision: The genes encoding blue, green, and red pigments. Science 232:193–210.

Nathans JN, Hogness DS (1984) Isolation and nucleotide sequence of the gene encoding human rhodopsin. Proc Natl Acad Sci USA 81:4851–4855.

Neel JV (1983) Frequency of spontaneous and induced point mutations in higher eukaryotes. J Hered 74:2–15.

Nelson K, Holmes LB (1989) Malformations due to presumed spontaneous mutations in newborn infants. N Engl J Med 320:19–23.

Neufeld EF, Muenzer J (1989) The mucopolysaccharidoses. In Scriver CR, Beaudet AL, Sly WS, Valle D (eds) The metabolic basis of inherited disease, 6th ed. McGraw-Hill, New York, pp. 1565–1587.

New MI, White PC, Pang S, et al (1989) The adrenal hyperplasias. In Scriver CJ, Beaudet AL, Sly W, Valle D (eds) The metabolic basis of inherited disease, 6th ed. McGraw-Hill, New York, pp. 1881–1917.

Nicholls RD, Knoll JH, Butler MG, et al (1989) Genetic imprinting suggested by maternal heterodisomy in nondeletion Prader-Willi syndrome. Nature 342:281–285.

Nienhuis AW, Maniatis T (1987) Structure and expression of globin genes in erythroid cells. In Stamatoyannopoulos G, Nienhuis AW, Leder P, Majerus PW (eds) The molecular basis of blood diseases. WB Saunders, Philadelphia, pp. 28–65.

Nora JJ (1968) Multifactorial inheritance hypothesis for the etiology of congenital heart diseases: The genetic-environmental interaction. Circulation 38:604–617.

Norio R, Nevanlinna HR, Perheentupa J (1973) Hereditary diseases in Finland: Rare flora in rare soil. Ann Clin Res 5:109–141.

Nourse J, Mellentin JD, Galili N, et al (1990) Chromosomal translocation t(1;19) results in synthesis of a homeobox fusion mRNA that codes for a potential chimeric transcription factor. Cell 60:535–545.

Nussbaum RL, Boggs BA, Beaudet AL, et al (1986) New mutation and prenatal diagnosis in ornithine transcarbamylase deficiency. Am J Hum Genet 38:149–158.

O

Okano Y, Wang T, Eisensmith RC, et al (1990a) Missense mutations associated with RFLP haplotypes 1 and 4 of the human phenylalanine hydroxylase gene. Am J Hum Genet 46:18–25.

Okano Y, Wang T, Eisensmith RC, et al (1990b) Correlation of mutant genotypes and clinical phenotypes of PKU in Caucasians. Vth International Congress of Inborn Errors of Metabolism, Abstract W4.3.

Orkin SH (1987) Disorders of hemoglobin synthesis: The thalassemias. In Stamatoyannopoulos G, Nienhuis AW, Leder P, Majerus PW (eds) The molecular basis of blood diseases. WB Saunders, Philadelphia, pp. 106–126.

P

Page DC, Fisher EMC, McGillivray B, et al (1990) Additional deletion in sex-determining region of human Y chromosome resolves paradox of X,t(Y;22) female. Nature 346:279–281.

Page DC, Mosher R, Simpson EM, et al (1987) The sex-determining region of the human Y chromosome encodes a zinc finger protein. Cell 51:1091–1104.

Painter TS (1921) The Y chromosome in mammals. Science 53:503–504.

Palmer MS, Sinclair AH, Berta P, et al (1989) Genetic evidence that ZFY is not the testis-determining factor. Nature 342:937–939.

Palmiter RD, Brinster RL (1986) Germ-line transformation of mice. Ann Rev Genet 20:465–499.

Palmiter RD, Norstedt G, Gelinas RE, et al (1983) Metallo-thionein-human GH fusion genes stimulate growth of mice. Science 222:809–814.

Pang S, Pollack MS, Marshall RN, Immken L (1990) Prenatal treatment of congenital adrenal hyperplasia due to 21-hydroxylase deficiency. N Engl J Med 322:111–115.

Park M, vande Woude GF (1989) Oncogenes: Genes associated with neoplastic disease. In Scriver CR, Beaudet AL, Sly WS, Valle D (eds), The metabolic basis of inherited disease, 6th ed. McGraw-Hill, New York, pp. 251–276.

Partridge TA, Morgan JE, Coulton GR, et al (1989) Conversion of mdx myofibres from dystrophin-negative to -positive by injection of normal myoblasts. Nature 337:176–179.

Patel PI, Framson PE, Caskey CT, et al (1986) Fine structure of the human hypoxanthine phosphoribosyltransferase gene. Mol Cell Biol 6:393–403.

Pauling L, Itano HA, Singer SJ, Wells IG (1949) Sickle cell anemia, a molecular disease. Science 110:543–548.

Paulson JR, Laemmli U (1977) The structure of histone-depleted metaphase chromosomes. Cell 12:817–828.

Pearson PL (1991) The Genome Data base (GDB), a human gene mapping repository. Nucl Acids Res 19:2237–2239.

Pellestor F, Sèle B, Jalbert H, Jalbert P (1989) Direct segregation analysis of reciprocal translocations: A study of 283 sperm karyotypes from four carriers. Am J Hum Genet 44:464–471.

Perry VH, Gordon S (1988) Macrophages and microglia in the nervous system. Trends Neurosci 11:273–277.

Petit C, de la Chapelle A, Levilliers J, et al (1987) An abnormal terminal X;Y interchange accounts for most but not all cases of human XX maleness. Cell 49:595–602.

Pettigrew AL, Gollin SM, Greenberg F, et al (1987) Duplication of proximal 15q as a cause of Prader-Willi syndrome. Am J Med Genet 28:791–802.

Pieters M, Geraedts JM, Meyer H, et al (1990) Human gametes and zygotes studied by non-radioactive in situ hybridization. Cytogenet Cell Genet 53:15–19.

Pinsky L, Kaufman M (1987) Genetics of steroid receptors and their disorders. Adv Hum Genet 16:299–472.

Ponder BAJ (1990) Inherited predisposition to cancer. Trends Genet 6:213–218.

Posselt AM, Barker CF, Tomaszewski JE, et al (1990) Induction of donor-specific unresponsiveness by intrathymic islet transplantation. Science 249:1293–1296.

Prockop DJ, Baldwin CT, Constantinou CD (1990) Mutations in Type I procollagen genes that cause osteogenesis imperfecta. Adv Hum Genet 19:105–132.

R

Race RR, Sanger R (1975) Blood groups in man, 6th ed. Blackwell, Oxford, England.

Rahmani Z, Blouin JL, Creau-Goldberg N, et al (1989) Critical role of the D21S55 region on chromosome 21 in the pathogenesis of Down syndrome. Proc Natl Acad Sci USA 86:5958–5962.

Ramsay M, Bernstein R, Zwane E, et al (1988) XX true hermaphroditism in southern African blacks: An enigma of primary sexual differentiation. Am J Hum Genet 43:4–13.

Rawlings CE, Wilkins RH, Cook WA, Burger C (1987) Segmental neurofibromatosis. Neurosurgery 20:946–949.

Ray PN, Belfall B, Duff C, et al (1985) Cloning of the breakpoint of an X;21 translocation associated with Duchenne muscular dystrophy. Nature 318:672–675.

Reed TE (1969) Caucasian genes in American Negroes. Science 165:76–78.

Reeders ST, Breuning MH, Davies KE, et al (1985) A highly polymorphic DNA marker linked to adult polycystic kidney disease on chromosome 16. Nature 317:542–544.

Reichardt JKV, Woo SLC (1991) Molecular basis of galactosemia: Mutations and polymorphisms in human galactose-1-phosphate uridyltransferase. Proc Natl Acad Sci USA 88:2633–2637.

Reik W (1989) Genomic imprinting and genetic disorders in man. Trends Genet 5:331–336.

Rey F, Berthelon M, Caillaud C, et al (1988) Clinical and molecular heterogeneity of phenylalanine hydroxylase deficiencies in France. Am J Hum Genet 43:914–921.

Rhoads GG, Jackson LG, Schlesselman SE, et al (1989) The safety and efficacy of chorionic villus sampling for early prenatal diagnosis of cytogenetic abnormalities. N Engl J Med 320:609–617.

Ricciuti FC, Gelehrter TD, Rosenberg LE (1976) X-chromosome inactivation in human liver: confirmation of X-linkage of ornithine transcarbamylase. Am J Hum Genet 28:332–338.

Rich DP, Anderson MP, Gregory RJ, et al (1990) Expression of cystic fibrosis transmembrane regulator corrects defective chloride channel regulation in cystic fibrosis airway epithelial cells. Nature 347:358–363.

Richards CS, Watkins SC, Hoffman EP, et al (1990) Skewed X inactivation in a female MZ twin results in Duchenne muscular dystrophy. Am J Hum Genet 46:672–681.

Ringe D, Petsko GA (1990) Cystic fibrosis: A transport problem? Nature 346:312–313.

Riordan JR, Rommens JR, Kerem B-S, et al (1989) Identification of the cystific fibrosis gene: Cloning and characterization of complementary DNA. Science 245:1066–1072.

Robinson A, Bender BGF, Linden MG (1989) Decisions following the intrauterine diagnosis of sex chromosome aneuploidy. Am J Med Genet 34:552–554.

Rodgers GP, Dover GJ, Noguchi CT, et al (1990) Hematologic responses of patients with sickle cell disease to treatment with hydroxyurea. N Engl J Med 322:1037–1045.

Rommens JR, Iannuzzi MC, Kerem B-S, et al (1989) Identification of the cystic fibrosis gene: Chromosome walking and jumping. Science 245:1059–1065.

Roscher AA, Hoefler S, Hoefler G, et al (1989) Genetic and phenotypic heterogeneity in disorders of peroxisome biogenesis—A complementation study involving cell lines from 19 patients. Pediat Res 26:67–72.

Rosen R, Morgan K (1990) Personal communication.

Rosenberg LE (1976) Vitamin-responsive inherited metabolic disorders. Adv Hum Genet 6:1–74.

Rosenberg LE (1980) Inborn errors of metabolism. In Bondy PK, Rosenberg LE (eds) Metabolic control and disease, 8th ed. WB Saunders, Philadelphia, pp. 73–102.

Rosenberg LE, Fenton WA (1989) Disorders of propionate and methylmalonate metabolism. In Scriver CR, Beaudet AL, Sly WS, Valle D (eds) The metabolic basis of inherited disease, 6th ed. McGraw-Hill, New York, pp. 821–844.

Rosenberg SA, Aebersold P, Cornetta K, et al (1990) Gene transfer into humans—Immunotherapy of patients with advanced melanoma, using tumor-infiltrating lymphocytes modified by retroviral gene transduction. N Engl J Med 323:570–578.

Rouyer F, Simmler MC, Page DC, Weissenbach J (1987) A sex chromosome rearrangement in a human XX male caused by Alu-Alu recombination. Cell 51:417–425.

Rowley JD (1973) A new consistent chromosomal abnormality in CML identified by quinacrine fluorescence and Giemsa staining. Nature 243:290–291.

Rudak E, Jacobs PA, Yanagimachi R (1978) Direct analysis of the chromosome constitution of human spermatozoa. Nature 174:911–913.

Ruddle FH (1984) The William Allan Memorial Award address: Reverse genetics and beyond. Am J Hum Genet 36:944–953.

Ruggeri ZM, Zimmerman TS (1987) Von Willebrand factor and von Willebrand disease. Blood 70:895–904.

S

Sadler JE (1989) Von Willebrand disease. *In* Scriver CR, Beaudet AL, Sly WS, Valle D (eds) The metabolic basis of inherited disease, 6th ed. McGraw-Hill, New York, pp. 2171–2187.

Sager R (1989) Tumor suppressor genes: The puzzle and the promise. Science 246:1406–1412.

Saiki RK, Scharf S, Faloona F, et al (1985) Enzymatic amplification of β-globin genomic sequences and restriction site analysis for diagnosis of sickle cell anemia. Science 230:1350–1354.

Sandhoff K, Conzelmann E, Neufeld EF, et al (1989) The G_{M2} gangliosidoses. *In* Scriver CR, Beaudet AL, Sly WS, Valle D (eds) The metabolic basis of inherited disease, 6th ed. McGraw-Hill, New York, pp. 1807–1839.

Sangiuolo F, Novelli S, Murru S, et al (1991) A serine to arginine (ATG to CTG) mutation in codon 549 of the CFTR gene in an Italian patient with severe cystic fibrosis. Genomics 9:788–789.

Santos MJ, Imanaka T, Shio H, et al (1988) Peroxisomal membrane ghosts in Zellweger syndrome—Aberrant organelle assembly. Science 239:1536–1538.

Schildkraut JM, Thompson WD (1988) Familial ovarian cancer: A population-based case-control study. Am J Epidemiol 128:456–466.

Schneider-Gadicke A, Beer-Romero P, Brown LG, et al (1989) ZFX has a gene structure similar to ZFY, the putative human sex determinant, and escapes X inactivation. Cell 57:1247–1258.

Scriver CR, Beaudet AL, Sly WS, Valle D (eds) (1989) The metabolic basis of inherited disease, 6th ed. McGraw-Hill, New York.

Scriver CR, Kaufman S, Woo SLC (1989) The hyperphenylalaninemias. *In* Scriver CR, Beaudet AL, Sly WS, Valle D (eds) The metabolic basis of inherited disease, 6th ed. McGraw-Hill, New York, pp. 495–546.

Segal S (1989) Disorders of galactose metabolism. *In* Scriver CR, Beaudet AL, Sly WS, Valle D (eds) The metabolic basis of inherited disease, 6th ed. McGraw-Hill, New York, pp. 453–480.

Shapiro LJ, Mohandas T, Weiss R, et al (1979) Non-inactivation of an X chromosome locus in man. Science 204:1224–1226.

Shoumatoff A (1985) The mountain of names: A history of the human family. Simon and Schuster, New York.

Shull RM, Breider MA, Constantinopoulos GC (1988) Long-term neurological effects of bone marrow transplantation in a canine lysosomal storage disease. Pediat Res 24:347–352.

Shull RM, Hastings NE, Selcer RR, et al (1987) Bone marrow transplantation in canine mucopolysaccharidosis I. J Clin Invest 79:435–443.

Sinclair AH, Berta P, Palmer MS, et al (1990) A gene from the human sex-determining region encodes a protein with homology to a conserved DNA-binding motif. Nature 346:240–244.

Sinha AA, Lopez MT, McDevitt HO (1990) Autoimmune diseases: The failure of self tolerance. Science 248:1380–1387.

Slack J, Evans KA (1966) The increased risk of death from ischaemic heart disease. J Med Genet 3:239–257.

Smithells RW, Sheppard S, Schorah CJ, et al (1980) Possible prevention of neural tube defects by periconceptional vitamin supplementation. Lancet 1:339–340.

Southern E (1975) Detection of specific sequences among DNA fragments separated by gel electrophoresis. J Mol Biol 98:503–517.

Spence JE, Perciaccante RG, Greig GM, et al (1988) Uniparental disomy as a mechanism for human genetic disease. Am J Hum Genet 42:217–226.

Spranger J, Benirschke K, Hall JG, et al (1982) Errors of morphogenesis: Concepts and terms. Recommendations of an international working group. J Pediatr 100:160–165.

Spritz RA, Jagadeeswaran P, Choudary PV, et al (1981) Base substitution in an intervening sequence of a β^+-thalassemic human globin gene. Proc Natl Acad Sci USA 78:2455–2459.

Stamatoyannopoulos G, Nienhuis AW (1987) Hemoglobin switching. *In* Stamatoyannopoulos G, Nienhuis AW, Leder P, Majerus PW (eds) The molecular basis of blood diseases. WB Saunders, Philadelphia, pp. 66–105.

Stanbridge EJ (1990) Identifying tumor suppressor genes in human colorectal cancer. Science 247:12–13.

Steele MW, Breg WR (1966) Chromosome analysis of human amniotic fluid cells. Lancet 1:383–385.

Stephens JC, Cavanaugh ML, Gradie MI, et al (1990) Mapping the human genome: Current status. Science 250:237–244.

Stewart GD, Hassold TJ, Berg A, et al (1988) Trisomy 21 (Down syndrome): Studying nondisjunction and meiotic recombination by using cytogenetic and molecular polymorphisms that span chromosome 21. Am J Hum Genet 42:227–236.

Stewart GD, Hassold TJ, Kurnit DM (1988) Trisomy 21: Molecular and cytogenetic studies of nondisjunction. Adv Hum Genet 17:99–140.

Strominger JL (1986) Biology of the human histocompatibility leukocyte antigen (HLA) system and a hypothesis regarding the generation of autoimmune diseases. J Clin Invest 77:1411–1415.

Stryer L (1981) Biochemistry, 2nd ed. WH Freeman, San Francisco.

Stunkard AJ, Harris JR, Pedersen NL, McClearn GE (1990) The body-mass index of twins who have been reared apart. N Engl J Med 322:1483–1487.

Swift M, Reitnauer PJ, Morrell D, et al (1987) Breast and other cancers in families with ataxia-telangiectasia. N Engl J Med 316:1289–1294.

T

Terasaki PI, Gjertson D, Bernoco D, et al (1978) Twins with two different fathers identified by HLA. N Engl J Med 299:590–592.

Therman E, Sarto GE, Patau K (1974) Apparently isodicentric but functionally monocentric X chromosome in man. Am J Hum Genet 26:83–92.

Thompson MW (1965) Genetic consequences of heteropyknosis of an X chromosome. Can J Genet Cytol 7:202–213.

Thomson G, Robinson WP, Kuhner HK, et al (1988) Genetic heterogeneity, modes of inheritance, and risk estimates for a joint study of Caucasians with insulin-dependent diabetes mellitus. Am J Hum Genet 43:799–816.

Todd JA, Bell JI, McDevitt HO (1987) HLA-DQ$_\beta$ gene contributes to susceptibility and resistance to insulin-dependent diabetes mellitus. Nature 329:599–604.

Trask B, van den Engh G, Mayall B, et al (1989) Chromosome hetermorphism quantified by high-resolution bivariate flow karyotyping. Am J Hum Genet 45:739–752.

Trent JM, Kaneko Y, Mitelman F (1989) Report of the committee on chromosomal changes in neoplasia. Human Gene Mapping 10: Tenth international workshop on human gene mapping. Cytogenet Cell Genet 51:533–562.

Triggs-Raine BL, Feigenbaum ASJ, Natowicz M, et al (1990) Screening for carriers of Tay-Sachs diseases among Ashkenazi Jews. N Engl J Med 323:6–12.

Tsui L-C (1990) Personal communication.

Tsui L-C, Buchwald M, Barker D, et al (1985) Cystic fibrosis locus defined by a genetically linked polymorphic DNA marker. Science 230:1054–1057.

Tsui L-C, Zengerling A, Willard HF, Buchwald M (1986) Mapping of the cystic fibrosis locus on chromosome 7. Cold Spring Harbor Symp Quant Biol 51:325–335.

V

Van Assendelft GB, Hanscombe O, Grosveld F, Greaves DR (1989). The β globin dominant control region activates homologous and heterologous promoters in a tissue-specific manner. Cell 56:969–977.

Vehar GA, Lawn RM, Tuddenham EGD, et al (1989) Factor VIII and factor V: Biochemistry and pathophysiology. In Scriver CR, Beaudet AL, Sly WS, Valle D (eds) The metabolic basis of inherited disease, 6th ed. McGraw-Hill, New York, pp. 2155–2170.

Verkerk A, Pieretti M, Sutcliffe JS, et al (in press) Identification of a gene (FMR-1) containing a CGG repeat coincident with a breakpoint cluster region exhibiting length variation in fragile X syndrome. Cell.

Vidaud D, Vidaud M, Plassa F, et al (1989) Father-to-son transmission of hemophilia A due to uniparental disomy. Am J Hum Genet 45:A226.

Viskochil D, Buchberg AM, Xu G, et al (1990) Deletions and a translocation interrupt a cloned gene at the neurofibromatosis type 1 locus. Cell 62:187–192.

Vogel F, Motulsky AG (1986) Human genetics, 2nd ed. Springer-Verlag, Berlin.

Voss R, Ben-Simon E, Avital A, et al (1989) Isodisomy of chromosome 7 in a patient with cystic fibrosis: Could uniparental disomy be common in humans? Am J Hum Genet 45:373–380.

W

Wald NJ, Cuckle HS (1987) Recent advances in screening for neural tube defects and Down syndrome. In Rodeck C (ed) Prenatal diagnosis. Baillière Tindal, London, pp. 649–676.

Wald NJ, Cuckle HS, Densem JW, et al (1988) Maternal serum screening for Down's syndrome in early pregnancy. Br Med J 297:883–887.

Wald NJ, Cuckle HS, Densem JW, et al (1988) Maternal serum unconjugated oestriol as an antenatal screening test for Down's syndrome. Br J Obstet Gynaecol 95:334–341.

Wallace DC (1989) Mitochondrial DNA mutations and neuromuscular disease. Trends Genet 5:9–13.

Wallace MR, Marchuk DA, Andersen LB, et al (1990) Type I neurofibromatosis gene: Identification of a large transcript disrupted in three NF1 patients. Science 249:181–186.

Wallis GA, Starman BJ, Zinn AB, Byers PH (1990) Variable expression of osteogenesis imperfecta in a nuclear family is explained by somatic mosaicism for a lethal point mutation in the α1(I) gene (COL1A1) of type I collagen in a parent. Am J Hum Genet 46:1034–1040.

Warburton D, Kline J, Stein Z, et al (1987) Does the karyotype of a spontaneous abortion predict the karyotype of a subsequent abortion?—Evidence from 273 women with two karyotyped spontaneous abortions. Am J Hum Genet 41:465–483.

Watkins WM (1980) Biochemistry and genetics of the ABO, Lewis, and P blood group systems. Adv Hum Genet 10:1–136.

Watson JD (1990) The human genome project. Science 248:44–49.

Watson JD, Crick FHC (1953) Molecular structure of nucleic acids—A structure for deoxyribose nucleic acid. Nature 171:737–738.

Weatherall DJ, Clegg JB (1981) The thalassemia syndromes, 3rd ed. Blackwell Scientific Publications, Oxford, England.

Weatherall DJ, Clegg JB, Higgs DR, et al (1989) The hemoglobinopathies. In Scriver CR, Beaudet AL, Sly WS, Valle D (eds) The metabolic basis of inherited disease. 6th ed. McGraw-Hill, New York, pp. 629–663.

Weinberg RA (1990) The retinoblastoma gene and cell growth control. Trends Biochem Sci 15:199–202.

Wewers M, Casolaro A, Sellers SE, et al (1987) Replacement therapy for alpha$_1$-antitrypsin deficiency associated with emphysema. N Engl J Med 316:1055–1062.

Wexler NS, Young AB, Tanzi RE, et al (1987) Homozygotes for Huntington's disease. Nature 326:194–197.

White C, Wyshak G (1964) Inheritance in human dizygotic twinning. N Engl J Med 271:1003–1005.

White MB, Amos J, Hsu JMC, et al (1990) A frame-shift mutation in the cystic fibrosis gene. Nature 344:665–667.

White R, Lalouel JM (1988) Sets of linked genetic markers for human chromosomes. Ann Rev Genet 22:259–279.

Whittaker M (1986) Cholinesterase. Karger, Basel.

WHO Working Group (1982) Hereditary anemias: Genetic basis, clinical features, diagnosis and treatment. Bull WHO 60:643.

Wiesmann UN, Lightbody J, Vasella F, Hershkowitz N (1971) Multiple enzyme deficiency due to enzyme leakage. N Engl J Med 285:1090–1091.

Williamson R, Bowcock A, Kidd KK, et al (1990) Report of the DNA committee and catalogues of cloned and mapped genes and DNA polymorphisms. Human Gene Mapping 10.5 (1990): Update to the Tenth International Workshop on Human Gene Mapping. Cytogenet Cell Genet 55:457–778.

Wolff JA, Malone RW, Williams P, et al (1990) Direct gene transfer into mouse muscle in vivo. Science 247:1465–1468.

Wong C, Dowling CE, Saiki RK, et al (1987) Characterization of β-thalassemia mutations using direct genomic sequencing of amplified single copy DNA. Nature 330:384–386.

Woo SLC, Lidsky AS, Guttler F, et al (1983) Cloned human phenylalanine hydroxylase gene allows prenatal diagnosis and carrier detection of classical phenylketonuria. Nature 306:151–155.

Wood WG (1976) Hemoglobin synthesis during normal fetal development. Br Med Bull 32:282–287.

Woolf LM, McBea MS, Woolf FM, et al (1975) Phenylketonuria as a balanced polymorphism: The nature of the heterozygote advantage. Ann Hum Genet 38:461–469.

Workshop on Population Screening for the Cystic Fibrosis Gene (1990) N Engl J Med 323:70–71.

Worton RG, Gillard EF (in press) Duchenne muscular dystrophy. *In* Conneally PM (ed) Molecular genetics in clinical medicine. Blackwell, Oxford, England.

Wyman AR, White R (1980) A highly polymorphic locus in human DNA. Proc Natl Acad Sci USA 77:6754–6758.

X

Xu G, O'Connell P, Viskochil D, et al (1990) The neurofibromatosis type 1 gene encodes a protein related to GAP. Cell 62:599–608.

Y

Yamamoto F, Clausen H, White T, et al (1990) Molecular genetic basis of the histo-blood group ABO system. Nature 345:229–233.

Yen PH, Li XM, Tsai SP, et al (1990) Frequent deletions of the human X chromosome short arm result from recombination between low copy repetitive elements. Cell 61:603–610.

Young BD, Ferguson-Smith MA, Sillar R, et al (1981) High resolution analysis of human peripheral lymphocyte chromosomes by flow cytometry. Proc Natl Acad Sci USA 78:7727–7731.

Youssoufian H, Kazazian HH, Philips DG, et al (1986) Recurrent mutations in hemophilia A: evidence for CpG dinucleotides as mutation hotspots. Nature 324:380–382.

Yu S, Pritchard M, Kremer E, et al (1991) Fragile X genotype characterized by an unstable region of DNA. Science 252:1179–1181.

Z

Zielenski J, Bozon D, Kerem B, et al (1991) Identification of mutations in the region spanning exons 1-8 of the cystic fibrosis gene. Genomics 10:229–235.

ANSWERS TO PROBLEMS

CHAPTER 2

1. a) *A* and *a*. b) i. At meiosis I. ii. At meiosis II.

2. a) 2. b) 2^4. c) 2^n.

3. $(1/2)^{23} \times (1/2)^{23}$; you would be female.

4. a) 23; 46; 92. b) 23; 23; 46. c) At fertilization; at S stage of the next cell cycle.

CHAPTER 3

1. There are several possible sequences because of the degeneracy of the genetic code. One possible sequence of the double-stranded DNA is

5' AAA AGA CAT CAT TAT CTA 3'
3' TTT T CT GTA GTA ATA GAT 5'

RNA polymerase "reads" the bottom (3' to 5') strand. The sequence of the resulting mRNA would be

5'AAA AGA CAU CAU UAU CUA 3'.

The mutants represent the following kinds of mutations:

    Mutant 1: single nucleotide substitution in fifth codon; e.g., UAU → UGU.
    Mutant 2: frameshift mutation, deletion in first nucleotide of third codon.
    Mutant 3: frameshift mutation, insertion of G between first and second codons.
    Mutant 4: in-frame deletion of three codons (nine nucleotides), beginning at the third base.

2. Chromosomes contain chromatin, consisting of nucleosomes. Chromosomes contain G bands that contain several thousand kilobase pairs of DNA (or several million base pairs) and hundreds of genes, each containing (usually) both introns and exons. The exons are a series of codons, each of which is three base pairs in length.

3. Chromosome 5 contains about 200 million base pairs of DNA and 3000 to 7000 genes. Band 5p15 is about one tenth to one fifteenth of the total chromosome length and, therefore, can be estimated to contain approximately 10 to 20 million base pairs of DNA and 200 to 700 genes. Even though these are gross estimates, the important concept to grasp is that chromosome bands potentially contain on the order of hundreds of genes.

CHAPTER 4

1. b) Autosomal recessive; 1/4.   c) About 1/180, about 10 times population risk.
   d) Betty, Barbara, Calvin, Cathy.

2. a) Heterozygous at each of two loci; e.g., *A/a B/b*.   b) The parents (Gilbert and Gisele, Horace and Hedy) are all homozygous for the *same* recessive allele for congenital deafness.

3. d, j, h, e, i, a, b, f, c, and g.

4. b) They are homozygous.   c) 100 percent; virtually zero if her partner is unaffected.
   d) 50 percent; virtually zero if her partner is unaffected.

5. All are possible except (c), which is unlikely if the parents are completely unaffected.

6. a) New mutation.   b) Near zero.   c) Near zero.   d) 50 percent.

CHAPTER 5

1. a) A gene deletion can be easily detected by DNA analysis, with either Southern blotting (with a DMD cDNA probe) or the polymerase chain reaction (with primers for a portion of the gene).   b) Northern blotting.   c) Indirect immunofluorescence, with dystrophin antibodies. See Figure 12–13. Western blotting would provide information on the abundance of dystrophin in these muscle specimens but would not reveal information regarding cellular localization.   d) Because the specific base pair change for which the fetus is at risk is known, a test with allele-specific oligonucleotides (ASOs) would be most useful.

2. The chief advantage of PCR is that much less DNA is required for an analysis than in Southern blotting. In addition, PCR is much faster and less expensive. Potential disadvantages include the fact that PCR can only "see" relatively short stretches of genomic DNA (in each assay), whereas Southern blotting can "examine" an entire gene. PCR is also much more sensitive to contamination by extraneous DNA. In comparison with biochemical assays, PCR has the same advantages of speed and sample economy. However, whereas biochemical assays can detect a range of mutations at a locus (including any unknown mutation that interferes with enzyme activity), PCR is best suited to examining specific, known mutations.

3. All except red blood cells.

4. Establishes the gene responsible for a given disorder; provides opportunity to determine the molecular basis of a disorder, through extensive laboratory research; provides immediate tools for diagnosis and genetic counseling.

5. The liver cDNA library would be a more appropriate starting point because (1) cDNA sequences are shorter than genomic genes, as a result of the absence of intronic and other flanking sequences from cDNAs, and therefore it is easier to obtain a significant portion of the coding sequences; and (2) particularly if the gene is expressed at high levels in liver, the desired cDNA clones may be present at a much higher frequency in the liver cDNA library (as high as 0.1 percent to 1 percent) than in a genomic library containing all sequences in the genome equally (in which any given gene represents ≪ 0.01 percent).

CHAPTER 6

1. There are a number of possible answers, including the following: a) Point mutation leading to an amino acid substitution critical for enzyme function. b) Nonsense mutation, leading to truncated, unstable protein that is rapidly degraded. c) Gene deletion or promoter mutation. d) Point mutation leading to an amino acid substitution in an area of the protein that is *not* critical for enzyme function, but which alters the overall charge of the protein. e) RNA splicing mutation, resulting in production of reduced levels of mature mRNA and thus reduced levels of GALT protein. f) Point mutation in a noncoding portion of the gene, resulting in change in a particular restriction enzyme recognition site.

2. 41 mutations/9 million alleles = 4.55×10^{-6}. Estimate is based on assumptions that ascertained cases result from new mutation, that the disease is fully penetrant, that all new mutants are liveborn (and ascertained), and that there is only a single locus at which mutations can lead to aniridia. If there are multiple loci, then the estimated rate is too high. If some mutations are not ascertained (because of lack of penetrance or death in utero), the estimated rate might be too low.

3. a) An X-linked restriction fragment length polymorphism. b) If polymorphism is due to a point mutation, then individuals of different genotypes would have indistinguishable patterns with a different restriction enzyme. However, if polymorphism is due to a 2-kb deletion/insertion, then the same polymorphism should be detected with any restriction enzyme that cleaves on either side of the deletion/insertion.

4. One way of determining this is to reverse the question and ask instead what proportion of individuals would be *homozygous*. For each allele, the frequency of homozygotes would be $.20 \times .20$, or .04. Thus $5 \times .04$, or 20 percent, of individuals would be homozygous for one of the five alleles. Therefore, 80 percent of individuals would be heterozygous at this locus.

5. *B/B*, .0001; *B/S*, .012; *B/O*, .0076; *S/S*, .372; *S/O*, .464; *O/O*, .144. Estimated lipoprotein(a) levels for the six genotypes will be 50, 35, 25, 20, 10, and 0 mg/dl, respectively. The *B/B* and *B/S* groups are at risk of premature coronary heart disease and include slightly more than 1 percent of this population.

CHAPTER 7

1. a) *a*, 0.1; *A*, 0.9. b) Same. c) $(0.18)^2$.

2. a) .02. b) $(.04)^2$ or about 1 in 600 (homozygotes do not reproduce). c) .0004. d) 1/4.

3. Only d) is in equilibrium. Selection for or against particular genotypes; nonrandom mating; recent migration.

4. a) Abby has a 2/3 chance of being a carrier. Andrew has about a 1/150 chance of being a carrier. Therefore, their risk of having an affected child is $2/3 \times 1/150 \times 1/4$, or 1/900. b) $2/3 \times 1/4 \times 1/4 = 1/24$. c) $2/3 \times 1/22 \times 1/4 = 1/132$; $2/3 \times 1/4 \times 1/4 = 1/24$.

5. a) Retinoblastoma, q = 1/50,000, 2pq = 1/25,000; Friedreich's ataxia, q = 1/158, 2pq = 1/79; choroideremia, q = 1/25,000, 2pq = 1/12,500. b) The autosomal dominant and X-linked disorders would increase rapidly, within one generation, to reach a new

balance; the autosomal recessive would increase also but only very slowly, because the vast majority of the mutant alleles are not subject to selection.

6. Approximately 1/25 and 1/300.

7. Because the high incidence appears to be due to a founder effect, most or all cases are descended from the one or more common founding ancestors; thus the mutant alleles are expected to be relatively homogeneous. For achondroplasia and Duchenne muscular dystrophy, because a large proportion of cases in each generation is the result of new mutation, the mutant alleles present in the population are heterogeneous. Color blindness, however, is relatively common; thus the mutant alleles would be expected to be more heterogeneous, having entered the population from a number of sources.

CHAPTER 8

1. The HD and MNSs loci map far apart on chromosome 4 and are thus unlinked, even though syntenic.

2. For HD, yes, because all evidence suggests that only one or at most a few different mutations are responsible for all cases. No new mutations have ever been documented. For NF1, no, because approximately half of all cases result from new mutations, which occur on a variety of different haplotypes.

3. Fragment 1 is present in hybrids II, III, IV, and VII, but absent in hybrids I, V, VI, and VIII. Fragment 2 cannot be mapped, because a mouse fragment of the same size is present in all hybrids, and the human and mouse fragments cannot be distinguished. Fragment 1 of the Q gene maps to chromosome 7.

4. The lod scores indicate that this polymorphism is closely linked to the polycystic kidney disease gene at an estimated distance of ~ 5 cM. The odds in favor of linkage at this distance compared to no linkage at all are $10^{25.85}$:1 (i.e., almost 10^{26}:1). The data in the second study indicate that there is *no* linkage between the disease gene and the polymorphism in this family. Thus there is genetic heterogeneity in this disorder, and linkage information can therefore be used for diagnosis only if there is prior evidence that the disease in that particular family is linked to the polymorphism.

5. Coppock's cataract seems to cosegregate with the "A" haplotype. There are no crossovers. A complete lod score analysis should be performed (see Lubsen et al., 1987). In addition, one might examine the gamma crystallin gene itself for mutations in affected persons, using one of many methods described in the text.

6. The phase in the mother is probably *B*-WAS, according to the genotype of the affected boy. This phase can be determined with 95 percent certainty, because there is a 5 percent chance that a crossover occurred in the meiosis leading to the affected boy. On the basis of this information, there is a $(.95 \times .95) + (.05 \times .05)$ chance that the fetus (who is male) will be *unaffected*.

7. This surprising result (assuming paternity is as stated) indicates that the mother has inherited the *A* allele (and the WAS allele) from her mother — that is, her phase is *A*-WAS, not *B*-WAS as surmised in question 6. Thus there must have been a crossover in the meiosis leading to the affected boy. To confirm this, one should examine polymorphisms on either side of this one on the X chromosome to make sure that the segregation patterns are consistent with a crossover. On the basis of this new information, there is now a 95 percent chance that the fetus in the current pregnancy is *affected*.

8. a) He must be heterozygous for the 7 and 9 kb alleles. b) The mother's phase is 12-disease and 9-normal. The father's phase must be 9-disease and 7-normal. This is determined by process of elimination, considering that the three children are known to be unaffected. c) From the phase information from (b), II.1 and II.3 are carriers. II.4 is not a carrier. d) The fetus will be affected. These conclusions are based on a number of assumptions, including that no crossovers have occurred, that the apparent father is indeed the father of all these children, and that the mutation occurs in the gene in which you think it occurs (i.e., that there is no unsuspected genetic heterogeneity).

9. This question is for open discussion. See text for possible answers.

CHAPTER 9

1. a) 46 chromosomes; male; one of the chromosome 18s has a shorter long arm than normal. b) To determine if the abnormality is de novo or inherited from a balanced carrier parent. c) 46 chromosomes, male, only one normal 7 and one normal 18, plus a reciprocal translocation between chromosomes 7 and 18. This is a balanced karyotype. For meiotic pairing and segregation, see text, particularly Figure 9–10. d) The 18q— chromosome is the der(18) translocation chromosome, 18pter → 18q12::7q35 → 7qter. The boy's karyotype is unbalanced; he is monosomic for the distal long arm of 18 and trisomic for the distal long arm of 7.

2. a) About 95 percent. b) No increased risk.

3. Postzygotic nondisjunction, in an early mitotic division. Although the clinical course cannot be predicted with complete accuracy, it is likely that she will be somewhat less severely affected than a nonmosaic trisomy 21 child.

4. a) Normal phenotype, but risk of Down syndrome offspring (see text). b) Abnormal phenotype (Down syndrome). c) Abnormal phenotype; will not reproduce. d) Abnormal phenotype in proband and ∼50 percent of offspring. e) Normal phenotype, but risk for unbalanced offspring (see text).

5. Mosaicism in a parent; theoretically, genetic factors also.

6. a) Not indicated. b) Fetal karyotyping indicated. At risk for trisomy 21, in particular. c) Karyotype indicated for child to determine if trisomy 21 or translocation Down syndrome. If translocation, then parental karyotypes are indicated. d) Not indicated, unless other clinical findings might suggest a contiguous gene syndrome. e) Karyotype indicated for the boys to rule out deletion of 17q12, in the vicinity of the NF1 gene, that might cause contiguous gene syndrome.

CHAPTER 10

1. Theoretically, X and XX gametes in equal proportions; expected XX, XY, XXX, and XXY offspring.

2. a) To determine whether presence of an X-linked recessive disorder in the girl is due to a chromosome defect, such as an X;autosome translocation or 45,X Turner syndrome, or to presence of a condition allowing a female phenotype in an XY person. See text. b) The break disrupts one copy of the hemophilia A (factor VIII) gene, and the normal X, as is usual with this type of translocation, is preferentially inactivated in most or all cells.

3. No. XYY can result only from meiosis II nondisjunction in the male, whereas XXY can result from nondisjunction at meiosis I in the male or at either division in the female.

4. Translocation of Y chromosome material containing the sex-determining region to the X chromosome.

5. 46,XY; testicular feminization (androgen insensitivity); the mother or child may be a new mutant, but if the mother is heterozygous, the usual X-linked risks apply.

6. 46,XX; autosomal recessive; prenatal diagnosis possible; need for clinical attention in neonatal period to determine sex and to forestall salt-losing crises.

7. a) None; the short arms of all acrocentric chromosomes are thought to be identical and contain multiple copies of rRNA genes. b) None if the deletion involves only heterochromatin. c) Cri du chat syndrome, severity depending on the amount of DNA deleted. d) Turner syndrome; the Xq− chromosome is preferentially inactivated in all cells (provided that the X inactivation center is not deleted), thus reducing the potential severity of such a deletion.

8. Question for discussion. See text for possible explanations.

CHAPTER 11

1. The pedigree should contain the following information: a) Hydrops fetalis is due to a total absence of α chains. b) The parents each must have the genotype $\alpha\alpha/--$. c) The $\alpha-$ genotype is very common in some populations, including Melanesians. Parents with this genotype cannot transmit a $--$ genotype to their offspring.

2. Except in isolated populations, patients with β-thalassemia will often be genetic compounds because there are usually many alleles present in a population in which β-thalassemia is common. In such populations, the chance that a patient is a true homozygote of a single allele is greater than it would be in a population in which thalassemia is rare. In the latter group, more "private mutations" might be expected (ones found solely or almost solely in a single pedigree). A patient is more likely to have identical alleles if he or she belongs to a geographical isolate with a high frequency of a single or a few alleles, or if his or her parents are consanguineous. See text in Chapter 7.

3. Three bands on the RNA blot could indicate, among other possibilities, that (a) one allele is producing two mRNAs, one normal in size and the other abnormal, and the other allele is producing one mRNA of abnormal size; (b) both alleles are making a normal-sized transcript and an abnormal transcript, but the aberrant ones are of different sizes; or (c) one allele is producing three mRNAs of different size, and the other allele is making no transcripts.

    Scenario (c) is highly improbable, if possible at all. Two mRNAs from a single allele could result from a splice defect that allows the normal mRNA to be made, but at reduced efficiency, while leading to the synthesis of another transcript of abnormal size, which results from either the incorporation of intron sequences in the mRNA or the loss of exon sequences from the mRNA. In this case, the other abnormal band comes from the other allele. A larger band from the other allele could result from a splice defect or an insertion, whereas a smaller band could be due to a splice defect or a deletion. Hb E is caused by an allele from which both a normal and a shortened transcript are made (see Fig. 11–17); the normal mRNA makes up 40 percent of the total β-globin mRNA, producing only a mild anemia.

4. These two mutations affect different globin chains. The expected offspring are 1/4 normal, 1/4 Hb M Saskatoon heterozygotes with methemoglobinemia, 1/4 Hb M Boston heterozygotes with methemoglobinemia, and 1/4 double heterozygotes with four Hb types: normal, both types of Hb M, and a type with abnormalities in both chains. In the double heterozygotes, the clinical consequences are unknown — probably more severe methemoglobinemia.

5. $2/3 \times 2/3 \times 1/4 = 1/9$.

6. 1/4.

7. 8, 1, 2, 7, 10, 4, 9, 5, 6, and 3.

CHAPTER 12

1. Three types of mutations that could explain a mutant protein that is 50 kilodaltons larger than the normal polypeptide are: (a) A mutation in the normal stop codon that allows translation to continue. (b) A splice mutation that results in the inclusion of intron sequences in the coding region. The intron sequences would have to be free of stop codons for sufficient length to allow the extra 50 kilodaltons of translation. (c) An insertion, with an open reading frame, into the coding sequence.

   For any of the above, approximately 500 extra residues would be added to the protein, if the average molecular weight of an amino acid is about 100. Five hundred amino acids would be encoded by 1500 nucleotides.

2. A nucleotide substitution that changes one amino acid residue to another should be termed a *putative mutation,* and possibly a *polymorphism,* unless (a) it has been demonstrated, through a functional assay of the protein, that the change impairs the function to a degree consistent with the phenotype of the patient, or (b) instead of or in addition to a functional assay, it can be demonstrated that the nucleotide change is found *only* on mutant chromosomes, which can be identified by haplotype analysis in the population of patients and their parents, and *not* on normal chromosomes in this population.

   The fact that the nucleotide change is only rarely observed in the normal population, and found with significantly higher frequency in a mutant population, is strong supportive evidence but not proof that the substitution is a mutation.

3. If Johnny has CF, the chances are about 0.85×0.85, or 70 percent, that he has a previously described mutation that could be readily identified by DNA analysis. His parents are from northern Europe; therefore, the probability that he is homozygous for the ΔF508 mutation is 0.7×0.7, or 50 percent, because about 70 percent of CF carriers in northern Europe have this mutation. If he does not have the ΔF508 mutation, he could certainly still have CF, because about 30 percent of the alleles (in the northern European population, at least) are not ΔF508. Steps to DNA diagnosis for CF include the following: (a) looking directly for the ΔF508 mutation; if not present, (b) looking for haplotypes to see which other mutations are most likely; (c) then looking directly for other mutations based on probabilities suggested by the haplotype data; (d) if all efforts to identify a mutation fail (or if time does not allow), performing linkage analysis with polymorphic DNA markers closely linked to CF.

4. James may have a new mutation on the X chromosome, because Joe inherited the same X chromosome from his mother, and in neither her nor Joe was the deletion present. If this is the case, there is no risk of recurrence. Alternatively, the mother may be a mosaic, and the mosaicism includes her germline. In this case, there is a definite risk that the mutant X

could be inherited by another son or passed to a carrier daughter. About 5 to 15 percent of cases of this type appear to be due to maternal germline mosaicism. Thus the risk is half of this figure for her male offspring, because the chance that a son will inherit the mutant X is $1/2 \times 5$ to 15 percent = 2.5 to 7.5 percent.

5. For DMD, as a classic X-linked recessive disease that is lethal in males, one third of cases are predicted to be new mutations. The large size of the gene is likely to account for the high mutation rate at this locus (i.e., it is a large target for mutation). The ethnic origin of the patient will have no effect on either of these phenomena.

6. The limited number of amino acids that have been observed to substitute for glycine in collagen mutants reflects the nature of the genetic code. Single nucleotide substitutions at the three positions of the glycine codons allow only a limited number of missense mutations. See Table 3–3.

7. Two bands of G6PD on electrophoresis of a red cell lysate (see Table 12–8) indicate that the woman has a different G6PD allele on each X chromosome and that each allele is being expressed in her red cell population. However, no single cell expresses both alleles, because of X inactivation. Males have only a single X chromosome and thus express only one G6PD allele. A female with two bands could have two normal alleles with different electrophoretic mobility, one normal allele and one mutant allele with different electrophoretic mobility, or two mutant alleles with different electrophoretic mobility.

 Because the two common deficiency alleles (A− and B−) migrate to the same position as the common normal activity alleles (A and B), the woman is unlikely to have a common deficiency allele at both loci. Apart from that, one cannot say much about the possible pathological significance of the two bands without measuring the enzymatic activity. If one of the alleles has low activity, then she would be at risk of hemolysis to the extent that the high activity allele is inactivated as a result of X inactivation.

8. The box in Chapter 12 entitled "Enzyme Deficiencies and Disease" lists the possible causes of loss of multiple enzyme activities: (a) They may share a cofactor whose synthesis or transport is defective. (b) They may share a subunit encoded by the mutant gene. (c) They may be processed by a common enzyme whose activity is critical to their becoming active. (d) They may normally be located in the same organelle, and a defect in the organelle's biological processes can affect all four enzymes. For example, they may not be imported normally into the organelle and may be degraded in the cytoplasm. Almost all enzymopathies are recessive (see text) and most genes are autosomal.

CHAPTER 13

1. Unresponsive patients may have mutations that drastically impair the synthesis of a functional gene product. Responsive patients may have mutations in the regulatory region of the gene. The effects of these mutations may be counteracted by the administration of interferon gamma. These mutations could be in the DNA binding site that responds to the interferon stimulus or in some other regulatory element that participates in the response to interferon gamma. Alternatively, responsive patients may produce a defective cytochrome *b* polypeptide that retains a small degree of residual function. The production of more of this mutant protein, in response to interferon gamma, increases the oxidase activity slightly but significantly.

2. An enzyme that is normally intracellular can function extracellularly if the substrate is in equilibrium between the intracellular and extracellular fluids and if the product is either

nonessential inside the cell or in a similar equilibrium state. Thus enzymes with substrates and products that do not fit these criteria would not be suitable for this strategy. This approach may not work for phenylalanine hydroxylase because of its need for tetrahydrobiopterin. However, if tetrahydrobiopterin could diffuse freely across the PEG layer around the enzyme, the administration of tetrahydrobiopterin orally may suffice. This strategy would not work for storage diseases because the substrate of the enzyme is trapped inside the lysosome. In Lesch-Nyhan syndrome, the most important pathological process is in the brain, and the enzyme in the extracellular fluid would not be able to cross the blood-brain barrier. Tay-Sachs disease could not be treated this way because of the nondiffusibility of the substrate from the lysosome.

3. Rhonda's mutations prevent the production of any LDL receptor. Thus the combination of a bile acid binding resin and a drug (e.g., lovastatin) to inhibit cholesterol synthesis would have no effect in increasing the synthesis of LDL receptors. The boy must have one or two mutant alleles that produce a receptor with some residual function, and the increased expression of these mutant receptors on the surface of the hepatocyte reduces the plasma LDL-bound cholesterol.

4. Unresponsive patients probably have alleles that do not make any protein, that decrease its cellular abundance in some other way (e.g., make an unstable protein), or that disrupt the conformation of the protein so extensively that its pyridoxal-phosphate binding site has no affinity for the cofactor, even at high concentrations.

   The answer to the second part of this question is less straightforward. The answer given here is based on the generalization that most patients with a rare autosomal recessive disease are likely to have two different alleles, which assumes that there is no mutational hotspot in the gene and that the patients are not descended from a "founder" and are not members of an ethnic group in whom the disease has a high frequency. In this context, (a) Tom is likely to have two alleles that are responsive; (b) First cousins with the same recessive disease are likely to share only one allele, so that Allan is likely to have one responsive allele that he shares with Tom and another allele that is either unresponsive or that responds more poorly to the cofactor than Tom's other allele.

5. a) You need both a promoter that will allow the synthesis of sufficient levels of the mRNA in the target tissue of choice and the phenylalanine hydroxylase cDNA. In reality, you also need a vector to deliver the "gene" into the cell, but this aspect of the problem has not been dealt with much in the book.   b) A phenylalanine hydroxylase "gene" will probably be effective in any tissue that had a good blood supply for the delivery of phenylalanine, and an adequate source of the cofactor of the enzyme, tetrahydrobiopterin. The promoter would have to be capable of driving transcription in the target tissue chosen for the treatment.   c) Any mutation that severely reduces the abundance of the protein in the cell but has no effect on transcription. This group includes those mutations that impair translation or that render the protein highly unstable. The thalassemias include examples of all these types.   d) Liver cells are capable of making tetrahydrobiopterin, whereas other cells may not be. The target cell for the gene transfer should thus be capable of making this cofactor; otherwise, the enzyme will not function unless the cofactor is administered in large amounts.   e) Human phenylalanine hydroxylase probably exists as a homodimer or homotrimer. In patients whose alleles produce a mutant polypeptide (vs. none at all), these alleles may manifest a dominant negative effect on the product of the transferred gene. This effect could be overcome by making a gene construct that produces more of the normal phenylalanine hydroxylase protein (thus diluting out the effect of the mutant polypeptide), or by transferring the gene into a cell type that does not normally express phenylalanine hydroxylase and that would therefore not be subject to the dominant negative effect.

CHAPTER 14

1. See text and glossary.

2. a) 1, MZ twin; 2, sib or DZ twin; 3, father, mother; 4, half-sib; 5, first cousin; 6, unrelated person. b) The organ of an MZ twin might be genetically susceptible to the same problem that led the recipient to need a transplant.

3. Involves splicing and rearrangement of genomic DNA, whereas splicing of introns and exons involves RNA.

4. Because of allelic exclusion, expression is from only one of the two alleles in each cell. In this regard, this is more similar to expression of X-linked genes, although the mechanisms of allelic exclusion and X inactivation are quite different. For most other (perhaps all other) autosomal loci, both alleles are expressed.

5. Nonrandom inactivation presumably reflects the differential survival of the two cell populations (with one or the other X active) in B or T cell lineages. Cells with the mutant gene on the active X are presumably at a great selective disadvantage in the lineage in which the particular gene product (currently unknown) plays a role. Thus only cells with the normal allele on the active X survive. For autosomal forms, X inactivation is presumably random, because both types of cell populations have equally functional X-linked gene products.

CHAPTER 15

1. a) Autosomal dominant. b) No increase in risk after two affected children, and so forth; see text.

2. Male-to-male transmission can disprove X linkage; other criteria of multifactorial inheritance can be examined, as in text.

3. For autosomal recessive but not for multifactorial inheritance, there is almost no chance that a parent will be affected; for other criteria, see text.

CHAPTER 16

1. Family history, DNA marker analysis, cytogenetic analysis, mutation identification; advise parents of the risk, but point out that a future child could be examined immediately after birth and at short intervals for some time to make sure that if tumors develop, they are detected and treated early.

2. Colorectal cancer seems to require a number of sequential mutations in several genes, a process that may take longer than a single mutation in the retinoblastoma gene. Age dependence may also reflect the number, timing, and rate of cell divisions in colon cells and in retinoblasts.

3. A cell line with i(17q) is monosomic for 17p and trisomic for 17q. Thus formation of the isochromosome leads to loss of heterozygosity for genes on 17p. This may be particularly important if one or more tumor-suppressor genes (such as p53) are present on 17p. In addition, a number of proto-oncogenes map to 17q. It is possible that increasing their dosage may confer a growth advantage on cells containing the i(17q).

4. The chief concern is the need to reduce radiation exposure to the lowest possible level because of the risk of cancer in children with this genetic defect.

5. Tumor progression from retinoma to retinoblastoma may require the loss of other tumor-suppressor genes or activated proto-oncogenes, or it may reflect the late (in the development of the retina) mutation of the second allele at the retinoblastoma locus.

6. Breast cancer appears to follow multifactorial inheritance. The empiric risk figures are consistent with a multifactorial model, with one or more dominant acting predisposition genes, in addition to nutritional and possibly environmental factors.

CHAPTER 17

1. a) Not a significant deviation from expectation; this suggests that ascertainment is unbiased. b) Excess of concordance in MZ pairs suggests importance of genetic factors in MS.

2. a) None; there would still be an even distribution of males and females at each birth order. b) A possible effect is a major drop in population as a result of a reduced number of females of reproductive age.

3. T, F, F, F, T, T, F, F, T, and F.

CHAPTER 18

1. a) Prior risk 1/4; posterior risk (2 normal brothers) 1/13. b) Zero.

2. a) Molly, 13/21; Molly's mother, 5/21; Norma and Nancy, 13/42; Olive and Odette, 13/84; Martha, 1/21; Nora and Nellie, 1/42; Maude, 5/42; Naomi, 5/84.   b) To have a 2 percent risk of having an affected son, a woman must have an 8 percent chance of being a carrier; thus Martha, Nora, and Nellie would not qualify, since their carrier risk is less than 8 percent.

3. $(1/2)^{13}$; $(1/2)^{13} \times 2$. (This answer is the chance of 13 consecutive male births or 13 consecutive female births, before any children are born.)

4. a) 10μ; 18μ; 90 percent; 45 percent. b) 3μ; 4μ. c) 14.7 percent.

5. 6, 8, 7, 5, 4, 2, 9, 1, 10, and 3.

6. a) The prior risk that either Ira or Margie is a CF carrier is 2/3; therefore, the probability that both are carriers is $2/3 \times 2/3 = 4/9$. b) Their risk of having an affected child in any pregnancy is $1/4 \times 4/9 = 1/9$. c) Bayesian analysis is carried out as follows:

	Both Carriers	Not Both Carriers
Prior risk for Ira and Margie	4/9	5/9
Conditional probability (3 normal children)	$(3/4)^3$	1
Joint probability	$4/9 \times (3/4)^3 = 3/16 = .19$	$5/9 = .56$
Posterior probability	$.19/(.19 + .56) = \sim 1/4$	$.56/.75 = \sim 3/4$

Thus the chance that Ira and Margie's next child will be affected is $1/4 \times 1/4 = 1/16$.

8. a) Yes; autosomal recessive, autosomal dominant (new mutation), X-linked recessive, chromosomal disorder, or multifactorial. b) This increases suspicion that the disorder is

autosomal recessive. c) This fact certainly supports the likelihood that the problem has a genetic explanation. The pedigree pattern would be consistent with autosomal recessive inheritance only if the sister's husband were carrying the same defect (possible if he is from the same village, for example). An X-linked recessive pattern (particularly if the affected children are all boys) or a chromosome defect ought to be considered. The mother and her son should be karyotyped.

9. The woman is mistaken. She has a 1/2 risk of passing the mutant NF1 gene to her offspring. The fact that she is probably a new mutant only reduces the recurrence risk elsewhere in the family.

CHAPTER 19

1. c, e, f, j, d, h, g, b, i, and a.

2. No, the child can have only Down syndrome or monosomy 21, which is almost always lethal. Thus they should receive counseling not to attempt pregnancy but to consider other alternatives for having children.

3. No, the problem could be maternal cell contamination.

4. MSAFP level is relatively high when the fetus has an open neural tube defect and relatively low when the fetus has Down syndrome.

5. a) Drop quickly to zero; very little effect. b) Drop quickly to the level sustained by new mutations (about half). c) Drop quickly to the level sustained by new mutations (very low).

6. a) About 15 percent. (See Table 1–2.) b) At least 50 percent are chromosomally abnormal. c) No, prenatal diagnosis or karyotyping of the parents would be indicated only after three such abortions, provided that there are no other indications, such as advanced maternal age.

7. a) Allele 1. b) Carrier. c) Homozygous normal. d) Expected to be extremely rare, because galactosemia is well known to be due to mutations in the GALT gene.

8. Question for discussion. See text for examples and discussion.

G-BANDING PATTERNS

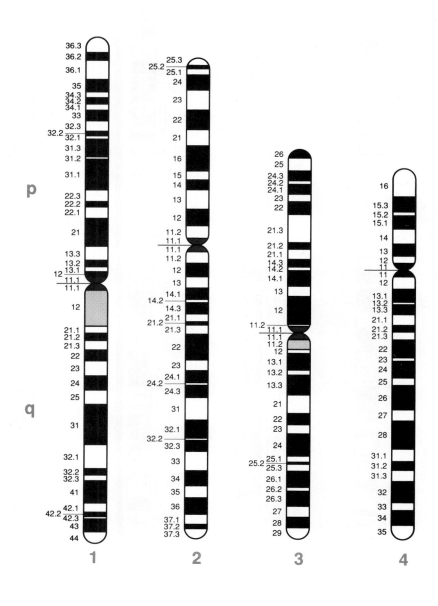

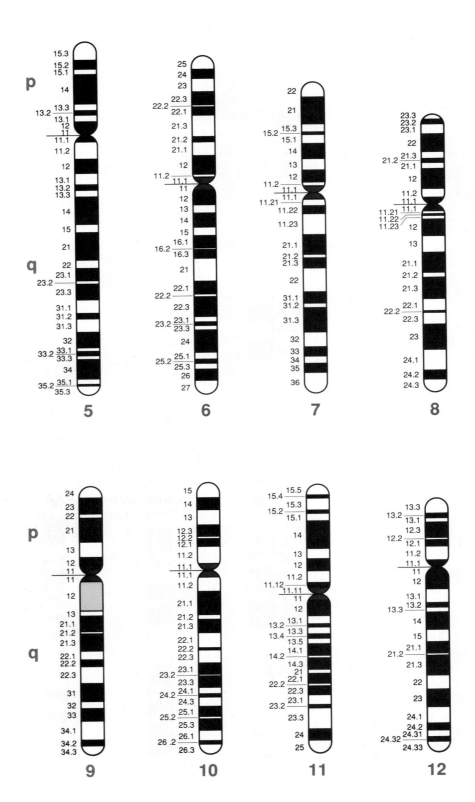

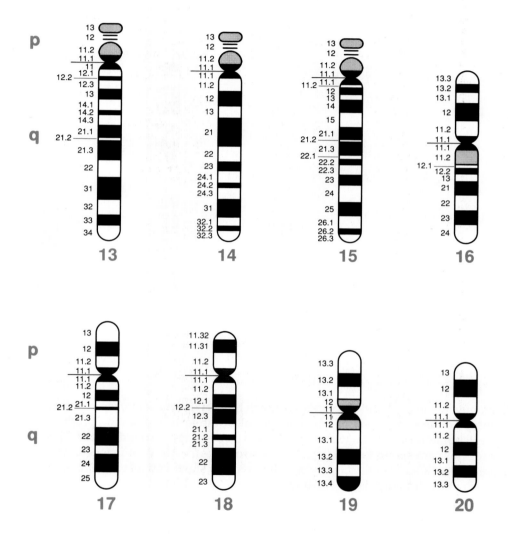

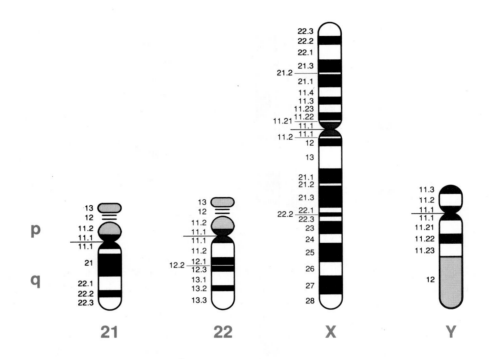

Diagrams showing G-banding patterns for each human chromosome, representing a haploid karyotype of approximately 550 bands, typical of the level of banding produced in most clinical laboratories. Dark regions correspond to bands that stain darkly with G banding, and light regions correspond to light G bands. Centromeres (primary constrictions) are indicated by darkly speckled regions. Lightly speckled regions show variable staining and are often positions of heteromorphisms. (Redrawn from ISCN, 1985.)

Appendix II

THE CHI-SQUARE TEST OF SIGNIFICANCE

The chi-square test is a measure of the significance of a particular data set in comparison with an expected value and is applicable to many problems in genetics because it requires, not that the data be more or less normally distributed, but only that the numbers in the different categories be known. The calculation of chi-square (χ^2) is quite simple. If O is the observed number in each category and E is the number in that category expected on the basis of the hypothesis being tested, then chi-square is the square of the difference between O and E, divided by E, summed over all the categories; in other terms:

$$\chi^2 = \Sigma\left[\frac{(O - E)^2}{E}\right]$$

The probability associated with a given value of chi-square can be obtained from tables originally prepared by R. A. Fisher and reprinted in many textbooks. To use these tables, it is necessary to know the number of degrees of freedom available—that is, the number of values that can be randomly assigned while the total is left unchanged. (For example, if one is comparing the number of boys and girls in a sample of 1000 consecutive live-born infants, there is only one degree of freedom, because once one class is known, then the other is known, because they must sum to 1000.) A value of chi-square associated with a probability of less than .05 is considered to be significant—that is, to indicate a significant disagreement between the observed data and the hypothesis. The table at the end of this appendix shows examples of significant chi-square values at the .05 and .01 levels of significance, for different degrees of freedom.

Example 1. To illustrate the use of the chi-square test in a different sample from that quoted in Chapter 7, we begin by determining that in the sample, the frequency of M is .57 and the frequency of N is .43, using the method given in the chapter. Then we compare the observed and expected values as follows:

Class	Observed	Expected	$\frac{(O - E)^2}{E}$
M	600	461	41.9
MN	419	696	110.2
N	400	262	72.7
Total	1419	1419	224.8

The chi-square value for these data is 224.8. There is one degree of freedom (calculated as the number of phenotypes minus the number of alleles). These data are significantly different from those predicted by Hardy-Weinberg equilibrium, with $p \ll .01$ (that is, there is far less than a 1 percent chance that these data would be obtained if Hardy-Weinberg equilibrium theory is being followed).

Example 2. A series of patients with congenital pyloric stenosis (see Chapter 15) includes 25 boys and 5 girls. Does this distribution differ from the expected $1:1$ sex ratio?

Sex	Observed	Expected	$\frac{(O-E)^2}{E}$
Boys	25	15	6.7
Girls	5	15	6.7
Total	30	30	13.4

The chi-square value for these data is 13.4. According to the table below, this value would occur by chance with a probability $< .01$. Thus the observed excess of boys in this series is statistically significant.

Examples of Significant Chi-Square Values

Degrees of Freedom	Significance Level	
	0.05	*0.01*
1	3.84	6.64
2	5.99	9.21
10	18.31	23.21

Appendix III

TABLE OF LOD SCORES FOR GENETIC LINKAGE ANALYSIS

Lod scores for families of 1 to 7 children, for both phase-known and phase-unknown pedigrees. If phase-known, the number of recombinant (R) and nonrecombinant (NR) children is given. If phase-unknown, the number of children of each type is given (Z score). For families with more than 7 children, lod scores can be determined from the addition of lod scores from smaller entries (e.g., lod scores for 9 children equal lod scores for 7 children plus lod scores for 2 children).

References

Smith SM, Penrose LS, Smith CAB (1961) Mathematical tables for research workers in human genetics. Churchill, London.

Smith CAB (1968) Linkage scores and corrections in simple two- and three-generation families. Ann Hum Genet 32:127–150.

Children Tested		Recombination Fraction						
Number	Distribution	0.00	0.01	0.02	0.03	0.04	0.05	0.075
1	1 NR:0 R	0.301	0.297	0.292	0.288	0.283	0.279	0.267
	0 NR:1 R	−∞	−1.699	−1.398	−1.222	−1.097	−1.000	−0.824
2	2 NR:0 R	0.602	0.593	0.585	0.576	0.567	0.558	0.534
	1 NR:1 R	−∞	−1.402	−1.106	−0.934	−0.814	−0.721	−0.557
	0 NR:2 R	−∞	−3.398	−2.796	−2.444	−2.194	−2.000	−1.648
	Z 2:0	0.301	0.292	0.284	0.275	0.266	0.258	0.236
	Z 1:1	−∞	−1.402	−1.106	−0.934	−0.814	−0.721	−0.557
3	3 NR:0 R	0.903	0.890	0.877	0.863	0.850	0.837	0.802
	2 NR:1 R	−∞	−1.106	−0.813	−0.646	−0.530	−0.442	−0.290
	1 NR:2 R	−∞	−3.101	−2.504	−2.156	−1.911	−1.721	−1.381
	0 NR:3 R	−∞	−5.097	−4.194	−3.666	−3.291	−3.000	−2.472
	Z 3:0	0.602	0.589	0.576	0.562	0.549	0.533	0.501
	Z 2:1	−∞	−1.402	−1.106	−0.934	−0.814	−0.721	−0.557
4	4 NR:0 R	1.204	1.187	1.169	1.151	1.133	1.116	1.069
	3 NR:1 R	−∞	−0.809	−0.521	−0.358	−0.247	−0.163	−0.022
	2 NR:2 R	−∞	−2.805	−2.211	−1.868	−1.627	−1.442	−1.113
	1 NR:3 R	−∞	−4.800	−3.902	−3.378	−3.007	−2.721	−2.205
	0 NR:4 R	−∞	−6.796	−5.592	−4.887	−4.388	−4.000	−3.296
	Z 4:0	0.903	0.886	0.868	0.850	0.832	0.814	0.768
	Z 3:1	−∞	−1.110	−0.822	−0.659	−0.547	−0.464	−0.321
	Z 2:2	−∞	−2.805	−2.211	−1.868	−1.627	−1.442	−1.113
5	5 NR:0 R	1.505	1.483	1.461	1.439	1.417	1.395	1.336
	4 NR:1 R	−∞	−0.512	−1.229	−1.071	0.036	0.116	0.245
	3 NR:2 R	−∞	−2.508	−1.919	−1.580	−1.344	−1.163	−0.846
	2 NR:3 R	−∞	−4.504	−3.609	−3.090	−2.724	−2.442	−1.937
	1 NR:4 R	−∞	−6.499	−5.300	−4.600	−4.104	−3.721	−3.028
	0 NR:5 R	−∞	−8.495	−6.990	−6.109	−5.485	−5.000	−4.120
	Z 5:0	1.204	1.182	1.160	1.138	1.115	1.093	1.035
	Z 4:1	−∞	−0.813	−0.530	−0.372	−0.265	−0.186	−0.056
	Z 3:2	−∞	−2.805	−2.211	−1.868	−1.627	−1.442	−1.113
6	6 NR:0 R	1.806	1.780	1.754	1.727	1.700	1.674	1.603
	5 NR:1 R	−∞	−0.216	0.063	0.217	0.320	0.395	0.511
	4 NR:2 R	−∞	−2.211	−1.627	−1.292	−1.061	−0.884	−0.579
	3 NR:3 R	−∞	−4.207	−3.317	−2.802	−2.441	−2.163	−1.670
	2 NR:4 R	−∞	−6.203	−5.007	−4.312	−3.821	−3.442	−2.761
	1 NR:5 R	−∞	−8.198	−6.697	−5.821	−5.201	−4.721	−3.852
	0 NR:6 R	−∞	−10.194	−8.388	−7.331	−6.581	−6.000	−4.943
	Z 6:0	1.505	1.479	1.453	1.426	1.399	1.371	1.302
	Z 5:1	−∞	−0.517	−0.238	−0.084	0.019	0.093	0.211
	Z 4:2	−∞	−2.512	−1.928	−1.593	−1.361	−1.185	−0.877
	Z 3:3	−∞	−4.207	−3.317	−2.802	−2.441	−2.164	−1.670
7	7 NR:0 R	2.107	2.077	2.046	2.015	1.983	1.953	1.870
	6 NR:1 R	−∞	0.081	0.356	0.505	0.603	0.674	0.779
	5 NR:2 R	−∞	−1.915	−1.335	−1.005	−0.777	−0.605	−0.312
	4 NR:3 R	−∞	−3.910	−3.025	−2.514	−2.158	−1.884	−1.403
	3 NR:4 R	−∞	−5.906	−4.715	−4.024	−3.538	−3.163	−2.494
	2 NR:5 R	−∞	−7.902	−6.405	−5.534	−4.918	−4.442	−3.585
	1 NR:6 R	−∞	−9.897	−8.095	−7.043	−6.298	−5.721	−4.676
	0 NR:7 R	−∞	−11.893	−9.786	−8.553	−7.678	−7.000	−5.767
	Z 7:0	1.806	1.776	1.745	1.714	1.682	1.650	1.569
	Z 6:1	−∞	−0.220	0.055	0.204	0.302	0.371	0.478
	Z 5:2	−∞	−2.216	−1.636	−1.306	−1.078	−0.907	−0.613
	Z 4:3	−∞	−4.207	−3.317	−2.802	−2.441	−2.164	−1.670

Recombination Fraction									
0.10	*0.125*	*0.15*	*0.175*	*0.20*	*0.25*	*0.30*	*0.35*	*0.40*	*0.45*
0.255	0.243	0.230	0.217	0.204	0.176	0.146	0.114	0.079	0.041
−0.699	−0.602	−0.523	−0.456	−0.398	−0.301	−0.222	−0.155	−0.097	−0.046
0.511	0.486	0.460	0.435	0.408	0.352	0.292	0.228	0.158	0.082
−0.444	−0.359	−0.293	−0.238	−0.194	−0.125	−0.076	−0.041	−0.018	−0.005
−1.398	−1.204	−1.046	−0.912	−0.796	−0.602	−0.444	−0.310	−0.194	−0.092
0.215	0.194	0.173	0.153	0.134	0.097	0.064	0.037	0.017	0.004
−0.444	−0.359	−0.292	−0.238	−0.914	−0.125	−0.076	−0.041	−0.018	−0.004
0.765	0.729	0.690	0.652	0.612	0.528	0.438	0.342	0.237	0.123
−0.189	−0.116	−0.063	−0.021	0.010	0.051	0.070	0.073	0.061	0.036
−1.143	−0.961	−0.816	−0.694	−0.592	−0.426	−0.298	−0.196	−0.115	−0.051
−2.097	−1.806	−1.569	−1.368	−1.194	−0.903	−0.666	−0.465	−0.291	−0.138
0.465	0.429	0.393	0.356	0.318	0.243	0.170	0.104	0.049	0.013
−0.444	−0.359	−0.292	−0.238	−0.194	−0.125	−0.076	−0.041	−0.018	−0.004
1.020	0.972	0.920	0.870	0.816	0.704	0.584	0.456	0.316	0.164
0.066	0.127	0.167	0.197	0.214	0.227	0.216	0.187	0.140	0.077
−0.888	−0.718	−0.586	−0.477	−0.388	−0.250	−0.152	−0.082	−0.036	−0.010
−1.842	−1.563	−1.339	−1.150	−0.990	−0.727	−0.520	−0.351	−0.212	−0.097
−2.796	−2.408	−2.092	−1.824	−1.592	−1.204	−0.888	−0.620	−0.388	−0.184
0.720	0.671	0.621	0.570	0.517	0.409	0.298	0.190	0.094	0.025
−0.229	−0.165	−0.119	−0.085	−0.060	−0.028	−0.011	−0.003	−0.001	−0.000
−0.887	−0.718	−0.585	−0.477	−0.388	−0.250	−0.151	−0.082	−0.035	−0.009
1.275	1.215	1.150	1.087	1.020	0.880	0.730	0.570	0.395	0.205
0.321	0.370	0.397	0.414	0.418	0.403	0.362	0.301	0.219	0.118
−0.633	−0.475	−0.356	−0.259	−0.184	−0.074	−0.006	0.032	0.043	0.031
−1.587	−1.320	−1.109	−0.933	−0.786	−0.551	−0.374	−0.237	−0.133	−0.056
−2.541	−2.165	−1.862	−1.606	−1.388	−1.028	−0.742	−0.506	−0.309	−0.143
−3.495	−3.010	−2.615	−2.280	−1.990	−1.505	−1.110	−0.775	−0.485	−0.230
0.975	0.914	0.851	0.787	0.720	0.581	0.436	0.288	0.149	0.042
0.022	0.070	0.099	0.117	0.124	0.118	0.095	0.063	0.031	0.008
−0.887	−0.718	−0.585	−0.477	−0.388	−0.250	−0.151	−0.082	−0.035	−0.009
1.530	1.458	1.380	1.305	1.224	1.056	0.876	0.684	0.474	0.246
0.576	0.613	0.627	0.631	0.622	0.579	0.508	0.415	0.298	0.159
−0.378	0.232	−0.126	−0.042	0.020	0.102	0.140	0.146	0.122	0.072
−1.332	−1.077	−0.879	−0.715	−0.582	−0.375	−0.228	−0.123	−0.054	−0.015
−2.286	−1.922	−1.632	−1.389	−1.184	−0.852	−0.596	−0.392	−0.230	−0.102
−3.240	−2.767	−2.385	−2.062	−1.786	−1.329	−0.964	−0.661	−0.406	−0.189
−4.194	−3.612	−3.138	−2.736	−2.388	−1.806	−1.332	−0.930	−0.582	−0.276
1.231	1.157	1.082	1.004	0.924	0.756	0.578	0.393	0.211	0.061
0.276	0.312	0.329	0.331	0.323	0.284	0.222	0.149	0.076	0.021
−0.673	−0.524	−0.412	−0.324	−0.254	−0.153	−0.087	−0.044	−0.018	−0.004
−1.331	−1.077	−0.877	−0.715	−0.582	−0.375	−0.227	−0.123	−0.053	−0.013
1.785	1.701	1.610	1.522	1.428	1.232	1.022	0.798	0.553	0.287
0.831	0.833	0.857	0.849	0.826	0.755	0.654	0.529	0.377	0.200
−0.123	0.011	0.104	0.175	0.224	0.278	0.286	0.260	0.201	0.113
−1.077	−0.834	−0.649	−0.498	−0.378	−0.199	−0.082	−0.009	0.025	0.026
−2.031	−1.679	−1.402	−1.171	−0.980	−0.676	−0.450	−0.278	−0.151	−0.061
−2.985	−2.524	−2.155	−1.845	−1.582	−1.153	−0.818	−0.547	−0.327	−0.148
−3.939	−3.369	−2.908	−2.518	−2.184	−1.630	−1.186	−0.816	−0.503	−0.235
−4.893	−4.212	−3.661	−3.192	−2.786	−2.107	−1.554	−1.085	−0.679	−0.322
1.486	1.400	1.312	1.221	1.128	0.932	0.723	0.502	0.278	0.084
0.532	0.555	0.559	0.548	0.526	0.456	0.360	0.247	0.131	0.037
−0.422	−0.289	−0.192	−0.121	−0.070	−0.007	0.019	0.022	0.014	0.004
−1.331	−1.077	−0.877	−0.715	−0.582	−0.375	−0.227	−0.123	−0.053	−0.013

Data from Smith et al. (1961), Smith (1968).

Appendix IV

THE MORBID ANATOMY OF THE HUMAN GENOME

This appendix contains schematic diagrams of the 24 types of human chromosome that indicate the location of genetic disorders for which the mutation has been mapped to a specific site. In some instances, the disease phenotype was mapped by finding linkage to a marker (as described in Chapter 8) or by finding a specific chromosomal change (see Chapters 9 and 10). In other instances, the disorder was located by virtue of mapping the normal gene, combined with the presumption or proof that the given disorder represents a mutation in that structural gene (e.g., Tay-Sachs disease at the hexosaminidase A locus on chromosome 15). Cancers are, in selected instances, included when a specific chromosomal change or locus has been implicated in the particular disorder (see Chapter 16).

The appendix was provided by Victor A. McKusick (The Johns Hopkins Hospital, Baltimore) and is updated continually, on the basis of human gene mapping information published in the literature or presented at the annual Human Gene Mapping International Workshops. Updated versions of The Morbid Anatomy of the Human Genome (*On-Line Mendelian Inheritance in Man;* McKusick, 1990), as well as complete catalogs of human genes and human DNA, are available on-line from the Genome Data Base (maintained at The Johns Hopkins University School of Medicine, Baltimore) (Pearson, 1991). Catalogs are also published annually (Human Gene Mapping 10, 1989; Human Gene Mapping 10.5, 1990).

References

Human Gene Mapping 10 (1989) Tenth International Workshop on Human Gene Mapping. Cytogenet Cell Genet 51:1–1148.

Human Gene Mapping 10.5 (1990) Update to the Tenth International Workshop on Human Gene Mapping. Cytogenet Cell Genet 55:1–785.

McKusick VA (1990) Mendelian inheritance in man: Catalogs of autosomal dominant, autosomal recessive, and X-linked phenotypes, 9th ed. Johns Hopkins University Press, Baltimore.

Pearson PL (1991) The Genome Data Base (GDB), a human gene mapping repository. Nucl Acids Res 19:2237–2239.

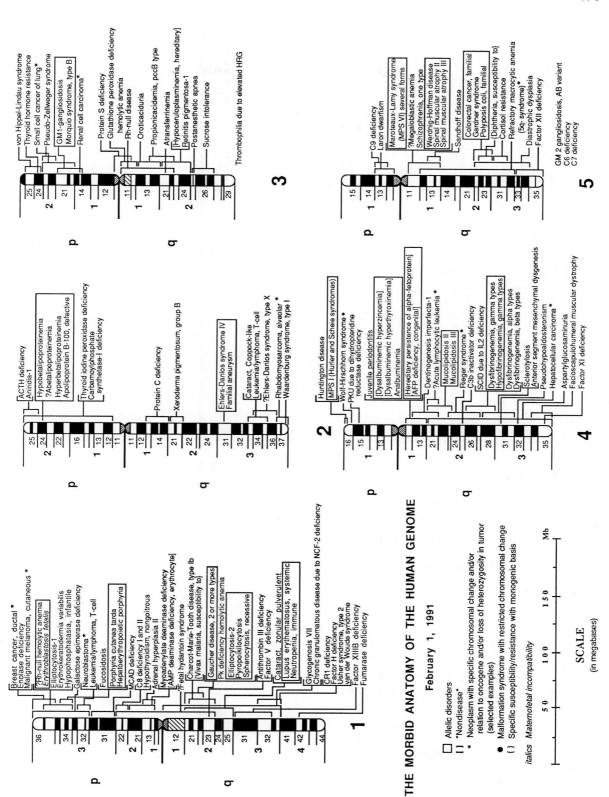

THE MORBID ANATOMY OF THE HUMAN GENOME

February 1, 1991

☐ Allelic disorders

⟮ ⟯ "Nondisease"

* Neoplasm with specific chromosomal change and/or relation to oncogene and/or loss of heterozygosity in tumor (selected examples)

● Malformation syndrome with restricted chromosomal change

{ } Specific susceptibility/resistance with monogenic basis

italics *Maternofetal incompatibility*

SCALE
(in megabases)

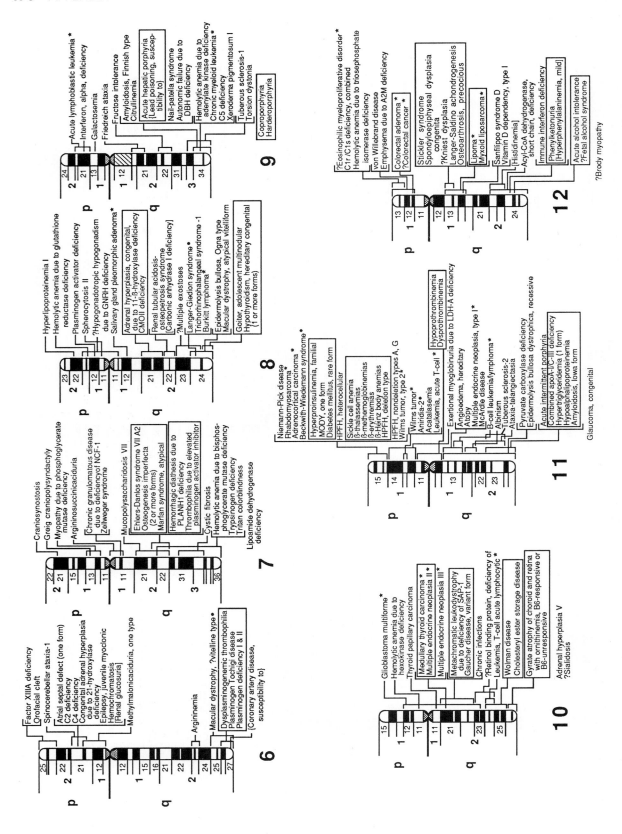

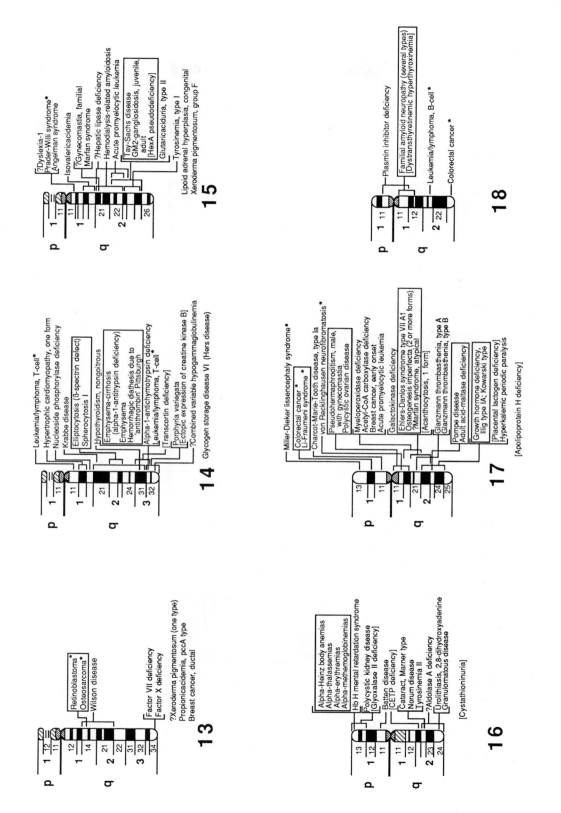

13

Retinoblastoma *
Osteosarcoma *
Wilson disease
Factor VII deficiency
Factor X deficiency
?Xeroderma pigmentosum (one type)
Propionicacidemia, pccA type
Breast cancer, ductal

14

Leukemia/lymphoma, T-cell *
Hypertrophic cardiomyopathy, one form
Nucleoside phosphorylase deficiency
Krabbe disease
Elliptocytosis (β-spectrin defect)
Spherocytosis I
Hypothyroidism, nongoitrous
Emphysema-cirrhosis (alpha-1-antitrypsin deficiency)
Emphysema
Hemorrhagic diathesis due to 'antithrombin' Pittsburgh
Alpha-1-antichymotrypsin deficiency
Leukemia/lymphoma, T-cell *
Transcortin deficiency
Porphyria variegata
[Ectopic expression of creatine kinase B]
?Combined variable hypogammaglobulinemia
Glycogen storage disease VI (Hers disease)

15

?Dyslexia-1
Prader-Willi syndrome •
Angelman syndrome
Isovalericacidemia
?Gynecomastia, familial
Marfan syndrome
?Hepatic lipase deficiency
Hemodialysis-related amyloidosis
Acute promyelocytic leukemia
Tay-Sachs disease
GM2-gangliosidosis, juvenile, adult
[HexA pseudodeficiency]
Glutaricaciduria, type II
Tyrosinemia, type I
Lipoid adrenal hyperplasia, congenital
Xeroderma pigmentosum, group F

16

Alpha-Heinz body anemias
Alpha-thalassemias
Alpha-erythremias
Alpha-methemoglobinemias
Hb H mental retardation syndrome
Polycystic kidney disease
[Glyoxalase II deficiency]
Batten disease
[CETP deficiency]
Cataract, Marner type
Norum disease
Tyrosinemia II
?Aldolase A deficiency
Urolithiasis, 2,8-dihydroxyadenine
Granulomatous disease
[Cystathioninuria]

17

Miller-Dieker lissencephaly syndrome •
Colorectal cancer *
Li-Fraumeni syndrome *
Charcot-Marie-Tooth disease, type Ia
von Recklinghausen neurofibromatosis *
Pseudohermaphroditism, male, with gynecomastia
Myeloperoxidase deficiency
Acetyl-CoA carboxylase deficiency
Breast cancer, early onset
Acute promyelocytic leukemia
?Marfan syndrome, atypical
Polycystic ovarian disease
Galactokinase deficiency
Ehlers-Danlos syndrome type VII A1
Osteogenesis imperfecta, (2 or more forms)
[Acanthocytosis, 1 form]
Glanzmann thrombasthenia, type A
Glanzmann thrombasthenia, type B
Pompe disease
Adult acid-maltase deficiency
Growth hormone deficiency, IIIg type IA; Kowarski type
Placental lactogen deficiency
Hyperkalemic periodic paralysis
[Apolipoprotein H deficiency]

18

Plasmin inhibitor deficiency
Familial amyloid neuropathy (several types)
[Dystransthyretinemic hyperthyroxinemia]
Leukemia/lymphoma, B-cell *
Colorectal cancer *

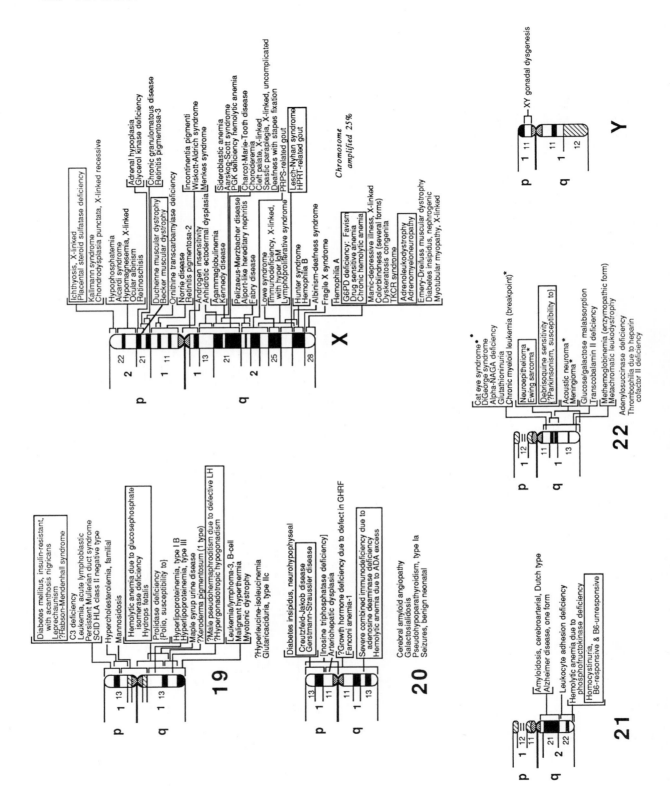

INDEX

Note: Numbers in *italics* refer to illustrations; numbers followed by t indicate tables.